Future Directions in Pc

Marilyn P. Safir • Helene S. Wallach
Albert "Skip" Rizzo
Editors

Future Directions in Post-Traumatic Stress Disorder

Prevention, Diagnosis, and Treatment

Springer

Editors
Marilyn P. Safir
Department of Psychology
University of Haifa
Haifa, Israel

Helene S. Wallach
Department of Psychology
University of Haifa
Haifa, Israel

Albert "Skip" Rizzo
University of Southern California Institute
for Creative Technologies
Department of Psychiatry and School of
Gerontology
Los Angeles, CA, USA

ISBN 978-1-4899-7521-8 ISBN 978-1-4899-7522-5 (eBook)
DOI 10.1007/978-1-4899-7522-5
Springer New York Heidelberg Dordrecht London

Library of Congress Control Number: 2014954586

Printed on acid-free paper

Springer is part of Springer Science+Business Media (www.springer.com)

Introduction

The seeds for this volume took fruit as a result of a grant from the Israel Science Foundation awarded to Marilyn Safir and Helene Wallach, to organize an international conference on PTSD. Israel seemed to be an extremely appropriate setting for such an international meeting because of the unusually high numbers of traumatic situations existing for Israeli residents which, unfortunately, create a natural laboratoryto study PTSD.

Israel, while a crossroad between Asia, Africa, and Europe, is very isolated, as during most of its existence it has been at war with the countries that surround it: Lebanon, Syria, Jordan, and Egypt. The UN passed a resolution in 1947 to split Palestine into two separate national entities: a Jewish Israel and an Arab Palestine. Following this resolution, Israel declared its independence (1948) as the homeland of the Jewish people. A war between Israel and the neighboring Arab countries resulted from rejection of these developments. Although peace treaties were signed with Egypt and Jordan, in the 1980s and 1990s, hostilities have continued between Israel and the surrounding Arab states, as well as with Palestinians living in territories Israel occupied following the 1967 war. Israel has also come under rocket attack twice from Iraq. An additional and relevant influence on life in Israel is the impact of WWII and the loss of six million Jews in the Holocaust. Furthermore, Israel's population was more than tripled by an influx of Jewish refugees in an extremely short time following WWII. Thus, the trauma of the Holocaust in Europe, and the trauma of expulsion of Jews from Islamic countries, where they had been living for centuries, has been added to this mix.

An additional factor in Israelis' exposure to trauma is the country's small physical area (about the size of the State of Delaware). Thus battles on its borders are never far from the home front. In addition, the home front has often come under terrorist attacks in all its major cities, as well as missile attacks in Northern Israel from Lebanon and from Gaza to Southern and Central Israel. This compounds the trauma of the missile attacks from Iraq that affected a wide spread of the population, including the center of the country.

We present this summary, as most Israelis have been, if not directly exposed to these various traumatic events, are at least acquainted with others who have been. Thus, Israeli clinicians and researchers have been working with a wide range of individuals who suffer from PTSD, from combat veterans to civilians of all ages, as well as Holocaust survivors. As a result, there is a wide range of research being done as well as various treatment programs for PTSD throughout Israel.

We were fortunate to receive this grant from the Israel Science Foundation to organize an international research conference at the Israel Institute for Advanced Studies at Hebrew University. The conference, which we co-chaired, was entitled Future Directions in PTSD: Prevention, Diagnosis and Treatment. The major conference goal was to invite an international group of researchers and clinicians in the forefront of PTSD research and treatment to establish an interdisciplinary and international dialogue between all those participating in the conference. The conference was held in Jerusalem in October, 2009. In addition to more than 30 lectures, there were roundtable discussions and poster sessions that were open to the professional public. There were over 100 participants. Having the conference in Israel (unfortunately, an environment conducive to PTSD), and accessible to the professional public, enabled and encouraged interactions among local and international participants, furthering dialogue and research. This dialogue focused on three important areas: prevention, diagnosis, and treatment.

As a result of these interactions, it became obvious that a book covering these topics would be desirable. Safir, Wallach, and Albert "Skip" Rizzo took upon themselves to edit such a volume. The idea was presented to Springer whose Health and Behavior editor, Janice Stern, was very open and enthusiastic about this idea.

While a number of chapter authors also participated in the conference, each chapter was specifically written for this volume. However, we decided that the volume should focus on future directions in PTSD. Only minorities of individuals who are exposed to traumatic events develop chronic PTSD. Thus, much current research is being done to identify those factors that cause individuals to be vulnerable or resistant to developing PTSD.

The authors of the chapters in the first section of this volume (Protective and Risk Factors for PTSD) examine the protective and risk factors that may protect or make individuals vulnerable to developing PTSD. Marina Bar-Shai and Ehud Klein have written two excellent chapters in which they give a broad overview of vulnerability and predictors of vulnerability to PTSD: from the perspective of *Psychosocial and demographic risk and resilience factors and Neurobiological and genetic risk factors*. Gal Richter-Levin, Omer Horovitz, and M. Michael Tsoory, in their chapter, *The early adolescent or "juvenile stress" translational animal model of posttraumatic stress disorder*, present research in which they develop an animal model to explain vulnerability and resilience to PTSD. The fourth chapter in this section was written by Mario Mikulincer, Phillip R. Shaver, and Zahava Solomon. In this chapter, *An attachment perspective on traumatic and posttraumatic reactions*, the authors examine the vast body of research on attachment and development of PTSD. The last chapter in this section, *Delayed-onset PTSD in Israel veterans: correlates, clinical picture, and controversy*, was written by Danny Horesh, Zahava

Solomon, Giora Keinan, and Tsachi Ein-Dor. They have followed a large group of Israeli combat veterans over a 20-year period. They identified soldiers who developed PTSD one year, two years, and 20 years following the Lebanon War. These veterans were matched with combat veterans who did not develop PTSD. Comparing these groups, they attempt to determine what factors may have predisposed veterans to develop PTSD at the varying time periods and what "protected" the combat veterans who did not develop PTSD.

The second section of this volume focuses on preventing PTSD. Exposure to trauma is widespread, but as we previously mentioned, only a minority of those exposed to trauma develop chronic symptoms of PTSD. Our authors discuss the possibilities of preventing PTSD from varying viewpoints, but examine various early approaches to prevent individuals exposed to trauma from developing PTSD. Megan C. Kearns, Alex O. Rothbaum, Cole G. Youngner, Mark S. Burton, Alexander McCarthy, and Barbara Olasov Rothbaum have focused on *Cutting edge research on prevention of PTSD*. The second two chapters present research that has been carried out in Israel. Danny Brom, Naomi L. Baum, and Ruth Pat-Horencyk focus on a school-based program for children, in their chapter *Systems of care for traumatized populations as a means for preventing PTSD*, and Sara A. Freedman and Arieh Y. Shalev present an early intervention program as a means of preventing PTSD, in their chapter *Prevention better than cure? How early interventions can prevent PTSD*.

Our third section on diagnosing PTSD is composed of two chapters. Chapter 9, by Lennis Echterling, Anne L. Stewart, and Thomas Field, presents a very complete historical overview of the *Evolution of DSM diagnosis for PTSD*. They begin with earliest diagnoses and the varying discussions and disputes about non-adaptive responses to trauma, and follow the evolution of the diagnosis through to latest definitions in the DSM-5. Asaf Gilboa, in his chapter *Functional neuroanatomy of PTSD: Developmental cytoarchitectonic trends, memory systems and control process*, demonstrates the possibility of diagnosing PTSD through a neurological approach. He attempts to identify differences in function of patients with PTSD and controls, employing the latest neuroimaging procedures, with a major emphasis on the amygdala.

The last half of this volume focuses on treatment of PTSD. The section on the development of evidence-based treatment for PTSD presents the two treatments that are the most widely research-based therapies currently employed for PTSD. The first of these treatments is prolonged exposure which is presented by Nitsa Nacasch, Lilach Rachamim, and Edna B. Foa in *The psychopathology and evidence-based treatment for posttraumatic stress disorder: PE*. Kathleen Chard and Kristen H. Walter present a newer but also strongly research-supported treatment, *Cognitive processing therapy: Beyond the basics (CPT)*. The last chapter in this section, *Interpersonal therapy for PTSD*, described by Alexandra Klein Rafaeli and John C. Markowitz, presents the newest therapeutic approach currently undergoing examination and comparison with PE and CPT.

Our next group of authors focuses on modifications of PTSD treatment. An important modification that rapidly incorporated into evidenced-based treatment is the use of virtual reality (VR) to replace in vitro or in vivo exposure. Thus, Azucena Garcia Palacios, Cristina Botella, Rosa Banos, Veronica Guillen, and Maria Vicenta Navarro present *A rationale for the use of VR in the treatment of PTSD*. Greg M. Reger, Albert A. Rizzo, and Gregory A. Gahm continue by describing the *Development and dissemination of virtual reality exposure therapy for combat-related PTSD*. Albert Rizzo, JoAnn Difede, Barbara Rothbaum, J. Galen Buckwalter, J. Martin Daughtry, and Greg Reger continue with their chapter on *Virtual reality as a tool for delivering PTSD exposure therapy*. Karen Seal presents *Mental health problems and treatment utilization of Iraq and Afghanistan veterans enrolled in Department of Veterans Affairs healthcare*. The largest group suffering from PTSD, and who have been studied and whose treatments were followed, are the many veterans who are treated by the United States Veterans Administration. Current research on a large civilian population (victims of 9/11) has been the focus of Megan Olden, Brittany Mello, Judith Cukor, Katarzyna Wyka, Nimali Jayasinghe, and JoAnn Difede's research on the implementation *of Evidence-based assessment, treatment, and research programs following the World Trade Center disaster on September 11, 2001*—probably the most worldwide viewed disaster, both through media presentation as it occurred and following the attacks. Burton S. Marks, Cole G. Youngner, Alexander J. McCarthy, Alex O. Rothbaum, and Barbara Olasov Rothbaum present their cutting-edge research on the employment of pharmaceutical aids in *Enhancing exposure therapy using D-cycloserine* (*DCS*).

To round out this volume, we thought it important to present a case study and case discussion, in which we would ask our different treatment experts to analyze a single case of a patient with PTSD and to present a treatment plan, so that you—the reader—could examine the similarities and difference between the different treatment programs and perhaps decide which treatment might be the treatment of choice. Nitsa Nacasch, Lilach Rachamim, and Edna B. Foa, who discuss the case from the point of view of PE, prepared the case presentation. Kathleen Chard employed *CPT*, Barbara Rothbaum—*VR* combined with *DCS, and* Alexandra Klein-Rafaeli—*IPT*. In the final chapter, Helene Wallach has taken the task of tying up and summarizing the current status of PTSD treatment. We hope that you have found this volume informative and innovative.

Haifa, Israel — Marilyn P. Safir
Haifa, Israel — Helene S. Wallach
Los Angeles, CA — Albert "Skip" Rizzo

Contents

Contributors

Rosa Baños Ciber Fisiopatología Obesidad y Nutrición CIBERobn, CB06/03, Instituto Salud Carlos III, Madrid, Spain

Universitat de Valencia, Valencia, Spain

Marina Bar-Shai Department of Psychiatry, Rambam Health Care Campus, Haifa, Israel

Faculty of Medicine, Technion IIT, Haifa, Israel

Naomi L. Baum The Israel Center for the Treatment of Psychotrauma, Herzog Hospital, Jerusalem, Israel

Cristina Botella Ciber Fisiopatología Obesidad y Nutrición CIBERobn, CB06/03 Instituto Salud Carlos III, Universitat Jaume I, Castellon, Spain

Ciber Fisiopatología Obesidad y Nutrición CIBERobn, CB06/03 Instituto Salud Carlos III, Madrid, Spain

Danny Brom The Israel Center for the Treatment of Psychotrauma, Herzog Hospital, Jerusalem, Israel

J. Galen Buckwalter Institute for Creative Technologies, University of Southern California, Los Angeles, CA, USA

Mark S. Burton Emory University School of Medicine, Atlanta, GA, USA

Kathleen M. Chard Trauma Recovery Center, Cincinnati VA Medical Center – Ft. Thomas Division, Ft. Thomas, KY, USA

PTSD & Anxiety Disorders Clinic, Cincinnati VA Medical Center, Ft. Thomas, KY, USA

Department of Psychiatry and Behavioral Neuroscience, University of Cincinnati College of Medicine, Cincinnati, OH, USA

Cincinnati VA Medical Center, Cincinnati, OH, USA

Beth E. Cohen Department of Medicine, University of California, San Francisco, San Francisco, CA, USA

Department Psychiatry, University of California, San Francisco, CA, USA

General Internal Medicine, San Francisco VA Medical Center, San Francisco, CA, USA

Judith Cukor Psychiatry Department, Weill Correll Medical College, New York, NY, USA

J. Martin Daughtry Department of Music, New York University, New York, NY, USA

JoAnn Difede Psychiatry Department, Weill Cornell Medical College, New York, NY, USA

Lennis G. Echterling James Madison University, Harrisonburg, VA, USA

Tsachi Ein-Dor School of Psychology, Interdisciplinary Center (IDC), Herzliya, Israel

Thomas A. Field James Madison University, Harrisonburg, VA, USA

Edna B. Foa Center for Treatment and Study of Anxiety, University of Pennsylvania, Philadelphia, PA, USA

Sara A. Freedman Department of Psychiatry, Center for Traumatic Stress, Hadassah University Hospital, Jerusalem, Israel

School of Social Work, Bar Ilan University, Ramat Gan, Israel

Gregory A. Gahm National Center for Telehealth and Technology, Joint Base Lewis-McChord, Tacoma, WA, USA

Azucena García-Palacios Universitat Jaume I, Castellon, Spain

Ciber Fisiopatología Obesidad y Nutrici6n CIBERobn, CB06/03 Instituto Salud Carlos III, Madrid, Spain

Asaf Gilboa The Rotman Research Institute at Baycrest, Toronto, ON, Canada

Heart and Stroke Foundation Canadian Partnership for Stroke Recovery, Toronto, ON, Canada

Department of Psychology, University of Toronto, Toronto, ON, Canada

Verónica Guillén Universitat Jaume I, Castellon, Spain

Centro Clínico PREVI, València, Spain

Danny Horesh Department of Psychology, Bar Ilan University, Ramat Gan, Israel

Department of Psychiatry, New York University, School of Medicine, New York, NY, USA

Omer Horovitz Department of Psychology, University of Haifa, Haifa, Israel

Nimali Jayasinghe Psychiatry Department, Weill Correll Medical College, New York, NY, USA

Megan C. Kearns Emory University School of Medicine, Atlanta, GA, USA

Giora Keinan Department of Psychology, Tel Aviv University, Tel Aviv, Israel

Ehud Klein Department of Psychiatry, Rambam Health Care Campus, Haifa, Israel

Faculty of Medicine, Technion IIT, Haifa, Israel

Shira Maguen Department of Medicine, University of California, San Francisco, CA, USA

Department Psychiatry, University of California, San Francisco, CA, USA

General Internal Medicine, San Francisco VA Medical Center, San Francisco, CA, USA

John C. Markowitz New York State Psychiatric Institute, New York, NY, USA

Columbia University College of Physicians & Surgeons, New York, NY, USA

Alexander J. McCarthy Emory University School of Medicine, Atlanta, GA, USA

Brittany Mello Sol Price School of Public Policy, University of Southern California, Los Angeles, CA, USA

Mario Mikulincer School of Psychology, Interdisciplinary Center (IDC) Herzliya, Herzliya, Israel

Nitsa Nacasch Brill Community Mental Health Center, Tel Aviv, Israel

Maria Vicenta Navarro University of Washington, Seattle, WA, USA

Megan Olden Psychiatry Department, Weill Correll Medical College, New York, NY, USA

Ruth Pat-Horenczy The Israel Center for the Treatment of Psychotrauma, Herzog Hospital, Jerusalem, Israel

Lilach Rachamim Interdisciplinary Center, Herzliya, Israel

Schneider Children's Medical Center of Israel, Petah Tikva, Israel

Alexandra Klein Rafaeli The Ruth and Allen Ziegler Student Services Division, Tel Aviv University, Tel Aviv, Israel

The New School of Psychotherapy, Israel

Greg M. Reger National Center for Telehealth and Technology, Joint Base Lewis-McChord, Tacoma, WA, USA

VA Puget Sound Health Care System, Seattle, WA, USA

Gal Richter-Levin Department of Psychology, University of Haifa, Haifa, Israel

The "Sagol" Department of Neurobiology, University of Haifa, Haifa, Israel

The Institute for the Study of Affective Neuroscience (ISAN), University of Haifa, Haifa, Israel

Albert A. Rizzo Institute for Creative Technologies, University of Southern California, Playa Vista, CA, USA

Barbara Olasov Rothbaum Emory University School of Medicine, Emory University, Atlanta, GA, USA

Alex O. Rothbaum Virtually Better, Inc., Decatur, GA, USA

Karen H. Seal Department of Medicine, University of California, San Francisco, CA, USA

Department Psychiatry, University of California, San Francisco, CA, USA

General Internal Medicine, San Francisco VA Medical Center, San Francisco, CA, USA

Arieh Y. Shalev Department of Psychiatry, Center for Traumatic Stress, Hadassah University Hospital, Jerusalem, Israel

Phillip R. Shaver Department of Psychology, UC Davis, Davis, CA, USA

Zahava Solomon Bob Shapell School of Social Work, Tel-Aviv University, Tel Aviv, Israel

Anne L. Stewart James Madison University, Harrisonburg, VA, USA

M. Michael Tsoory Department of Veterinary Resources, Weizmann Institute of Science, Rehovot, Israel

Helene S. Wallach Department of Psychology, University of Haifa, Haifa, Israel

Kristen H. Walter Veterans Medical Research Foundation, VA San Diego Healthcare System, San Diego, CA, USA

Cincinnati VA Medical Center, Cincinnati, OH, USA

Katarzyna Wyka Public Health Department, Hunter College, City University of New York, New York, USA

Cole G. Youngner Emory University School of Medicine, Atlanta, GA, USA

Part I
Protective and Risk Factors for PTSD

Chapter 1
Vulnerability to PTSD: Psychosocial and Demographic Risk and Resilience Factors

Marina Bar-Shai and Ehud Klein

Introduction

According to the DSM-IV, posttraumatic stress disorder (PTSD) is defined as the development of symptoms following exposure to an extreme traumatic event, in which an individual experienced an actual or perceived threat of death, or serious injury, or threat to one's physical integrity; or witnessed an event that involved an actual or perceived threat of death, serious bodily injury, or threat to the physical integrity of another individual. Symptoms are characterized as belonging to one of three independent, but often interconnected, clusters. *Re-experiencing* symptoms involve spontaneous, uncontrollable intrusions of the traumatic memory that may manifest themselves as nightmares or memory flashbacks. These intrusions are typically associated with marked physiological responses. *Avoidance* symptoms are best described as individuals' efforts to distance themselves from trauma-related stimuli, such as television news and fireworks (for combat-related PTSD) or crowds and public transportation vehicles (for civilian trauma-related PTSD). The avoidance cluster may also include emotional and social withdrawal behaviors. *Hyperarousal* symptoms include robust physiological reactions such as irritability, hypervigilance, and exaggerated startle response. PTSD is unique with respect to acute stress disorder (ASD) or normal recovery from a traumatic experience in that the aforementioned symptoms must persist for at least 1 month to meet the criteria for a diagnosis of PTSD. Exposure to trauma can also result in a posttraumatic "syndrome" characterized by a diagnosis of PTSD *and* comorbidity with major depressive disorder (MDD), generalized anxiety disorder (GAD), as well as somatic symptoms, dissociation, and substance abuse (Pervanidou, 2008).

M. Bar-Shai, M.D., Ph.D. • E. Klein, M.D. (✉)
Department of Psychiatry, Rambam Health Care Campus, Haifa, Israel

Faculty of Medicine, Technion IIT, Haifa, Israel
e-mail: m_bar-shai@rambam.health.gov.il; e_klein@rambam.health.gov.il

M.P. Safir et al. (eds.), *Future Directions in Post-Traumatic Stress Disorder*,
DOI 10.1007/978-1-4899-7522-5_1

The lifetime prevalence of PTSD, as assessed in several community-based studies, is estimated at 3–8 % (Creamer, Burgess, & McFarlane, 2001). Exposure to trauma in itself is not sufficient for subsequent development of PTSD. Moreover, the traumatic symptoms may at times improve or disappear altogether within a few months after the traumatic event, suggesting a self-limited process similar to spontaneous recovery from a depressive episode (Zohar, Juven-Wetzler, Myers, & Fostick, 2008).

Consequently, the currently held view is that the event itself is only one of several determinants responsible for the transition from a normal response to PTSD. It is currently assumed that PTSD is an abnormal response to a severe traumatic event, developing only in a percentage of people who are exposed. Therefore, predisposing and vulnerability factors may determine who will develop PTSD following exposure to a traumatic event. Accordingly, considerable research has been devoted to the identification of predictors and risk factors that may increase the likelihood of developing PTSD following exposure to a traumatic event. These factors may be classified in three temporal domains: *pre-traumatic*, *peri-traumatic*, and *posttraumatic* factors.

Pre-traumatic factors exist prior to the traumatic event and are viewed as predisposing, vulnerability factors in those exposed, such as previous experiences of traumatic events, history of psychiatric disorder, personality traits, and demographic variables (McFarlane, 2000). *Peri-traumatic* factors are those linked to the actual traumatic occurrence. Certain characteristics of a situation are associated with greater stress responses. These include the intensity or severity of the stressor and controllability of the stressor, the degree of exposure, the magnitude of the initial response, the presence of physical injury, and dissociation (Ozer, Best, Lipsey, & Weiss, 2003), as well as features that determine the nature of the cognitive responses or appraisals. *Posttraumatic* factors are related to the long-term course of the trauma response, including the coping abilities of the survivors and their support network (Ozer et al., 2003).

Although little is known about predictive factors of PTSD and the immediate response to the trauma, the symptoms that were found to be associated with higher frequency of PTSD include, among others, a significant panic-like response, pronounced distress, dissociative response, and past history of anxiety or depression (McFarlane, 2000). These symptoms may reflect the intensity or severity of the current experience, a preexisting individual trait, or sensitization from prior trauma exposure. Factors associated with the development of symptoms of PTSD and mental health disorders include injury, damage to property, loss of resources, bereavement, and perceived threat to life (McNally, 2003). Stress-related outcomes also vary according to personal and environmental factors. *Personal risk factors* for the development of depression, anxiety, or PTSD after a serious life event, disaster, or trauma include prior psychiatric history, neuroticism, female gender, and other socio-demographic variables (McNally, 2003). There is also some evidence that the relationship between personality and environmental adversity may be bidirectional (Kendler, Gardner, & Prescott, 2003). Levels of neuroticism, emotionality, and reactivity correlate with poor interpersonal relationships as well as "event proneness."

Protective factors that have been identified include, but are not limited to, coping, resources (e.g., social support, self-esteem, optimism), and finding meaning. For example, those with social support fare better after a natural disaster (Madakasira & O'Brien, 1987) or after myocardial infarction (Clarke, Frasure-Smith, Lesperance, & Bourassa, 2000). Attaching meaning to the event is another protective factor against the development of PTSD, even when horrific torture has occurred. Left-wing political activists who were tortured by Turkey's military regime had lower rates of PTSD than did non-activists who were arrested and tortured by the police (Basoglu et al., 1994).

Finally, human beings are resilient and, in general, are able to cope with adverse situations. An illustration is provided by a study of a nationally representative sample of Israelis following 19 months of ongoing exposure to the Palestinian intifada. Despite considerable distress, most Israelis reported adapting to the situation without substantial mental health symptoms or impairment (Hobfoll et al., 2008).

The scope of the current chapter focuses on the psychobiological and demographic vulnerability and resilience factors of PTSD.

Pre-traumatic Risk Factors

Trauma timing, type, and severity seem to modify genetic risk in PTSD. Individuals whose first trauma occurs in childhood as opposed to adolescence or adulthood are at particularly high risk of developing the disorder (Ozer et al., 2003). One of the strongest predictors of exposure to traumatic events has consistently been prior exposure (Testa, VanZile-Tamsen, & Livingston, 2007). Multiple previous events had a stronger effect than a single previous event. Previous events involving assaultive violence—single or multiple, in childhood, were associated with a higher risk of PTSD in adulthood (Breslau, Chilcoat, Kessler, & Davis, 1999). In particular, victims of childhood sexual abuse are at increased risk of being raped later in life (Widom, 1999). The conditional risk of developing PTSD is higher for interpersonal violence events, such as rape, than for other types of traumatic events (e.g., sudden unexpected death) (Breslau, Chilcoat, Kessler, Peterson, & Lucia, 1999). A dose–response relation between severity of exposure and conditional risk of developing PTSD also has been well documented (Kessler, Sonnega, Bromet, Hughes, & Nelson, 1995).

Depression is an additional variable identified as a risk factor for subsequent exposure (Breslau, Davis, Peterson, & Schultz, 1997), potentially via a diminished cognitive capacity with which to detect perpetrators and/or make decisions to avoid risk. The low motivation and energy levels characteristic of depression may also inhibit escape from dangerous situations or abusive relationships.

Overall study findings suggest that different types of PTSD symptoms play different roles in predicting exposure to different types of traumatic events. Re-experiencing symptoms, in particular, appeared to play an important role in predicting subsequent violent assault or rape by a non-intimate perpetrator, though such symptoms did not predict intimate partner violence. These findings were, thus, consistent with those of Orcutt, Erickson, and Wolfe (2002), who found re-experiencing symptoms are more important than other symptom clusters in predicting subsequent trauma exposure of any type.

Previous or Concurrent Psychiatric Morbidity

A positive family history of psychiatric disorders is a consistent risk factor for development of PTSD (Ozer et al., 2003). Preexisting psychiatric disorders, particularly conduct disorder, major depression, and nicotine dependence, also increase PTSD risk (Breslau, 2002). Twin studies have demonstrated that genetic influences common to major depression, generalized anxiety disorder, panic disorder, or substance dependence account for up to 60 % of the genetic variance in PTSD (Koenen et al., 2005). Variants implicated in PTSD also have been associated with other psychiatric conditions (Caspi et al., 2003).

PTSD is highly comorbid with other psychiatric illnesses, including mood disorders such as major depressive disorder (Kessler et al., 1995). It has been suggested that susceptibility to anxiety disorders is associated with increased risk for mood disorders and vice versa (Dilsaver, Akiskal, Akiskal, & Benazzi, 2006). It has been demonstrated that preexisting depression is a risk factor to experience a traumatic event as well as to develop PTSD after trauma exposure (Breslau, Davis, Peterson, & Schultz, 2000). In addition, the development of depression after a traumatic event is more frequent in individuals with PTSD as compared with traumatized individuals without PTSD (Breslau et al., 2000). The accumulating literature suggests common genetic susceptibility factors for the development of PTSD and major depression. For example, Koenen, Moffitt, Poulton, Martin, and Caspi (2007) calculated that a majority of the genetic variance in PTSD is the result of comorbid major depression (Koenen, 2007). In addition, the homozygous S polymorphism of the serotonin transporter has been associated with both PTSD and major depression (Caspi et al., 2003).

Gender

It has been frequently demonstrated that women show a greater propensity to develop PTSD following any traumatic event (Testa et al., 2007). Thus, it has been proposed that women may be more vulnerable to aberrant hypothalamus–pituitary–adrenal (HPA) axis responses to stress. For instance, basal cortisol was examined in healthy men and women and following acute exposure to stressors. Among healthy participants, men had higher basal cortisol levels than women. In response to acute stressors, such as carbon dioxide or noise, respectively, cortisol levels were comparable between men and women or higher among women. Cortisol levels were also examined among those with PTSD. Men who have motor vehicle accident-related PTSD demonstrate more aberrant cortisol function, than do their female counterparts. Although these sex differences in cortisol seem to vary with type of stress exposure and/or pathophysiological status of the individual, other hormones may influence cortisol response (Paris et al., 2010).

Furthermore, studies of civilians typically find that female gender is a risk factor for PTSD. In contrast, police and military studies often find no gender differences in PTSD. A study compared female police officers and female civilians on several variables including trauma exposure, peri-traumatic emotional distress, current somatization, and cumulative PTSD symptoms. It was found that despite greater exposure to assaultive violence in the officer group, female civilians reported significantly more severe PTSD symptoms. Elevated PTSD symptoms in female civilians were explained by significantly more intense peri-traumatic emotional distress. However, it was demonstrated that female officers showed a stronger direct relationship between peri-traumatic emotional distress and current somatization. These findings suggest that apparent gender differences in PTSD may result from differences in peri-traumatic emotionality, which influence subsequent PTSD and somatization symptoms. Therefore, emotionality may be more important than biological sex in understanding gender differences in PTSD (Lilly, Pole, Best, Metzler, & Marmar, 2009).

Ethnic and Cultural Aspects

A number of reviews (Fothergill, Maestas, & Darlington, 1999) observed that being a member of an ethnic minority increased the likelihood of developing adverse outcomes following a disaster. Brewin, Andrews, and Valentine (2000) in a meta-analysis of 22 studies with 8,165 subjects confirmed minority status as a risk factor for PTSD following major disasters. In studies assessing the impact of the 9/11 terrorist attacks, Stein et al. (2004) reported more persistent distress in non-whites. Ford, Adams, and Dailey (2005) and Chu, Seery, Ence, Holman, and Cohen-Silver (2006) found Hispanic ethnicity to be a risk factor in reporting psychological problems. Rubin, Brewin, Greenberg, Simpson, and Wessely (2005) reported that being non-white as well as Muslim predicted substantial distress following the 2005 bombing in London. A number of studies have also found that being part of the Arab minority in Israel, during times of ongoing terrorism, is a risk factor. Compared to Jews, Musallam, Ginzburg, Lev-Shalem, and Solomon (2005) found more distress in Arab-Israeli students; Somer et al. (2006) found more PTSD and depression in Arabs in ethnically mixed towns, and Hobfoll, Canetti-Nisim, and Johnson (2006) found more posttraumatic symptomatology in a large sample of urban Arabs compared to Jews.

A number of reasons have been proposed as to why minorities are more at risk for mental health sequelae following traumatic exposure. For example, minorities often have higher exposure rates (Beals et al., 2002) and live in at-risk areas.

They often have high mortality, morbidity and injury rates (Hobfoll et al., 2006), and less health care following disasters (Ford, 2005). Empirical studies suggest that minorities may have higher risk perceptions, more motion focused coping (Chu et al., 2006), less behavioral adaptation to terror (Goltz, Russell, & Bourque, 1992), and less psychological resources (Zeidner, Klingman, & Itskowitz, 1993), all conducive to more distress. Economic and social–political factors such as less education and economic resources (Goltz et al., 1992), closed and overburdened social networks (Kaniasty & Norris, 1993), acculturation stress (Perilla, Norris, & Lavizzio, 2002), racism (Loo, Fairbank, & Chemtob, 2005), and political stress may also compound the burden on these populations. However, following 19 months of terrorism, Arab Israelis and Jewish Israelis reacted similarly. This is in line with a number of previous studies that have also found no (Adams & Boscarino, 2005) or only minor differences in the way most minorities reacted in the aftermath of the 9/11 events (Galea et al., 2003). One might assume an equalizing mechanism, whereby national or community stress impacts in a way that overshadows certain risk factors usually closely associated with traumatic reactions such as ethnicity (Somer, Ruvio, Soref, & Sever, 2005), education (Lewin, Carr, & Webster, 1998), and socioeconomic status (Kaniasty & Norris, 1995). This situation changed over 44 months of terror. In the Jewish population some symptoms worsened, some remained unchanged, and others improved. In the Arab population, outcome measures worsened significantly. These results suggest that traumatic events may impact over time differentially in minorities and majorities (Palinkas, Petterson, Russell, & Downs, 2004). Resilience eroding factors such as dual allegiance, feelings of political and social oppression, and internal pressure to actively support terrorist activities may have elevated the Arab population's level of stress to a point where available material, societal, and psychological resources become inadequate to meet the threat of terror.

Further, issues about the impact of traumatic experiences on minority soldiers and veterans have been initially raised in the context of the Vietnam era studies.

Findings from the American troops in Operation Desert Storm, who were of a more diverse ethnicity than in previous military operations, supported findings from studies of Vietnam veterans that ethnic minorities are more vulnerable to traumatic stress following war-zone duty (Sutker, Davis, Uddo, & Ditta, 1995). Veterans from ethnic minority backgrounds may have different experiences during service, such as higher levels of combat stressors (MacDonald, Chamberlain, & Long, 1997) and exposure to adverse race-related events (Loo et al., 2005), as well as added difficulties in the readjustment period following discharge (Brende, 1983).

Personality Characteristics

Breslau (2002) noted, "Personality traits of neuroticism and extroversion, early conduct problems, a family history of psychiatric disorders, and preexisting psychiatric disorders are associated with increased risk for exposure to traumatic events".

Thus, a portion of the psychopathology observed following trauma may simply represent an extension of preexisting risk factors for exposure (Zeidner et al., 1993).

A prospective study examined constitutional and contextual factors leading to the development of PTSD in a cohort of children aged 3–5 years, who were followed into adulthood. Constitutional factors were defined as within-individual capacities, such as childhood cognitive ability, early temperament and behavior, and juvenile mental disorders. Contextual factors were defined as aspects of the child's social environment, such as maternal depression, poverty, and residential instability.

It has been shown that childhood IQ assessed as early as age 5 was inversely associated with risk for developing PTSD by age 32. No association was found between PTSD and other neurodevelopmental factors assessed in this cohort, including number of perinatal insults or gross motor skills in childhood. This suggested that the IQ-PTSD association was specific to cognitive ability and not a marker of broader neurodevelopmental deficits. Lower childhood IQ was not associated with increased risk of later trauma exposure. The authors have posited that individuals with greater cognitive ability are better able to translate their traumatic event into a narrative and make meaning out of it, both of which are thought to be important in recovery from PTSD (Koenen et al., 2007).

It was also found that children characterized as exhibiting externalizing temperament and behavior, defined as having difficult temperaments aged 3–5 or manifesting antisocial behavior and hyperactivity aged 5–11, were at increased risk of developing PTSD (Koenen et al., 2007). This increased risk was explained, in part, by an association between externalizing and increased risk of trauma exposure. However, even among the trauma exposed, externalizing increased risk of PTSD. One explanation for this association is that externalizing tendencies might interfere with tolerating the emotions (e.g., fear) necessary for processing the traumatic event, and thus impede recovery. Anger, which is a characteristic of individuals with externalizing tendencies, has been associated with reduced likelihood of recovery from PTSD, both in treatment settings (Koenen et al., 2007) and in the community (Koenen et al., 2007).

Only 15 % of the trauma exposed with no juvenile mental disorder history developed PTSD. In contrast, 41 % of those with one juvenile diagnosis and 48 % of those with two or more developed PTSD. This effect was not specific to any one juvenile diagnosis. The longitudinal findings of this study also suggest that characteristics of the child's early social context may sensitize them to the adverse effects of later trauma. Specifically, children raised in poverty were predisposed to developing PTSD by age 32 when exposed to a traumatic event, as compared with children of high socioeconomic status. Residential instability, defined as moving three or more times before age 11, was also a strong contributor to PTSD risk. Other factors that contributed to the development of PTSD were maternal depression and parent changes before age 11. It was speculated that these factors—poverty, residential instability, maternal depression, and caregiver changes—result in an unpredictable and uncontrollable environments that have adverse life course effects.

Childhood adversity in human studies is associated with HPA axis dysregulation in adulthood (Watson et al., 2007). Thus, HPA axis dysregulation is a potential biological mechanism linking the association between an unpredictable and uncontrollable childhood environment and the later development of PTSD.

To summarize: developmental factors may be useful in identifying individuals who are at high risk and should be monitored more carefully for persistent symptoms. Identification of high-risk groups is particularly important in natural and human-made disasters where large numbers of individuals are trauma exposed but resources are limited for follow-up. A better understanding of the role of developmental factors in PTSD may also help inform resiliency training for persons in professions with a high probability of trauma exposure, such as the military, police, firefighters, or other first responders. Finally, prevention efforts aimed at addressing some of these developmental capacities, such as externalizing temperament and behavior or at improving conditions of childhood adversity, may ultimately reduce risk of PTSD.

Peri-traumatic Factors

Nature of traumatic event (severity, duration, man-made vs. natural).

It has been demonstrated that cognitive factors play a large role in the onset, severity, and outcome of PTSD following sexual assault (Koss & Figueredo, 2004). These factors include mental defeat and confusion, negative appraisal of emotions and symptoms, avoidance, and perceived negative responses from others (Dunmore, Clark, & Ehlers, 1999). If the survivor of sexual assault believes that others have failed to react in a positive and supportive manner, there is a greater risk of PTSD (Dunmore et al., 1999).

Perceiving events as uncontrollable is much more distressing than controllable events. Therefore, with uncontrollable events such as sexual assault, survivors attempt to attribute blame to behavioral, dispositional, or vicarious causes (Frazier, 2003). Behavioral self-blame is potentially adaptive as it promotes the belief that negative outcomes can be avoided in the future. However, dispositional self-blame attributes the traumatic event to one's personality and this attitude does not give a sense of future control (Frazier, 2003). Vicarious control refers to the perception that some other person or entity had control over the occurrence of that event (Frazier, 2003). Attributing blame in any of these ways focuses on the past and is associated with poorer outcomes in PTSD.

Duration of exposure made a small, significant contribution to clinical status in the immediate aftermath of trauma among women who had experienced violent sexual assault (McHugh & Treisman, 2007). These findings are consistent with the emerging viewpoint that severe and persistent post-trauma problems represent a failure to recover from common and often transient reactions (McHugh & Treisman, 2007). Within this framework, an early temporal relationship between objective indexes of event magnitude and initial posttraumatic reactions may be observed. Solely, a simple dose–response model, on the other hand, may not explain longer-term outcomes. Instead, a variety of factors influence an individual's ability to adjust in the aftermath of trauma: pre-incident psychiatric vulnerability, subjective appraisals, alterations in cognitive schema, and post-incident social and situational concerns.

Severity of Initial Reaction

It has been postulated that the severity of initial reaction to stress may be predictive of subsequent development of PTSD (Goltz et al., 1992). Thus, it was demonstrated that a significant portion of injured traffic accident victims manifested PTSD one year after the event. Development of PTSD at one year can be predicted as early as 1 week after the accident, on the basis of the existence and severity of early PTSD-related symptoms. However, the first 3 months following the accident appear to be the critical period for the development of PTSD (Koren, Arnon, & Klein, 1999). This study examined the prevalence of peri-traumatic and persistent panic symptoms following trauma. Panic attacks were experienced by 77 % of participants during their trauma, and 47 % reported recurrent panic attacks post-trauma. Individuals suffering from Acute Stress Disorder (ASD) demonstrated more panic symptoms during and after their trauma than those not diagnosed with ASD. Posttraumatic panic was most strongly associated with anxiety sensitivity. There is increasing evidence that panic attacks play a role in psychopathological response to trauma. A significant proportion of people with panic disorder report a history of trauma (Nixon & Bryant, 2003). Moreover, two-thirds of trauma survivors report panic attacks within the previous 2 weeks (Nixon & Bryant, 2003). There is also evidence that people with PTSD display elevated levels of anxiety sensitivity (Nixon & Bryant, 2003). ASD is a useful framework in which to investigate the role of panic in post-traumatic stress because ASD describes acute responses to trauma that are strongly predictive of chronic PTSD (Nixon & Bryant, 2003).

Memory of the Traumatic Event

Memory of the traumatic event (MTE) is considered a central component of trauma-related disorders, including PTSD. It has been suggested that the psychopathology of PTSD is closely related to abnormal memory processes, namely, that in PTSD patients, traumatic events create pathogenic ("toxic") memories. These memories, rather than the events themselves, are responsible for generating the characteristic symptoms of the disorder. Traumatic memories share both explicit and implicit features and are believed to be processed differently than ordinary memories (Brewin, 2001). This results in a failure to organize the traumatic event into a coherent verbally represented narrative (Brewin, 2001). The abnormal nature of traumatic memories is considered to be a central feature of PTSD. This is manifested by two well-documented and seemingly contradictory observations of traumatized individuals: hypermnesic symptoms, such as re-experiencing, intrusive thoughts, nightmares, and flashbacks, on the one hand, and impaired memory for certain aspects of the traumatic event in the form of amnesia and delayed recall, on the other hand. Furthermore, it appears that traumatic memories tend to be disorganized and fragmented. Patients with PTSD provide less coherent memories, exhibiting extra repetitions and nonconsecutive memory chunks (Halligan, Michael, Clark, & Ehlers, 2003). Their memories are characterized by dissociation and sensory verbal representation, namely, frequent use of sensory symbols. These abnormal features of memory (i.e., repetition and nonconsecutive chunks) were found to predict PTSD severity (Halligan et al., 2003) as well as to contribute to the preservation of PTSD, by interfering with processing and resolution of the traumatic memory (Ehlers & Clark, 2000). On the other hand, Foa, Molnar, and Cashman (1995) found that participants who exhibited a decrease in narrative fragmentation over time reported a reduction in trauma-related anxiety.

Preclinical and clinical data suggest that amnesia of the traumatic event is associated with a decreased prevalence of PTSD. Clinical data include following up on traumatic brain injury and examination of the frequency of PTSD in individuals with amnesia as compared to non-amnesic patients. Klein, Caspi, and Gil (2003) examined 120 patients with mild traumatic brain injury. Patients' memory of the traumatic event was recorded (24-h post-trauma), and they were assessed for PTSD symptoms 1 week, 3 months, and 6 months later. Rates of PTSD 6 months following the traumatic event were found to be significantly lower in patients with no memory of the traumatic event (6 % PTSD) than in patients with memory of the event (23 % PTSD).

Along these lines, psychological defense mechanisms which mimic amnesia (such as repression) might be predicted as useful. Indeed, a study of repressive coping styles after myocardial infarction revealed this to be the case (Ginzburg, Solomon, & Bleich, 2002). In this study, 116 myocardial infarction patients were assessed for repressive coping style within a week of their myocardial infarction. These patients were divided into four groups: high anxious, low anxious, defensive, and repressors. Patients were also assessed at this point for symptoms of ASD, and for symptoms of PTSD at 7 months. The repressor group displayed fewer symptoms of both ASD and PTSD, implying that repression is indeed useful in buffering against the potential consequences of trauma.

Dissociation

Dissociation is a common feature of PTSD (van der Kolk et al., 1996). It involves disruptions in, and fragmentation of, the usually integrated functions of consciousness, memory, identity, body awareness, and perception of the self and the environment (American Psychiatric Association, 1994). Alterations in memory encoding and storage occur in dissociation, leading to fragmentation and compartmentalization of memory and impairments in memory retrieval (Spiegel & Cardena, 1991). Chronic psychological, sexual, and physical trauma as well as emotional neglect, including parental psychological unavailability, has been etiologically related to dissociation (Loewenstein & Putnam, 2004). Even though dissociative symptoms are often observed following exposure to chronic psychological trauma, acute traumatic events can also lead to dissociative experiences, often referred to as peri-traumatic dissociation. For example, a number of studies of individuals experiencing danger or life threat have shown specific peri-traumatic dissociative changes, including alterations in time sense, perception, attentional focus, and awareness of pain among others (Morgan et al., 2001). In addition, depersonalization has been described in a significant percentage of individuals facing acute life threat (Ironson et al., 1997). Information related to traumatic experiences is often differently encoded in these altered states, resulting in decreased access to information about the trauma, once the person returns to his or her baseline state. This may give a subjective sense of "compartmentalization" of the trauma and lead to cognitive fragmentation or emotional detachment from the experience. The cost of this detachment may be avoidance of necessary cognitive and affective processing of trauma in its aftermath (Spiegel & Cardena, 1991). Acute dissociative responses to psychological trauma have been found to predict the development of chronic PTSD (Marmar et al., 1994). Moreover, a chronic pattern of dissociation in response to reminders of the original trauma and minor stressors develops in persons who experience acute dissociative responses to psychological trauma (Butler, Duran, Jasiukaitis, Koopman, & Spiegel, 1996).

Immediate peri-traumatic dissociative responses have been noted in police and emergency personnel attending to catastrophes (Marmar et al., 1999), as well as fire victims (Koopman, Classen, & Spiegel, 1994), victims of earthquakes (Cardena & Spiegel, 1993), and combat soldiers (Marmar et al., 1994). Dissociative responses to trauma have also been correlated with increased dissociative response to reminders of trauma (Bremner et al., 1998), increased dissociative responses to subsequent traumas and stressors, and long-term PTSD and dissociative pathology (Bremner & Brett, 1997). Prospective studies in healthy military personnel have also revealed that severe stress leads to heightened dissociation (Morgan et al., 2001).

Bremner (1999) has hypothesized that there may be two subtypes of acute trauma response that represent unique pathways to chronic stress-related psychopathology: one is primarily dissociative, and the other predominantly intrusive and hyperaroused. Data from neuroimaging studies have shown that two subtypes of response can persist in persons with chronic PTSD and are associated with distinct patterns of neural activation upon exposure to reminders of traumatic events (Lanius, Bluhm, Lanius, & Pain, 2006). It should be noted that these response patterns are not completely distinct, and that individual patients with PTSD may show both response patterns either simultaneously, or at different time points. However, PTSD patients with prolonged traumatic experiences, such as chronic childhood abuse or combat trauma, often show a clinical syndrome that is characterized by chronic symptoms of dissociation (Pervanidou, 2008) as opposed to patients who have suffered from more acute traumatic experiences.

Psychobiological responses to recalling traumatic experiences can differ significantly among patients with chronic PTSD (Breslau, Davis, Andreski, Peterson, &

Schultz, 1997). Approximately 70 % of patients had subjective experiences of reliving their traumatic experience and showed an increase in heart rate while recalling the traumatic memory (Lanius et al., 2006). The other 30 % of PTSD subjects had a dissociative response. The latter predominantly involved subjective states of depersonalization and derealization with no significant concomitant increase in heart rate (Hopper, Frewen, van der Kolk, & Lanius, 2007).

Terr (1991) proposed two types of traumatic experiences. Type I trauma refers to traumatic conditions that result from single traumatic experiences and include predominantly full and vividly detailed memories, cognitive reappraisals, and misperceptions. In contrast, Type II trauma was hypothesized to be associated with long-standing or repeated exposure to extreme stressors, and includes dissociation, denial and numbing, states of self-hypnosis, and rage. Further support for these hypotheses comes from a study by van der Kolk et al. (1996) which, as part of a DSM-IV field trial, examined a sample of 395 traumatized treatment-seeking subjects and 125 non-treatment-seeking subjects who had been exposed to traumatic experiences. Results showed that participants who had suffered early-onset interpersonal abuse (age ≤14 years) had significantly higher percentages of endorsements of dissociative symptoms than participants with late-onset interpersonal abuse and disaster survivors. Moreover, subjects with dissociative symptoms continued to suffer from dissociation even after they no longer met criteria for PTSD. This suggests that severe, chronic dissociative symptoms develop in response to early-onset interpersonal violence.

More recently, Ginzburg et al. (2006) employed signal detection analyses to identify high and low dissociation PTSD subgroups in a sample of 122 women who were seeking treatment for childhood sexual abuse. Specifically, three PTSD symptoms, including hypervigilance, sense of foreshortened future, and sleep difficulties, discriminated between high and low dissociation subgroups. In addition, Zucker, Spinazzola, Blaustein, and van der Kolk (2006) examined differences in dissociative symptoms in subjects with PTSD, versus subjects with PTSD who also met criteria for disorders of extreme stress not otherwise specified. Criteria for disorders of extreme stress not otherwise specified were developed to characterize traumatized individuals who suffer "complex" forms of PTSD-related multiple episodes of trauma over several developmental epochs, with symptoms of dissociation, emotion dysregulation, somatization, altered relationships and attachments, and alterations in systems of meaning (Cash, 1993). Subjects with both PTSD and disorders of extreme stress not otherwise specified exhibited chronic symptoms of dissociation, as evidenced by higher scores on the Dissociative Experiences Scale, than participants who were suffering from PTSD only. Prospective longitudinal studies have shown that trauma leads to heightened dissociation in children (Putnam, Helmers, Horowitz, & Trickett, 1995). Cross-sectional studies have also consistently show a heightened level of dissociation in children whose trauma histories have been objectively confirmed compared to non-traumatized children (Valentino, Cicchetti, Rogosch, & Toth, 2008).

Vietnam combat veterans with PTSD ($N=40$) scored significantly higher on all five aspects of dissociation as measured by the clinician administered SCID-D (Steinberg, Rounsaville, & Cicchetti, 1990) compared to Vietnam veterans without

PTSD (Bremner, Steinberg, Southwick, Johnson, & Charney, 1993). In fact, the symptom with the greatest difference between PTSD and non-PTSD patients was amnesia. Furthermore, prospective, longitudinal research showed that individuals presenting to emergency rooms resulting from acute assaults and with ASD retrieved fewer specific autobiographical memories than those without ASD 2 weeks post-assault (Kleim & Ehlers, 2008). In addition, reduced memory specificity at 2 weeks predicted PTSD at 6 months over and above what could be predicted by initial diagnoses and symptom severity.

Studies in combat-related PTSD also point to a dissociative subtype of PTSD. Taxometric analyses in a sample of 316 Vietnam veterans consistently revealed a taxon/subtype (subgroup identified by scores that are discontinuous with a dimensional distribution) of highly dissociative individuals. The dissociative subtype of PTSD was also associated with more severe PTSD (Creamer et al., 2001). Furthermore, Putnam et al. (1996) examined whether mean dissociation scores, as measured by the Dissociative Experiences Scale, resulted from uniform distributions of scores in a group of 166 predominantly combat-related PTSD patients. Results showed that the diagnostic group's mean Dissociative Experiences Scale scores were a function of the proportion of subjects within the group who were high dissociators, thus suggesting the existence of a distinct dissociative subtype. An earlier study of Vietnam veterans also reported that chronic dissociative symptoms are an important element of long-term psychological responses to combat trauma, which is often repetitive in nature (Bremner et al., 1992).

Exposure-based treatments for PTSD (Institute of Medicine, 2007) have the strongest empirical support and involve repeated imaginary and in vivo exposure to trauma-related stimuli. However, exposure treatments should be used with caution in patients with significant emotional over modulation, such as dissociative and numbing symptoms. Foa and Kozak (1986) have suggested that such symptoms can prevent emotional engagement with trauma-related information and thus reduce treatment effectiveness (Jaycox, Foa, & Morral, 1998). In fact, a more recent study (Waelde, Silvern, & Fairbank, 2005) suggests that levels of dissociation are an important negative predictor of psychotherapy outcome in patients with borderline personality disorder, a disorder that has often been associated with childhood abuse (Ball & Links, 2009). Therefore, it is crucial, before commencing exposure-based treatments, to assess levels of dissociative psychopathology and to provide interventions to reduce dissociative symptomatic responses to trauma-related stimuli. Failure to do so may lead to an actual increase in PTSD and related symptoms, including dissociation, emotional dysregulation, and an increase in the patient's overall distress and functional impairment.

Degree of Perceived Threat to Life and of Helplessness

As far as psychological mechanisms are concerned, the most direct hypothesis is that bodily injury intensifies the perceived threat to one's life or physical integrity during the trauma. According to the literature (Shalev, 1992), trauma survivors' perceived level of danger is a better predictor of PTSD than the objective severity of the traumatic event. However, this hypothesis may be overly simplistic due to data (Koren, Norman, Cohen, Berman, & Klein, 2005), suggesting that the heightened level of perceived threat is not directly correlated with the severity of injury. These findings suggest that the effect of bodily injury on perceived threat is moderated by other factors, such as sense of control and the ability to effectively function and cope during the traumatic event (Asmundson, Coons, Taylor, & Katz, 2002).

It has been suggested that the feelings of helplessness during exposure to a traumatic event may result in increased severity of PTSD symptoms (Campbell, 1990) while a significant role in the setting of trauma may be protective.

During the 5-week-long second Lebanon war in the summer of 2006, the Rambam Medical Center, the largest hospital and main trauma center for Northern Israel, provided emergency treatment to 850 injured people and additional 350 people with acute stress reactions. In addition, for the first time in its history, the hospital operated under direct fire, with about 45 missiles falling within a radius of 500 meters from the hospital. The hospital was not protected and the staff worked long hours under extreme stress. The rates and severity of PTSD symptoms among hospital workers operating under fire while treating war-related injured patients, and the level of functioning in real time, were assessed by the Posttraumatic Stress Disorder Scale (PSS). It was demonstrated that 10.2 % of the participants met the symptom and severity threshold for a probable diagnosis of PTSD. However, only 3 % reported significant distress and impaired level of functioning (DSM-IV-TR criteria for acute PTSD). Administration workers and nurses reported higher number of PS compared to paramedical staff and physicians (significant role effect). There were no significant differences on PS severity and rates of probable PTSD, between personnel who had direct exposure to injured or traumatized casualties (secondary traumatization) and those who did not. These findings suggest that hospital workers operating under prolonged life-threatening conditions are at low to moderate risk for PTSD. However, they do not support an incremental effect of secondary traumatic exposure. The majority of medical personnel treating injured traumatized patients under fire adapted to the stressful situation without significant impact on their functioning and coping. Role seems to be an important moderator of vulnerability suggesting that intervention and prevention programs should be targeted those at risk (Koren et al., 2009).

Posttraumatic Factors

Social support plays a large role in the onset, severity, and outcome of PTSD after sexual assault (Koss & Figueredo, 2004). Thus, it was demonstrated that if the survivor of sexual assault believes that others have failed to react in a positive and supportive manner, there is a greater risk of PTSD (Chivers-Wilson, 2006).

In general, numerous studies have shown that social support following a traumatic event is negatively associated with PTSD symptoms (Ozer et al., 2003).

Based on 11 studies (combined $n = 3{,}537$), Ozer et al. (2003) report the average weighted correlation between perceived social support and PTSD symptoms to be −.28.

Historically, most studies in this area have examined the effect of PTSD on combat veterans' romantic relationships and family functioning. Results suggest increased stress, more marital dysfunction, and greater difficulties with parenting among families of veterans with PTSD relative to those without (Jordan et al., 1992). In an effort to explore this issue more closely, Riggs, Byrne, Weathers, and Litz (1998) considered the association between PTSD symptom clusters (re-experiencing, avoidance/numbing, and physiological hyperarousal) and self-reported marital quality in 50 Vietnam veterans and their romantic partners. Results suggested that avoidance and numbing symptoms showed the strongest negative correlation with marital quality in this sample, relative to the other two symptoms clusters.

Depression

One study examined the separate influences of PTSD symptoms and depression on interpersonal functioning with friends, romantic partners, and family. These findings suggested that hyperarousal symptoms are the most salient among PTSD symptom clusters in their negative effect on interpersonal functioning. However, depression appears to be a more robust factor in interviewer-assessed interpersonal strain, relative to PTSD symptoms. The findings suggest that emotional numbing, depression, and to a lesser extent, hyperarousal symptoms are the more salient symptoms in their negative effect on perceived social support (Testa et al., 2007).

Alcohol and Substance Abuse

Substance use disorders (SUDs) have been found to be associated with numerous co-occurring difficulties, including mood and anxiety disorders (Conway, Compton, Stinson, & Grant, 2006), as well as high rates of traumatic exposure. Indeed, as many as 95 % of individuals with SUDs report a history of traumatic exposure (Ford, Hawke, Alessi, Ledgerwood, & Petry, 2007), with rates of current diagnoses of PTSD ranging from approximately 20–60 % among samples of substance users in inpatient or outpatient treatment (Jacobsen, Southwick, & Kosten, 2001). In addition, separate from PTSD, elevated rates of posttraumatic stress (PTS) symptoms have been found among substance users exposed to potentially traumatic events (PTEs) (Sullivan & Holt, 2008). Further, a particularly strong association has been found among PTSD, PTS symptoms, and illicit drug use, including both crack/cocaine and heroin use (Sullivan & Holt, 2008).

High rates of co-occurrence between PTS and SUDs have led researchers to suggest that the experience of PTS symptoms and substance abuse may be functionally related (Stewart & Conrod, 2003). One prominent hypothesis concerning the functional relationship between PTS and SUDs focuses on the notion that substance use may operate as a form of self-medication among individuals experiencing symptoms of PTS following exposure to a PTE. Specifically, among PTE-exposed individuals, substance use may function to modulate or escape aversive PTS symptoms (Chilcoat & Breslau, 1998). Extant data on the temporal relationship between PTS and SUDs provide support for the self-medication hypothesis. For example, Chilcoat and Breslau (1998) found that whereas a PTSD diagnosis greatly increased risk for subsequent development of a drug use disorder, a drug use disorder did not increase risk for traumatic exposure or PTSD. Likewise, Wasserman, Havassy, and Boles (1997) found that 69 % of cocaine-dependent inpatients with PTSD indicated that their PTSD developed prior to their cocaine dependence, consistent with findings that 86 % of a sample of cocaine-dependent individuals with PTSD reported that a worsening of their PTS symptoms was associated with an increase in cocaine use and 64 % reported that an improvement in PTS symptoms was associated with a decrease in cocaine use (Back, Brady, Jaanimagi, & Jackson, 2006). In examining the longitudinal course of PTS symptoms and substance use among Vietnam veterans, Bremner, Southwick, Darnell, and Charney (1996) demonstrated that increases in both licit (i.e., alcohol) and illicit (i.e., heroin, marijuana, and cocaine) substance abuse paralleled a worsening of PTS symptoms. However, veterans reported that alcohol, heroin, benzodiazepines, and marijuana were useful in managing the hyperarousal symptoms of PTSD, and alcohol and heroin were also useful in reducing the severity of re-experiencing symptoms. Moreover, findings indicate that alcohol- and cocaine-dependent individuals with PTSD are more likely to report that their substance use is motivated by the experience of aversive internal states, compared with those without PTSD (Waldrop, Back, Verduin, & Brady, 2007). Finally, experimental studies of the interplay between PTSD symptoms and substance use have demonstrated that the severity of PTSD symptoms predicts cravings in response to trauma-related imaginary cues among alcohol- and cocaine-dependent individuals with PTSD (Saladin et al., 2003).

Indeed, preliminary research generally suggests a positive association between hyperarousal and re-experiencing PTSD symptoms and use of substances that have a depressant or anxiolytic effect (e.g., alcohol, prescription anxiolytic medications) (Stewart, Conrod, Pihl, & Dongier, 1999), as well as positive associations between illicit drug use in general and re-experiencing, avoidance/emotional numbing, and hyperarousal PTS symptoms (Sullivan & Holt, 2008). Further, although both Shipherd, Stafford, and Tanner (2005) and Sullivan and Holt (2008) did not find evidence for associations between particular PTSD symptom clusters and alcohol use, Saladin, Brady, Dansky, and Kilpatrick (1995) found higher levels of hyperarousal symptoms among inpatients with PTSD and alcohol dependence than among those with PTSD and cocaine dependence, suggesting that hyperarousal symptoms may be more strongly associated with substances that have a depressant, rather than a stimulant, effect. Likewise, Najavits et al. (2003) found that a restricted range of affect and feelings of detachment (both considered to be emotional numbing symptoms of PTSD) were two of the most prominent PTSD symptoms reported by patients with cocaine dependence. Despite preliminary evidence for an association between particular PTSD symptom clusters and use of specific substances that could counter those symptoms, none of these studies have examined the unique associations between particular PTSD symptom clusters and specific substances (both licit and illicit).

In another study (Tull, Gratz, Aklin, & Lejuez, 2010), results demonstrated a unique association between severity of hyperarousal symptoms and a dependence on heroin. Given that heroin functions to dampen central nervous system activity, individuals with a history of trauma exposure and subsequent PTSD symptoms may be motivated to use heroin as a way of alleviating or escaping hyperarousal symptoms in particular.

Interestingly, avoidance symptoms were also found to be related (albeit inversely) to heroin dependence. Although unexpected, these findings are consistent with those of Stewart et al. (1999), who found a small positive association between avoidance symptoms and prescription analgesic dependence. One possible explanation for these findings is that hyperarousal symptoms may become a conditioned stimulus for drug-seeking behavior due to past experiences in which heroin was successful in reducing those hyperarousal symptoms. Consequently, motivations to diminish hyperarousal symptoms and subsequent drug-seeking behavior may override the desire to avoid trauma-related cues, thus establishing an inverse relationship between avoidance symptoms and heroin dependence (consistent with animal models of drug-seeking behavior; e.g., Di Ciano & Everitt, 2003). Another possibility is that heroin use may decrease avoidance symptoms of PTSD. Specifically, as individuals increase their use of heroin, they may have less of a need for other strategies to avoid internal or external experiences associated with a traumatic event, resulting in a reduction in their reported PTSD-related avoidance symptoms. Finally, given that heroin use has been found to be associated with social isolation (McNamee, Mirin, Kuehnle, & Meyer, 1976), it is also possible that the regular use of heroin may limit exposure to trauma-related cues, thereby reducing the opportunity and/or need for avoidance behaviors.

Conversely, no evidence was found for a specific relationship between any of the PTSD symptom clusters and crack/cocaine or alcohol dependence. Although contrary to the hypothesized relationship between emotional numbing symptoms and crack/cocaine dependence (and the findings of Najavits et al., 2003), findings of an absence of a relationship between PTSD symptoms and crack/cocaine dependence are consistent with past studies indicating stronger relationships between PTSD symptoms and substances that have an anxiolytic/depressant effect than between PTSD symptoms and cocaine use (e.g., Saladin et al., 1995). Likewise, whereas alcohol, heroin, marijuana, opiates, and benzodiazepines were identified as being helpful in reducing severity of PTSD symptoms among Vietnam veterans, cocaine was not (Bremner et al., 1996). Given that cocaine use results in heightened central nervous system activity, it might be expected that individuals experiencing PTSD symptoms such as hyperarousal may be motivated to avoid substances that would further increase arousal. Indeed, Bremner et al. (1996) found that cocaine use was associated with a worsening of PTSD symptoms among Vietnam veterans.

Yet, there is previous research which demonstrated that cocaine-dependent individuals report a functional relationship between their PTS symptoms and cocaine use, indicating that an increase in their cocaine use corresponds with a worsening of their PTSD symptoms (Back et al., 2006). This suggests that crack/cocaine use may not be motivated by the experience of PTSD symptoms per se, but instead by the desire to escape unpleasant emotions (e.g., shame, guilt, sadness) associated with the experience of PTS symptoms (Waldrop et al., 2007). Of course, it is also possible that cocaine use among trauma-exposed individuals with PTSD symptoms may be motivated by factors other than expectancies focused on the alleviation of distress. One factor worth investigating in the future may be impulsivity, as separate lines of research demonstrate that both individuals with PTSD (Kotler, Iancu, Efroni, & Amir, 2001) and cocaine-dependent (vs. heroin-dependent) individuals (Bornovalova, Daughters, Hernandez, Richards, & Lejuez, 2005) exhibit heightened levels of impulsivity.

Alcohol abuse is negatively associated with health, and alcohol misuse may mediate the relationship between PTSD and functional health outcomes. In a study of 151 U.S. veterans (136 men and 15 women) of the wars in Iraq and Afghanistan, 39.1 % screened positive for PTSD and 26.5 % screened positive for hazardous drinking. PTSD symptoms and hazardous drinking were significantly correlated with each other and with health functioning. Hazardous drinking was found to partially mediate the relationship between PTSD and functional mental health, but not physical health (McDevitt-Murphy et al., 2010).

Guilt Feelings and Shame

Veterans of various service eras ($N = 174$) completed an Internet survey about combat exposure, PTSD symptoms, depression, guilt, and meaning in life. Results of a hierarchical regression indicated that younger age; higher levels of combat exposure, depression, and guilt; and lower meaning in life predicted greater PTSD severity (Owens, Steger, Whitesell, & Herrera, 2009).

A 2010 study examined the degree to which combat-related guilt mediated the relations between exposure to combat-related abusive violence and both PTSD and major depressive disorder (MDD) in Vietnam Veterans (Marx et al., 2010). Results revealed that combat-related guilt partially mediated the association between exposure to combat-related abusive violence and PTSD, but completely mediated the association with MDD, with overall combat exposure held constant in the model. Follow-up analyses showed that, when comparing those participants who actually participated in combat-related abusive violence with those who only observed it, combat-related guilt completely mediated the association between participation in abusive violence and both PTSD and MDD. Moreover, when comparing those participants who observed combat-related abusive violence with those who had no exposure at all to it, combat-related guilt completely mediated the association between observation of combat-related abusive violence and MDD, but only partially mediated the association with PTSD (Marx et al., 2010). These findings suggest that guilt may be a mechanism through which abusive violence is related to PTSD and MDD among combat-deployed veterans.

Another prospective longitudinal study examined the course of PTSD symptoms in mothers of children with burns between one and 11 years following the burn event, the role of burn severity, and feelings of guilt on this course (Bakker, Van Loey, Van Son, & Van der Heijden, 2010). Self-reported PTSD symptoms of 48 mothers were measured with the Impact of Event Scale. Guilt feelings were assessed during an in-depth interview two years following the burn event. Eleven years after the burn event, mothers marked their child's scars on a drawing at the present time. Over a period of 10 years, maternal PTSD symptoms decreased. Multiple regression analysis showed that the interaction between guilt and burn severity predicted the course of PTSD. Although PTSD symptoms substantially decreased through the years, a subset of mothers, in particular mothers who felt guilty about the burn event and whose children had more extensive permanent scarring, seemed at risk for longer-term PTSD (Bakker et al., 2010).

In a web-based survey in 2010, in which nonclinical participants identified an event associated with shame or guilt and completed questionnaire measures of shame, guilt, PTSD, and depression. Shame predicted depression and PTSD symptoms. There was no association between guilt and psychological symptoms after controlling statistically for the effects of shame. The results suggest shame is capable of eliciting the intrusive and distressing memories characteristic of PTSD (Robinaugh & McNally, 2010).

Cognitive theory suggests that PTSD is caused by traumatic experiences being processed in a way that causes ongoing current threat. Shame might contribute to the creation/maintenance of ongoing current threat as it attacks an individual's psychological integrity. A correlational design was used to investigate some of the factors that might contribute to a shame response within a PTSD sample. It was shown that individuals with PTSD who report higher levels of shame were more prone to engage in self-critical thinking and less prone to engage in self-reassuring thinking than individuals with PTSD who reported lower levels of shame (Harman & Lee, 2010).

Litigation and Compensation

There is a substantial body of literature supporting the view that access to health compensation—notably health care cover and income support—is associated with poor recovery after injury. In one study in 2010, the motor vehicle accident-compensable group did have significantly higher levels of anxiety than the non-compensable group, but this appeared to be explained by the level of stress experienced in dealing with the compensation agency. Stress in dealing with compensation agencies can arise from having to undergo numerous assessments, delays in receiving funds, and the often adversarial relationship between client and organization. The study suggests that stressful interactions of this kind can affect mental health outcomes (O'Donnell, Creamer, McFarlane, Silove, & Bryant, 2010).

In another study, data from outpatient and inpatient programs for the treatment of posttraumatic stress disorder and associated disorders in the US Department of Veterans Affairs were used to compare outcomes for veterans who were and were not seeking compensation. Outcome was measured as pre/post-improvement in symptoms and work performance over the course of one year after the initiation of treatment. No compensation-seeking effect was observed among outpatients, but a significant effect was found for some inpatients. The effect for inpatients was manifested essentially by patients in a program type which was designed to have an extremely long length of stay, thus triggering a virtually automatic increase in payments. Like outpatients, inpatients in programs with a moderate length of stay did not manifest a compensation-seeking effect on improvement. Although unable to provide a definitive explanation, the preponderance of the evidence favors overstatement of symptoms, rather than either the severity or the chronicity of the disorder, as the most likely explanation for the compensation-seeking effect that was observed. For patients treated in standard outpatient and short-stay inpatient programs, compensation does not seem to affect clinical outcomes adversely (Fontana & Rosenheck, 1998). These findings were further supported by the findings of DeViva and Bloem (2003), according to which compensation seeking was not related to assessment scores or exaggeration in a sample of PTSD patients.

An additional study examined changes in psychiatric status and use of mental health services after the adjudication of Department of Veterans Affairs (VA) disability claims for PTSD in a sample of 101 veteran claimants. After the PTSD claim determination, half the sample had filed or planned to file a claim for a rating increase or an appeal, and thus remained compensation seeking. It was demonstrated that psychiatric status did not improve and treatment dropout rates did not increase among veterans who were no longer compensation seeking after the claim determination (Sayer, Spoont, Nelson, Clothier, & Murdoch, 2008).

Finally, another study investigated the potential utility of file characteristics as predictors of chronic PTSD among 686 victims of violence in 2006 who had applied for state compensation with the Dutch Victim Compensation Fund (DVCF). Results indicated that approximately one out of two victims applying for state compensation in the Netherlands still had PTSD many years after victimization and claim settlement. Age, female sex, time since victimization, acquaintance with the perpetrator, violence-related hospitalization, and compensation for immaterial damage proved to be predictive of PTSD, although female sex and immaterial damage compensation failed to reach significance after adjusting for recalled peri-traumatic distress severity (Kunst, Winkel, & Bogaerts, 2010).

Summary

To summarize, the risk of developing PTSD after a traumatic experience depends on several vulnerability factors that may be classified into three distinct categories—pre-traumatic, peri-traumatic, and posttraumatic. Accordingly, while attempting to draw the profile of the high-risk patient for PTSD, the following factors should be included, among others: the history of previous trauma, the history of previous psychiatric disorder, female gender, ethnic minority, high severity of initial post-traumatic symptoms (ASR), associated body injury, "high-risk" traumatic event (man-made trauma), and peri-traumatic dissociation.

In contrast—various resilience factors may be protective and act to prevent the development of PTSD. Although resilience factors were generally not discussed in this chapter, future research should be designed to uncover resilience factors, in order to differentiate between high-risk and low-risk patients in order to identifying the patients at risk and to attempt to develop the strategies to prevent the development of PTSD.

References

Adams, R. E., & Boscarino, J. A. (2005). Differences in mental health outcomes among Whites, African Americans, and Hispanics following a community disaster. *Psychiatry, 68*(3), 250–265.

American Psychiatric Association. (1994). *Diagnostic and statistical manual of mental disorders (DSM-IV)* (4th ed.). Washington, DC: American Psychiatric Association.

Asmundson, G. J., Coons, M. J., Taylor, S., & Katz, J. (2002). PTSD and the experience of pain: Research and clinical implications of shared vulnerability and mutual maintenance models. *Canadian Journal of Psychiatry, 47*(10), 930–937.

Back, S. E., Brady, K. T., Jaanimagi, U., & Jackson, J. L. (2006). Cocaine dependence and PTSD: A pilot study of symptom interplay and treatment preferences. *Addictive Behaviors, 31*(2), 351–354.

Bakker, A., Van Loey, N. E., Van Son, M. J., & Van der Heijden, P. G. (2010). Brief report: Mothers' long-term posttraumatic stress symptoms following a burn event of their child. *Journal of Pediatric Psychology, 35*(6), 656–661.

Ball, J. S., & Links, P. S. (2009). Borderline personality disorder and childhood trauma: Evidence for a causal relationship. *Current Psychiatry Reports, 11*(1), 63–68.

Basoglu, M., Paker, M., Paker, O., Ozmen, E., Marks, I., Incesu, C., et al. (1994). Psychological effects of torture: A comparison of tortured with nontortured political activists in Turkey. *The American Journal of Psychiatry, 151*(1), 76–81.

Beals, J., Manson, S. M., Shore, J. H., Friedman, M., Ashcraft, M., Fairbank, J. A., et al. (2002). The prevalence of posttraumatic stress disorder among American Indian Vietnam veterans: Disparities and context. *Journal of Traumatic Stress, 15*(2), 89–97.

Bornovalova, M. A., Daughters, S. B., Hernandez, G. D., Richards, J. B., & Lejuez, C. W. (2005). Differences in impulsivity and risk-taking propensity between primary users of crack cocaine and primary users of heroin in a residential substance-use program. *Experimental and Clinical Psychopharmacology, 13*(4), 311–318.

Bremner, J. D. (1999). Acute and chronic responses to psychological trauma: Where do we go from here? *The American Journal of Psychiatry, 156*(3), 349–351.

Bremner, J. D., & Brett, E. (1997). Trauma-related dissociative states and long-term psychopathology in posttraumatic stress disorder. *Journal of Traumatic Stress, 10*(1), 37–49.

Bremner, J. D., Krystal, J. H., Putnam, F. W., Southwick, S. M., Marmar, C., Charney, D. S., et al. (1998). Measurement of dissociative states with the Clinician-Administered Dissociative States Scale (CADSS). *Journal of Traumatic Stress, 11*(1), 125–136.

Bremner, J. D., Southwick, S., Brett, E., Fontana, A., Rosenheck, R., & Charney, D. S. (1992). Dissociation and posttraumatic stress disorder in Vietnam combat veterans. *The American Journal of Psychiatry, 149*(3), 328–332.

Bremner, J. D., Southwick, S. M., Darnell, A., & Charney, D. S. (1996). Chronic PTSD in Vietnam combat veterans: Course of illness and substance abuse. *The American Journal of Psychiatry, 153*(3), 369–375.

Bremner, J. D., Steinberg, M., Southwick, S. M., Johnson, D. R., & Charney, D. S. (1993). Use of the Structured Clinical Interview for DSM-IV Dissociative Disorders for systematic assessment of dissociative symptoms in posttraumatic stress disorder. *The American Journal of Psychiatry, 150*(7), 1011–1014.

Brende, J. O. (1983). A psychodynamic view of character pathology in Vietnam combat veterans. *Bulletin of the Menninger Clinic, 47*(3), 193–216.

Breslau, N. (2002). Epidemiologic studies of trauma, posttraumatic stress disorder, and other psychiatric disorders. *Canadian Journal of Psychiatry, 47*(10), 923–929.

Breslau, N., Chilcoat, H. D., Kessler, R. C., & Davis, G. C. (1999). Previous exposure to trauma and PTSD effects of subsequent trauma: Results from the Detroit Area Survey of Trauma. *The American Journal of Psychiatry, 156*(6), 902–907.

Breslau, N., Chilcoat, H. D., Kessler, R. C., Peterson, E. L., & Lucia, V. C. (1999). Vulnerability to assaultive violence: Further specification of the sex difference in post-traumatic stress disorder. *Psychological Medicine, 29*(4), 813–821.

Breslau, N., Davis, G. C., Andreski, P., Peterson, E. L., & Schultz, L. R. (1997). Sex differences in posttraumatic stress disorder. *Archives of General Psychiatry, 54*(11), 1044–1048.

Breslau, N., Davis, G. C., Peterson, E. L., & Schultz, L. (1997). Psychiatric sequelae of posttraumatic stress disorder in women. *Archives of General Psychiatry, 54*(1), 81–87.

Breslau, N., Davis, G. C., Peterson, E. L., & Schultz, L. R. (2000). A second look at comorbidity in victims of trauma: The posttraumatic stress disorder-major depression connection. *Biological Psychiatry, 48*(9), 902–909.

Brewin, C. R. (2001). A cognitive neuroscience account of posttraumatic stress disorder and its treatment. *Behaviour Research and Therapy, 39*(4), 373–393.

Brewin, C. R., Andrews, B., & Valentine, J. D. (2000). Meta-analysis of risk factors for posttraumatic stress disorder in trauma-exposed adults. *Journal of Consulting and Clinical Psychology, 68*(5), 748–766.

Butler, L. D., Duran, R. E., Jasiukaitis, P., Koopman, C., & Spiegel, D. (1996). Hypnotizability and traumatic experience: A diathesis-stress model of dissociative symptomatology. *The American Journal of Psychiatry, 153*(7 Suppl), 42–63.

Campbell, J. C. (1990). Battered woman syndrome: A critical review. *Violence Update, 1*(4), 1, 4, 10–11.

Cardena, E., & Spiegel, D. (1993). Dissociative reactions to the San Francisco Bay Area earthquake of 1989. *The American Journal of Psychiatry, 150*(3), 474–478.

Cash, A. (1993). Sequelae of prolonged and repeated trauma: Evidence for a complex posttraumatic syndrome (DESNOS). In J. R. T. Davidson & E. B. Foa (Eds.), *Posttraumatic stress disorder: DSM-IV and beyond* (pp. 213–228). Washington, DC: American Psychiatric Press.

Caspi, A., Sugden, K., Moffitt, T. E., Taylor, A., Craig, I. W., Harrington, H., et al. (2003). Influence of life stress on depression: Moderation by a polymorphism in the 5-HTT gene. *Science, 301*(5631), 386–389.

Chilcoat, H. D., & Breslau, N. (1998). Investigations of causal pathways between PTSD and drug use disorders. *Addictive Behaviors, 23*(6), 827–840.

Chivers-Wilson, K. A. (2006). Sexual assault and posttraumatic stress disorder: A review of the biological, psychological and sociological factors and treatments. *McGill Journal of Medicine, 9*(2), 111–118.

Chu, T. Q., Seery, M. D., Ence, W. A., Holman, A., & Cohen-Silver, R. (2006). Ethnicity and gender in the face of a terrorist attack: A national longitudinal study of immediate responses and outcomes two years after September 11. *Basic Appl Soc Psychiatr Clin North Am, 28*, 200–224.

Clarke, S. P., Frasure-Smith, N., Lesperance, F., & Bourassa, M. G. (2000). Psychosocial factors as predictors of functional status at 1 year in patients with left ventricular dysfunction. *Research in Nursing and Health, 23*(4), 290–300.

Conway, K. P., Compton, W., Stinson, F. S., & Grant, B. F. (2006). Lifetime comorbidity of DSM-IV mood and anxiety disorders and specific drug use disorders: Results from the National Epidemiologic Survey on Alcohol and Related Conditions. *The Journal of Clinical Psychiatry, 67*(2), 247–257.

Creamer, M., Burgess, P., & McFarlane, A. C. (2001). Post-traumatic stress disorder: Findings from the Australian National Survey of Mental Health and Well-being. *Psychological Medicine, 31*(7), 1237–1247.

DeViva, J. C., & Bloem, W. D. (2003). Symptom exaggeration and compensation seeking among combat veterans with posttraumatic stress disorder. *Journal of Traumatic Stress, 16*(5), 503–507.

Di Ciano, P., & Everitt, B. J. (2003). Differential control over drug-seeking behavior by drug-associated conditioned reinforcers and discriminative stimuli predictive of drug availability. *Behavioral Neuroscience, 117*(5), 952–960.

Dilsaver, S. C., Akiskal, H. S., Akiskal, K. K., & Benazzi, F. (2006). Dose-response relationship between number of comorbid anxiety disorders in adolescent bipolar/unipolar disorders, and psychosis, suicidality, substance abuse and familiality. *Journal of Affective Disorders, 96*(3), 249–258.

Dunmore, E., Clark, D. M., & Ehlers, A. (1999). Cognitive factors involved in the onset and maintenance of posttraumatic stress disorder (PTSD) after physical or sexual assault. *Behaviour Research and Therapy, 37*(9), 809–829.

Ehlers, A., & Clark, D. M. (2000). A cognitive model of posttraumatic stress disorder. *Behaviour Research and Therapy, 38*(4), 319–345.

Foa, E. B., & Kozak, M. J. (1986). Emotional processing of fear: Exposure to corrective information. *Psychological Bulletin, 99*(1), 20–35.

Foa, E. B., Molnar, C., & Cashman, L. (1995). Change in rape narratives during exposure therapy for posttraumatic stress disorder. *Journal of Traumatic Stress, 8*(4), 675–690.

Fontana, A., & Rosenheck, R. (1998). Effects of compensation-seeking on treatment outcomes among veterans with posttraumatic stress disorder. *The Journal of Nervous and Mental Disease, 186*(4), 223–230.

Ford, J. D., Adams, M. L., & Dailey, W. F. (2005). Factors associated with receiving help and risk factors for disaster-related distress among Connecticut adults 5-15 months after the September 11th terrorist incident. *Social Psychiatry and Psychiatric Epidemiology, 40*, 1–10.

Ford, J. D., Hawke, J., Alessi, S., Ledgerwood, D., & Petry, N. (2007). Psychological trauma and PTSD symptoms as predictors of substance dependence treatment outcomes. *Behaviour Research and Therapy, 45*(10), 2417–2431.

Fothergill, A., Maestas, E. G., & Darlington, J. D. (1999). Race, ethnicity and disasters in the United States: A review of the literature. *Disasters, 23*(2), 156–173.

Frazier, P. A. (2003). Perceived control and distress following sexual assault: A longitudinal test of a new model. *Journal of Personality and Social Psychology, 84*(6), 1257–1269.

Galea, S., Vlahov, D., Resnick, H., Ahern, J., Susser, E., Gold, J., et al. (2003). Trends of probable post-traumatic stress disorder in New York City after the September 11 terrorist attacks. *American Journal of Epidemiology, 158*(6), 514–524.

Ginzburg, K., Koopman, C., Butler, L. D., Palesh, O., Kraemer, H. C., Classen, C. C., et al. (2006). Evidence for a dissociative subtype of post-traumatic stress disorder among help-seeking childhood sexual abuse survivors. *Journal of Trauma & Dissociation, 7*(2), 7–27.

Ginzburg, K., Solomon, Z., & Bleich, A. (2002). Repressive coping style, acute stress disorder, and posttraumatic stress disorder after myocardial infarction. *Psychosomatic Medicine, 64*(5), 748–757.

Goltz, J. D., Russell, L. A., & Bourque, L. B. (1992). Initial behavioral response to a rapid onset. Disaster: A case study. *The International Journal of Mass Emergencies and Disasters, 10*, 43–69.

Halligan, S. L., Michael, T., Clark, D. M., & Ehlers, A. (2003). Posttraumatic stress disorder following assault: The role of cognitive processing, trauma memory, and appraisals. *Journal of Consulting and Clinical Psychology, 71*(3), 419–431.

Harman, R., & Lee, D. (2010). The role of shame and self-critical thinking in the development and maintenance of current threat in post-traumatic stress disorder. *Clinical Psychology & Psychotherapy, 17*(1), 13–24.

Hobfoll, S. E., Canetti-Nisim, D., & Johnson, R. J. (2006). Exposure to terrorism, stress-related mental health symptoms, and defensive coping among Jews and Arabs in Israel. *Journal of Consulting and Clinical Psychology, 74*(2), 207–218.

Hobfoll, S. E., Canetti-Nisim, D., Johnson, R. J., Palmieri, P. A., Varley, J. D., & Galea, S. (2008). The association of exposure, risk, and resiliency factors with PTSD among Jews and Arabs exposed to repeated acts of terrorism in Israel. *Journal of Traumatic Stress, 21*(1), 9–21.

Hopper, J. W., Frewen, P. A., van der Kolk, B. A., & Lanius, R. A. (2007). Neural correlates of reexperiencing, avoidance, and dissociation in PTSD: Symptom dimensions and emotion dysregulation in responses to script-driven trauma imagery. *Journal of Traumatic Stress, 20*(5), 713–725.

Institute of Medicine. (2007). *Treatment of posttraumatic stress disorder: An assessment of the evidence*. Washington, DC: National Academies.

Ironson, G., Wynings, C., Schneiderman, N., Baum, A., Rodriguez, M., Greenwood, D., et al. (1997). Posttraumatic stress symptoms, intrusive thoughts, loss, and immune function after Hurricane Andrew. *Psychosomatic Medicine, 59*(2), 128–141.

Jacobsen, L. K., Southwick, S. M., & Kosten, T. R. (2001). Substance use disorders in patients with posttraumatic stress disorder: A review of the literature. *The American Journal of Psychiatry, 158*(8), 1184–1190.

Jaycox, L. H., Foa, E. B., & Morral, A. R. (1998). Influence of emotional engagement and habituation on exposure therapy for PTSD. *Journal of Consulting and Clinical Psychology, 66*(1), 185–192.

Jordan, B. K., Marmar, C. R., Fairbank, J. A., Schlenger, W. E., Kulka, R. A., Hough, R. L., et al. (1992). Problems in families of male Vietnam veterans with posttraumatic stress disorder. *Journal of Consulting and Clinical Psychology, 60*(6), 916–926.

Kaniasty, K., & Norris, F. H. (1993). A test of the social support deterioration model in the context of natural disaster. *Journal of Personality and Social Psychology, 64*(3), 395–408.

Kaniasty, K., & Norris, F. H. (1995). In search of altruistic community: Patterns of social support mobilization following Hurricane Hugo. *American Journal of Community Psychology, 23*(4), 447–477.

Kendler, K. S., Gardner, C. O., & Prescott, C. A. (2003). Personality and the experience of environmental adversity. *Psychological Medicine, 33*(7), 1193–1202.

Kessler, R. C., Sonnega, A., Bromet, E., Hughes, M., & Nelson, C. B. (1995). Posttraumatic stress disorder in the National Comorbidity Survey. *Archives of General Psychiatry, 52*(12), 1048–1060.

Kleim, B., & Ehlers, A. (2008). Reduced autobiographical memory specificity predicts depression and posttraumatic stress disorder after recent trauma. *Journal of Consulting and Clinical Psychology, 76*(2), 231–242.

Klein, E., Caspi, Y., & Gil, S. (2003). The relation between memory of the traumatic event and PTSD: Evidence from studies of traumatic brain injury. *Canadian Journal of Psychiatry, 48*(1), 28–33.

Koenen, K. C. (2007). Genetics of posttraumatic stress disorder: Review and recommendations for future studies. *Journal of Traumatic Stress, 20*(5), 737–750.

Koenen, K. C., Hitsman, B., Lyons, M. J., Niaura, R., McCaffery, J., Goldberg, J., et al. (2005). A twin registry study of the relationship between posttraumatic stress disorder and nicotine dependence in men. *Archives of General Psychiatry, 62*(11), 1258–1265.

Koenen, K. C., Moffitt, T. E., Poulton, R., Martin, J., & Caspi, A. (2007). Early childhood factors associated with the development of post-traumatic stress disorder: Results from a longitudinal birth cohort. *Psychological Medicine, 37*(2), 181–192.

Koopman, C., Classen, C., & Spiegel, D. (1994). Predictors of posttraumatic stress symptoms among survivors of the Oakland/Berkeley, Calif., firestorm. *The American Journal of Psychiatry, 151*(6), 888–894.

Koren, D., Arnon, I., & Klein, E. (1999). Acute stress response and posttraumatic stress disorder in traffic accident victims: A one-year prospective, follow-up study. *The American Journal of Psychiatry, 156*(3), 367–373.

Koren, D., Caspi, Y., Leiba, R., Bloch, D., Vexler, B., & Klein, E. (2009). Acute stress reactions among medical and non-medical personnel in a general hospital under missile attacks. *Depression and Anxiety, 26*(2), 123–128.

Koren, D., Norman, D., Cohen, A., Berman, J., & Klein, E. M. (2005). Increased PTSD risk with combat-related injury: A matched comparison study of injured and uninjured soldiers experiencing the same combat events. *The American Journal of Psychiatry, 162*(2), 276–282.

Koss, M. P., & Figueredo, A. J. (2004). Change in cognitive mediators of rape's impact on psychosocial health across 2 years of recovery. *Journal of Consulting and Clinical Psychology, 72*(6), 1063–1072.

Kotler, M., Iancu, I., Efroni, R., & Amir, M. (2001). Anger, impulsivity, social support, and suicide risk in patients with posttraumatic stress disorder. *The Journal of Nervous and Mental Disease, 189*(3), 162–167.

Kunst, M., Winkel, F. W., & Bogaerts, S. (2010). Prevalence and predictors of posttraumatic stress disorder among victims of violence applying for state compensation. *Journal of Interpersonal Violence, 25*(9), 1631–1654.

Lanius, R. A., Bluhm, R., Lanius, U., & Pain, C. (2006). A review of neuroimaging studies in PTSD: Heterogeneity of response to symptom provocation. *Journal of Psychiatric Research, 40*(8), 709–729.

Lewin, T. J., Carr, V. J., & Webster, R. A. (1998). Recovery from post-earthquake psychological morbidity: Who suffers and who recovers? *The Australian and New Zealand Journal of Psychiatry, 32*(1), 15–20.

Lilly, M. M., Pole, N., Best, S. R., Metzler, T., & Marmar, C. R. (2009). Gender and PTSD: What can we learn from female police officers? *Journal of Anxiety Disorders, 23*(6), 767–774.

Loewenstein, R. J., & Putnam, F. W. (2004). The dissociative disorders. In B. J. Kaplan & V. A. Sadock (Eds.), *Comprehensive textbook of psychiatry* (8th ed., Vol. 1, pp. 1844–1901). Baltimore: Lippincott Williams & Wilkins.

Loo, C. M., Fairbank, J. A., & Chemtob, C. M. (2005). Adverse race-related events as a risk factor for posttraumatic stress disorder in Asian American Vietnam veterans. *The Journal of Nervous and Mental Disease, 193*(7), 455–463.

MacDonald, C., Chamberlain, K., & Long, N. (1997). Race, combat, and PTSD in a community sample of New Zealand Vietnam War veterans. *Journal of Traumatic Stress, 10*(1), 117–124.

Madakasira, S., & O'Brien, K. F. (1987). Acute posttraumatic stress disorder in victims of a natural disaster. *The Journal of Nervous and Mental Disease, 175*(5), 286–290.

Marmar, C. R., Weiss, D. S., Metzler, T. J., Delucchi, K. L., Best, S. R., & Wentworth, K. A. (1999). Longitudinal course and predictors of continuing distress following critical incident exposure in emergency services personnel. *The Journal of Nervous and Mental Disease, 187*(1), 15–22.

Marmar, C. R., Weiss, D. S., Schlenger, W. E., Fairbank, J. A., Jordan, B. K., Kulka, R. A., et al. (1994). Peritraumatic dissociation and posttraumatic stress in male Vietnam theater veterans. *The American Journal of Psychiatry, 151*(6), 902–907.

Marx, B. P., Foley, K. M., Feinstein, B. A., Wolf, E. J., Kaloupek, D. G., & Keane, T. M. (2010). Combat-related guilt mediates the relations between exposure to combat-related abusive violence and psychiatric diagnoses. *Depression and Anxiety, 27*(3), 287–293.

McDevitt-Murphy, M. E., Williams, J. L., Bracken, K. L., Fields, J. A., Monahan, C. J., & Murphy, J. G. (2010). PTSD symptoms, hazardous drinking, and health functioning among U.S.OEF and OIF veterans presenting to primary care. *Journal of Traumatic Stress, 23*(1), 108–111.

McFarlane, A. C. (2000). Posttraumatic stress disorder: A model of the longitudinal course and the role of risk factors. *The Journal of Clinical Psychiatry, 61*(Suppl 5), 15–20. discussion 21–23.

McHugh, P. R., & Treisman, G. (2007). PTSD: A problematic diagnostic category. *Journal of Anxiety Disorders, 21*(2), 211–222.

McNally, R. J. (2003). Progress and controversy in the study of posttraumatic stress disorder. *Annual Review of Psychology, 54*, 229–252.

McNamee, H. B., Mirin, S. M., Kuehnle, J. C., & Meyer, R. E. (1976). Affective changes in chronic opiate use. *The British Journal of Addiction to Alcohol and Other Drugs, 71*(3), 275–280.

Morgan, C. A., 3rd, Hazlett, G., Wang, S., Richardson, E. G., Jr., Schnurr, P., & Southwick, S. M. (2001). Symptoms of dissociation in humans experiencing acute, uncontrollable stress: A prospective investigation. *The American Journal of Psychiatry, 158*(8), 1239–1247.

Musallam, N., Ginzburg, K., Lev-Shalem, L., & Solomon, Z. (2005). The psychological effects of Intifada Al Aqsa: Acute stress disorder and distress in Palestinian-Israeli Students. *The Israel Journal of Psychiatry and Related Sciences, 42*, 96–105.

Najavits, L. M., Runkel, R., Neuner, C., Frank, A. F., Thase, M. E., Crits-Christoph, P., et al. (2003). Rates and symptoms of PTSD among cocaine-dependent patients. *Journal of Studies on Alcohol, 64*(5), 601–606.

National Center for Post Traumatic Stress Disorder. (2005). Epidemiological facts about PTSD – A National Center for PTSD Fact Sheet, from http://www.ncptsd.va.gov/facts/general/fs_epidemiological.html

Nixon, R. D., & Bryant, R. A. (2003). Peritraumatic and persistent panic attacks in acute stress disorder. *Behaviour Research and Therapy, 41*(10), 1237–1242.

O'Donnell, M. L., Creamer, M. C., McFarlane, A. C., Silove, D., & Bryant, R. A. (2010). Does access to compensation have an impact on recovery outcomes after injury? *The Medical Journal of Australia, 192*(6), 328–333.

Orcutt, H. K., Erickson, D. J., & Wolfe, J. (2002). A prospective analysis of trauma exposure: The mediating role of PTSD symptomatology. *Journal of Traumatic Stress, 15*(3), 259–266.

Owens, G. P., Steger, M. F., Whitesell, A. A., & Herrera, C. J. (2009). Posttraumatic stress disorder, guilt, depression, and meaning in life among military veterans. *Journal of Traumatic Stress, 22*(6), 654–657.

Ozer, E. J., Best, S. R., Lipsey, T. L., & Weiss, D. S. (2003). Predictors of posttraumatic stress disorder and symptoms in adults: A meta-analysis. *Psychological Bulletin, 129*(1), 52–73.

Palinkas, L. A., Petterson, J. S., Russell, J. C., & Downs, M. A. (2004). Ethnic differences in symptoms of post-traumatic stress after the Exxon Valdez oil spill. *Prehospital and Disaster Medicine, 19*(1), 102–112.

Paris, J. J., Franco, C., Sodano, R., Freidenberg, B., Gordis, E., Anderson, D. A., et al. (2010). Sex differences in salivary cortisol in response to acute stressors among healthy participants, in recreational or pathological gamblers, and in those with posttraumatic stress disorder. *Hormones and Behavior, 57*(1), 35–45.

Perilla, J. L., Norris, F. H., & Lavizzio, E. A. (2002). Ethnicity, culture and disaster response: Identifying and explaining ethnic differences in PTSD six months after Hurricane Andrew. *J Soc Clin Psychol Psychother, 21*, 20–45.

Pervanidou, P. (2008). Biology of post-traumatic stress disorder in childhood and adolescence. *Journal of Neuroendocrinology, 20*(5), 632–638.

Putnam, F. W., Carlson, E. B., Ross, C. A., Anderson, G., Clark, P., Torem, M., et al. (1996). Patterns of dissociation in clinical and nonclinical samples. *The Journal of Nervous and Mental Disease, 184*(11), 673–679.

Putnam, F. W., Helmers, K., Horowitz, L. A., & Trickett, P. K. (1995). Hypnotizability and dissociativity in sexually abused girls. *Child Abuse and Neglect, 19*(5), 645–655.

Riggs, D. S., Byrne, C. A., Weathers, F. W., & Litz, B. T. (1998). The quality of the intimate relationships of male Vietnam veterans: Problems associated with posttraumatic stress disorder. *Journal of Traumatic Stress, 11*(1), 87–101.

Robinaugh, D. J., & McNally, R. J. (2010). Autobiographical memory for shame or guilt provoking events: Association with psychological symptoms. *Behaviour Research and Therapy, 48*(7), 646–652.

Rubin, G. J., Brewin, C. R., Greenberg, N., Simpson, J., & Wessely, S. (2005). Psychological and behavioural reactions to the bombings in London on 7 July 2005: Cross sectional survey of a representative sample of Londoners. *BMJ, 331*(7517), 606.

Saladin, M. E., Brady, K. T., Dansky, B. S., & Kilpatrick, D. G. (1995). Understanding comorbidity between PTSD and substance use disorders: Two preliminary investigations. *Addictive Behaviors, 20*(5), 643–655.

Saladin, M. E., Drobes, D. J., Coffey, S. F., Dansky, B. S., Brady, K. T., & Kilpatrick, D. G. (2003). PTSD symptom severity as a predictor of cue-elicited drug craving in victims of violent crime. *Addictive Behaviors, 28*(9), 1611–1629.

Sayer, N. A., Spoont, M., Nelson, D. B., Clothier, B., & Murdoch, M. (2008). Changes in psychiatric status and service use associated with continued compensation seeking after claim determinations for posttraumatic stress disorder. *Journal of Traumatic Stress, 21*(1), 40–48.

Shalev, A. Y. (1992). Posttraumatic stress disorder among injured survivors of a terrorist attack. Predictive value of early intrusion and avoidance symptoms. *The Journal of Nervous and Mental Disease, 180*(8), 505–509.

Shipherd, J. C., Stafford, J., & Tanner, L. R. (2005). Predicting alcohol and drug abuse in Persian Gulf War veterans: What role do PTSD symptoms play? *Addictive Behaviors, 30*(3), 595–599.

Somer, E., Maguen, S., Or-Chen, K., & Litz, B. T. (2007). Managing terror: Differences between Jews and Arabs in Israel. *International Journal of Psychology, 42*, 1–9.

Somer, E., Ruvio, A., Soref, E., & Sever, I. (2005). Terrorism, distress and coping: High versus low impact regions and direct versus indirect civilian exposure. *Anxiety, Stress, and Coping, 18*, 165–182.

Spiegel, D., & Cardena, E. (1991). Disintegrated experience: The dissociative disorders revisited. *Journal of Abnormal Psychology, 100*(3), 366–378.

Stein, B. D., Elliott, M. N., Jaycox, L. H., Collins, R. L., Berry, S. H., Klein, D. J., et al. (2004). A national longitudinal study of the psychological consequences of the September 11, 2001 terrorist attacks: Reactions, impairment, and help-seeking. *Psychiatry, 67*(2), 105–117.

Steinberg, M., Rounsaville, B., & Cicchetti, D. V. (1990). The Structured Clinical Interview for DSM-III-R Dissociative Disorders: Preliminary report on a new diagnostic instrument. *The American Journal of Psychiatry, 147*(1), 76–82.

Stewart, S. H., & Conrod, P. J. (2003). Psychosocial models of functional associations between posttraumatic stress disorder and substance use disorder. In P. Ouimette & P. J. Brown (Eds.), *Trauma and substance abuse: Causes, consequences, and treatment of comorbid disorders* (pp. 29–55). Washington, DC: American Psychological Association.

Stewart, S. H., Conrod, P. J., Pihl, R. O., & Dongier, M. (1999). Relations between posttraumatic stress symptom dimensions and substance dependence in a community-recruited sample of substance-abusing women. *Psychology of Addictive Behaviors, 13*, 78–88.

Sullivan, T. P., & Holt, L. J. (2008). PTSD symptom clusters are differentially related to substance use among community women exposed to intimate partner violence. *Journal of Traumatic Stress, 21*(2), 173–180.

Sutker, P. B., Davis, J. M., Uddo, M., & Ditta, S. R. (1995). Assessment of psychological distress in Persian Gulf troops: Ethnicity and gender comparisons. *Journal of Personality Assessment, 64*(3), 415–427.

Terr, L. C. (1991). Childhood traumas: An outline and overview. *The American Journal of Psychiatry, 148*(1), 10–20.

Testa, M., VanZile-Tamsen, C., & Livingston, J. A. (2007). Prospective prediction of women's sexual victimization by intimate and nonintimate male perpetrators. *Journal of Consulting and Clinical Psychology, 75*(1), 52–60.

Tull, M. T., Gratz, K. L., Aklin, W. M., & Lejuez, C. W. (2010). A preliminary examination of the relationships between posttraumatic stress symptoms and crack/cocaine, heroin, and alcohol dependence. *Journal of Anxiety Disorders, 24*(1), 55–62.

Valentino, K., Cicchetti, D., Rogosch, F. A., & Toth, S. L. (2008). Memory, maternal representations, and internalizing symptomatology among abused, neglected, and nonmaltreated children. *Child Development, 79*(3), 705–719.

van der Kolk, B. A., Pelcovitz, D., Roth, S., Mandel, F. S., McFarlane, A., & Herman, J. L. (1996). Dissociation, somatization, and affect dysregulation: The complexity of adaptation of trauma. *The American Journal of Psychiatry, 153*(7 Suppl), 83–93.

Waelde, L. C., Silvern, L., & Fairbank, J. A. (2005). A taxometric investigation of dissociation in Vietnam veterans. *Journal of Traumatic Stress, 18*(4), 359–369.

Waldrop, A. E., Back, S. E., Verduin, M. L., & Brady, K. T. (2007). Triggers for cocaine and alcohol use in the presence and absence of posttraumatic stress disorder. *Addictive Behaviors, 32*(3), 634–639.

Wasserman, D. A., Havassy, B. E., & Boles, S. M. (1997). Traumatic events and post-traumatic stress disorder in cocaine users entering private treatment. *Drug and Alcohol Dependence, 46*(1–2), 1–8.

Watson, S., Owen, B. M., Gallagher, P., Hearn, A. J., Young, A. H., & Ferrier, I. N. (2007). Family history, early adversity and the hypothalamic-pituitary-adrenal (HPA) axis: Mediation of the vulnerability to mood disorders. *Neuropsychiatric Disease and Treatment, 3*(5), 647–653.

Widom, C. S. (1999). Posttraumatic stress disorder in abused and neglected children grown up. *The American Journal of Psychiatry, 156*(8), 1223–1229.

Zeidner, M., Klingman, A., & Itskowitz, R. (1993). Children's affective reactions and coping under threat of missile attack: A semiprojective assessment procedure. *Journal of Personality Assessment, 60*(3), 435–457.

Zohar, J., Juven-Wetzler, A., Myers, V., & Fostick, L. (2008). Post-traumatic stress disorder: Facts and fiction. *Current Opinion in Psychiatry, 21*(1), 74–77.

Zucker, M., Spinazzola, J., Blaustein, M., & van der Kolk, B. A. (2006). Dissociative symptomatology in posttraumatic stress disorder and disorders of extreme stress. *Journal of Trauma & Dissociation, 7*(1), 19–31.

Chapter 2
Neurobiological Risk Factors and Predictors of Vulnerability and Resilience to PTSD

Marina Bar-Shai and Ehud Klein

Introduction

Risk factors for PTSD may be classified in three temporal domains: pre-traumatic, peri-traumatic, and posttraumatic factors.

Pre-traumatic factors predispose an individual to developing PTSD. These include various neurobiological, anatomic, and genetic variables. Peri-traumatic factors are those linked to the actual traumatic occurrence and reflect greater stress responses. Posttraumatic factors are related to the long-term course of the trauma response, including the coping abilities of the survivors and their support network (Ozer, Best, Lipsey, & Weiss, 2003). Currently, the vast majority of the posttraumatic risk factors that have been delineated are psychosocial and not biological. The scope of the current chapter focuses on neurobiological and genetic vulnerability and resilience factors of PTSD.

Pre-traumatic Risk Factors

Neurobiological Factors

Much attention in PTSD research has focused on the two predominant biological systems involved in stress responses: the noradrenergic system and the corticotrophin releasing hormone (CRH) stress response. Under normal conditions, in the presence of a stressor, the sympathetic nervous system is activated, causing

M. Bar-Shai, M.D., Ph.D. • E. Klein, M.D. (✉)
Department of Psychiatry, Rambam Health Care Campus, Haifa, Israel

Faculty of Medicine, Technion IIT, Haifa, Israel
e-mail: m_bar-shai@rambam.health.gov.il; e_klein@rambam.health.gov.il

M.P. Safir et al. (eds.), *Future Directions in Post-Traumatic Stress Disorder*,
DOI 10.1007/978-1-4899-7522-5_2

norepinephrine (NE) to be released from the locus ceruleus (LC). This in turn produces a number of physiological responses, such as vasoconstriction of peripheral blood flow, increased blood flow to the heart, increased respiratory rate, and pupillary dilation—the so-called "fight or flight" response. However, there is a large body of evidence that suggests this functioning is altered, and there may, in fact, be hyperactive noradrenergic function in PTSD.

The amygdala has received particular attention in research into emotional memory. Cahill and McGaugh (1996) used positron emission tomography (PET) to demonstrate that enhanced activity in the amygdala during viewing of emotionally arousing films influenced subsequent recall of the arousing material, although this was not true of neutral material. Subsequently, research has shown that both the emotional valence of the stimulus and the level of arousal at the time of encoding into memory appear to be important factors in the process of memory consolidation (Zald, 2003). As such, in the presence of an emotionally arousing stimulus, sensory information received by the basolateral nucleus of the amygdala (BLA) is amalgamated along with information from other brain structures to form an emotional association with memory of the stimulus. Input from the BLA is then transmitted, via the central nucleus of the amygdala, to other neural structures, including the hypothalamus, effecting motor, and autonomic responses. In this way, the amygdala plays a critical role in fear conditioning, by creating the association that links a potential threat to a fear response.

The amygdala is also thought to modulate consolidation of emotional memories in the hippocampus, and this process is significantly influenced by the noradrenergic system. In a pivotal study by Cahill, Prins, Weber, and McGaugh (1994), administration of a central β-adrenergic antagonist (propranolol) prior to viewing a series of emotional slides resulted in selectively impairing effects on recall of emotional material; recall of neutral material was unaffected. Building on this, van Stegeren et al. (2005) conducted a functional magnetic resonance imaging (fMRI) study, comparing memory retrieval in a group of healthy controls that received either propranolol or placebo prior to viewing emotional and neutral pictures. van Stegeren et al. demonstrated that, following placebo administration, amygdala activation increased in response to emotional pictures, but this response decreased following propranolol, suggesting that NE is an important modulator of amygdala activation. As such, enhanced noradrenergic activity seen in patients with PTSD may act to increase amygdala activation, intensifying the fear conditioning process, which may partially explain why these individuals avoid thoughts, feelings, or physical triggers that remind them of the trauma. Increased amygdala activation with acquisition of fear responses, and a failure of the medial prefrontal cortex to properly mediate extinction, is hypothesized to underlie symptoms of PTSD.

Interestingly, resilience to PTSD may be associated with relatively decreased amygdala activation (Osuch, Willis, Bluhm, Ursano, & Drevets, 2008), and amygdala lesions may reduce the occurrence of PTSD (Armony, Corbo, Clement, & Brunet, 2005). In support of the potential role of amygdala in PTSD, some studies have reported that amygdala activation is positively correlated with PTSD symptom severity (Dickie, Brunet, Akerib, & Armony, 2008). Similarly, response to cognitive-behavioral treatment is associated with a decrease in amygdala activation (Peres et al., 2007), and relatively higher pre-treatment amygdala activation is predictive of a less favorable response to cognitive-behavioral therapy (Bryant et al., 2008).

One study using positron emission tomography (PET) and [^{11}C]-carfentanil reported diminished mu-opioid receptor binding in the extended amygdala in trauma-exposed individuals with and without PTSD (Liberzon et al., 2007). Another study found decreased [^{11}C]-flumazenil binding in the left amygdala in PTSD subjects compared with trauma-exposed control participants, consistent with altered gamma amino-butyric acid (GABA)ergic function in this disorder (Geuze et al., 2008).

As mentioned above, another critical brain structure implicated in PTSD is the hippocampus, which has an essential role in the formation and retrieval of episodic and declarative memories. The hippocampus is linked reciprocally to the amygdala and is subject to altered noradrenergic function via NE's actions on the amygdala. A review of evidence from animal studies showed that chronic stress was associated with dendritic atrophy in the CA3 region of the hippocampus and the medial prefrontal cortex (mPFC), as well as decreased neurogenesis (Kuroda & McEwen, 1998). One commonly cited observation in individuals with PTSD is a finding of decreased hippocampal volumes, which was initially postulated to reflect atrophy secondary to chronic stress and glucocorticoid overexposure. More recently, however, Kasai et al. (2008) employed an impressively designed twin study of brain morphometrics and PTSD. In the latter study, two classifications of twin pairs were used. One classification included sets of twins in which one twin was combat-exposed in Vietnam and diagnosed with PTSD, while his co-twin was unexposed to combat and did not have PTSD (co-twin was termed "high risk"). The second classification included sets of twins in which one twin was combat-exposed in Vietnam and did not have PTSD while his co-twin was not exposed to combat and did not have PTSD (co-twin termed "low risk"). Combat-exposed twins with PTSD had less gray matter volume in the hippocampus, pregenual anterior cingulate cortex, and bilateral insular regions compared to combat-exposed twins without PTSD. In addition, a Diagnosis by Exposure interaction revealed less gray matter volume in the pregenual anterior cingulate cortex of combat-exposed PTSD twins compared to the other three twin groups (Kasai et al., 2008). This finding suggests that lower gray matter volume is a consequence of combat stress exposure and subsequent PTSD and not of genetic factors.

Some functional neuroimaging studies have reported decreased hippocampal activation during symptomatic states (Bremner et al., 1999) and during memory tasks that involve neutral or emotional stimuli (Moores et al., 2008). One study in 2010 found reduced glucose metabolic rate in the hippocampus at rest (Molina, Isoardi, Prado, & Bentolila, 2010), and another reported that successful treatment was related to increased hippocampal activation (Peres et al., 2007). Other studies, however, have reported increased activation in the hippocampus in PTSD (Werner et al., 2009) or a positive correlation between hippocampal activation and PTSD symptom severity (Shin et al., 2004).

Hippocampal volumes have been inversely associated with verbal memory deficits (Bremner et al., 1995), combat exposure severity (Gurvits et al., 1996), dissociative symptom severity (Bremner et al., 2003), depression severity (Villarreal et al., 2002), and PTSD symptom severity (Bremner et al., 2003). Spectroscopy studies have reported decreased *N*-acetyl aspartate (NAA) in the hippocampus, often interpreted as consistent with decreased neuronal integrity (Ham et al., 2007). Furthermore, NAA levels in the pregenual ACC were negatively correlated with the severity of reexperiencing symptoms (Ham et al., 2007). The results of some studies suggest that hippocampal volumes may increase following treatment with serotonin reuptake inhibitors (Bossini et al., 2007).

With regard to neurochemistry, one PET study found decreased [^{11}C]-flumazenil binding in the hippocampus (as well as thalamus and cortical areas) suggesting diminished benzodiazepine–GABA function in the hippocampus in PTSD (Geuze et al., 2008).

Although not originally included in early neurocircuitry models, the dorsal anterior cingulated cortex (dACC) and insular cortex may have a role in PTSD as well. Recent studies have suggested that the dACC is hyperresponsive in PTSD, perhaps underlying exaggerated fear learning. The findings of several studies suggest diminished volumes or gray matter densities in the ACC in PTSD (Kasai et al., 2008), and smaller ACC volumes have been associated with greater PTSD symptom severity (Woodward et al., 2006). Enhanced resting metabolic activity in the dACC/MCC appears to represent a familial risk factor for developing PTSD after exposure to psychological trauma (Shin et al., 2009).

Functional neuroimaging studies of PTSD have reported decreased activation or failure to activate the medial prefrontal cortex (mPFC) (including the right ACC, medial frontal gyrus, and subcallosal cortex) during traumatic script-driven imagery (Shin et al., 2004), the presentation of trauma-related stimuli (Hou et al., 2007), and negative, non-traumatic stimuli (Phan, Britton, Taylor, Fig, & Liberzon, 2006). Furthermore, mPFC activation appears to be inversely correlated with PTSD symptom severity (Dickie et al., 2008) and positively correlated with pre-scan cortisol levels (Liberzon et al., 2007). Finally, increased mPFC activation following treatment has been positively associated with symptomatic improvement (Felmingham et al., 2007).

Relative to comparison groups, increased activation in the insular cortex has been found in PTSD during script-driven imagery (Lanius et al., 2007), fear conditioning and extinction (Bremner et al., 2005), the retrieval of emotional or neutral stimuli (Whalley, Rugg, Smith, Dolan, & Brewin, 2009), aversive smells and painful stimuli (Geuze et al., 2007), and the performance of an emotional Stroop task (Shin et al., 2001). Insular cortex activation has been found to be positively correlated with measures of symptom severity (Osuch et al., 2001) and post-scan plasma adrenocorticotropic hormone levels (Liberzon et al., 2007). Although greater insular activation in PTSD has been confirmed by a recent voxel-wise meta-analysis (Etkin & Wager, 2007), a few studies have reported either no group differences in insular activation or relatively decreased activation in PTSD (Moores et al., 2008).

Genetic Factors

Several major genotypes have been linked either to risk for developing, or resilience to, PTSD following trauma exposure (Broekman, Olff, & Boer, 2007). Prior candidate gene association studies have identified genes related to the HPA axis, the ascending brainstem LC noradrenergic system, and the limbic amygdalar frontal pathway that mediates fear processing (Charney, Shin, & Phelps, 2006). Within the latter anatomical systems, association studies have implicated the serotonin, dopamine, glucocorticoid receptor (GR), GABA, apolipoprotein (APO), brain-derived neurotrophic factor (BDNF), and neuropeptide Y (NPY) systems in the genetic contribution to the onset of PTSD symptoms following a traumatic event.

Early evidence of a genetic contribution to development of PTSD following trauma exposure came in the form of familial transmission studies (Davidson, Tupler, Wilson, & Connor, 1998), followed by twin studies. Moreover, twin studies suggested a heritability component for susceptibility to experience trauma as well as for the development of PTSD symptoms following a trauma event (True et al., 1993). Later twin studies identified potential biomarkers for PTSD such as hippocampal volume (Gilbertson et al., 2002) and altered acoustic startle responses (Orr et al., 2003). Thus, examination of 3,000–4,000 twin pairs from the Vietnam Twin Registry revealed that approximately 32–35 % of the variance of PTSD symptoms could be attributed to inherited influences upon exposure to combat (Chantarujikapong et al., 2001).

Furthermore, psychiatric morbidity in families has been identified as a risk factor for PTSD. Early work by Davidson et al. (1998) demonstrated that alcohol, depression, and anxiety disorders were commonly reported by first-degree family members of probands with PTSD. In addition, work by Yehuda and Bierer (2008) as well as Yehuda, Bell, Bierer, and Schmeidler (2008) showed that parental PTSD is a significant risk factor for PTSD in children. For example, PTSD diagnosis was more frequent in adult offspring of Holocaust survivors with PTSD when compared to offspring of Holocaust survivors without PTSD (Yehuda et al., 2008). Neuroendocrine analyses of offspring of Holocaust-exposed parents with PTSD have revealed lower urinary and salivary cortisol levels and increased plasma cortisol suppression, following low dose dexamethasone administration, compared to children of survivors without PTSD (Yehuda & Bierer, 2008). Similarly, the offspring of mothers with PTSD, who were pregnant at the time of the 9/11 terrorist attacks, also exhibit lower cortisol levels (Brand, Engel, Canfield, & Yehuda, 2006). The negative correlation between offspring cortisol levels and maternal PTSD suggests that epigenetic mechanisms contribute to the intergenerational transmission of PTSD risk.

Dysregulation of brain serotonergic systems has been implicated in the pathophysiology of PTSD (Davis, Clark, Kramer, Moeller, & Petty, 1999). Studies have suggested that serotonin transporter (SERT) genetic polymorphisms contribute to an individual's response to a traumatic event (Lee et al., 2005). The SERT gene, mapped to chromosome 17q11.1–q12, contains a polymorphism (5HTTLPR) within the promoter region such that there is a long L allele and a short S allele

(Heils et al., 1996). SERT expression at the presynaptic membrane and 5-HT uptake activity is significantly greater in carriers of the long allele when compared to carriers of the short allele (Heils et al., 1996).

The data from the 2004 Florida Hurricanes study showed that low expression (s) variant of the 5-HTTLPR increased risk of post-hurricane PTSD, but only under high stress conditions of high hurricane exposure and low social support (Koenen et al., 2009). It was further investigated whether rs4606, a single nucleotide polymorphism (SNP) of regulator of G-protein signaling 2 (RGS2), and low social support moderated risk for post-hurricane and lifetime PTSD. This polymorphism was associated with lifetime PTSD symptoms under conditions of lifetime exposure to a traumatic event (other than the current hurricane) and low social support (Koenen et al., 2009). It was also demonstrated that county-level crime rate and percent unemployment modified the association between the 5-HTTLPR genotype and PTSD; low expression allele carriers (s) were at increased risk for PTSD in high environmental stress conditions (high unemployment; high crime), and were at decreased risk for PTSD in low-risk environments (low unemployment, low crime) (Koenen et al., 2009). These findings underscored the importance of the interactions between genes and the environment to produce the symptoms of PTSD. Sayin et al. (2010) observed a positive association between the s allele and severity of PTSD and hyperarousal symptoms. In a prospective study of emergency department physical trauma patients, Thakur, Joober, and Brunet (2009) found that 5-HTTLPR was not significantly associated with initial risk for PTSD diagnosis. To examine the variant's association with PTSD chronicity, the authors compared participants continuing to evidence PTSD at 12 months with those who no longer met criteria for PTSD at 12 months. Findings supported excess l/l genotypes in chronic PTSD patients compared with a group of acute PTSD patients and exposed nonpatients. The results of this study suggest that predictors of onset may differ from predictors of chronicity. Additionally, the 5-HTTLPR polymorphism has been found to be triallelic in that a third functional allele L_G, has been identified (Nakamura, Ueno, Sano, & Tanabe, 2000). Accordingly, investigations that have examined only the insertion/deletion may have included less transcriptionally efficient variants in their "l" allele groups. Yet another serotonergic polymorphism, a G → A substitution (rs6311) in serotonin receptor 2A (5-HT2A), was examined in a sample of Koreans by Lee, Kwak, Paik, Kang, and Lee (2007) and in a sample of Americans by Mellman et al. (2009). Both reported an increased risk of PTSD associated with the G allele, although Lee et al. (2007) observed this effect only among women.

The increasingly prevalent finding of an interaction between the 5-HTTLPR polymorphism and stressful life events as a vulnerability factor to depressive illnesses (Caspi et al., 2003) has spurred further explorations of this interaction with other psychiatric illnesses. Stein, Schork, and Gelernter (2008) investigated the relationship between the 5-HTTLPR polymorphism, childhood maltreatment, and anxiety sensitivity (AS). AS has been defined as the fear of anxiety-related symptoms such that an individual who fears his/her symptoms will lead to an adverse event (e.g., cardiac arrest) (Bernstein & Zvolensky, 2007). In the aforementioned study, Stein et al. found a significant association between childhood maltreatment, as measured by the Childhood Trauma Questionnaire (CTQ), and 5-HTTLPR genotype. More specifically, homozygotes with the S allele who also had a higher degree of maltreatment exhibited higher AS scores compared to heterozygotes and homozygous L carriers. Based on this association, the authors of the Stein study suggest that anxiety sensitivity may represent an intermediate phenotype for anxiety, depression, and their comorbidity (Stein et al., 2008). Xie et al. (2009) observed a significant interaction between variation in 5-HTTLPR and adult and/or child trauma for risk of lifetime PTSD. More specifically, increased risk of PTSD was evidenced in "s" allele carriers who experienced childhood and adulthood trauma. Moreover, some fMRI studies found increased amygdala reactivity to fearful stimuli in healthy subjects carrying the S allele (Hariri et al., 2002).

PTSD pathophysiology may also reflect altered dopaminergic and noradrenergic neurotransmission (Glover et al., 2003). Genetic variants of the dopamine beta-hydroxylase gene (DBH) represent a likely candidate for examinations of genetic contributions to anxiety disorders, because of the role this enzyme plays in converting dopamine to norepinephrine as part of catecholamine synthesis (Bloom, 1982). Plasma DBH activity is regulated by genetic factors (Mustapic et al., 2007). More specifically, individual differences in DBH activity (approximately 35–52 % of the variance) are influenced by an SNP in the 5′ flanking region of DBH-1021C/T variant (rs1611115) (Zabetian et al., 2001). Mustapic et al. (2007) suggest that genotype-mediated plasma DBH activity may serve as a biomarker for an individual's response to trauma (i.e., vulnerability to developing PTSD).

Several studies examined the association between SNPs of the dopamine receptor D2 (DRD2) region and chronic PTSD, for instance (Voisey et al., 2009). A number of studies such as (Comings, Muhleman, & Gysin, 1996) found a positive association between risk and a SNP commonly known as *TaqIA* within the coding region of the ankyrin repeat and kinase domain containing 1 (ANKK1) gene, located downstream of DRD2. Some studies examined a variable number tandem repeat (VNTR) in a dopamine transporter gene (DAT1), and both reported an increased risk of PTSD with nine 40-bp repeats compared with ten repeats despite differences in traumatic exposure across studies (Segman et al., 2002). Finally, a VNTR in the gene encoding the dopamine receptor D4 (DRD4) was examined in relation to PTSD diagnosis and symptoms within 3 months of exposure to a flood (Dragan & Oniszczenko, 2009). Findings supported significantly higher levels of avoidance/numbing symptoms in carriers of the long (seven or eight repeats) allele, as well as higher levels of PTSD symptoms as measured by a questionnaire indexing the intensity of PTSD symptoms.

In general, these genetic association studies have revealed that (1) it is unlikely that specific anxiety disorders are associated with a single genetic variant, (2) there is a complex interaction between genetic and environmental factors, and (3) many of the identified genetic polymorphisms are in the regulatory promoter regions and not necessarily in the coding regions (Smoller, Gardner-Schuster, & Covino, 2008). Thus, future investigations aimed at identifying genetic contributions to PTSD should examine multiple susceptibility loci (including total genome analyses) (Shalev & Segman, 2008) and should employ expanded gene X environment (GxE) investigations.

Increased HPA axis reactivity (Ham et al., 2007) and elevated GR sensitivity (Yehuda, Golier, Yang, & Tischler, 2004) have been recurrently demonstrated in patients with PTSD. In particular, the experience of child abuse appears to pathologically alter the function of the HPA axis (Heim, Newport, Mletzko, Miller, & Nemeroff, 2008). Depressed patients who have a history of childhood adversity show elevated secretion of adrenocorticotropic hormone (ACTH) and cortisol in response to a laboratory stress test (Heim et al., 2000), as well as with neuroendocrine challenge tests including the dexamethasone-corticotropin-releasing factor (CRF) test (Heim et al., 2008). More recently reported data (McGowan et al., 2009) identified epigenetic regulation of glucocorticoid receptors (GR) in postmortem tissue from individuals with a history of child abuse. These data indicate that trauma exposure during childhood persistently alters the endogenous stress response, acting principally upon CRH and its downstream effectors, suggesting that a GxE interaction at this locus may be important in mediating the effects of childhood trauma exposure on adult risk for depression.

One study examined a population that reported high levels of exposure to childhood physical, sexual, and emotional abuse. Fifteen SNPs spanning 57 kb of the CRH receptor1 (CRHR1) were examined. Significant GxE interactions with multiple individual SNPs were identified, as well as with a common haplotype spanning intron 1 of the CRHR1 locus that modify adult risk of depression in the presence of childhood trauma exposure. Specific CRHR1 polymorphisms (rs7209436, rs110402, and rs242924) appeared to moderate the effect of child abuse on the risk for adult depressive symptomatology but did not influence risk for adult posttraumatic stress symptomatology. These data suggest that a GxE interaction is important for the expression of depressive symptoms in adults with CRHR1 risk or protective alleles who have a history of child abuse (Amstadter et al., 2010).

FKBP5 is a co-chaperone component of the GR heterocomplex (Binder, 2009) that plays a key role in the regulation of GR sensitivity and hence the expression of glucocorticoid-responsive genes by virtue of its participation in an ultrashort, intracellular negative feedback loop regulating GR activity (Vermeer, Hendriks-Stegeman, van der Burg, van Buul-Offers, & Jansen, 2003). Clinical research has identified FKBP5 alleles associated with variation in GR resistance in depressed patients (Binder et al., 2004) that are also associated with elevated peri-traumatic dissociation in medically injured children (Koenen et al., 2005), a psychological response to trauma which is predictive of PTSD risk in adults (Ozer et al., 2003). The level of FKBP5 expression in peripheral blood mononuclear cells at 4 months post-trauma exposure is predictive of PTSD diagnosis in trauma survivors (Segman et al., 2005). Most recently, gene expression analysis from a study of subjects with PTSD following the World Trade Center Attacks found that FKBP5 showed reduced expression in PTSD, consistent with enhanced GR responsiveness (Yehuda, 2009). Further, FKBP5 polymorphisms were examined in association with level of adult PTSD symptomatology (Binder et al., 2008). This cross-sectional study examined genetic and psychological risk factors for PTSD using a verbally presented survey, combined with SNP genotyping, in a randomly chosen sample of nonpsychiatric clinic patients who experienced significant levels of childhood abuse as well as non-child abuse trauma. It was shown that although FKBP5 SNPs did not directly predict PTSD outcome, or interact with level of non-child abuse trauma to predict PTSD, four SNPs in the FKBP5 locus significantly interacted with the severity of child abuse to predict level of adult PTSD (Binder et al., 2008).

One possible explanation for these findings is that a critical period exists for the normative development of a theoretic emotional regulatory system. It has been proposed that during sufficiently supported childhood development, an amygdala-dependent emotional circuit develops that is able to appropriately differentiate threatening from nonthreatening environmental stimuli. In contrast, when child abuse is combined with these biological risk factors, amygdala development may be altered through interactions of elevated stress/cortisol and genetic risk/resilience factors such as described with variation in FKBP5 or CRHR1. This developmental interaction may lead to an amygdala-dependent emotional circuit that is always primed for stress responsiveness. In the case of child maltreatment with combined genetic risk, this emotion circuit is unable to appropriately differentiate threat. Thus, in the presence of an adult trauma these individuals may be at a higher risk for PTSD or other trauma-related psychopathology, such as depression.

No significant associations were reported between chronic PTSD and variation in genes encoding glucocorticoid receptor (GCCR) (Bachmann et al., 2005), neuropeptide Y (NPY) (Lappalainen et al., 2002), or BDNF (Zhang et al., 2006).

Lu et al. (2008) reported a significant association between lifetime PTSD and one of four SNPs in CNR1 (cannabinoid receptor 1) among parents and a haplotype of two CNR1 SNPs among parents of youth with attention-deficit/hyperactivity disorder.

Significant G × E interactions for risk of PTSD were reported in studies of GABRA2 (γ-aminobutyric acid A receptor, α2) (Nelson et al., 2009) and COMT (catechol-*O*-methyltransferase) (Breslau, Davis, Peterson, & Schultz, 2000). Several variants of GABRA2 interacted with composite lifetime history of trauma exposure (Nelson et al., 2009), while a well-characterized amino acid substitution (Val158Met) in *COMT* interacted with the number of traumatic event types (Kolassa, Kolassa, Ertl, Papassotiropoulos, & De Quervain, 2010). A single study examined the association between the commonly investigated *APOE* variation and PTSD symptoms among PTSD veterans (Freeman, Roca, Guggenheim, Kimbrell, & Griffin, 2005). The *APOE* ε2 allele was associated with higher reexperiencing scores (Freeman et al., 2005).

HPA Axis

The HPA axis and immune system communicate in a complex feedback system that can be disrupted following the experience of a traumatic event. Children who experienced permanent or long-term separations from parents, or parental death, have been found to have increases in basal salivary cortisol concentrations (Pfeffer, Altemus, Heo, & Jiang, 2007) and cortisol nonsuppression in the dexamethasone-suppression test (Weller, Weller, Fristad, & Bowes, 1990), but decreased morning cortisol concentrations are seen in some cases of separation (Flinn, Quinlan, Decker, Turner, & England, 1996) and in studies of institutionalized children (Gunnar, Morison, Chisholm, & Schuder, 2001). Two more recent studies of university students with less severe forms of loss have found attenuation of the cortisol response to CRH stimulation in subjects with a childhood history of parental divorce,(Bloch, Peleg, Koren, Aner, & Klein, 2007) and a decreased awakening cortisol response in students with a history of either parental separation/divorce or death of a very close friend or relative (Meinlschmidt & Heim, 2005). It was found that childhood parental loss was associated with increased cortisol responses to the Dex/CRH test. It was also demonstrated that patients with major depressive episode (MDE) had the highest plasma cortisol levels and patients with MDE+PTSD, the levels were the lowest, with healthy volunteers (HVs) having intermediate levels compared with the other two groups. Furthermore, there was a significant increase in cortisol after dl-fenfluramine administration in each of the three groups of patients, but hormonal response to dl-fenfluramine failed to discriminate between MDE, MDE+PTSD, and HVs. The findings did not detect a relationship between suicidal behavior and HPA function regardless of comorbid PTSD (Oquendo et al., 2003).

Domestic violence survivors with a sole diagnosis of PTSD show a very strong hypersuppression of cortisol following administration of a low (0.5 mg) dexamethasone dose (Yehuda et al., 1993). In particular, these findings lend support to the idea of a dysregulation in the HPA axis, and perhaps to enhanced negative feedback inhibition in PTSD (Yehuda, 2002).

Lower levels of cortisol and altered HPA axis functioning have been observed in traumatized women without PTSD (Ganzel et al., 2007). In PTSD patients, female gender was associated with lower cortisol levels in a meta-analysis (Meewisse, Reitsma, de Vries, Gersons, & Olff, 2007). In addition, lower waking salivary cortisol levels have been reported in samples of men and women with PTSD (Wessa, Rohleder, Kirschbaum, & Flor, 2006).

Women with PTSD demonstrated significantly elevated cortisol levels compared to abused women without PTSD when exposed to personalized scripts of childhood abuse, with the greatest magnitude of elevations during and shortly after exposure to the trauma scripts. During recovery, cortisol levels in the PTSD group dropped significantly to a level similar to the non-PTSD group. Taken together, these findings are consistent with findings of increased negative feedback sensitivity (Elzinga, Schmahl, Vermetten, van Dyck, & Bremner, 2003).

Comorbid MDD may further alter cortisol levels in PTSD subjects. PTSD participants with comorbid MDD exhibited lower plasma cortisol levels compared to participants with only MDD (Oquendo et al., 2003), and lower continuous plasma levels compared to healthy subjects (Yehuda, Teicher, Trestman, Levengood, & Siever, 1996), and also lower urinary levels in those women with lifetime PTSD and comorbid MDD compared to controls (Young & Breslau, 2004). Following stimulation with dexamethasone and CRH, PTSD+MDD subjects exhibited lower levels of adrenocorticotropin hormone compared to PTSD-MDD subjects (de Kloet et al., 2008).

In healthy subjects, delta sleep activity peaks in the first half of the night and is temporally associated with the nadir of cortisol output (Steiger, 2002). Multiple studies have shown that increased hypothalamic CRF release is associated with disturbed sleep and particularly with decreased delta sleep activity (Neylan et al., 2003). In turn, treatment with a CRF receptor antagonist increased delta sleep in depressed patients (Held et al., 2004). It was demonstrated that PTSD subjects had diminished ACTH response and a less pronounced decrease of delta sleep to an indirect CRF challenge with metyrapone (Neylan et al., 2003). Further, PTSD subjects had significantly less delta sleep, but no significant differences in total sleep time, sleep maintenance, rapid eye movements (REM) sleep latency, or REM density compared to control subjects. By blocking the last step of cortisol synthesis, metyrapone acutely reduces cortisol levels and attenuates cortisol-mediated feedback inhibition at the pituitary, hypothalamus, and hippocampus, while increasing the release of hypothalamic CRF. Therefore, an attenuated increase of ACTH and a diminished decrease of delta sleep after metyrapone in subjects with PTSD could be explained by chronic increased CRF activity and downregulated CRF receptors.

The evidence supporting the role of increased hypothalamic CRF associated with decreased delta sleep includes the following: (1) hypercortisolemic depression is associated with increased hypothalamic CRF and decreased delta sleep (Steiger, 2002), (2) there is a strong inverse relationship between delta sleep and pulsatile cortisol release (Vgontzas et al., 1999), (3) exogenous cortisol infusion, which reduces CRF in the hypothalamus, increases delta sleep (Friess, Tagaya, Grethe, Trachsel, & Holsboer, 2004), (4) metyrapone administration, which leads to an increase in hypothalamic CRF, causes a decrease in delta sleep (Neylan et al., 2003), and (5) rats with genetically reduced hypothalamic CRF spent more time in delta sleep than genetically intact rats (Opp, 1997).

The mechanism by which CRF might decrease delta sleep is not known. One possible explanation is that an increase in hypothalamic CRF release effects other brain areas involved in sleep or arousal. This possibility is supported by studies showing that not only extrahypothalamic CRF neurons but also neurons from the hypothalamus (Valentino, Page, Van Bockstaele, & Aston-Jones, 1992) project to the LC, which may be a point of integration between neurohormonal and neurotransmitter CRF systems (Koob, 1999). It is possible that stimulation of the LC by way of CRF neurons from the hypothalamus is of sufficient magnitude to affect delta sleep. However, other constituents that parallel cortisol release from the adrenal gland, such as dehydroepiandrosterone (DHEA), could be involved in sleep regulation. Consistent with this hypothesis, DHEA has been associated with sleep.

DHEA and DHEA sulphate ester (DHEA-S) are produced by the adrenal cortex and under normal conditions DHEA levels are closely correlated with cortisol. However, an imbalance of cortisol/DHEA secretion may occur when an individual experiences chronic stress (Raison & Miller, 2003). DHEA-S is more abundant than DHEA in plasma and saliva, and exerts effects at glutamate and GABA receptors that may contribute to PTSD symptoms. DHEA also modulates actions of the immune system, resulting in reduced Th1 immune activities, similar to cortisol (Schuld et al., 2000). Higher DHEA levels among participants with PTSD have been reported (Olff, de Vries, Guzelcan, Assies, & Gersons, 2007), as well as higher DHEA-S (Rasmusson et al., 2004); however a lower level was reported in traumatized individuals that were highly comorbid with MDD and PTSD (Kanter et al., 2001). DHEA administration has been shown to reduce MDD symptoms in depressed individuals (Hsiao, 2006), indicating a possible mechanism for symptom improvement. DHEA levels following HPA axis stimulation were inversely related to negative mood among women with chronic PTSD such that higher levels of depressive symptoms were related to lower production of DHEA (Rasmusson et al., 2004). Sondergaard, Hansson, and Theorell (2002) reported that DHEA levels were lower in participants with PTSD and MDD compared to participants with PTSD and no MDD.

Activation of the Immune System

Indicators of immune activation have been observed in studies of individuals suffering from PTSD. These include increased circulating inflammatory markers, increased reactivity to antigen skin tests, lower natural killer cell activity, and lower total T lymphocyte counts. Certain pro-inflammatory cytokines are able to induce neurochemical and behavioral changes that resemble some key features of PTSD (Pace & Heim, 2010).

The majority of studies in adults with PTSD have reported increased pro-inflammatory cytokine levels in plasma including TNF-α (von Kanel et al., 2007), IL-1β (Spivak et al., 1997), IL-6 (Maes et al., 1999), IL-8 (Song, Zhou, Guan, & Wang, 2007), and stimulated levels of IL-6 (Rohleder, Joksimovic, Wolf, & Kirschbaum, 2004) and INFγ (Woods et al., 2005). Maes et al. (1999) also reported that IL-6 receptor levels were higher in individuals with PTSD and comorbid MDD compared to PTSD participants without MDD. In addition, salivary secretory IgA (sIgA), an immunoglobulin that protects mucosal surfaces from upper respiratory infection, was lower in chronically stressed persons (Ng et al., 2004) including women with PTSD (Woods et al., 2005), possibly resulting in exposure to additional antigens that require an inflammatory immune response.

Following a stressor, cortisol increases and results in suppression of Th1 cytokines by binding to glucocorticoid (GC) receptors in lymphocytes, resulting in downregulation of inflammatory activities (Raison & Miller, 2003). The immune system also affects HPA axis function in an effort to protect the individual. Th1 cytokines stimulate the HPA axis resulting in increased cortisol and a reduction in Th1 immune activities (Raison & Miller, 2003).

Rohleder et al. (2004) reported lower cortisol levels and greater whole blood IL-6 production in male and female Bosnian war refugees with PTSD, as did Pervanidou et al. (2007), who linked elevated evening cortisol and morning serum IL-6 with PTSD development in children following a motor vehicle accident. Together, these studies provide evidence of insufficient glucocorticoid signaling in PTSD sufferers, such that impaired feedback regulation of stress responses and HPA axis activity may be linked to greater pro-inflammatory immune responsiveness (Raison & Miller, 2003).

Other studies have shown IL-6 to be correlated with depression in individuals with PTSD (Miller, Sutherland, Hutchison, & Alexander, 2001) and the level of the IL-6 receptor to be significantly higher in individuals with PTSD and MDD compared to PTSD without MDD (Maes et al., 1999).

Peri-traumatic Factors

These factors reflect stress response during and immediately following the traumatic event.

Physical Injury

Desborough found that surgery-associated tissue injury results in activation of the HPA axis and that increased plasma concentrations of cortisol can be detected shortly following the start of surgery (Desborough, 2000). These findings suggest that tissue injury elicits a hypothalamic endocrine response, independent of the context in which it was inflicted (Shavit et al., 2005). Thus, it is plausible to assume that concurrent physical and psychological stresses may have an additive effect on HPA-axis activity, especially among people with hypersensitive cortisol receptors. The additive effects of injury and trauma on cortisol release may raise the likelihood that an overactive negative feedback pathway will eventually lead to suboptimal HPA-axis activity and prolongation of the stress response.

Substance P, a peptide known as neurokinin 1, has been implicated in transmitting sensory pain impulses to receptors in the spinal cord, and from there to the brain. Moreover, elevated Substance P levels have been shown to be related to persistent and intense regional pain after minor injury or surgery (Schinkel et al., 2006). Thus, it is possible that Substance P increases the risk for PTSD by prolonging the stressful effects of chronic and intense pain.

Intense bodily pain, with its accompanying neurobiological and psychological effects, can be an integral part of the posttraumatic experience for critically injured trauma survivors. Under certain circumstances, physical pain may even be a powerful enough stressor to serve as the primary cause of PTSD (Schreiber & Galai-Gat, 1993). The co-occurrence of PTSD, and chronic pain in particular, has been well documented in the literature (Gayle Beck, Gudmundsdottir, & Shipherd, 2003). The overlap between regulation of pain and emotion lends credence to the theory that pain may be a stimulus for PTSD. By the same token, hyperarousal, stress intolerance, and selective attention typical of PTSD may aggravate pain (Buchwald, Goldberg, Noonan, Beals, & Manson, 2005). The modest correlations between pain and injury severity suggest that the effect of injury on pain is moderated by multiple mechanisms, such as attentional bias, pain sensitivity, anxiety sensitivity, and depression (Asmundson, Coons, Taylor, & Katz, 2002).

Endogenous opioids, which inhibit pain and reduce panic, are secreted after prolonged exposure to severe stress. Siegfried, Frischknecht, and Nunes de Souza (1990) showed that both excessive endogenous opioids and NE affect the storage of experience in explicit memory. Based on these findings, it has been proposed that the dissociative reactions in people responding to trauma may be analogous to the opioid-mediated analgesia that occurs in animals after prolonged exposure to severe uncontrollable stress (van der Kolk, Greenberg, Boyd, & Krystal, 1985). In support of this hypothesis, research has shown that as late as two decades after the original trauma, individuals with PTSD developed opioid-mediated analgesia in response to a stimulus resembling the traumatic stressor (Pitman, van der Kolk, Orr, & Greenberg, 1990). Moreover, they showed that change in pain perception was the best predictor of PTSD. While the exact nature of the relationship between increased levels of endogenous opioids and PTSD symptoms is not fully understood, it is reasonable to postulate that the enhanced risk for PTSD following injury is mediated, at least in part, by increased levels of endogenous opioids. Preliminary support for this hypothesis comes from a study (Nishith, Griffin, & Poth, 2002) that compared battered and non-battered traumatized women. The study found that the presence of stress-induced analgesia in battered women 1-month post-trauma predicted an increase in the severity of PTSD 3 months later (Nishith et al., 2002).

The secretion of pro-inflammatory cytokines is suppressed by glucocorticoids and stimulated by catecholamines. As previously mentioned, patients with PTSD commonly have decreased cortisol levels and increased catecholamine levels (Baker et al., 2001). Thus, low glucocorticoid signaling among injured PTSD-prone individuals may result in elevated levels of pro-inflammatory cytokines (Raison & Miller, 2003). Elevated levels of cytokines may contribute to PTSD by increasing anxiety, depression, and sleep disturbances. Baker et al. (2001) found elevated cerebrospinal fluid concentrations of interleukin-6 in patients with PTSD versus normal controls. Finally, higher levels of interleukin-6 may also explain the higher frequency of physical complaints in PTSD patients (Baker, Mendenhall, Simbartl, Magan, & Steinberg, 1997).

As far as psychological mechanisms are concerned, the most direct hypothesis is that bodily injury intensifies the perceived threat to one's life or physical integrity during the trauma. According to the literature (Shalev, 1992), the perceived level of danger by trauma survivors is a better predictor of PTSD than the objective severity of the traumatic event. However, this hypothesis may be overly simplistic due to data suggesting that the heightened level of perceived threat is not directly correlated with the severity of injury (Koren, Norman, Cohen, Berman, & Klein, 2005). These findings suggest that the effect of bodily injury on perceived threat is moderated by other factors, such as sense of control and the ability to effectively function and cope during the traumatic event.

Disfigured trauma survivors may be more likely to exhibit avoidant behaviors due to self-consciousness about their appearance, or in response to negative reactions from others about their appearance. One study involving female patients with burn injuries or digital amputation found that the degree of cosmetic disfigurement correlated with symptoms of avoidance and emotional numbing (Fukunishi, 1999).

Hospitalization, and ensuing medical procedures, may constitute secondary stressors that can increase the risk for PTSD, even in patients who were not highly traumatized by the initial traumatic event. For example, increased levels of disturbing memories have been found in patients hospitalized in intensive care units for medical conditions that were not caused by traumatic events (Buchwald et al., 2005).

Traumatic Brain Injury

Traumatic brain injury (TBI) is commonly associated with loss of consciousness or impaired memory (retrograde amnesia) and thus potentially serves as a natural model for the study of memory and its role in the development of PTSD. Some of the studies that focused on TBI have provided evidence that traumatic events involving TBI are associated with reduced prevalence of PTSD, consistent with the view that TBI and PTSD are incompatible. It has been suggested (Gil, Caspi, Ben-Ari, Koren, & Klein, 2005) that amnesia for the traumatic event minimizes the possibility of establishing any cognitive representation of the trauma, thus reducing the likelihood of intrusive symptoms.

However, several studies suggest that PTSD is fairly prevalent among TBI patients. These studies indicate that loss of consciousness may not guarantee protection from trauma-related intrusive memories or PTSD (Ohry, Rattok, & Solomon, 1996). Although head injury seemed to be associated with reduced frequency of fear, helplessness, and intrusive memories 1-month post-trauma, there was no difference in the likelihood of a diagnosis of PTSD between trauma survivors with and without head injury at 6-month follow-up (Bryant & Harvey, 1998).

A similar trend was observed in a study that explored the relationship between mild TBI, amnesia, and PTSD among 307 consecutive admissions to a Level one Trauma Center (Creamer, O'Donnell, & Pattison, 2005). This highlights the fact that both ASD and PTSD may develop following trauma despite amnesia for the event.

In another study, Gil et al. (2005) examined the relationship between memory of traumatic event (MTE) and subsequent development of PTSD in a prospective design. One hundred twenty subjects, hospitalized for observation after sustaining a mild TBI, were assessed immediately after the trauma and were followed up for 6 months. The results yielded a bimodal distribution of MTE, with most participants reporting either very good MTE or total lack of MTE. Overall, 14 % of the participants met full criteria for PTSD at 6 months. However, participants with MTE were significantly more likely to develop PTSD than those without MTE, with the difference attributable primarily to the reexperiencing cluster. MTE within the first 24 h was a strong predictor of PTSD 6 months after the traumatic event. However, it should be noted that, albeit less frequently, PTSD was nonetheless present even in the absence of explicit memory of the event, indicating that TBI and PTSD are not mutually exclusive, even in the absence of MTE.

A possible mechanism to account for findings that PTSD occurs without explicit memory of the event is that emotionally charged traumatic memories are initially processed via brain circuits that bypass cortical structures and are mediated primarily through the amygdala and related brain structures, resulting in the formation of implicit (unconscious) memories. In addition, stress-induced secretion of glucocorticoids, which have been shown to impair hippocampal functioning, may disrupt the formation of explicit memory (LeDoux, 1998).

One may question whether "deliberate disruption" of MTE might prove therapeutically beneficial in trauma survivors. It may be predicted that psychological interventions which enhance the traumatic memory may produce less favorable outcome. Indeed, a single-session debriefing—a session that often leads to reconstruction of the trauma—was found to be associated with a less positive outcome when compared with nonintervention. A randomized controlled trial in which some traffic accident victims were given a single 1-h debriefing intervention, and others no intervention, was followed up after 4 months and again after 3 years. At 4 months, the intervention group was found to have marginally (though mostly nonsignificantly) poorer outcome (Hobbs, Mayou, Harrison, & Worlock, 1996). Measures of psychiatric symptoms, travel anxiety, and level of functioning were all significantly worse for patients in the intervention group at 3-year follow-up (Mayou, Ehlers, & Hobbs, 2000).

Sijbrandij, Olff, Reitsma, Carlier, and Gersons (2006) carried out a further study on debriefing, in which trauma survivors were given emotional debriefing, educational debriefing, or no intervention, 2 weeks after the traumatic event. Follow-up was carried out at several time intervals following the intervention. This study showed that although scores on PTSD, anxiety, and depression measures decreased over time, there was no significant difference between the groups on any of the measures. It seems as if, in line with the "amnestic hypothesis," psychological interventions that interfere with the amnesia/repression process should not be routinely used, as this may impede the powerful spontaneous recovery process. This line of reasoning also suggests that pharmacological intervention, that is associated with a decrease in consolidation of the traumatic memory, might be beneficial and vice versa—interventions that are associated with enhancing the traumatic memory would be associated with a worse outcome.

Early administration of benzodiazepines (BNZ) was found to be associated with a less favorable outcome in two small studies (Mellman, Bustamante, David, & Fins, 2002), (Gelpin, Bonne, Peri, Brandes, & Shalev, 1996). Data supporting this trend was also found in the animal model of PTSD. In this study (Matar, Cohen, Kaplan, & Zohar, 2006), although both early and late administrations of BNZ (alprazolam) were associated with decreased anxiety in the short term, only the early BNZ group displayed an increase in PTSD-like behavior (as expressed by the anxiety scale) when the rats were exposed a month later to the traumatic cue. One possible explanation for these sequelae of early BNZ administration might be related to its effect on the HPA axis; BNZ abolishes the cortisol response and, therefore, might attenuate the natural response—increased cortisol levels, an increase associated with a decrease in the fear index (Soravia et al., 2006).

The only medications with specific indication for PTSD are selective serotonin reuptake inhibitors (SSRIs). However, they were only tested several months (and in many cases years) after exposure. Would early administration of SSRIs immediately after exposure have a preventive effect? The potential role of SSRIs in hippocampal neurogenesis (Santarelli et al., 2003) along with open naturalistic clinical observations enabled examination of this question in a PTSD animal model (Matar et al., 2006). Results were quite promising and suggested that early administration of SSRI (sertraline, in this case) was associated with a significant decrease in PTSD-like behavior.

Other possible interventions that might be considered for PTSD prophylaxis are the use of medications that act to suppress catecholamine activity of sympathetic arousal, such as proponalol and guanfacine. A double-blind study examined the severity of acute PTSD symptoms among subjects who received propranolol 40 mg (believed to interfere with memory consolidation) 6-h post-trauma compared with severity of symptoms among participants who received placebos (Pitman et al., 2002). Results showed that the experimental group tended to exhibit lower levels of PTSD symptoms 10 days following the traumatic event. If further corroborated, these findings could support the notion that not only does lack of MTE protect against development of PTSD, but that pharmacologically induced disruption of consolidation of traumatic memories can be therapeutically beneficial for some trauma survivors.

Early Activation of Specific Genes

Gene expression profiling during the triggering and development of PTSD may be informative of its onset and course. Strategies for discovering multiple susceptibility loci may stem from studies such as that conducted by Levi et al. (2005). They examined peripheral gene expression and identified a cluster of differential genes 4 months following a traumatic event, a time frame consistent with the development of a pathological disease state. The differentiated clusters identified in this study included those that are related to amygdala activity, apoptosis, and neural plasticity. The authors suggest that these clusters, if replicable, may represent a starting point from which future whole genome studies can be initiated.

PTSD is associated with decreased activity in the dorsolateral prefrontal cortex (DLPFC), the brain region that regulates working memory and preparation and selection of fear responses. DLPFC, including Brodmann area 46 (BA46), is one of the three regions of prefrontal cortex, which regulates working memory and execution of fear responses (Cohen et al., 2004). This brain region has been correlated with structural and functional alterations and treatment response in patients with PTSD. In children with PTSD symptoms, decreased volume of gray matter in the DLPFC is correlated with increased functional impairment (Cohen et al., 2004). Adult patients with PTSD core symptoms (i.e., re-experiencing, avoidance) were markedly improved by treatment with 10-Hz repetitive transcranial magnetic stimulation over the right DLPFC (Cohen et al., 2004).

One possibility is that functional and structural changes in the brain may result from mitochondria-centered responses to repeated or chronic harmful stresses

(Manoli et al., 2007). Mitochondrial dysfunctions are increasingly recognized as key components in stress-related mental disorders (Manoli et al., 2007). Human brain DLPFC including BA46 is involved in regulation of working memory and preparation and selection of fear responses, and has been correlated with both structural and functional alterations and treatment response of patients with PTSD (Cohen et al., 2004). In one study (Su et al., 2008), the authors applied human mitochondria-focused cDNA microarrays (hMitChip3) to PTSD brain samples and have successfully identified expression signatures, canonical pathways, molecular networks, and drug targets of neurological disease- and psychological/psychiatric disorder-related genes that are dysregulated in the DLPFC BA46. These results indicate mitochondrial dysfunction is involved in neuronal function and survival in the DLPFC BA46, and may prove useful for development of methods for diagnosis, prevention, and treatment of PTSD (Su et al., 2008). Moreover, unsupervised clusters of 12 DLPFC BA46 RNA samples, based solely on expression similarities of informative 800 mitochondria-focused genes, clearly distinguish PTSD brains from controls. Demonstration that a highly significant number of oxidative phosphorylation genes were dysregulated in PTSD brains' BA46, strongly suggests the presence of at least energy deficiency in this brain region (Su et al., 2008).

Early Sleep Disturbances

Historically, sleep problems have been conceptualized as a secondary symptom of PTSD (Hefez, Metz, & Lavie, 1987). However, recent accounts have suggested that sleep problems may be central to the PTSD syndrome (Spoormaker & Montgomery, 2008). A wealth of data suggests sleep problems are correlated with traumatic event exposure and PTSD (Pillar, Malhotra, & Lavie, 2000). For example, sleep problems were the most prevalent symptom among individuals who survived the 1995 Hanshin earthquake in Japan (Kato, Asukai, Miyake, Minakawa, & Nishiyama, 1996) and among survivors of the Holocaust (Kuch & Cox, 1992). The relation between traumatic event exposure and sleep problems is particularly pronounced among persons who do not recover from initial symptomatic reactions to such exposure, including persons with PTSD (Mellman & Hipolito, 2006). Individuals with PTSD, compared to those without, report greater trouble initiating (41 % and 13 %, respectively) and maintaining (47 % and 18 % respectively) sleep (Ohayon & Shapiro, 2000).

REM sleep is the sleep stage associated with dreaming and consolidation of memories (Maquet, 2001). REM density is a measure of the frequency of rapid eye movements during REM sleep, which typically increases over the course of sleep. Sleep efficiency refers to the ratio between total time asleep and the amount of time spent in bed. In one study, all traumatic event-exposed participants had lower sleep efficiency, increased sleep latency, shorter REM time, and longer REM latency, in comparison with controls (Hefez et al., 1987).

Mellman, David, Kulick-Bell, Hebding, and Nolan (1995) tested the role of sleep in recovery from recent traumatic event exposure in hurricane survivors.

Sleep assessments measured current sleep problems, as well as retrospectively reported sleep problems before being exposed to a hurricane. Objective measures of sleep (polysomnography) were administered to (1) a subgroup of hurricane victims with psychiatric diagnoses and (2) a healthy comparison group not affected by the hurricane. In terms of pre-hurricane sleep problems, results indicated those with the highest levels of bad dreams, global severity of sleep problems, sleep disturbances, and awakenings had greater levels of active psychiatric morbidity (including PTSD). These data coalesce to suggest that sleep problems prior to a traumatic event may increase the likelihood to develop PTSD (Mellman et al., 1995). Dagan, Lavie, and Bleich (1991) conducted a study on awakening thresholds (i.e., decibel level of a tone presented during stage 3/4 of sleep required to awaken the individual) of individuals with and without PTSD as a result of participation in the First Lebanon War. All participants' sleep problems, 4–6 years posttraumatic event, were evaluated via polysomnography. Findings revealed that those with PTSD had increased awakening thresholds in comparison to controls. This finding suggests those with PTSD may experience greater depth of sleep, and, therefore, more difficulty in waking (Dagan et al., 1991).

Taken together, these studies demonstrate that exposure to traumatic events alone can result in sleep problems, regardless of recovery from the event.

Klein, Koren, Arnon, and Lavie (2002) explored the development of sleep problems after relatively recent traumatic event exposure. Sleep problems were monitored via polysomnography among traffic accident victims with PTSD for up to 1 year after the traumatic event. Results demonstrated no significant differences in self-reported or polysomnographic assessments of sleep between those with and without PTSD. Overall, results suggested only marginal differences in self-reported sleep problems between those with and without PTSD.

This research team, in another study with a larger sample size, (Koren, Arnon, Lavie, & Klein, 2002) prospectively examined self-reported insomnia symptoms among motor vehicle accident victims over a 1-year period. Results indicated that a quarter of original accident victims developed PTSD by the 12-month follow-up. In comparison, none of the control group met diagnostic criteria for PTSD throughout the study. Furthermore, results indicated the presence of insomnia symptoms at 1-month assessment, and subsequent assessments significantly predicted the development of PTSD at the 12-month follow-up. These data suggest that sleep problems occur shortly after a traumatic event and indicate an increased likelihood of developing PTSD.

Mellman, Pigeon, Nowell, and Nolan (2007) conducted a study investigating the role of REM sleep and PTSD symptoms after recent traumatic event exposure. Results indicated that subjective insomnia ratings and nightmares were greatest among the PTSD group (compared to the sub-threshold and control groups). Furthermore, REM duration was negatively correlated with severity of PTSD symptoms and subjective insomnia ratings.

It was further demonstrated that traumatic event exposure alone, relative to the presence of PTSD and no-traumatic event exposure, predicted increased sleep problems, including greater frequency of awakenings and lower rates of arousal during REM sleep (Mellman, Bustamante, Fins, Pigeon, & Nolan, 2002). Moreover, REM fragmentation 1-month post-traumatic event was positively correlated with development of PTSD symptoms by 6 months posttraumatic event (Mellman, Bustamante, Fins et al., 2002), and decreased REM duration is negatively correlated with PTSD symptom severity (Mellman et al., 2007).

Researchers have theorized why sleep problems may interfere with recovery from traumatic event exposure. First, it has been hypothesized that disruptions in REM sleep may interfere with the integration of new associations into traumatic event-related memory (e.g., safety-related learning) (Mellman, Bustamante, Fins et al., 2002), thereby preventing emotional processing critical to recovery from a traumatic event (Brewin, Dalgleish, & Joseph, 1996). Second, it is possible that sleep problems impair daytime coping, resulting in increased avoidance of traumatic event-related cues, thereby preventing the extinction of learned fear of traumatic event-related cues (Rothbaum, Foa, Riggs, Murdock, & Walsh, 1992). Third, pairing of fear experienced during a nightmare, with cognitive cues of a traumatic event present during the nightmare, may further sensitize persons to traumatic event cues (Rothbaum et al., 1992). Fourth, experimental studies have suggested sleep deprivation generally increases anxiety (Sagaspe et al., 2006), which may maintain elevated posttraumatic stress symptoms, by virtue of maintenance of relatively elevated basal levels of anxiety. Furthermore, it also is possible that substance abuse subsequent to sleep problems after a traumatic event may interfere with healthy recovery. Indeed, studies suggest that people with PTSD may use substances to self-medicate sleep problems (Nishith, Resick, & Mueser, 2001) and negative affect (Kaysen et al., 2007). Prospective research is emerging, suggesting that substance use in the wake of traumatic event exposure may potentiate the development of PTSD (van der Velden, Kleber, & Koenen, 2008). Finally, the role of gender must be considered in relationship between sleep and PTSD. Evidence indicates women are more likely to have sleep problems (Soares, 2005) and develop PTSD (Breslau & Anthony, 2007).

Early Changes in Cardiovascular Activity

Rise in catecholamine levels during stress response leads to increases in heart rate, blood pressure, and a blood glucose level. Several converging lines of evidence suggest that increased sympathetic activity and subsequently elevated levels of plasma catecholamines are related to increased risk for PTSD. Some studies (Buckley & Kaloupek, 2001) have found that shortly after trauma exposure, individuals who develop PTSD have higher heart rates on average than individuals who do not. Similarly, it has been shown that people with PTSD have elevated levels of plasma norepinephrine (NE) at rest and experience significant increases in plasma NE when exposed to trauma-related stimuli (Schoenfeld, Marmar, & Neylan, 2004).

Given the role of catecholamines in memory formation, it has been postulated that excessive adrenergic activation in the immediate aftermath of a traumatic event may enhance memory consolidation of the event (Shalev et al., 1998) and increase the probability that an individual will experience intrusive recollections (Yehuda, Bryant, Marmar, & Zohar, 2005).

Few studies to date have investigated physiological responses to trauma reminders soon after trauma. Elsesser, Sartory, and Tackenberg (2004) found that chronic PTSD patients and recent trauma survivors who met criteria for ASD 6 weeks following trauma showed heart rate acceleration to individualized trauma-related pictures, whereas non-traumatized controls and survivors without ASD showed heart rate deceleration. Blanchard et al. (1996) studied survivors of motor vehicle accidents (MVA) around 2 and a half months following trauma and found heart rate responses to audiotaped individualized scripts describing the participants' accident, but not responses to other stressors, distinguished survivors with PTSD from those without PTSD and nontraumatized controls. These results are in line with the notion that in the initial months after trauma, PTSD is characterized by strong learned fear responses to reminders of the trauma.

There is also preliminary evidence that heart rate responses (HRR) to trauma reminders can be used to predict the chronicity of PTSD. Elsesser, Sartory, and Tackenberg (2005) found that greater HRR to the individualized trauma-related pictures predicted PTSD symptoms 3 months after trauma. Kleim, Wilhelm, Glucksman, and Ehlers (2010) found that HRR to guided imagery of the trauma at 2 weeks predicted PTSD severity at 6 months following trauma in female but not male assault survivors.

Another study in 2010 (Suendermann, Ehlers, Boellinghaus, Gamer, & Glucksman, 2010) also explored whether skin conductance responses to trauma reminders are related to PTSD in assault or MVA survivors. Skin conductance responses (SCR) were chosen for this study because SCR are widely used as a measure of conditioned emotional responses in laboratory studies (Orr et al., 2000) and because SCR has been shown to differentiate between people with chronic PTSD and controls in some, but not all idiographic trauma cue studies (Pole, 2007). This study also examined whether HRR to trauma reminders are related to the participants' emotional and cognitive responses during the trauma, in particular to the degree of peri-traumatic fear and dissociation. These responses have been shown to predict PTSD (Nixon, Bryant, Moulds, Felmingham, & Mastrodomenico, 2005).

It was demonstrated that trauma survivors with PTSD exhibit heightened HRR to standardized trauma-related pictures compared to survivors without PTSD as early as 1 month following trauma. This result supports the hypothesis that in PTSD, learned fear responses acquired during the trauma generalize to stimuli that resemble the original traumatic situation, so that more and more situations trigger fear and physiological arousal (Keane, Zimering, & Caddell, 1985).

In a cohort of patients with TBI, some of whom had developed PTSD (Bryant, Marosszeky, Crooks, & Gurka, 2004), PTSD patients had higher HR levels than non-PTSD patients. The intriguing aspect of these findings is that PTSD patients were amnesic of their trauma, and they only met criteria for PTSD; despite no intrusive memories or nightmares of the trauma, they reported psychological distress or physiological reactivity in response to trauma-related cues. One interpretation of this finding is that these patients experienced fear conditioning at a level that did not require awareness of the trauma experienced. The conditioned fear response involves the central nucleus of the amygdala stimulating sympathetic activation, which can be reflected in increased HR and need not involve cortical regions associated with conscious awareness (LeDoux, Iwata, Cicchetti, & Reis, 1988). Overall, these data may suggest that fear-conditioned responses during trauma can occur in the absence of awareness. Lack of this difference 1 month following trauma accords with one previous prospective study of HR and PTSD (Shalev et al., 1998), and is consistent with evidence of a lack of elevated baseline HR in chronic PTSD (Pitman, 1990). It is possible that adrenergic activation in the acute, rather than the chronic, phase is important in overconsolidation of trauma memories and the contribution to subsequent PTSD.

Summary

To summarize, the risk of developing PTSD after a traumatic experience depends on several vulnerability factors that may be classified into three distinct categories—pre-traumatic, peri-traumatic, and posttraumatic vulnerability factors. Accordingly, while attempting to draw the profile of the high-risk patient for PTSD, the following factors should be included, among others: small hippocampus, previously altered HPA axis, vulnerable genetic profile, associated body injury, increased post-trauma noradrenergic activity.

Some protective factors that have been identified include, but are not limited to, coping, resources (e.g., social support, self-esteem, optimism), and finding meaning. Finally, human beings are resilient and in general are able to cope with adverse situations. Therefore, discovering possible resilience factors may assist in identifying the patients at risk and may contribute to developing the strategies to prevent the development of PTSD.

References

Amstadter, A. B., Nugent, N. R., Yang, B. Z., Miller, A., Siburian, R., Moorjani, P., et al. (2010). Corticotrophin-releasing hormone type 1 receptor gene (CRHR1) variants predict posttraumatic stress disorder onset and course in pediatric injury patients. *Disease Markers, 30*(2–3), 89–99.

Armony, J. L., Corbo, V., Clement, M. H., & Brunet, A. (2005). Amygdala response in patients with acute PTSD to masked and unmasked emotional facial expressions. *The American Journal of Psychiatry, 162*(10), 1961–1963.

Asmundson, G. J., Coons, M. J., Taylor, S., & Katz, J. (2002). PTSD and the experience of pain: Research and clinical implications of shared vulnerability and mutual maintenance models. *Canadian Journal of Psychiatry, 47*(10), 930–937.

Bachmann, A. W., Sedgley, T. L., Jackson, R. V., Gibson, J. N., Young, R. M., & Torpy, D. J. (2005). Glucocorticoid receptor polymorphisms and post-traumatic stress disorder. *Psychoneuroendocrinology, 30*(3), 297–306.

Baker, D. G., Ekhator, N. N., Kasckow, J. W., Hill, K. K., Zoumakis, E., Dashevsky, B. A., et al. (2001). Plasma and cerebrospinal fluid interleukin-6 concentrations in posttraumatic stress disorder. *Neuroimmunomodulation, 9*(4), 209–217.

Baker, D. G., Mendenhall, C. L., Simbartl, L. A., Magan, L. K., & Steinberg, J. L. (1997). Relationship between posttraumatic stress disorder and self-reported physical symptoms in Persian Gulf War veterans. *Archives of Internal Medicine, 157*(18), 2076–2078.

Bernstein, A., & Zvolensky, M. J. (2007). Anxiety sensitivity: Selective review of promising research and future directions. *Expert Review of Neurotherapeutics, 7*(2), 97–101.

Binder, E. B. (2009). The role of FKBP5, a co-chaperone of the glucocorticoid receptor in the pathogenesis and therapy of affective and anxiety disorders. *Psychoneuroendocrinology, 34*(Suppl 1), S186–S195.

Binder, E. B., Bradley, R. G., Liu, W., Epstein, M. P., Deveau, T. C., Mercer, K. B., et al. (2008). Association of FKBP5 polymorphisms and childhood abuse with risk of posttraumatic stress disorder symptoms in adults. *JAMA, 299*(11), 1291–1305.

Binder, E. B., Salyakina, D., Lichtner, P., Wochnik, G. M., Ising, M., Putz, B., et al. (2004). Polymorphisms in FKBP5 are associated with increased recurrence of depressive episodes and rapid response to antidepressant treatment. *Nature Genetics, 36*(12), 1319–1325.

Blanchard, E. B., Hickling, E. J., Buckley, T. C., Taylor, A. E., Vollmer, A., & Loos, W. R. (1996). Psychophysiology of posttraumatic stress disorder related to motor vehicle accidents: Replication and extension. *Journal of Consulting and Clinical Psychology, 64*(4), 742–751.

Bloch, M., Peleg, I., Koren, D., Aner, H., & Klein, E. (2007). Long-term effects of early parental loss due to divorce on the HPA axis. *Hormones and Behavior, 51*(4), 516–523.

Bloom, A. S. (1982). Effect of delta9-tetrahydrocannabinol on the synthesis of dopamine and norepinephrine in mouse brain synaptosomes. *The Journal of Pharmacology and Experimental Therapeutics, 221*(1), 97–103.

Bossini, L., Tavanti, M., Lombardelli, A., Calossi, S., Polizzotto, N. R., Galli, R., et al. (2007). Changes in hippocampal volume in patients with post-traumatic stress disorder after sertraline treatment. *Journal of Clinical Psychopharmacology, 27*(2), 233–235.

Brand, S. R., Engel, S. M., Canfield, R. L., & Yehuda, R. (2006). The effect of maternal PTSD following in utero trauma exposure on behavior and temperament in the 9-month-old infant. *The Annals of the New York Academy of Sciences, 1071*, 454–458.

Bremner, J. D., Narayan, M., Staib, L. H., Southwick, S. M., McGlashan, T., & Charney, D. S. (1999). Neural correlates of memories of childhood sexual abuse in women with and without posttraumatic stress disorder. *The American Journal of Psychiatry, 156*(11), 1787–1795.

Bremner, J. D., Randall, P., Scott, T. M., Bronen, R. A., Seibyl, J. P., Southwick, S. M., et al. (1995). MRI-based measurement of hippocampal volume in patients with combat-related posttraumatic stress disorder. *The American Journal of Psychiatry, 152*(7), 973–981.

Bremner, J. D., Vermetten, E., Schmahl, C., Vaccarino, V., Vythilingam, M., Afzal, N., et al. (2005). Positron emission tomographic imaging of neural correlates of a fear acquisition and extinction paradigm in women with childhood sexual-abuse-related post-traumatic stress disorder. *Psychological Medicine, 35*(6), 791–806.

Bremner, J. D., Vythilingam, M., Vermetten, E., Southwick, S. M., McGlashan, T., Nazeer, A., et al. (2003). MRI and PET study of deficits in hippocampal structure and function in women with childhood sexual abuse and posttraumatic stress disorder. *The American Journal of Psychiatry, 160*(5), 924–932.

Breslau, N., & Anthony, J. C. (2007). Gender differences in the sensitivity to posttraumatic stress disorder: An epidemiological study of urban young adults. *Journal of Abnormal Psychology, 116*(3), 607–611.

Breslau, N., Davis, G. C., Peterson, E. L., & Schultz, L. R. (2000). A second look at comorbidity in victims of trauma: The posttraumatic stress disorder-major depression connection. *Biological Psychiatry, 48*(9), 902–909.

Brewin, C. R., Dalgleish, T., & Joseph, S. (1996). A dual representation theory of posttraumatic stress disorder. *Psychological Review, 103*(4), 670–686.

Broekman, B. F., Olff, M., & Boer, F. (2007). The genetic background to PTSD. *Neuroscience and Biobehavioral Reviews, 31*(3), 348–362.

Bryant, R. A. (2008). Disentangling mild traumatic brain injury and stress reactions. *The New England Journal of Medicine, 358*(5), 525–527.

Bryant, R. A., Felmingham, K., Kemp, A., Das, P., Hughes, G., Peduto, A., et al. (2008). Amygdala and ventral anterior cingulate activation predicts treatment response to cognitive behaviour therapy for post-traumatic stress disorder. *Psychological Medicine, 38*(4), 555–561.

Bryant, R. A., & Harvey, A. G. (1998). Relationship between acute stress disorder and posttraumatic stress disorder following mild traumatic brain injury. *The American Journal of Psychiatry, 155*(5), 625–629.

Bryant, R. A., Marosszeky, J. E., Crooks, J., & Gurka, J. A. (2004). Elevated resting heart rate as a predictor of posttraumatic stress disorder after severe traumatic brain injury. *Psychosomatic Medicine, 66*(5), 760–761.

Buchwald, D., Goldberg, J., Noonan, C., Beals, J., & Manson, S. (2005). Relationship between posttraumatic stress disorder and pain in two American Indian tribes. *Pain Medicine, 6*(1), 72–79.

Buckley, T. C., & Kaloupek, D. G. (2001). A meta-analytic examination of basal cardiovascular activity in posttraumatic stress disorder. *Psychosomatic Medicine, 63*(4), 585–594.

Cahill, L., & McGaugh, J. L. (1996). The neurobiology of memory for emotional events: Adrenergic activation and the amygdala. *Proceedings of the Western Pharmacology Society, 39*, 81–84.

Cahill, L., Prins, B., Weber, M., & McGaugh, J. L. (1994). Beta-adrenergic activation and memory for emotional events. *Nature, 371*(6499), 702–704.

Caspi, A., Sugden, K., Moffitt, T. E., Taylor, A., Craig, I. W., Harrington, H., et al. (2003). Influence of life stress on depression: Moderation by a polymorphism in the 5-HTT gene. *Science, 301*(5631), 386–389.

Chantarujikapong, S. I., Scherrer, J. F., Xian, H., Eisen, S. A., Lyons, M. J., Goldberg, J., et al. (2001). A twin study of generalized anxiety disorder symptoms, panic disorder symptoms and post-traumatic stress disorder in men. *Psychiatry Research, 103*(2–3), 133–145.

Charney, D. S., Shin, L. M., & Phelps, E. A. (2006). Neurocircuitry models of posttraumatic stress disorder and extinction: Human neuroimaging research – Past, present, and future. *Biological Psychiatry, 60*, 376–382.

Cohen, H., Kaplan, Z., Kotler, M., Kouperman, I., Moisa, R., & Grisaru, N. (2004). Repetitive transcranial magnetic stimulation of the right dorsolateral prefrontal cortex in posttraumatic stress disorder: A double-blind, placebo-controlled study. *The American Journal of Psychiatry, 161*(3), 515–524.

Comings, D. E., Muhleman, D., & Gysin, R. (1996). Dopamine D2 receptor (DRD2) gene and susceptibility to posttraumatic stress disorder: A study and replication. *Biological Psychiatry, 40*(5), 368–372.

Creamer, M., O'Donnell, M. L., & Pattison, P. (2005). Amnesia, traumatic brain injury, and posttraumatic stress disorder: A methodological inquiry. *Behaviour Research and Therapy, 43*(10), 1383–1389.

Dagan, Y., Lavie, P., & Bleich, A. (1991). Elevated awakening thresholds in sleep stage 3-4 in war-related post-traumatic stress disorder. *Biological Psychiatry, 30*(6), 618–622.

Davidson, J. R., Tupler, L. A., Wilson, W. H., & Connor, K. M. (1998). A family study of chronic post-traumatic stress disorder following rape trauma. *Journal of Psychiatric Research, 32*(5), 301–309.

Davis, L. L., Clark, D. M., Kramer, G. L., Moeller, F. G., & Petty, F. (1999). D-fenfluramine challenge in posttraumatic stress disorder. *Biological Psychiatry, 45*(7), 928–930.

de Kloet, C., Vermetten, E., Lentjes, E., Geuze, E., van Pelt, J., Manuel, R., et al. (2008). Differences in the response to the combined DEX-CRH test between PTSD patients with and without co-morbid depressive disorder. *Psychoneuroendocrinology, 33*(3), 313–320.

Desborough, J. P. (2000). The stress response to trauma and surgery. *British Journal of Anaesthesia, 85*(1), 109–117.

Dickie, E. W., Brunet, A., Akerib, V., & Armony, J. L. (2008). An fMRI investigation of memory encoding in PTSD: Influence of symptom severity. *Neuropsychologia, 46*(5), 1522–1531.

Dragan, W. L., & Oniszczenko, W. (2009). The association between dopamine D4 receptor exon III polymorphism and intensity of PTSD symptoms among flood survivors. *Anxiety, Stress, and Coping, 22*(5), 483–495.

Elsesser, K., Sartory, G., & Tackenberg, A. (2004). Attention, heart rate, and startle response during exposure to trauma-relevant pictures: A comparison of recent trauma victims and patients with posttraumatic stress disorder. *Journal of Abnormal Psychology, 113*(2), 289–301.

Elsesser, K., Sartory, G., & Tackenberg, A. (2005). Initial symptoms and reactions to trauma-related stimuli and the development of posttraumatic stress disorder. *Depression and Anxiety, 21*(2), 61–70.

Elzinga, B. M., Schmahl, C. G., Vermetten, E., van Dyck, R., & Bremner, J. D. (2003). Higher cortisol levels following exposure to traumatic reminders in abuse-related PTSD. *Neuropsychopharmacology, 28*(9), 1656–1665.

Etkin, A., & Wager, T. D. (2007). Functional neuroimaging of anxiety: A meta-analysis of emotional processing in PTSD, social anxiety disorder, and specific phobia. *The American Journal of Psychiatry, 164*(10), 1476–1488.

Felmingham, K., Kemp, A., Williams, L., Das, P., Hughes, G., Peduto, A., et al. (2007). Changes in anterior cingulate and amygdala after cognitive behavior therapy of posttraumatic stress disorder. *Psychological Science, 18*(2), 127–129.

Flinn, M. V., Quinlan, R. J., Decker, S. A., Turner, M. T., & England, B. G. (1996). Male-female differences in effects of parental absence on glucocorticoid stress response. *Human Nature, 7*(2), 125–162.

Freeman, T., Roca, V., Guggenheim, F., Kimbrell, T., & Griffin, W. S. (2005). Neuropsychiatric associations of apolipoprotein E alleles in subjects with combat-related posttraumatic stress disorder. *The Journal of Neuropsychiatry and Clinical Neurosciences, 17*(4), 541–543.

Friess, E., Tagaya, H., Grethe, C., Trachsel, L., & Holsboer, F. (2004). Acute cortisol administration promotes sleep intensity in man. *Neuropsychopharmacology, 29*(3), 598–604.

Fukunishi, I. (1999). Relationship of cosmetic disfigurement to the severity of posttraumatic stress disorder in burn injury or digital amputation. *Psychotherapy and Psychosomatics, 68*(2), 82–86.

Ganzel, B. L., Eckenrode, J. J., Kim, P., Wethington, E., Horowitz, E., & Temple, E. (2007). Salivary cortisol levels and mood vary by lifetime trauma exposure in a sample of healthy women. *Journal of Traumatic Stress, 20*(5), 689–699.

Gayle Beck, J., Gudmundsdottir, B., & Shipherd, J. C. (2003). PTSD and emotional distress symptoms measured after a motor vehicle accident: Relationships with pain coping profiles. *Journal of Psychopathology and Behavioral Assessment, 25*(4), 219–227.

Gelpin, E., Bonne, O., Peri, T., Brandes, D., & Shalev, A. Y. (1996). Treatment of recent trauma survivors with benzodiazepines: A prospective study. *The Journal of Clinical Psychiatry, 57*(9), 390–394.

Geuze, E., van Berckel, B. N., Lammertsma, A. A., Boellaard, R., de Kloet, C. S., Vermetten, E., et al. (2008). Reduced GABAA benzodiazepine receptor binding in veterans with post-traumatic stress disorder. *Molecular Psychiatry, 13*(1), 74–83, 73.

Geuze, E., Westenberg, H. G., Jochims, A., de Kloet, C. S., Bohus, M., Vermetten, E., et al. (2007). Altered pain processing in veterans with posttraumatic stress disorder. *Archives of General Psychiatry, 64*(1), 76–85.

Gil, S., Caspi, Y., Ben-Ari, I. Z., Koren, D., & Klein, E. (2005). Does memory of a traumatic event increase the risk for posttraumatic stress disorder in patients with traumatic brain injury? A prospective study. *The American Journal of Psychiatry, 162*(5), 963–969.

Gilbertson, M. W., Shenton, M. E., Ciszewski, A., Kasai, K., Lasko, N. B., Orr, S. P., et al. (2002). Smaller hippocampal volume predicts pathologic vulnerability to psychological trauma. *Nature Neuroscience, 5*(11), 1242–1247.

Glover, D. A., Powers, M. B., Bergman, L., Smits, J. A., Telch, M. J., & Stuber, M. (2003). Urinary dopamine and turn bias in traumatized women with and without PTSD symptoms. *Behavioural Brain Research, 144*(1–2), 137–141.

Gunnar, M. R., Morison, S. J., Chisholm, K., & Schuder, M. (2001). Salivary cortisol levels in children adopted from romanian orphanages. *Development and Psychopathology, 13*(3), 611–628.

Gurvits, T. V., Shenton, M. E., Hokama, H., Ohta, H., Lasko, N. B., Gilbertson, M. W., et al. (1996). Magnetic resonance imaging study of hippocampal volume in chronic, combat-related posttraumatic stress disorder. *Biological Psychiatry, 40*(11), 1091–1099.

Ham, B. J., Chey, J., Yoon, S. J., Sung, Y., Jeong, D. U., Ju Kim, S., et al. (2007). Decreased N-acetyl-aspartate levels in anterior cingulate and hippocampus in subjects with post-traumatic stress disorder: A proton magnetic resonance spectroscopy study. *The European Journal of Neuroscience, 25*(1), 324–329.

Hariri, A. R., Mattay, V. S., Tessitore, A., Kolachana, B., Fera, F., Goldman, D., et al. (2002). Serotonin transporter genetic variation and the response of the human amygdala. *Science, 297*(5580), 400–403.

Hefez, A., Metz, L., & Lavie, P. (1987). Long-term effects of extreme situational stress on sleep and dreaming. *The American Journal of Psychiatry, 144*(3), 344–347.

Heils, A., Teufel, A., Petri, S., Stober, G., Riederer, P., Bengel, D., et al. (1996). Allelic variation of human serotonin transporter gene expression. *Journal of Neurochemistry, 66*(6), 2621–2624.

Heim, C., Newport, D. J., Heit, S., Graham, Y. P., Wilcox, M., Bonsall, R., et al. (2000). Pituitary-adrenal and autonomic responses to stress in women after sexual and physical abuse in childhood. *JAMA, 284*(5), 592–597.

Heim, C., Newport, D. J., Mletzko, T., Miller, A. H., & Nemeroff, C. B. (2008). The link between childhood trauma and depression: Insights from HPA axis studies in humans. *Psychoneuroendocrinology, 33*(6), 693–710.

Held, K., Kunzel, H., Ising, M., Schmid, D. A., Zobel, A., Murck, H., et al. (2004). Treatment with the CRH1-receptor-antagonist R121919 improves sleep-EEG in patients with depression. *Journal of Psychiatric Research, 38*(2), 129–136.

Hobbs, M., Mayou, R., Harrison, B., & Worlock, P. (1996). A randomised controlled trial of psychological debriefing for victims of road traffic accidents. *BMJ, 313*(7070), 1438–1439.

Hou, C., Liu, J., Wang, K., Li, L., Liang, M., He, Z., et al. (2007). Brain responses to symptom provocation and trauma-related short-term memory recall in coal mining accident survivors with acute severe PTSD. *Brain Research, 1144*, 165–174.

Hsiao, C. C. (2006). Difference in pre- and post-treatment plasma DHEA levels were significantly and positively correlated with difference in pre- and post-treatment Hamilton depression scores following successful therapy for major depression. *Psychoneuroendocrinology, 31*(7), 839–846.

Kanter, E. D., Wilkinson, C. W., Radant, A. D., Petrie, E. C., Dobie, D. J., McFall, M. E., et al. (2001). Glucocorticoid feedback sensitivity and adrenocortical responsiveness in posttraumatic stress disorder. *Biological Psychiatry, 50*(4), 238–245.

Kasai, K., Yamasue, H., Gilbertson, M. W., Shenton, M. E., Rauch, S. L., & Pitman, R. K. (2008). Evidence for acquired pregenual anterior cingulate gray matter loss from a twin study of combat-related posttraumatic stress disorder. *Biological Psychiatry, 63*(6), 550–556.

Kato, H., Asukai, N., Miyake, Y., Minakawa, K., & Nishiyama, A. (1996). Post-traumatic symptoms among younger and elderly evacuees in the early stages following the 1995 Hanshin-Awaji earthquake in Japan. *Acta Psychiatrica Scandinavica, 93*(6), 477–481.

Kaysen, D., Dillworth, T. M., Simpson, T., Waldrop, A., Larimer, M. E., & Resick, P. A. (2007). Domestic violence and alcohol use: Trauma-related symptoms and motives for drinking. *Addictive Behaviors, 32*(6), 1272–1283.

Keane, T. M., Zimering, R. T., & Caddell, J. M. (1985). A behavioral formulation of posttraumatic stress disorder in Vietnam veterans. *Behavior Therapist, 8*, 9–12.

Kleim, B., Wilhelm, F. H., Glucksman, E., & Ehlers, A. (2010). Sex differences in heart rate responses to script-driven imagery soon after trauma and risk of posttraumatic stress disorder. *Psychosomatic Medicine, 72*(9), 917–924.

Klein, E., Koren, D., Arnon, I., & Lavie, P. (2002). No evidence of sleep disturbance in post-traumatic stress disorder: A polysomnographic study in injured victims of traffic accidents. *The Israel Journal of Psychiatry and Related Sciences, 39*(1), 3–10.

Koenen, K. C., Aiello, A. E., Bakshis, E., Amstadter, A. B., Ruggiero, K. J., Acierno, R., et al. (2009). Modification of the association between serotonin transporter genotype and risk of posttraumatic stress disorder in adults by county-level social environment. *American Journal of Epidemiology, 169*(6), 704–711.

Koenen, K. C., Saxe, G., Purcell, S., Smoller, J. W., Bartholomew, D., Miller, A., et al. (2005). Polymorphisms in FKBP5 are associated with peritraumatic dissociation in medically injured children. *Molecular Psychiatry, 10*(12), 1058–1059.

Kolassa, I. T., Kolassa, S., Ertl, V., Papassotiropoulos, A., & De Quervain, D. J. (2010). The risk of posttraumatic stress disorder after trauma depends on traumatic load and the catechol-o-methyltransferase Val(158)Met polymorphism. *Biological Psychiatry, 67*(4), 304–308.

Koob, G. F. (1999). Corticotropin-releasing factor, norepinephrine, and stress. *Biological Psychiatry, 46*(9), 1167–1180.

Koren, D., Arnon, I., Lavie, P., & Klein, E. (2002). Sleep complaints as early predictors of post-traumatic stress disorder: A 1-year prospective study of injured survivors of motor vehicle accidents. *The American Journal of Psychiatry, 159*(5), 855–857.

Koren, D., Norman, D., Cohen, A., Berman, J., & Klein, E. M. (2005). Increased PTSD risk with combat-related injury: A matched comparison study of injured and uninjured soldiers experiencing the same combat events. *The American Journal of Psychiatry, 162*(2), 276–282.

Kuch, K., & Cox, B. J. (1992). Symptoms of PTSD in 124 survivors of the Holocaust. *The American Journal of Psychiatry, 149*(3), 337–340.

Kuroda, Y., & McEwen, B. S. (1998). Effect of chronic restraint stress and tianeptine on growth factors, growth-associated protein-43 and microtubule-associated protein 2 mRNA expression in the rat hippocampus. *Brain Research. Molecular Brain Research, 59*(1), 35–39.

Lanius, R. A., Frewen, P. A., Girotti, M., Neufeld, R. W., Stevens, T. K., & Densmore, M. (2007). Neural correlates of trauma script-imagery in posttraumatic stress disorder with and without comorbid major depression: A functional MRI investigation. *Psychiatry Research, 155*(1), 45–56.

Lappalainen, J., Kranzler, H. R., Malison, R., Price, L. H., Van Dyck, C., Rosenheck, R. A., et al. (2002). A functional neuropeptide Y Leu7Pro polymorphism associated with alcohol dependence in a large population sample from the United States. *Archives of General Psychiatry, 59*(9), 825–831.

LeDoux, J. (1998). Fear and the brain: Where have we been, and where are we going? *Biological Psychiatry, 44*(12), 1229–1238.

LeDoux, J. E., Iwata, J., Cicchetti, P., & Reis, D. J. (1988). Different projections of the central amygdaloid nucleus mediate autonomic and behavioral correlates of conditioned fear. *The Journal of Neuroscience, 8*(7), 2517–2529.

Lee, H., Kwak, S., Paik, J., Kang, R., & Lee, M. (2007). Association between serotonin 2A receptor gene polymorphism and posttraumatic stress disorder. *Psychiatry Investigation, 4*, 104–108.

Lee, H. J., Lee, M. S., Kang, R. H., Kim, H., Kim, S. D., Kee, B. S., et al. (2005). Influence of the serotonin transporter promoter gene polymorphism on susceptibility to posttraumatic stress disorder. *Depression and Anxiety, 21*(3), 135–139.

Levi, A., Kohn, Y., Kanyas, K., Amann, D., Pae, C. U., Hamdan, A., et al. (2005). Fine mapping of a schizophrenia susceptibility locus at chromosome 6q23: Increased evidence for linkage and reduced linkage interval. *European Journal of Human Genetics, 13*(6), 763–771.

Liberzon, I., Taylor, S. F., Phan, K. L., Britton, J. C., Fig, L. M., Bueller, J. A., et al. (2007). Altered central micro-opioid receptor binding after psychological trauma. *Biological Psychiatry, 61*(9), 1030–1038.

Lu, A. T., Ogdie, M. N., Jarvelin, M. R., Moilanen, I. K., Loo, S. K., McCracken, J. T., et al. (2008). Association of the cannabinoid receptor gene (CNR1) with ADHD and post-traumatic stress disorder. *American Journal of Medical Genetics Part B: Neuropsychiatric Genetics, 147B*(8), 1488–1494.

Maes, M., Lin, A. H., Delmeire, L., Van Gastel, A., Kenis, G., De Jongh, R., et al. (1999). Elevated serum interleukin-6 (IL-6) and IL-6 receptor concentrations in posttraumatic stress disorder following accidental man-made traumatic events. *Biological Psychiatry, 45*(7), 833–839.

Manoli, I., Alesci, S., Blackman, M. R., Su, Y. A., Rennert, O. M., & Chrousos, G. P. (2007). Mitochondria as key components of the stress response. *Trends in Endocrinology and Metabolism, 18*(5), 190–198.

Maquet, P. (2001). The role of sleep in learning and memory. *Science, 294*(5544), 1048–1052.

Matar, M. A., Cohen, H., Kaplan, Z., & Zohar, J. (2006). The effect of early poststressor intervention with sertraline on behavioral responses in an animal model of post-traumatic stress disorder. *Neuropsychopharmacology, 31*(12), 2610–2618.

Mayou, R. A., Ehlers, A., & Hobbs, M. (2000). Psychological debriefing for road traffic accident victims. Three-year follow-up of a randomised controlled trial. *The British Journal of Psychiatry, 176*, 589–593.

McGowan, P. O., Sasaki, A., D'Alessio, A. C., Dymov, S., Labonte, B., Szyf, M., et al. (2009). Epigenetic regulation of the glucocorticoid receptor in human brain associates with childhood abuse. *Nature Neuroscience, 12*(3), 342–348.

Meewisse, M. L., Reitsma, J. B., de Vries, G. J., Gersons, B. P., & Olff, M. (2007). Cortisol and post-traumatic stress disorder in adults: Systematic review and meta-analysis. *The British Journal of Psychiatry, 191*, 387–392.

Meinlschmidt, G., & Heim, C. (2005). Decreased cortisol awakening response after early loss experience. *Psychoneuroendocrinology, 30*(6), 568–576.

Mellman, T. A., Alim, T., Brown, D. D., Gorodetsky, E., Buzas, B., Lawson, W. B., et al. (2009). Serotonin polymorphisms and posttraumatic stress disorder in a trauma exposed African American population. *Depression and Anxiety, 26*(11), 993–997.

Mellman, T. A., Bustamante, V., David, D., & Fins, A. I. (2002). Hypnotic medication in the aftermath of trauma. *The Journal of Clinical Psychiatry, 63*(12), 1183–1184.

Mellman, T. A., Bustamante, V., Fins, A. I., Pigeon, W. R., & Nolan, B. (2002). REM sleep and the early development of posttraumatic stress disorder. *The American Journal of Psychiatry, 159*(10), 1696–1701.

Mellman, T. A., David, D., Kulick-Bell, R., Hebding, J., & Nolan, B. (1995). Sleep disturbance and its relationship to psychiatric morbidity after Hurricane Andrew. *The American Journal of Psychiatry, 152*(11), 1659–1663.

Mellman, T. A., & Hipolito, M. M. (2006). Sleep disturbances in the aftermath of trauma and posttraumatic stress disorder. *CNS Spectrums, 11*(8), 611–615.

Mellman, T. A., Pigeon, W. R., Nowell, P. D., & Nolan, B. (2007). Relationships between REM sleep findings and PTSD symptoms during the early aftermath of trauma. *Journal of Traumatic Stress, 20*(5), 893–901.

Miller, R. J., Sutherland, A. G., Hutchison, J. D., & Alexander, D. A. (2001). C-reactive protein and interleukin 6 receptor in post-traumatic stress disorder: A pilot study. *Cytokine, 13*(4), 253–255.

Molina, M. E., Isoardi, R., Prado, M. N., & Bentolila, S. (2010). Basal cerebral glucose distribution in long-term post-traumatic stress disorder. *The World Journal of Biological Psychiatry, 11*(2 Pt 2), 493–501.

Moores, K. A., Clark, C. R., McFarlane, A. C., Brown, G. C., Puce, A., & Taylor, D. J. (2008). Abnormal recruitment of working memory updating networks during maintenance of trauma-neutral information in post-traumatic stress disorder. *Psychiatry Research, 163*(2), 156–170.

Mustapic, M., Pivac, N., Kozaric-Kovacic, D., Dezeljin, M., Cubells, J. F., & Muck-Seler, D. (2007). Dopamine beta-hydroxylase (DBH) activity and -1021C/T polymorphism of DBH gene in combat-related post-traumatic stress disorder. *American Journal of Medical Genetics Part B: Neuropsychiatric Genetics, 144B*(8), 1087–1089.

Nakamura, M., Ueno, S., Sano, A., & Tanabe, H. (2000). The human serotonin transporter gene linked polymorphism (5-HTTLPR) shows ten novel allelic variants. *Molecular Psychiatry, 5*(1), 32–38.

Nelson, E. C., Agrawal, A., Pergadia, M. L., Lynskey, M. T., Todorov, A. A., Wang, J. C., et al. (2009). Association of childhood trauma exposure and GABRA2 polymorphisms with risk of posttraumatic stress disorder in adults. *Molecular Psychiatry, 14*(3), 234–235.

Neylan, T. C., Lenoci, M., Maglione, M. L., Rosenlicht, N. Z., Metzler, T. J., Otte, C., et al. (2003). Delta sleep response to metyrapone in post-traumatic stress disorder. *Neuropsychopharmacology, 28*(9), 1666–1676.

Ng, V., Koh, D., Mok, B., Lim, L. P., Yang, Y., & Chia, S. E. (2004). Stressful life events of dental students and salivary immunoglobulin A. *International Journal of Immunopathology and Pharmacology, 17*(2 Suppl), 49–56.

Nishith, P., Griffin, M. G., & Poth, T. L. (2002). Stress-induced analgesia: Prediction of posttraumatic stress symptoms in battered versus nonbattered women. *Biological Psychiatry, 51*(11), 867–874.

Nishith, P., Resick, P. A., & Mueser, K. T. (2001). Sleep difficulties and alcohol use motives in female rape victims with posttraumatic stress disorder. *Journal of Traumatic Stress, 14*(3), 469–479.

Nixon, R. D., Bryant, R. A., Moulds, M. L., Felmingham, K. L., & Mastrodomenico, J. A. (2005). Physiological arousal and dissociation in acute trauma victims during trauma narratives. *Journal of Traumatic Stress, 18*(2), 107–113.

Ohayon, M. M., & Shapiro, C. M. (2000). Sleep disturbances and psychiatric disorders associated with posttraumatic stress disorder in the general population. *Comprehensive Psychiatry, 41*(6), 469–478.

Ohry, A., Rattok, J., & Solomon, Z. (1996). Post-traumatic stress disorder in brain injury patients. *Brain Injury, 10*(9), 687–695.

Olff, M., de Vries, G. J., Guzelcan, Y., Assies, J., & Gersons, B. P. (2007). Changes in cortisol and DHEA plasma levels after psychotherapy for PTSD. *Psychoneuroendocrinology, 32*(6), 619–626.

Opp, M. R. (1997). Rat strain differences suggest a role for corticotropin-releasing hormone in modulating sleep. *Physiology and Behavior, 63*(1), 67–74.

Oquendo, M. A., Echavarria, G., Galfalvy, H. C., Grunebaum, M. F., Burke, A., Barrera, A., et al. (2003). Lower cortisol levels in depressed patients with comorbid post-traumatic stress disorder. *Neuropsychopharmacology, 28*(3), 591–598.

Orr, S. P., Metzger, L. J., Lasko, N. B., Macklin, M. L., Hu, F. B., Shalev, A. Y., et al. (2003). Physiologic responses to sudden, loud tones in monozygotic twins discordant for combat exposure: Association with posttraumatic stress disorder. *Archives of General Psychiatry, 60*(3), 283–288.

Orr, S. P., Metzger, L. J., Lasko, N. B., Macklin, M. L., Peri, T., & Pitman, R. K. (2000). De novo conditioning in trauma-exposed individuals with and without posttraumatic stress disorder. *Journal of Abnormal Psychology, 109*(2), 290–298.

Osuch, E. A., Benson, B., Geraci, M., Podell, D., Herscovitch, P., McCann, U. D., et al. (2001). Regional cerebral blood flow correlated with flashback intensity in patients with posttraumatic stress disorder. *Biological Psychiatry, 50*(4), 246–253.

Osuch, E. A., Willis, M. W., Bluhm, R., Ursano, R. J., & Drevets, W. C. (2008). Neurophysiological responses to traumatic reminders in the acute aftermath of serious motor vehicle collisions using [15O]-H2O positron emission tomography. *Biological Psychiatry, 64*(4), 327–335.

Ozer, E. J., Best, S. R., Lipsey, T. L., & Weiss, D. S. (2003). Predictors of posttraumatic stress disorder and symptoms in adults: A meta-analysis. *Psychological Bulletin, 129*(1), 52–73.

Pace, T. W., & Heim, C. M. (2010). A short review on the psychoneuroimmunology of posttraumatic stress disorder: From risk factors to medical comorbidities. *Brain, Behavior, and Immunity, 25*(1), 6–13.

Peres, J. F., Newberg, A. B., Mercante, J. P., Simao, M., Albuquerque, V. E., Peres, M. J., et al. (2007). Cerebral blood flow changes during retrieval of traumatic memories before and after psychotherapy: A SPECT study. *Psychological Medicine, 37*(10), 1481–1491.

Pervanidou, P., Kolaitis, G., Charitaki, S., Margeli, A., Ferentinos, S., Bakoula, C., et al. (2007). Elevated morning serum interleukin (IL)-6 or evening salivary cortisol concentrations predict posttraumatic stress disorder in children and adolescents six months after a motor vehicle accident. *Psychoneuroendocrinology, 32*(8–10), 991–999.

Pfeffer, C. R., Altemus, M., Heo, M., & Jiang, H. (2007). Salivary cortisol and psychopathology in children bereaved by the September 11, 2001 terror attacks. *Biological Psychiatry, 61*(8), 957–965.

Phan, K. L., Britton, J. C., Taylor, S. F., Fig, L. M., & Liberzon, I. (2006). Corticolimbic blood flow during nontraumatic emotional processing in posttraumatic stress disorder. *Archives of General Psychiatry, 63*(2), 184–192.

Pillar, G., Malhotra, A., & Lavie, P. (2000). Post-traumatic stress disorder and sleep-what a nightmare! *Sleep Medicine Reviews, 4*(2), 183–200.

Pitman, R. K., Orr, S. P., Forgue, D. F., Altman, B., de Jong, J. B., & Herz, L. R. (1990). Psychophysiologic response to combat imagery in Vietnam Veterans with post-traumatic stress disorder vs. other anxiety disorders. *Journal of Abnormal Psychology, 99*, 49–54.

Pitman, R. K., Sanders, K. M., Zusman, R. M., Healy, A. R., Cheema, F., Lasko, N. B., et al. (2002). Pilot study of secondary prevention of posttraumatic stress disorder with propranolol. *Biological Psychiatry, 51*(2), 189–192.

Pitman, R. K., van der Kolk, B. A., Orr, S. P., & Greenberg, M. S. (1990). Naloxone-reversible analgesic response to combat-related stimuli in posttraumatic stress disorder. A pilot study. *Archives of General Psychiatry, 47*(6), 541–544.

Pole, N. (2007). The psychophysiology of posttraumatic stress disorder: A meta-analysis. *Psychological Bulletin, 133*(5), 725–746.

Raison, C. L., & Miller, A. H. (2003). When not enough is too much: The role of insufficient glucocorticoid signaling in the pathophysiology of stress-related disorders. *The American Journal of Psychiatry, 160*(9), 1554–1565.

Rasmusson, A. M., Vasek, J., Lipschitz, D. S., Vojvoda, D., Mustone, M. E., Shi, Q., et al. (2004). An increased capacity for adrenal DHEA release is associated with decreased avoidance and negative mood symptoms in women with PTSD. *Neuropsychopharmacology, 29*(8), 1546–1557.

Rohleder, N., Joksimovic, L., Wolf, J. M., & Kirschbaum, C. (2004). Hypocortisolism and increased glucocorticoid sensitivity of pro-Inflammatory cytokine production in Bosnian war refugees with posttraumatic stress disorder. *Biological Psychiatry, 55*(7), 745–751.

Rothbaum, B. O., Foa, E. B., Riggs, D. S., Murdock, T., & Walsh, W. (1992). A prospective examination of post-traumatic stress disorder in rape victims. *Journal of Traumatic Stress, 5*, 455–475.

Sagaspe, P., Sanchez-Ortuno, M., Charles, A., Taillard, J., Valtat, C., Bioulac, B., et al. (2006). Effects of sleep deprivation on Color-Word, Emotional, and Specific Stroop interference and on self-reported anxiety. *Brain and Cognition, 60*(1), 76–87.

Santarelli, L., Saxe, M., Gross, C., Surget, A., Battaglia, F., Dulawa, S., et al. (2003). Requirement of hippocampal neurogenesis for the behavioral effects of antidepressants. *Science, 301*(5634), 805–809.

Sayin, A., Kucukyildirim, S., Akar, T., Bakkaloglu, Z., Demircan, A., Kurtoglu, G., et al. (2010). A prospective study of serotonin transporter gene promoter (5-HTT gene linked polymorphic region) and intron 2 (variable number of tandem repeats) polymorphisms as predictors of trauma response to mild physical injury. *DNA and Cell Biology, 29*(2), 71–77.

Schinkel, C., Gaertner, A., Zaspel, J., Zedler, S., Faist, E., & Schuermann, M. (2006). Inflammatory mediators are altered in the acute phase of posttraumatic complex regional pain syndrome. *The Clinical Journal of Pain, 22*(3), 235–239.

Schoenfeld, F. B., Marmar, C. R., & Neylan, T. C. (2004). Current concepts in pharmacotherapy for posttraumatic stress disorder. *Psychiatric Services, 55*(5), 519–531.

Schreiber, S., & Galai-Gat, T. (1993). Uncontrolled pain following physical injury as the core-trauma in post-traumatic stress disorder. *Pain, 54*(1), 107–110.

Schuld, A., Mullington, J., Friess, E., Hermann, D. M., Galanos, C., Holsboer, F., et al. (2000). Changes in dehydroepiandrosterone (DHEA) and DHEA-sulfate plasma levels during experimental endotoxinemia in healthy volunteers. *The Journal of Clinical Endocrinology and Metabolism, 85*(12), 4624–4629.

Segman, R. H., Cooper-Kazaz, R., Macciardi, F., Goltser, T., Halfon, Y., Dobroborski, T., et al. (2002). Association between the dopamine transporter gene and posttraumatic stress disorder. *Molecular Psychiatry, 7*(8), 903–907.

Segman, R. H., Shefi, N., Goltser-Dubner, T., Friedman, N., Kaminski, N., & Shalev, A. Y. (2005). Peripheral blood mononuclear cell gene expression profiles identify emergent post-traumatic stress disorder among trauma survivors. *Molecular Psychiatry, 10*(5), 500–513, 425.

Shalev, A. Y. (1992). Posttraumatic stress disorder among injured survivors of a terrorist attack. Predictive value of early intrusion and avoidance symptoms. *The Journal of Nervous and Mental Disease, 180*(8), 505–509.

Shalev, A. Y., Sahar, T., Freedman, S., Peri, T., Glick, N., Brandes, D., et al. (1998). A prospective study of heart rate response following trauma and the subsequent development of posttraumatic stress disorder. *Archives of General Psychiatry, 55*(6), 553–559.

Shalev, A. Y., & Segman, R. H. (2008). Commentary: Biological findings in PTSD – Too much or too little? *Progress in Brain Research, 167*, 187–199.

Shavit, Y., Weidenfeld, J., DeKeyser, F. G., Fish, G., Wolf, G., Mayburd, E., et al. (2005). Effects of surgical stress on brain prostaglandin E2 production and on the pituitary-adrenal axis: Attenuation by preemptive analgesia and by central amygdala lesion. *Brain Research, 1047*(1), 10–17.

Shin, L. M., Lasko, N. B., Macklin, M. L., Karpf, R. D., Milad, M. R., Orr, S. P., et al. (2009). Resting metabolic activity in the cingulate cortex and vulnerability to posttraumatic stress disorder. *Archives of General Psychiatry, 66*(10), 1099 1107.

Shin, L. M., Orr, S. P., Carson, M. A., Rauch, S. L., Macklin, M. L., Lasko, N. B., et al. (2004). Regional cerebral blood flow in the amygdala and medial prefrontal cortex during traumatic imagery in male and female Vietnam veterans with PTSD. *Archives of General Psychiatry, 61*(2), 168–176.

Shin, L. M., Shin, P. S., Heckers, S., Krangel, T. S., Macklin, M. L., Orr, S. P., et al. (2004). Hippocampal function in posttraumatic stress disorder. *Hippocampus, 14*(3), 292–300.

Shin, L. M., Whalen, P. J., Pitman, R. K., Bush, G., Macklin, M. L., Lasko, N. B., et al. (2001). An fMRI study of anterior cingulate function in posttraumatic stress disorder. *Biological Psychiatry, 50*(12), 932–942.

Siegfried, B., Frischknecht, H. R., & Nunes de Souza, R. L. (1990). An ethological model for the study of activation and interaction of pain, memory and defensive systems in the attacked mouse. Role of endogenous opioids. *Neuroscience and Biobehavioral Reviews, 14*(4), 481–490.

Sijbrandij, M., Olff, M., Reitsma, J. B., Carlier, I. V., & Gersons, B. P. (2006). Emotional or educational debriefing after psychological trauma. Randomised controlled trial. *The British Journal of Psychiatry, 189*, 150–155.

Smoller, J. W., Gardner-Schuster, E., & Covino, J. (2008). The genetic basis of panic and phobic anxiety disorders. *American Journal of Medical Genetics. Part C: Seminars in Medical Genetics, 148C*(2), 118–126.

Soares, C. N. (2005). Insomnia in women: An overlooked epidemic? *Archives of Women's Mental Health, 8*(4), 205–213.

Sondergaard, H. P., Hansson, L. O., & Theorell, T. (2002). Elevated blood levels of dehydroepiandrosterone sulphate vary with symptom load in posttraumatic stress disorder: Findings from a longitudinal study of refugees in Sweden. *Psychotherapy and Psychosomatics, 71*(5), 298–303.

Song, Y., Zhou, D., Guan, Z., & Wang, X. (2007). Disturbance of serum interleukin-2 and interleukin-8 levels in posttraumatic and non-posttraumatic stress disorder earthquake survivors in northern China. *Neuroimmunomodulation, 14*(5), 248–254.

Soravia, L. M., Heinrichs, M., Aerni, A., Maroni, C., Schelling, G., Ehlert, U., et al. (2006). Glucocorticoids reduce phobic fear in humans. *Proceedings of the National Academy of Sciences of the United States of America, 103*(14), 5585–5590.

Spivak, B., Shohat, B., Mester, R., Avraham, S., Gil-Ad, I., Bleich, A., et al. (1997). Elevated levels of serum interleukin-1 beta in combat-related posttraumatic stress disorder. *Biological Psychiatry, 42*(5), 345–348.

Spoormaker, V. I., & Montgomery, P. (2008). Disturbed sleep in post-traumatic stress disorder: Secondary symptom or core feature? *Sleep Medicine Reviews, 12*(3), 169–184.

Steiger, A. (2002). Sleep and the hypothalamo-pituitary-adrenocortical system. *Sleep Medicine Reviews, 6*(2), 125–138.

Stein, M. B., Schork, N. J., & Gelernter, J. (2008). Gene-by-environment (serotonin transporter and childhood maltreatment) interaction for anxiety sensitivity, an intermediate phenotype for anxiety disorders. *Neuropsychopharmacology, 33*(2), 312–319.

Su, Y. A., Wu, J., Zhang, L., Zhang, Q., Su, D. M., He, P., et al. (2008). Dysregulated mitochondrial genes and networks with drug targets in postmortem brain of patients with posttraumatic stress disorder (PTSD) revealed by human mitochondria-focused cDNA microarrays. *International Journal of Biological Sciences, 4*(4), 223–235.

Suendermann, O., Ehlers, A., Boellinghaus, I., Gamer, M., & Glucksman, E. (2010). Early heart rate responses to standardized trauma-related pictures predict posttraumatic stress disorder: A prospective study. *Psychosomatic Medicine, 72*(3), 301–308.

Thakur, G. A., Joober, R., & Brunet, A. (2009). Development and persistence of posttraumatic stress disorder and the 5-HTTLPR polymorphism. *Journal of Traumatic Stress, 22*(3), 240–243.

True, W. R., Rice, J., Eisen, S. A., Heath, A. C., Goldberg, J., Lyons, M. J., et al. (1993). A twin study of genetic and environmental contributions to liability for posttraumatic stress symptoms. *Archives of General Psychiatry, 50*(4), 257–264.

Valentino, R. J., Page, M., Van Bockstaele, E., & Aston-Jones, G. (1992). Corticotropin-releasing factor innervation of the locus coeruleus region: Distribution of fibers and sources of input. *Neuroscience, 48*(3), 689–705.

van der Kolk, B., Greenberg, M., Boyd, H., & Krystal, J. (1985). Inescapable shock, neurotransmitters, and addiction to trauma: Toward a psychobiology of post traumatic stress. *Biological Psychiatry, 20*(3), 314–325.

van der Velden, P. G., Kleber, R. J., & Koenen, K. C. (2008). Smoking predicts posttraumatic stress symptoms among rescue workers: A prospective study of ambulance personnel involved in the Enschede Fireworks Disaster. *Drug and Alcohol Dependence, 94*(1–3), 267–271.

van Stegeren, A. H., Goekoop, R., Everaerd, W., Scheltens, P., Barkhof, F., Kuijer, J. P., et al. (2005). Noradrenaline mediates amygdala activation in men and women during encoding of emotional material. *NeuroImage, 24*(3), 898–909.

Vermeer, H., Hendriks-Stegeman, B. I., van der Burg, B., van Buul-Offers, S. C., & Jansen, M. (2003). Glucocorticoid-induced increase in lymphocytic FKBP51 messenger ribonucleic acid expression: A potential marker for glucocorticoid sensitivity, potency, and bioavailability. *The Journal of Clinical Endocrinology and Metabolism, 88*(1), 277–284.

Vgontzas, A. N., Mastorakos, G., Bixler, E. O., Kales, A., Gold, P. W., & Chrousos, G. P. (1999). Sleep deprivation effects on the activity of the hypothalamic-pituitary-adrenal and growth axes: Potential clinical implications. *Clinical Endocrinology, 51*(2), 205–215.

Villarreal, G., Hamilton, D. A., Petropoulos, H., Driscoll, I., Rowland, L. M., Griego, J. A., et al. (2002). Reduced hippocampal volume and total white matter volume in posttraumatic stress disorder. *Biological Psychiatry, 52*(2), 119–125.

Voisey, J., Swagell, C. D., Hughes, I. P., Morris, C. P., van Daal, A., Noble, E. P., et al. (2009). The DRD2 gene 957C>T polymorphism is associated with posttraumatic stress disorder in war veterans. *Depression and Anxiety, 26*(1), 28–33.

von Kanel, R., Hepp, U., Kraemer, B., Traber, R., Keel, M., Mica, L., et al. (2007). Evidence for low-grade systemic proinflammatory activity in patients with posttraumatic stress disorder. *Journal of Psychiatric Research, 41*(9), 744–752.

Weller, E. B., Weller, R. A., Fristad, M. A., & Bowes, J. M. (1990). Dexamethasone suppression test and depressive symptoms in bereaved children: A preliminary report. *The Journal of Neuropsychiatry and Clinical Neurosciences, 2*(4), 418–421.

Werner, N. S., Meindl, T., Engel, R. R., Rosner, R., Riedel, M., Reiser, M., et al. (2009). Hippocampal function during associative learning in patients with posttraumatic stress disorder. *Journal of Psychiatric Research, 43*(3), 309–318.

Wessa, M., Rohleder, N., Kirschbaum, C., & Flor, H. (2006). Altered cortisol awakening response in posttraumatic stress disorder. *Psychoneuroendocrinology, 31*(2), 209–215.

Whalley, M. G., Rugg, M. D., Smith, A. P., Dolan, R. J., & Brewin, C. R. (2009). Incidental retrieval of emotional contexts in post-traumatic stress disorder and depression: An fMRI study. *Brain and Cognition, 69*(1), 98–107.

Woods, A. B., Page, G. G., O'Campo, P., Pugh, L. C., Ford, D., & Campbell, J. C. (2005). The mediation effect of posttraumatic stress disorder symptoms on the relationship of intimate partner violence and IFN-gamma levels. *American Journal of Community Psychology, 36*(1–2), 159–175.

Woodward, S. H., Kaloupek, D. G., Streeter, C. C., Martinez, C., Schaer, M., & Eliez, S. (2006). Decreased anterior cingulate volume in combat-related PTSD. *Biological Psychiatry, 59*(7), 582–587.

Xie, P., Kranzler, H. R., Poling, J., Stein, M. B., Anton, R. F., Brady, K., et al. (2009). Interactive effect of stressful life events and the serotonin transporter 5-HTTLPR genotype on posttraumatic stress disorder diagnosis in 2 independent populations. *Archives of General Psychiatry, 66*(11), 1201–1209.

Yehuda, R. (2002). Current status of cortisol findings in post-traumatic stress disorder. *The Psychiatric Clinics of North America, 25*(2), 341–368, vii.

Yehuda, R. (2009). Status of glucocorticoid alterations in post-traumatic stress disorder. *The Annals of the New York Academy of Sciences, 1179*, 56–69.

Yehuda, R., Bell, A., Bierer, L. M., & Schmeidler, J. (2008). Maternal, not paternal, PTSD is related to increased risk for PTSD in offspring of Holocaust survivors. *Journal of Psychiatric Research, 42*(13), 1104–1111.

Yehuda, R., & Bierer, L. M. (2008). Transgenerational transmission of cortisol and PTSD risk. *Progress in Brain Research, 167*, 121–135.

Yehuda, R., Bryant, R., Marmar, C., & Zohar, J. (2005). Pathological responses to terrorism. *Neuropsychopharmacology, 30*(10), 1793–1805.

Yehuda, R., Golier, J. A., Yang, R. K., & Tischler, L. (2004). Enhanced sensitivity to glucocorticoids in peripheral mononuclear leukocytes in posttraumatic stress disorder. *Biological Psychiatry, 55*(11), 1110–1116.

Yehuda, R., Southwick, S. M., Krystal, J. H., Bremner, D., Charney, D. S., & Mason, J. W. (1993). Enhanced suppression of cortisol following dexamethasone administration in posttraumatic stress disorder. *The American Journal of Psychiatry, 150*(1), 83–86.

Yehuda, R., Teicher, M. H., Trestman, R. L., Levengood, R. A., & Siever, L. J. (1996). Cortisol regulation in posttraumatic stress disorder and major depression: A chronobiological analysis. *Biological Psychiatry, 40*(2), 79–88.

Young, E. A., & Breslau, N. (2004). Cortisol and catecholamines in posttraumatic stress disorder: An epidemiologic community study. *Archives of General Psychiatry, 61*(4), 394–401.

Zabetian, C. P., Anderson, G. M., Buxbaum, S. G., Elston, R. C., Ichinose, H., Nagatsu, T., et al. (2001). A quantitative-trait analysis of human plasma-dopamine beta-hydroxylase activity: Evidence for a major functional polymorphism at the DBH locus. *The American Journal of Human Genetics, 68*(2), 515–522.

Zald, D. H. (2003). The human amygdala and the emotional evaluation of sensory stimuli. *Brain Research. Brain Research Reviews, 41*(1), 88–123.

Zhang, H., Ozbay, F., Lappalainen, J., Kranzler, H. R., van Dyck, C. H., Charney, D. S., et al. (2006). Brain derived neurotrophic factor (BDNF) gene variants and Alzheimer's disease, affective disorders, posttraumatic stress disorder, schizophrenia, and substance dependence. *American Journal of Medical Genetics. Part B: Neuropsychiatric Genetics, 141B*(4), 387–393.

Chapter 3
The Early Adolescent or "Juvenile Stress" Translational Animal Model of Posttraumatic Stress Disorder

Gal Richter-Levin, Omer Horovitz, and M. Michael Tsoory

Introduction

Criterion A of posttraumatic stress disorder (PTSD) in the fourth edition of American Psychiatric Association Diagnostic and Statistical Manual of Mental Disorders (DSM-IV-TR) is the exposure to a traumatic experience, in which both of the following have been present:

(a) The person has experienced, witnessed, or been confronted with an event or events that involve actual or threatened death or serious injury, or a threat to the physical integrity of oneself or others.
(b) The person's response involved intense fear, helplessness, or horror.

This view holds a hidden assumption—that PTSD is induced by exposure to the traumatic event. This view has influenced attempts to develop valid animal models of PTSD. Various attempts to develop a translational model focused on the question of what may be an effective experimental trauma that could induce a PTSD state in the animal. However, this view ignored the well-known fact about PTSD, i.e., that

G. Richter-Levin (✉)
Department of Psychology, University of Haifa, Haifa, Israel

The "Sagol" Department of Neurobiology, University of Haifa, Haifa, Israel

The Institute for the Study of Affective Neuroscience (ISAN), University of Haifa, Haifa, Israel
e-mail: galrichterlevin@gmail.com

O. Horovitz
Department of Psychology, University of Haifa, Haifa, Israel
e-mail: horovitz.omer@gmail.com

M.M. Tsoory
Department of Veterinary Resources, Weizmann Institute of Science, Rehovot, Israel
e-mail: Michael.Tsoory@weizmann.ac.il

M.P. Safir et al. (eds.), *Future Directions in Post-Traumatic Stress Disorder*,
DOI 10.1007/978-1-4899-7522-5_3

only a certain percentage of people exposed to a traumatic experience will eventually develop PTSD. Reported numbers may vary between 5 and 30 %, but the reality remains that regardless of the type of trauma or the severity we attribute to it, most people exposed to a traumatic event will not develop PTSD. This is a significant characteristic of the phenomenon, which indicates that the trauma may be a necessary but not a sufficient condition to induce PTSD, and that additional factors should be considered in the effort to elucidate the core of the disorder. Furthermore, when attempting to develop an effective translational animal model of PTSD, these factors should be taken into consideration.

Several factors have been proposed as contributing to vulnerability, or to resilience in face of an exposure to a significant traumatic challenge. They include genetic background, developmental factors, and proximal factors, such as the quality and amount of sleep, social relations, and stress load just before exposure to the trauma. Until recently, relatively little was done to incorporate such factors in animal models of PTSD.

In psychiatric literature, childhood adversities have been suggested as a risk factor for developing PTSD later in life. Several years ago, we have set out to develop a rodent model of PTSD that would include exposure to stress in a parallel developmental period—the postweaning, prepuberty, or early adolescence period—and reexposure to stress in adulthood. The assumption was straightforward; if indeed a risk factor, animals exposed to childhood adversities would exhibit stronger and longer lasting responses to a stressful experience in adulthood.

This chapter summarizes several years of research in developing this model as an effective platform for studying the neurobiology of PTSD.

Stress-Related Disorders

Recent years have witnessed a growing interest in the effects of adversities such as terror attacks, natural disasters, car accidents, and other traumatic life events on brain functions and risk for psychiatric illness (Yehuda, 2002).

Stress may be broadly defined as any form of threat (real or inferred) to the physiological or psychological integrity of an individual which results in physiological and/or behavioral responses (Kalueff & Tuohimaa, 2004). While some individuals find stressful situations interesting, challenging or even strengthening, others exhibit maladaptive responses, which in turn, may result in psychological and/or physiological pathology. Of these maladaptive responses to stressful events, mood and anxiety disorders are most common, particularly depression and PTSD (Nemeroff, 1999).

It is estimated that in a given year in the adult US population, approximately 9.5 % (20.9 million individuals) will suffer from a mood disorder and about 18.1 % (40 million individuals) will suffer from an anxiety disorder (Kessler, Berglund et al., 2005); furthermore, mood disorders often co-occur with anxiety disorders (Kessler, Chiu, Demler, Merikangas, & Walters, 2005).

Factors that play an important role in the intensity of the response to a certain stressful experience include "event-related factors" such as the degree of controllability, predictability, the actual perceived threat, the relative success of attempts to minimize injury to oneself or others, and the actual loss (Yehuda, 2002) but also "personal factors" like genetic background, gender, and previous exposure to stressors, particularly exposure to stressors early in life (Anisman & Matheson, 2005; Arborelius, Owens, Plotsky, & Nemeroff, 1999; Heim & Nemeroff, 2001; Horovitz, Tsoory, Hall, Jacobson-Pick, & Richter-Levin, 2012; Levine, 2005; Nemeroff, 2004a; Nemeroff et al., 2006; Piccinelli & Wilkinson, 2000). Here we will focus on stress early in life as a risk factor for stress-related disorders, and particularly PTSD, later in life.

Stress Early in Life

Freud was amongst the first to highlight the importance of early life experiences in shaping an individual's mental functions for the rest of his/her life (Freud, 1987). This emphasis on the importance of early developmental experiences still holds and with it the notion that stress early in life may induce a vulnerability to the effects of stress later in life, possibly by inducing a persistent sensitization in stress-responsive neural circuits, which augments the consequences of later adverse experiences (Agid, Kohn, & Lerer, 2000; Heim & Nemeroff, 2001; Nemeroff, 2004b).

Across species, including humans, the early adolescent or juvenile brain is considered to be a transition phase, differing markedly both anatomically and neurochemically from that of newborns, weanlings, or adults. Preteens and adolescent humans have enhanced stress perception and responses. Stressful life events during this period have been suggested as being associated with later socio-emotional maladaptive behaviors, and to represent a significant risk factor for the later development of stress-related psychopathologies (Maughan & McCarthy, 1997; Spear, 2004).

There is increasing evidence that the adolescent brain is particularly vulnerable to effects of stress. Recently Casey, Getz, and Galvan (2008) addressed human adolescent brain development and suggested that during adolescence a unique imbalance exists between levels of activity in subcortical regions and cortical regions. Based on both preclinical evidence and brain imaging studies of children, adolescents, and adults, it appears that during adolescence, subcortical activity is relatively higher than cortical activity. It was suggested that these findings may indicate that during the processing of negative emotional information, this bias between unregulated and prominent subcortical activity (e.g., limbic regions) and a relatively reduced activity in the prefrontal cortex may relate to the emergence of affective disorders during adolescence (Casey et al., 2008).

Many studies in humans point to late childhood and early adolescence as periods of particular vulnerability development of psychopathologies later in life (Maercker, Michael, Fehm, Becker, & Margraf, 2004; Pynoos, Steinberg, & Piacentini, 1999). The net consequence of stress in the juvenile/adolescent brain that has been suggested is the sensitization of the emotional brain to the effects of later life stress, increasing the likelihood of depression and anxiety (Agid et al., 2000; Anisman & Matheson, 2005; Costello et al., 2002; Gregory et al., 2007; Heim & Nemeroff, 2001; Levine, 2005; Maughan & McCarthy, 1997; Nemeroff, 2004a; Nemeroff et al., 2006; Spear, 2004). However, it is important to note that some epidemiological studies suggest that stress early in life, but at different developmental stages, may result in the development of different psychopathologies. Childhood trauma (under the age of 12 years) was found to increase the risk of developing major depression, while trauma during adolescence was associated with a greater predisposition to PTSD (Maercker et al., 2004), suggesting challenging maturing mechanisms of emotional or mood regulation at different developmental phases may predispose to different psychopathologies later in life (Maercker et al., 2004; Pynoos et al., 1999).

Animal Models of Stress Early in Life

Many of the rodent early life stress (ELS) models focus on the perinatal preweaning period and involve some form of maternal deprivation or separation (Kehoe, Shoemaker, Arons, Triano, & Suresh, 1998; Levine, Huchton, Wiener, & Rosenfeld, 1991; Ogawa et al., 1994; Plotsky, Thrivikraman, & Meaney, 1993; Rosenfeld, Wetmore, & Levine, 1992; van Oers, de Kloet, & Levine, 1998; Vazquez, Van Oers, Levine, & Akil, 1996; von Hoersten, Dimitrijevic, Markovic, & Jankovic, 1993), producing acute and long-term effects that vary with the pups' age (Levine, 1994). For example, prolonged early maternal separation attenuated rates of synaptic development in the hippocampus, which was evident only after sexual maturation (Andersen & Teicher, 2004). Evidence from ELS animal models suggests persistent changes in the function of brain regions pivotal to the meditation of stress and emotion, which are similar to the neurobiological alterations found in patients suffering from depression or anxiety disorders (Nemeroff, 2004a). For example, these studies have demonstrated that stressful experiences which occur during critical periods of brain development (perinatal to preweaning) persistently change the responses to stressors at both the behavioral level and the endocrine levels, the response of the hypothalamic–pituitary–adrenal (HPA) axis, thereby increasing the vulnerability to mood and anxiety disorders later in life (Nemeroff, 2004a; Wang et al., 2011, 2012). Likewise, other studies indicated that a brief separation of pups from their dams during early development enhances adrenocorticotropic hormone (ACTH) and corticosterone (CORT) secretion in response to a stressor in adulthood (Anisman, Zaharia, Meaney, & Merali, 1998), while also reducing the number/density of pituitary corticotrophin-releasing factor (CRF) binding sites, possibly relating to increased CRF release in response to the stressor in adulthood (Nemeroff, 2004b). Accumulating evidence has thus raised the possibility that ELS induces a sensitization of stress response mechanisms that may be due to altered limbic functioning, thereby augmenting the consequences of stressors later in life (Nemeroff, 2004a, 2004b).

However the brain's development continues well after the preweaning period, and substantial maturation processes like myelination continue with varying dynamics well into puberty (Hamano et al., 1998). The ongoing maturational changes render the postweaning brain susceptible to the harmful effects of stress. Prolonged postweaning isolation rearing compromises the development and function of central aminergic neurotransmission, which is associated with altered behaviors in adulthood (Lapiz et al., 2001; Muchimapura, Fulford, Mason, & Marsden, 2002; Muchimapura, Mason, & Marsden, 2003).

The Postweaning Pre-puberty (Juvenile) Stress Model

While most ELS rodent models focus on the perinatal to preweaning periods (for a review see: Sanchez, Ladd, & Plotsky, 2001), recent work in our laboratory and others, focused on an alternative period in the rat ontology, "juvenility" (~28 days), the earlier phase of the adolescent/postweaning to the prepubertal period (Avital, Ram, Maayan, Weizman, & Richter-Levin, 2006; Avital & Richter-Levin, 2005; Horovitz et al., 2012; Ilin & Richter-Levin, 2009; Jacobson-Pick, Elkobi, Vander, Rosenblum, & Richter-Levin, 2008; Jacobson-Pick & Richter-Levin, 2012; Tsoory, Cohen, & Richter-Levin, 2007; Tsoory, Guterman, & Richter-Levin, 2008; Tsoory & Richter-Levin, 2006; Tsoory, Vouimba et al., 2008). This period is likely to relate closely to human childhood, a developmental period known to be relevant to the pathogenesis of a range of psychiatric disorders (Lapiz et al., 2001; Muchimapura et al., 2002, 2003). The rationale behind the "Juvenile Stress" model is that this is expected to induce long-term alterations in stress responsiveness, by exposing rats to stressors during juvenility, thus augmenting the consequences of additional exposure to stressors in adulthood.

A brief exposure to "Juvenile Stress" compromised the ability of rats to cope with stressors in adulthood. The result of exposure to the same stressor in adulthood was more severe and longer lasting if the stressor was presented on the background of previous exposure to the "Juvenile Stress" (Avital et al., 2006; Avital & Richter-Levin, 2005; Brydges, Hall, Nicolson, Holmes, & Hall, 2012; Horovitz et al., 2012; Ilin & Richter-Levin, 2009; Jacobson-Pick et al., 2008; Tsoory et al., 2007; Tsoory, Guterman, et al., 2008; Tsoory & Richter-Levin, 2006; Tsoory, Vouimba, et al., 2008). For example, startle reflex response was higher in adult rats exposed to elevated platform stress in adulthood compared to control, unexposed rats. However, the startle response of rats exposed to the same stress in adulthood but on the background of pre-exposure to "Juvenile" stress was yet significantly higher than that of animals exposed only to the stress in adulthood (Avital & Richter-Levin, 2005). The exacerbation of the effects of the adulthood stress by the "Juvenile Stress" was evident at the behavioral level (Avital et al., 2006; Avital & Richter-Levin, 2005; Brydges et al., 2012; Horovitz et al., 2012; Tsoory et al., 2007; Tsoory & Richter-Levin, 2006), but correlations were found at the physiological (Cohen et al., 2007; Yee, Plassmann, & Fuchs, 2011; Yee, Schwarting, Fuchs, & Wöhr, 2012), biochemical (Bazak et al., 2009; Jacobson-Pick et al., 2008; Jacobson-Pick & Richter-Levin, 2012; Tsoory, Guterman, & Richter-Levin, 2010; Tsoory, Guterman, et al., 2008; Tsoory, Vouimba, et al., 2008), and electrophysiological (Maggio & Segal, 2011) levels. For example, the induction of long-term potentiation (LTP) in the CA1 area of the hippocampus was suppressed by the exposure to forced swim stress in adult rats, when tested 1 day after the exposure, but this ability to induce plasticity was completely recovered within 1 week. However, adult animals exposed to the same stressor but on the background of a history of exposure to "Juvenile" stress exhibited impaired LTP even 1 week after the exposure to the stress in adulthood (Maggio & Segal, 2011).

However, even though early exposure to stress predisposes individuals to the development of both mood and anxiety disorders later in life (Heim & Nemeroff, 2001; Nemeroff, 1999; Nemeroff, 2004a, 2004b; Yehuda, 2002), individual differences are found in the response to the adulthood stress.

Individual Differences in the Response to Stress

In this respect, it is of significance that there is a significant difference between the way a psychiatric disorder is diagnosed in humans and the way it is conducted in the animal models. In humans, the diagnosis of PTSD is given only when an individual exhibits a certain number of symptoms from each of three quite well-defined symptom clusters over a certain period of time. Yet in animal studies, irrespective of the study design/model or of the stress paradigm, results are presented, discussed, and conceptualized as involving the entire exposed population versus controls, although in practice, the exposed animals display a diverse range of responses. In order to more closely approximate the animal model approach to contemporary understanding of the clinical condition, a novel approach was conceived that enables segregating the study animals into groups according to the degree of their response to the trauma (Cohen et al., 2004).

The profiling of animals as "affected" or "non-affected" was based on the cutoff behavioral criteria (CBC) analysis approach, developed by Cohen, Zohar, and Matar (2003). By integrating different levels of responses patterns, classification criteria are formed in a similar manner to that used in clinical diagnosis procedures to form psychopathological symptom clusters; thus sets of classification criteria, representing inclusion and exclusion criteria, produce distinct patterns of stress-induced indices. The "CBC" analysis maximizes the accuracy of the animals' classifications and minimizes the likelihood of including "false-positives," by making sure that each animal that meets both sets of criteria (inclusion and exclusion) is defined as "affected" or "unaffected." The validity of the criteria is affirmed by ascertaining that the vast majority of "unexposed" animals are found within the "unaffected" category and only a minority with the "affected." Employing a version of that novel analysis approach, we were able to demonstrate a similar individual dissociation in animal models, as in humans (Lanius, Frewen, Vermetten, & Yehuda, 2010; Lanius,

Vermetten, et al., 2010), for those animals that demonstrate more anxious symptoms and those that exhibit more depressive symptoms (Horovitz et al., 2012; Tsoory et al., 2007; Tsoory & Richter-Levin, 2006). Examining the impact of "Juvenile Stress" on learning under stressful conditions in adulthood, we compared the effects of pre-exposure to stress at "juvenility" on the ability of animals to acquire a two-way shuttle avoidance task (TWS hereafter) in adulthood (PNDs 59–60). In this task, in which a tone precedes a foot shock, animals first learn to escape the shock by shuttling to the other compartment, but later may learn to avoid the shock completely by shuttling already when the predictive tone comes up. Only very rarely would an animal exhibit a response failure, i.e., will not move to the other compartment until the end of the session. While control animals have learned to effectively avoid the shock, animals pre-exposed to "Juvenile" stress were impaired. Interestingly, some animals were impaired in avoidance because they did not make the shift from escaping to avoiding, despite high rates of escape responses, but about a third of the pre-exposed animals demonstrated high rates of response failure (Tsoory & Richter-Levin, 2006). High escape rates with impaired avoidance was termed "anxious" behavior while high response failure, which is a form of learned helplessness, was termed "depressive" (Tsoory, 2006). In another study we compared the effects of pre-exposure to stress at "juvenility" (PNDs 27–29) or "adolescence" (PNDs 33–35). While among adult adolescence-stressed rats only "anxious" animals were observed, comprising 50 % of the animals, and none conformed to the "depressive" profile, juvenile-stressed rats tested in adulthood exhibited either "anxious" or "depressive" pattern of behavior (Tsoory et al., 2007).

We have further developed the methodology of profiling altered behavioral responses in several ways. First, while in the original "CBC" methodology the lowest 25th percentile was compared with the highest 25th percentile (Cohen et al., 2004), the comparison group we believe should be used is the averaged performance of the control group for each behavioral variable. Second, and probably a most important modification is the implementation of separate male/female comparison groups (Horovitz et al., 2012).

Gender/Sex Differences

Women are more prone than men to mood disorders, particularly depression (Garde, 2007; Gater et al., 1998; Noble, 2005) and anxiety disorders, including PTSD and generalized anxiety disorder (GAD) (Bekker & van Mens-Verhulst, 2007; Gater et al., 1998; Tolin & Foa, 2006). In addition to the different prevalence's of mood and anxiety disorders in men and women, there is evidence for gender-dependent differences in the response to psychotropic medications between men and women as well (Gorman, 2006; Yonkers, Kando, Cole, & Blumenthal, 1992). These differences suggest that gender-dependent differences in neuroanatomy and neurophysiology might underlie some of the observed differences in the prevalence and symptom profiles of mood and anxiety disorders between men and women.

Consistent with this hypothesis, differences between the genders were reported in several components of the central nervous system. Cahill (2006) for example noted gender differences in hippocampal structure and functions. These gender differences included the adrenergic, serotonergic, cholinergic, and cholecystokinin systems; anatomical structure; relative size (adjusted for total brain size); reactivity to stressors; as well as the effects of CORT and Benzodiazepines.

Men and women may also react differentially to stress. Melchior et al. (2007) found that young men and women from a well-characterized birth cohort differed in the extent to which low work support affected their response to work-related stress in adulthood. While the overall vulnerability to the effects of work-related stress was comparable in men and women, the impact of multiple stressors appeared to be significantly higher in men than in women.

While both men and women may develop the standard symptoms of a disorder, there are differences between the genders in both prevalence and symptom profiles. Women suffer from both depression and anxiety at significantly greater rates than men do; additionally, women exhibit higher rates of comorbid depression and anxiety disorders, and a threefold higher prevalence of atypical depression (Halbreich & Kahn, 2007). Therefore, Halbreich and Kahn (2007) suggested that the heterogeneity of symptoms and course of various disorders subtypes imply distinct etiological factors operating in the two genders.

There is a controversy among epidemiologists about the prevalence of psychiatric disorders among the genders and its etiological relevance. Since women in Western societies are diagnosed with major depression and with some anxiety disorders about twice as often as men (for a review see: Piccinelli & Wilkinson, 2000), it has been frequently argued that "womanhood" per se is a risk factor (Nemeroff et al., 2006). However, others like Melchior et al. (2007) suggested a more complex relationship between the specific stressors and their psychiatric consequences in men and women. In a meta-analysis of studies that compared the effects of specific traumatic events on the likelihood of men and women to develop PTSD, Tolin and Foa (2006) found that after controlling for different rates of exposure, almost all stressors produced more PTSD in women. However, childhood sexual abuse and adult sexual assault appeared to produce PTSD in similar odds ratios in men and women, with some indications that men are more vulnerable than women to the effects of childhood sexual abuse.

Gender-specific mood disturbances, including premenstrual dysphoric disorder, postpartum depression, and perimenopausal mood disturbance, were suggested to contribute to this bias (for a review see: Gater et al., 1998). However a complementary explanation was suggested by Garde (2007), that relates to differences in the repertoire of symptoms presented, leading to differential diagnosis. For example, depression is characterized in more in women as feelings of hopelessness and helplessness, whereas among men it is characterized as being irritable, angry, and discouraged (Garde, 2007).

In a recent study, in which we have included, in addition to the TWS also measures of exploratory behavior and unhedonia, we were able to demonstrate that the recurrent exposure to "Juvenile + Adulthood Stress," resulted in similar rates of "affected" rats among both sexes, but that the sexes differed in the profile of "symptoms."

While most of the male rats were found to exhibit comorbid (anxious and depressive symptoms), female rats exhibited mainly depressive symptoms (Horovitz et al., 2012). These findings are in agreement with Garde's conception (Garde, 2007), indicating our model has validity also in that respect.

While most rodent studies studying the consequences of exposure to stress employed male rats, those that did use females attributed some of the stress effects as dependent on the female estrus cycle, particularly on the gonadal hormones progesterone and estradiol, in the development of stress-induced behavioral despair or "learned helplessness" (Jenkins, Williams, Kramer, Davis, & Petty, 2001). However, a study which assessed male and female rats' ability to learn a difficult escape task following pre-exposure to either "controllable stress" (escaping mild footshocks) or "uncontrollable stress" (having no escape option from mild footshocks), indicated no involvement of gonadal hormones for either sex in behavioral despair (Dalla, Edgecomb, Whetstone, & Shors, 2008). Most males in the uncontrollable condition did not learn to escape following pre-exposure to "uncontrollable stress," whereas females learnt to escape irrespectively of pre-exposure conditions, i.e., controllable or uncontrollable stress. Moreover, since neither ovariectomy of females nor castration of males (at the age of 2–3 months) abolished the evident sex differences in helplessness behavior, the authors suggested that these behaviors do not depend on the presence of sex hormones in adulthood (Dalla et al., 2008). Dalla et al. (2008) suggested that although the estrus cycle does have a direct impact on females' behaviors, affecting their ability to cope with stress (Bekker & van Mens-Verhulst, 2007; Garde, 2007; Gater et al., 1998; Noble, 2005; Tolin & Foa, 2006) by interacting with both the stressful event's characteristics and the individual's traits, it appears that some of the effects of exposure to the stressor may overshadow the underlying effects of the different estrus cycle stages.

To conclude, it is suggested that in preclinical research that attempts to model stress-related psychopathologies, the establishment of different control groups for each of the sexes may be instrumental in setting "sex/gender-specific" criteria in order to better profile the animals. A similar gender-specific profiling approach may also be beneficial for human pathology diagnosis. This possibility should at least be considered, in association with the consideration of promoting also "sex/gender-specific" therapeutic interventions.

Acknowledgment "This research was funded by the Institute for the Study of Affective Neuroscience, University of Haifa, which was endowed by the Hope for Depression Research Foundation, and by a DoD Award 10071009 to GRL."

References

Agid, O., Kohn, Y., & Lerer, B. (2000). Environmental stress and psychiatric illness. *Biomedicine and Pharmacotherapy, 54*(3), 135–141.

American Psychiatric Association. (1994). *Diagnostic and statistical manual of mental disorders (DSM IV)* (4th ed.). Washington, DC: APA.

Andersen, S. L., & Teicher, M. H. (2004). Delayed effects of early stress on hippocampal development. *Neuropsychopharmacology, 29*, 1988–1993.
Anisman, H., & Matheson, K. (2005). Stress, depression, and anhedonia: Caveats concerning animal models. *Neuroscience and Biobehavioral Reviews, 29*(4–5), 525–546.
Anisman, H., Zaharia, M. D., Meaney, M. J., & Merali, Z. (1998). Do early-life events permanently alter behavioral and hormonal responses to stressors? *International Journal of Developmental Neuroscience, 16*(3–4), 149–164.
Arborelius, L., Owens, M. J., Plotsky, P. M., & Nemeroff, C. B. (1999). The role of corticotropin-releasing factor in depression and anxiety disorders. *The Journal of Endocrinology, 160*(1), 1–12.
Avital, A., Ram, E., Maayan, R., Weizman, A., & Richter-Levin, G. (2006). Effects of early-life stress on behavior and neurosteroid levels in the rat hypothalamus and entorhinal cortex. *Brain Research Bulletin, 68*(6), 419–424.
Avital, A., & Richter-Levin, G. (2005). Exposure to juvenile stress exacerbates the behavioural consequences of exposure to stress in the adult rat. *The International Journal of Neuropsychopharmacology, 8*(2), 163–173.
Bazak, N., Kozlovsky, N., Kaplan, Z., Matar, M., Golan, H., Zohar, J., et al. (2009). Pre-pubertal stress exposure affects adult behavioral response in association with changes in circulating corticosterone and brain-derived neurotrophic factor. *Psychoneuroendocrinology, 34*(6), 844–858.
Bekker, M. H., & van Mens-Verhulst, J. (2007). Anxiety disorders: Sex differences in prevalence, degree, and background, but gender-neutral treatment. *Gender Medicine, 4*(Suppl B), S178–S193.
Brydges, N. M., Hall, L., Nicolson, R., Holmes, M. C., & Hall, J. (2012). The effects of juvenile stress on anxiety, cognitive bias and decision making in adulthood: A rat model. *PLoS One, 7*(10), e48143.
Cahill, L. (2006). Why sex matters for neuroscience. *Nature Reviews. Neuroscience, 7*(6), 477–484.
Casey, B. J., Getz, S., & Galvan, A. (2008). The adolescent brain. *Developmental Review, 28*(1), 62–77.
Cohen, H., Zohar, J., & Matar, M. (2003). The relevance of differential response to trauma in an animal model of posttraumatic stress disorder. *Biological Psychiatry, 53*(6), 463–473.
Cohen, H., Zohar, J., Matar, M. A., Zeev, K., Loewenthal, U., & Richter-Levin, G. (2004). Setting apart the affected: The use of behavioral criteria in animal models of post traumatic stress disorder. *Neuropsychopharmacology, 29*(11), 1962–1970.
Costello, E. J., Pine, D. S., Hammen, C., March, J. S., Plotsky, P. M., Weissman, M. M., et al. (2002). Development and natural history of mood disorders. *Biological Psychiatry, 52*(6), 529–542.
Dalla, C., Edgecomb, C., Whetstone, A. S., & Shors, T. J. (2008). Females do not express learned helplessness like males do. *Neuropsychopharmacology, 33*(7), 1559–1569.
Freud, S. (1987). The origin and development of psychoanalysis. By Sigmund Freud, 1910. *The American Journal of Psychology, 100*(3–4), 472–488.
Garde, K. (2007). Depression – Gender differences. *Ugeskrift for Laeger, 169*(25), 2422–2425.
Gater, R., Tansella, M., Korten, A., Tiemens, B. G., Mavreas, V. G., & Olatawura, M. O. (1998). Sex differences in the prevalence and detection of depressive and anxiety disorders in general health care settings: Report from the World Health Organization Collaborative Study on Psychological Problems in General Health Care. *Archives of General Psychiatry, 55*(5), 405–413.
Gorman, J. M. (2006). Gender differences in depression and response to psychotropic medication. *Gender Medicine, 3*(2), 93–109.
Gregory, A. M., Caspi, A., Moffitt, T. E., Koenen, K., Eley, T. C., & Poulton, R. (2007). Juvenile mental health histories of adults with anxiety disorders. *The American Journal of Psychiatry, 164*(2), 301–308.
Halbreich, U., & Kahn, L. S. (2007). Atypical depression, somatic depression and anxious depression in women: Are they gender-preferred phenotypes? *Journal of Affective Disorders, 102*(1–3), 245–258.

Heim, C., & Nemeroff, C. B. (2001). The role of childhood trauma in the neurobiology of mood and anxiety disorders: Preclinical and clinical studies. *Biological Psychiatry, 49*(12), 1023–1039.

Horovitz, O., Tsoory, M. M., Hall, J., Jacobson-Pick, S., & Richter-Levin, G. (2012). Post-weaning–pre-pubertal ('juvenile') stress: A model of induced predisposition to stress-related disorders. *Neuroendocrinology, 95*, 56–64.

Horovitz, O., Tsoory, M. M., Yovell, Y., & Richter-Levin, G. (2014). A rat model of pre-puberty (Juvenile) stress-induced predisposition to stress-related disorders: Sex similarities and sex differences in effects and symptoms. *World Journal of Biological Psychiatry, 15*(1), 36–48.

Ilin, Y., & Richter-Levin, G. (2009). Enriched environment experience overcomes learning deficits and depressive-like behavior induced by juvenile stress. *PLoS One, 4*(1), e4329.

Jacobson-Pick, S., Elkobi, A., Vander, S., Rosenblum, K., & Richter-Levin, G. (2008). Juvenile stress-induced alteration of maturation of the GABAA receptor alpha subunit in the rat. *The International Journal of Neuropsychopharmacology, 11*(7), 891–903.

Jacobson-Pick, S., & Richter-Levin, G. (2012). Short- and long-term effects of juvenile stressor exposure on the expression of GABAA receptor subunits in rats. *Stress, 15*(4), 416–424.

Jenkins, J. A., Williams, P., Kramer, G. L., Davis, L. L., & Petty, F. (2001). The influence of gender and the estrous cycle on learned helplessness in the rat. *Biological Psychology, 58*, 147–158.

Kalueff, A. V., & Tuohimaa, P. (2004). Experimental modeling of anxiety and depression. *Acta Neurobiologiae Experimentalis (Warsaw), 64*(4), 439–448.

Kehoe, P., Shoemaker, W. J., Arons, C., Triano, L., & Suresh, G. (1998). Repeated isolation stress in the neonatal rat: Relation to brain dopamine systems in the 10-day-old rat. *Behavioral Neuroscience, 112*, 1466–1474.

Kessler, R. C., Berglund, P., Demler, O., Jin, R., Merikangas, K. R., & Walters, E. E. (2005). Lifetime prevalence and age-of-onset distributions of DSM-IV disorders in the National Comorbidity Survey Replication. *Archives of General Psychiatry, 62*(6), 593–602.

Kessler, R. C., Chiu, W. T., Demler, O., Merikangas, K. R., & Walters, E. E. (2005). Prevalence, severity, and comorbidity of 12-month DSM-IV disorders in the National Comorbidity Survey Replication. *Archives of General Psychiatry, 62*(6), 617–627.

Lanius, R. A., Frewen, P. A., Vermetten, E., & Yehuda, R. (2010). Fear conditioning and early life vulnerabilities: Two distinct pathways of emotional dysregulation and brain dysfunction in PTSD. *European Journal of Psychotraumatology, 1*. doi:10.3402/ejpt.v1i0.5467.

Lanius, R. A., Vermetten, E., Loewenstein, R. J., Brand, B., Schmahl, C., Bremner, J. D., et al. (2010). Emotion modulation in PTSD: Clinical and neurobiological evidence for a dissociative subtype. *The American Journal of Psychiatry, 167*(6), 640–647.

Lapiz, M. D., Fulford, A., Muchimapura, S., Mason, R., Parker, T., & Marsden, C. A. (2001). Influence of postweaning social isolation in the rat on brain development, conditioned behaviour and neurotransmission. Rossiiskii fiziologicheskii zhurnal imeni I.M. *Sechenova, 87*, 730–775.

Levine, S. (1994). The ontogeny of the hypothalamic–pituitary–adrenal axis. The influence of maternal factors. *Annals of the New York Academy of Sciences, 746*, 275–288 (discussion pp. 289–293).

Levine, S. (2005). Developmental determinants of sensitivity and resistance to stress. *Psychoneuroendocrinology, 30*(10), 939–946.

Levine, S., Huchton, D. M., Wiener, S. G., & Rosenfeld, P. (1991). Time course of the effect of maternal deprivation on the hypothalamic–pituitary–adrenal axis in the infant rat. *Developmental Psychobiology, 24*, 547–558.

Maercker, A., Michael, T., Fehm, L., Becker, E. S., & Margraf, J. (2004). Age of traumatisation as a predictor of posttraumatic stress disorder or major depression in young women. *British Journal of Psychiatry, 184*, 482–487.

Maggio, N., & Segal, M. (2011). Persistent changes in ability to express long-term potentiation/depression in the rat hippocampus after juvenile/adult stress. *Biological Psychiatry, 69*(8), 748–753.

Maughan, B., & McCarthy, G. (1997). Childhood adversity and psychosocial disorders. *British Medical Bulletin, 53*(1), 156–169.

Melchior, M., Caspi, A., Milne, B. J., Danese, A., Poulton, R., & Moffitt, T. E. (2007). Work stress precipitates depression and anxiety in young, working women and men. *Psychological Medicine, 37*(8), 1119–1129.
Muchimapura, S., Fulford, A. J., Mason, R., & Marsden, C. A. (2002). Isolation rearing in the rat disrupts the hippocampal response to stress. *Neuroscience, 112*, 697–705.
Muchimapura, S., Mason, R., & Marsden, C. A. (2003). Effect of isolation rearing on pre- and post-synaptic serotonergic function in the rat dorsal hippocampus. *Synapse, 47*, 209–217.
Nemeroff, C. B. (1999). The preeminent role of early untoward experience on vulnerability to major psychiatric disorders: The nature-nurture controversy revisited and soon to be resolved. *Molecular Psychiatry, 4*(2), 106–108.
Nemeroff, C. B. (2004a). Neurobiological consequences of childhood trauma. *The Journal of Clinical Psychiatry, 65*(1), 18–28.
Nemeroff, C. B. (2004b). Early-life adversity, CRF dysregulation, and vulnerability to mood and anxiety disorders. *Psychopharmacology Bulletin, 38*(1), 14–20.
Nemeroff, C. B., Bremner, J. D., Foa, E. B., Mayberg, H. S., North, C. S., & Stein, M. B. (2006). Posttraumatic stress disorder: A state-of-the-science review. *Journal of Psychiatric Research, 40*(1), 1–21.
Noble, R. E. (2005). Depression in women. *Metabolism, 54*(5–1), 49–52.
Ogawa, T., Mikuni, M., Kuroda, Y., Muneoka, K., Mori, K. J., & Takahashi, K. (1994). Periodic maternal deprivation alters stress response in adult offspring: Potentiates the negative feedback regulation of restraint stress-induced adrenocortical response and reduces the frequencies of open field-induced behaviors. *Pharmacology, Biochemistry, and Behavior, 49*, 961–967.
Piccinelli, M., & Wilkinson, G. (2000). Gender differences in depression. Critical review. *The British Journal of Psychiatry, 177*, 486–492.
Plotsky, P. M., Thrivikraman, K. V., & Meaney, M. J. (1993). Central and feedback regulation of hypothalamic corticotropin-releasing factor secretion. *Ciba Foundation Symposium, 172*, 59–75 (discussion pp. 75–84).
Pynoos, R. S., Steinberg, A. M., & Piacentini, J. C. (1999). A developmental psychopathology model of childhood traumatic stress and intersection with anxiety disorders. *Biological Psychiatry, 46*, 1542–1554.
Rosenfeld, P., Wetmore, J. B., & Levine, S. (1992). Effects of repeated maternal separations on the adrenocortical response to stress of preweanling rats. *Physiology and Behavior, 52*, 787–791.
Sanchez, M. M., Ladd, C. O., & Plotsky, P. M. (2001). Early adverse experience as a developmental risk factor for later psychopathology: Evidence from rodent and primate models. *Development and Psychopathology, 13*(3), 419–449.
Spear, L. P. (2004). Adolescent brain development and animal models. *Annals of the New York Academy of Sciences, 1021*, 23–26.
Tolin, D. F., & Foa, E. B. (2006). Sex differences in trauma and posttraumatic stress disorder: A quantitative review of 25 years of research. *Psychological Bulletin, 132*(6), 959–992.
Tsoory, M., Cohen, H., & Richter-Levin, G. (2007). Juvenile stress induces a predisposition to either anxiety or depressive-like symptoms following stress in adulthood. *European Neuropsychopharmacology, 17*(4), 245–256.
Tsoory, M., Guterman, A., & Richter-Levin, G. (2008). Exposure to stressors during juvenility disrupts development-related alterations in the PSA-NCAM to NCAM expression ratio: Potential relevance for mood and anxiety disorders. *Neuropsychopharmacology, 33*(2), 378–393.
Tsoory, M. M., Guterman, A., & Richter-Levin, G. (2010). "Juvenile stress" alters maturation-related changes in expression of the neural cell adhesion molecule L1 in the limbic system: Relevance for stress-related psychopathologies. *Journal of Neuroscience Research, 88*(2), 369–380.
Tsoory, M., & Richter-Levin, G. (2006). Learning under stress in the adult rat is differentially affected by 'juvenile' or 'adolescent' stress. *The International Journal of Neuropsychopharmacology, 9*(6), 713–728.

Tsoory, M. M., Vouimba, R. M., Akirav, I., Kavushansky, A., Avital, A., & Richter-Levin, G. (2008). Amygdala modulation of memory-related processes in the hippocampus: Potential relevance to PTSD. *Progress in Brain Research, 167*, 35–51.

van Oers, H. J., de Kloet, E. R., & Levine, S. (1998). Early vs. late maternal deprivation differentially alters the endocrine and hypothalamic responses to stress. *Brain Research. Developmental Brain Research, 111*, 245–252.

Vazquez, D. M., Van Oers, H., Levine, S., & Akil, H. (1996). Regulation of glucocorticoid and mineralocorticoid receptor mRNAs in the hippocampus of the maternally deprived infant rat. *Brain Research, 731*, 79–90.

von Hoersten, S., Dimitrijevic, M., Markovic, B. M., & Jankovic, B. D. (1993). Effect of early experience on behavior and immune response in the rat. *Physiology and Behavior, 54*, 931–940.

Wang, X. D., Labermaier, C., Holsboer, F., Wurst, W., Deussing, J. M., Müller, M. B., et al. (2012). Early-life stress-induced anxiety-related behavior in adult mice partially requires forebrain corticotropin-releasing hormone receptor 1. *The European Journal of Neuroscience, 36*(3), 2360–2367.

Wang, X. D., Rammes, G., Kraev, I., Wolf, M., Liebl, C., Scharf, S. H., et al. (2011). Forebrain CRF_1 modulates early-life stress-programmed cognitive deficits. *The Journal of Neuroscience, 31*(38), 13625–13634.

Yee, N., Plassmann, K., & Fuchs, E. (2011). Juvenile stress impairs body temperature regulation and augments anticipatory stress-induced hyperthermia responses in rats. *Physiology and Behavior, 104*(3), 408–416.

Yee, N., Schwarting, R. K., Fuchs, E., & Wöhr, M. (2012). Juvenile stress potentiates aversive 22-kHz ultrasonic vocalizations and freezing during auditory fear conditioning in adult male rats. *Stress, 15*(5), 533–544.

Yehuda, R. (2002). Post-traumatic stress disorder. *The New England Journal of Medicine, 346*(2), 108–114.

Yonkers, K. A., Kando, J. C., Cole, J. O., & Blumenthal, S. (1992). Gender differences in pharmacokinetics and pharmacodynamics of psychotropic medication. *The American Journal of Psychiatry, 149*(5), 587–595.

Chapter 4
An Attachment Perspective on Traumatic and Posttraumatic Reactions

Mario Mikulincer, Phillip R. Shaver, and Zahava Solomon

Attachment theory (Bowlby, 1973, 1980, 1982) is one of the most fruitful contemporary frameworks for understanding emotion regulation and mental health. Adult attachment research has provided strong evidence for the anxiety-buffering function, of what Bowlby called the attachment behavioral system, and for the importance of individual differences in attachment in shaping psychological resilience, distress management, coping with stress, and adjustment (see Mikulincer & Shaver, 2007a, for a review). In this chapter, we present an attachment perspective on emotional problems resulting from traumatic events. Following a brief overview of attachment theory's basic concepts, we focus on the implications of the theory for emotion regulation and mental health in general and for traumatic reactions and posttraumatic stress disorder (PTSD) in particular. We review research findings showing that attachment insecurities—called attachment anxiety and avoidance in the theory—are associated with the severity of PTSD symptoms, and that the sense of attachment security has a healing effect on these symptoms. We also review recent findings regarding the reciprocal, recursive, amplifying cycle of PTSD symptoms and attachment insecurities over time.

M. Mikulincer (✉)
School of Psychology, Interdisciplinary Center (IDC) Herzliya, P.O. Box 167, Herzliya 46150, Israel
e-mail: Mario@idc.ac.il

P.R. Shaver, Ph.D.
Department of Psychology, UC Davis, One Shields Avenue, Davis, CA 95616-8686, USA
e-mail: prshaver@ucdavis.edu

Z. Solomon
Bob Shapell School of Social Work, Tel-Aviv University, Tel Aviv 69978, Israel
e-mail: Solomon@post.tau.ac.il

M.P. Safir et al. (eds.), *Future Directions in Post-Traumatic Stress Disorder*, DOI 10.1007/978-1-4899-7522-5_4

Overview of Attachment Theory

According to attachment theory (Bowlby, 1973, 1980, 1982), human beings are born with a psychobiological system (the *attachment behavioral system*) that motivates them to seek proximity to supportive others (*attachment figures*) in times of need for the sake of gaining a sense of safety and security. However, although every human being is born with this propensity to seek support and rely on others as a source of protection and security, people differ in the way their attachment system functions, primarily as a result of their history of interactions with attachment figures (Bowlby, 1973). Interactions with figures who are available, sensitive, and responsive in times of need promote effective support-seeking strategies and encourage the development of a stable sense of security. This sense of security includes implicit beliefs that the world is generally safe, that other people are "well-intentioned and kind-hearted" (Hazan & Shaver, 1987), that one is valued, loved, understood, accepted, and cared for by others, and that one can explore the environment with interest and engage rewardingly with other people. These beliefs are associated with and rooted in positive mental representations of self and others, which Bowlby (1973) called *internal working models*. These models shape a person's expectations for future interactions with the same or other relationship partners over time, especially in times of need.

Unfortunately, when a person's attachment figures have not been reliably available, sensitive, and supportive, he or she has not learned that seeking proximity to others relieves distress. Moreover, the person is not likely to have developed a core sense of security. Rather, negative working models of self (as not sufficiently lovable) and others (as unaccepting, unreliable, and unresponsive if not downright abusive or cruel) are formed, and affect-regulation strategies other than confident proximity seeking are developed. These *secondary attachment strategies* are called "anxious" and "avoidant" in attachment theory. According to the theory, individual differences in working models and distress-regulation strategies eventually become trait-like attachment "styles" or orientations—characteristic patterns of relational expectations, emotions, and behavior (Fraley & Shaver, 2000).

Beginning with Ainsworth, Blehar, Waters, and Wall's (1978) studies of infant attachment, and then followed by hundreds of developmental studies of children and social psychological studies of adults (reviewed by Mikulincer & Shaver, 2003, 2007a), researchers have found that attachment orientations can be measured along the two roughly orthogonal dimensions already mentioned: attachment-related anxiety and attachment-related avoidance (Brennan, Clark, & Shaver, 1998). A person's position on the attachment anxiety dimension indicates the degree to which he or she worries that a partner will not be responsive in times of need and is afraid of being rejected or abandoned, partly because of his or her own self-doubts and self-criticism. A person's position on the avoidance dimension indicates the extent to which he or she distrusts relationship partners' goodwill and their capacity to help, and the extent to which he or she defensively strives to maintain independence and emotional distance from partners. People who score low on both dimensions are said to be secure with respect to attachment (Brennan et al., 1998). In extreme cases, attachment insecurities can result in a "disorganized" attachment pattern—a mixture of contradictory approach and avoidance tendencies or a form of psychological and behavioral paralysis (Simpson & Rholes, 2002). A person's location in this two-dimensional space can be measured with reliable and valid self-report scales (e.g., Brennan et al., 1998) and is associated in theoretically predictable ways with many aspects of relationship quality and psychological adjustment (see Mikulincer & Shaver, 2007a, for a review).

Although attachment orientations are initially formed in relationships with primary caregivers (usually parents) during infancy and childhood (Bowlby, 1982), as confirmed by several decades-long longitudinal studies (reviewed in Cassidy & Shaver, 2008), Bowlby (1988) also claimed that meaningful interactions with later attachment figures (e.g., friends, romantic partners) can alter the sense of security and move a person from one region of the two-dimensional space (defined by anxiety by avoidance) to another. Moreover, although attachment orientations are often conceptualized as single, stable, global patterns, they may also be considered in terms of the most accessible working models at a given moment, selected from a complex network of many episodic, context-specific, and relationship-anchored memories and schemas (Mikulincer & Shaver, 2003). Research indicates that a person's sense of attachment security can change, subtly or dramatically, depending on naturally occurring or experimentally induced contexts (Mikulincer & Shaver, 2007b; Shaver & Mikulincer, 2008), making it possible to study the psychological and relational effects of both experimentally primed senses of security or insecurity and actual partners' sensitivity and responsiveness.

Individual differences in attachment anxiety and avoidance reflect both a person's sense of attachment security and the ways in which he or she deals with stress and distress (Mikulincer & Shaver, 2003, 2007a). People who score low on these dimensions are generally secure, hold positive representations of self and others, tend to employ constructive and effective distress management strategies, and generally engage comfortably and rewardingly in intimate relationships and in exploration of many aspects of the physical, social, and cultural environment. In contrast, people who score high on either attachment anxiety or avoidance, or both, suffer from a variety of insecurities, including doubts about their safety and lovability and about other people's intentions and goodwill. Insecure people tend to use secondary attachment and emotion-regulation strategies that we, following Cassidy and Kobak (1988), call "hyperactivation" or "deactivation" of the attachment behavioral system in an effort to cope with threats.

People who score high on attachment anxiety rely on hyperactivating strategies—that is, energetic attempts to achieve proximity, support, and love combined with a lack of confidence that these resources will be provided, and with feelings of sadness or anger when they are in fact not provided (Cassidy & Kobak, 1988). Hyperactivating strategies include attempts to elicit a partner's involvement, care, and support through begging, complaining, clinging, and attempting to control a partner (Davis, Shaver, & Vernon, 2003); overdependence on relationship partners as sources of protection (Shaver & Hazan, 1993); and perception of the self as relatively helpless at regulating emotion (Mikulincer & Shaver, 2003). These strategies also include exaggeration of threats, intensification of distress, and rumination on distress-eliciting thoughts as means of upregulating the attachment system and eliciting others' attention, care, and support (Shaver & Mikulincer, 2002). These reactions stem from relationships in which an attachment figure is sometimes responsive but unreliably so, placing the needy person on a partial reinforcement schedule that rewards exaggeration of threats and persistence in proximity-seeking attempts until an attachment figure is perceived to be adequately available and supportive.

In contrast, people who score high on attachment-related avoidance tend to keep their attachment systems downregulated, to avoid the frustration and pain of being unlovable and rejected. This goal is achieved through deactivating strategies that include avoidance of dependence on close relationship partners and maintenance of emotional distance from others. These tendencies are supplemented by what Bowlby (1982) called compulsive self-reliance, a defensive stance that decreases attachment-system activation by denying threats, failing to acknowledge distress, vulnerabilities, and personal weaknesses, and suppressing distress-eliciting thoughts. These strategies develop in relationships with attachment figures who disapprove of and punish bids for closeness and expressions of need (Ainsworth et al., 1978).

Attachment, Emotion Regulation, and Mental Health

According to attachment theory (Bowlby, 1982), the attachment system evolved because it increased safety (hence survival and the opportunity to reproduce) and taught vulnerable children how to regulate emotions effectively in times of stress and distress. This behavioral system is automatically activated by external threats or internal sources of distress, and when it functions appropriately and successfully, it leads to socially supported emotional stability. Optimal functioning is associated with a relational if-then script, which Waters and Waters (2006) called a *secure-base* script: "If I encounter an obstacle and/or become distressed, I can approach a significant other for help. He or she is likely to be available and supportive. I will experience relief and comfort as a result of proximity to this person, and I can then return to other activities." Once activated, this script guides behavior, but even by itself it can mitigate distress, promote optimism and hope, and help a person cope effectively with problems (Mikulincer, Shaver, Sapir-Lavid, & Avihou-Kanza, 2009).

Recently, adult attachment researchers have designed experimental procedures to examine these regulatory properties of the attachment system. For example, in a series of laboratory experiments, Mikulincer, Gillath, and Shaver (2002) showed that mental representations of attachment figures (e.g., names of security-enhancing attachment figures) are automatically activated in a person's mind when he or she is exposed to threatening stimuli, even unconsciously. Specifically, when a threat-related word (e.g., "death") was presented very briefly (i.e., subliminally) on a computer screen, participants were faster to detect the name of one of their attachment figures when it appeared on the screen and were slower to name the color in which such names were printed on the screen—an indication that the words had been automatically activated in memory (Mikulincer et al., 2002). In other words, threats, even when arising unconsciously, can automatically activate mental representations of security providers.

In another set of studies of what we call "security priming," Mikulincer, Hirschberger, Nachmias, and Gillath (2001) showed that activation of representations of security-enhancing attachment figures can automatically infuse a previously neutral stimulus with positive affect. For example, subliminal presentation of the names of people who were nominated by the participants as attachment figures, compared with mere acquaintances or close others who were not nominated as attachment figures, led to greater liking of previously unfamiliar stimuli. Moreover, subliminal exposure to names of attachment figures eliminated the detrimental effects that threats otherwise had on liking for previously neutral stimuli. These effects of security priming on positive affect have been replicated in subsequent studies (see Mikulincer & Shaver, 2007b, for a review). Combining our findings, we conclude that people automatically search for internal representations of security-enhancing attachment figures during times of stress, and mental activation of such representations results in positive affect that can facilitate effective coping and restore emotional equanimity. Moreover, people who generally feel safe and protected benefit from what we, following Fredrickson (2001), call a "broaden and build" cycle of attachment security (Mikulincer & Shaver, 2003), which supports psychological resilience and broadens skills and interests (by virtue of what Bowlby, 1969/1982, called the exploration behavioral system).

According to adult attachment theory (Mikulincer & Shaver, 2003, 2007a; Shaver & Mikulincer, 2002), although secondary attachment strategies (anxious hyperactivation and avoidant deactivation) are initially adaptive in the sense that they adjust a child's behavior to the requirements of an inconsistently available or consistently distant or unavailable attachment figure, they are maladaptive when used in later relationships in which support-seeking and relational interdependence could be rewarding and could help people to maintain a sense of well-being even in times of stress. These attachment strategies encourage repeated activation of negative working models of self and others that can interfere with social adjustment and mental health.

The early attachment experiences of insecure people (whether anxious, avoidant, or both) are characterized by unstable and inadequate distress regulation (Bowlby, 1973; Shaver & Hazan, 1993), which interferes with the development of inner resources necessary for coping successfully with stressors and maintaining mental health. This impairment is particularly likely to be noticed during prolonged, highly demanding stressful experiences that require active support-seeking and actual confrontation with a problem (Berant, Mikulincer, & Shaver, 2008). In such cases, anxious (hyperactivating) strategies may become extreme, damaging not only a person's own mental health but that of key relationship partners, and avoidant (deactivating) strategies can collapse, resulting in a marked decline in psychological functioning. These negative outcomes of attachment anxiety and avoidance have been documented in hundreds of cross-sectional and longitudinal studies (see Mikulincer & Shaver, 2007a, for a review).

Attachment, Trauma, and Posttraumatic Processes

The mental health implications of attachment insecurities are important for understanding individual differences in the way people react to traumatic events. Traumatic experiences such as rape, assault, car accidents, floods, war, and a host of other natural and man-made disasters disrupt a person's psychological stability and may place him or her at risk for serious emotional and adjustment problems. In some cases psychological well-being is maintained even during severe stress or is restored shortly after a traumatic experience ends. In other cases, however, attempted restoration of emotional stability fails. Studies of the psychosocial effects of traumatic events have identified posttraumatic stress disorder (PTSD) as the most common and debilitating outcome (see Ball & Stein, 2012, for a review). PTSD is characterized by repeated reexperiencing of a traumatic event (unwanted intrusion of trauma-related material into conscious thoughts, mental images, and dreams), numbing of responsiveness to or reduced involvement with the external world (trauma-related avoidance responses), and a variety of autonomic, affective, and cognitive signs of hyperarousal (American Psychiatric Association, 1994).

As with other stressful experiences, we would expect the attachment behavioral system to be automatically activated when a person is exposed to traumatic events. According to Horowitz (1982), a person's state of mind when undergoing trauma includes overwhelming shock and intense feelings of panic, vulnerability, helplessness, and exhaustion. Such a state of mind should automatically activate the attachment system, impelling a person to search for external or internalized attachment figures who can protect him or her from trauma. This attachment-system activation is likely to be experienced as an intense cry for help.

When internal or external sources of support can be mobilized during a traumatic event, the traumatized person can maintain psychological well-being despite the external challenge, thereby making PTSD less likely when the trauma subsides. A secure person's mental cry for help during trauma should result in mobilization of internal representations of security-providing attachment figures and/or actual external sources of support. As a result, the secure person is likely to activate optimistic and hopeful representations of self and others, rely on constructive strategies of affect regulation, deal effectively with the trauma, and restore emotional balance. In other words, the sense of attachment security should act, at least to some extent, as a protective shield against the formation of emotional problems, including PTSD, following trauma.

In contrast, disruptions in the sense of attachment security may prevent maintenance or restoration of emotional equanimity during and following trauma, thereby contributing to PTSD formation. In such cases, a traumatized person may fail to find inner representations of security or external sources of support and comfort, which then interferes with the regulation of distress. This regulatory failure may initiate a cascade of psychological processes, including strong feelings of loneliness and rejection as well as negative working models of self and others, intensification of distress, and reliance on less effective (hyperactivating or deactivating) strategies of affect regulation, which may prevent resolution of the trauma and enhance the likelihood of prolonged PTSD. In other words, an insecure attachment orientation (anxious, avoidant, or both) can predispose a traumatized person to PTSD.

According to Horowitz (1982), the posttraumatic process is defined by two kinds of intrapsychic manifestations of PTSD: intrusion and avoidance. Intrusion refers to unwanted and uncontrollable thoughts, images, emotions, and nightmares related to the traumatic event. Avoidance refers to psychic numbing, denial of the significance and consequences of the traumatic event, and behavioral inhibition. The relative salience of intrusion versus avoidance is not constant (Horowitz, 1982). Intrusion is generally experienced immediately after the trauma, but the two states can alternate during the posttraumatic period until successful "working through" of the trauma is achieved, if in fact it is achieved.

Attachment insecurities are also important in regulating the intensity and frequency of posttraumatic intrusion and avoidance tendencies. Anxious hyperactivation can facilitate reactivation of, and mental rumination about, the traumatic experience and the frustrated cry for help, thereby encouraging intrusive responses. Avoidant deactivation predisposes a traumatized person to deny inner pain and avoid direct or symbolic confrontation with trauma reminders, thereby encouraging posttraumatic avoidance responses. As a result, an insecure attachment orientation (anxious, avoidant, or both) can intensify posttraumatic intrusion and avoidance tendencies. Moreover, contextual activation of mental representations of attachment anxiety or avoidance, due to symbolic or actual encounters with rejecting or unsupportive figures, during the posttraumatic period can further increase the likelihood of intrusive or avoidant responses.

Following this line of reasoning, infusions of attachment security during the posttraumatic period should reduce the intensity and frequency of intrusive and avoidant responses and lead to a successful working through of the trauma. Research has shown that the activation of mental representations of attachment security, due to symbolic or actual encounters with loving, accepting, caring, and supporting others (including a trustworthy and reliable therapist), results in feelings of lovability, hope, optimism, and self-esteem, and can move a person to a more secure location in the two-dimensional anxiety-by-avoidance space, and can activate more constructive and effective ways of managing distress (see Mikulincer & Shaver, 2007b; Shaver & Mikulincer, 2008, for reviews). In this way, activating a sense of security can help people work through trauma, with healing effects on PTSD symptoms.

So far in this chapter we have focused on the potential effects of attachment orientations on traumatic and posttraumatic responses. However, traumatic events and prolonged PTSD, which include mental reactivation of the trauma, can also have important effects on attachment orientations. Although attachment orientations are fairly stable over time (like many core personality traits), they can be altered by powerful experiences that affect a person's beliefs about the value of seeking help from attachment figures and the feasibility of attaining safety, protection, and comfort (e.g., Baldwin & Fehr, 1995; Davila & Cobb, 2004). Persistent and pervasive PTSD can increase a person's sense of helplessness and vulnerability and therefore heighten attachment insecurities, especially among individuals who entered a period of trauma with already existing attachment-related doubts and insecurities.

The constant mental reactivation of a trauma, particularly a man-made trauma that shatters one's trust in others' goodwill and one's sense of personal value and lovability, can gradually increase the strength of negative working models of self and other, thereby heightening attachment insecurities and reducing the likelihood of attaining a calmer, more secure mental state.

Thus, prolonged and pervasive PTSD may involve a reciprocal, recursive, amplifying cycle of reactivation of the trauma and attachment insecurities: Attachment worries and doubts can prevent successful working through of the trauma, and the resulting mental reactivation of the trauma can further erode the sense of security. Moreover, this gradual but persistent exacerbation of attachment insecurities during the posttraumatic period may lead to the disorganization of the attachment system and the disruption of the regulatory and healing benefits of attachment security. As a result, traumatized people with persistent and pervasive PTSD are likely to score high on both attachment anxiety and avoidance, may be less likely to activate security-related representations during threat exposure, and may be impervious to contextual augmentation of the sense of security. That is, activation of security-related representations may be less effective than might be expected in increasing positive affect and healing the symptoms of PTSD. For severely traumatized people, restoration of a sense of having a safe haven and a secure base may be a long, difficult, and complex process.

Our analysis of the role of attachment orientations in traumatic and posttraumatic processes can be summarized in four hypotheses. First, attachment insecurities will be associated with the formation of PTSD following traumatic events, with attachment anxiety being especially associated with posttraumatic intrusion tendencies and avoidant attachment being especially associated with posttraumatic avoidance tendencies. Second, mobilizing external sources of support and protection or activating internal representations of security during the posttraumatic period will help to reduce PTSD symptoms and facilitate working through the trauma. Third, persistent and pervasive PTSD will increase attachment insecurities over time, thereby contributing to a recursive, amplifying cycle of trauma reactivation and attachment-related worries and doubts. Fourth, persistent and pervasive PTSD will be associated with attachment-system disorganization and a disruption of the regulatory and healing powers of the sense of attachment security. In the following sections, we review empirical evidence for each of these hypotheses.

Are Attachment Insecurities Associated with PTSD?

The first systematic attempt to examine whether and how attachment insecurities are associated with PTSD symptoms focused on reactions of young adults to Iraqi Scud missile attacks on Israel during the 1991 Gulf War (Mikulincer, Florian, & Weller, 1993). In this study, Israeli undergraduates were approached 2 weeks after the end of the Gulf War and asked to complete self-report measures of attachment orientations and PTSD symptoms. Attachment anxiety was associated with more severe posttraumatic intrusion and avoidance symptoms, and avoidant attachment was associated with more severe posttraumatic avoidance responses (assessed with the *Impact of Events Scale*; Horowitz, Wilner, & Alvarez, 1979).

Subsequent studies have replicated this association between self-reported attachment insecurities and PTSD symptoms across different samples of adults who have been exposed to a variety of traumatic events. These samples include victims of childhood sexual or physical abuse (e.g., Alexander et al., 1998; Muller & Lemieux, 2000; Muller, Sicoli, & Lemieux, 2000; Roche, Runtz, & Hunter, 1999; Sandberg, 2010; Shapiro & Levendosky, 1999), civilians living under life-endangering conditions (e.g., Besser & Neria, 2010, 2012; Besser, Neria, & Haynes, 2009; Mikulincer, Horesh, Eilati, & Kotler, 1999), recruits in military training (Neria et al., 2001), prisoners of war (Dieperink, Leskela, Thuras, & Engdahl, 2001; Solomon, Ginzburg, Mikulincer, Neria, & Ohry, 1998; Zakin, Solomon, & Neria, 2003), war veterans (Dekel, Solomon, Ginzburg, & Neria, 2004; Ghafoori, Hierholzer, Howsepian, & Boardman, 2008; Renaud, 2008), Holocaust survivors (Cohen, Dekel, & Solomon, 2002), survivors of the 9/11 terror attacks (Fraley, Fazzari, Bonanno, & Dekel, 2006; Twaite & Rodriguez-Srednicki, 2004), security workers (e.g., Bogaerts, Daalder, Van Der Knaap, Kunst, & Buschman, 2008; Bogaerts, Kunst, & Winkel, 2009; Declercq & Willemsen, 2006), and victims of interpersonal violence (e.g., Elwood & Williams, 2007; Sandberg, Suess, & Heaton, 2010; Scott & Babcock, 2010). For example, Fraley et al. (2006) found that both attachment anxiety and avoidance, as assessed by self-report scales administered 7 months after the 9/11 terror attacks, predicted more severe PTSD symptoms 11 months later. Moreover, friends and relatives viewed attachment-anxious survivors as displaying decreased adjustment 7 months after the attacks.

Studies assessing attachment orientations with the *Adult Attachment Interview* (AAI; Main, Hesse, & Goldwyn, 2009) have produced a less consistent pattern of findings. As expected, Kanninen, Punamaki, and Qouta (2003) found that former Palestinian political prisoners who were classified as anxious or avoidant, based on the AAI, reported more severe PTSD symptoms than those who were classified as secure. However, Nye et al. (2008) and Harari et al. (2009) found no significant association between AAI classification and PTSD symptoms among combat veterans who were in treatment following a PTSD diagnosis. One study used the *Adult Attachment Projective Interview* (George & West, 2001), which is similar to a TAT, and found that attachment insecurities were associated with more PTSD symptoms at 1 and 3 months post-trauma in a sample of adults who were recruited in hospital emergency rooms (Benoit, Bouthillier, Moss, Rousseau, & Brunet, 2010).

The Healing Effects of Attachment Security

There is growing evidence that a sense of attachment security can have healing effects on people suffering from PTSD and can improve their response to treatment. For example, Forbes, Parslow, Fletcher, McHugh, and Creamer (2010) assessed the effectiveness of group-based treatment for combat-related PTSD and found that self-reports of attachment security predicted better treatment outcome and recovery from PTSD following treatment. In another psychotherapy-outcome study, Muller and Rosenkranz (2009) found that self-reports of attachment security increased during treatment in an inpatient program for adults with PTSD (as compared to a waitlist group), and this increase was maintained over 6 months following treatment. More important, these positive changes in attachment security were associated with a reduction in PTSD symptoms during and after treatment.

In two independent studies, Mikulincer, Shaver, and Horesh (2006) found direct evidence for the healing effects of attachment security. One study used a diary methodology and assessed Israelis' daily psychological reactions during 21 days of the 2003 US-Iraq war. Specifically, this study examined the effects of experiences of being comforted, supported, and connected to others (i.e., contextual activation of attachment security) during the 21-day period on daily PTSD symptoms. In addition, participants' global attachment orientations had been measured before the war. Global attachment insecurities were associated with more severe war-related PTSD across the 21-day period. In addition, contextual activation of the sense of attachment security (which we call "security priming") on a given day reduced the severity of war-related PTSD symptoms that day and the next day. Moreover, contextual security augmentation weakened the link between dispositional attachment anxiety and PTSD. That is, the feeling of being supported by others on a given day reduced anxiously attached individuals' PTSD symptoms. However, daily inductions of a sense of security did not reduce the detrimental effects of avoidant attachment on PTSD symptoms. It seems possible, therefore, that avoidant people's deactivating strategies continue to operate even when actual or symbolic attachment figures are supportive.

The second study focused on Palestinian terrorist attacks on Israeli cities and examined whether global and contextual attachment-related representations affect implicit responses to trauma (Mikulincer et al., 2006). These responses were assessed in terms of the cognitive accessibility of trauma-related mental representations in a Stroop color-naming task (Stroop, 1935). Accessibility was operationalized by the time taken to name the color in which a trauma-related word was printed: The longer the latencies for naming the colors of these words, the higher the implied accessibility of trauma-related thoughts, because such thoughts interfered with color naming. Previous studies have found longer reaction times for naming the colors of trauma-related words among people with PTSD (see Emilien et al., 2000; McNally, 1998, for reviews.)

Israeli undergraduates, who had previously reported their attachment orientations, completed a self-report scale tapping the severity of PTSD symptoms with regard to Palestinian terrorist attacks, and they were divided into two groups (PTSD, non-PTSD) according to the reported severity of their symptoms. On a later occasion they performed a Stroop color-naming task that included words connoting terror (e.g., Hamas, car bomb) as well as negatively valenced words not related to terror and some emotionally neutral words. On each trial, participants were subliminally primed with an attachment-security word (the Hebrew word for "being loved"), a positively valenced but attachment-unrelated word (success), or a neutral word (hat).

The results replicated previous findings concerning the accessibility of trauma-related thoughts among people suffering from PTSD symptoms: Participants in the PTSD group took longer, on average, to name the colors in which terror-related words were presented (indicating greater mental availability of the words) than participants in the non-PTSD group. In addition, higher scores on attachment anxiety and avoidance scales were associated with longer color-naming latencies for terror words among people with PTSD symptoms. More important, there was evidence that contextual activation of attachment security had a healing effect on implicit PTSD responses. Specifically, subliminal priming of attachment-security representations lowered the color-naming latencies of terror-related words among people who suffered from PTSD symptoms and countered the effects of attachment anxiety on these color-naming latencies. However, security priming failed to reduce the association between avoidant attachment and implicit PTSD responses. That is, the link between avoidance and longer color-naming responses for terror words was found even in the security priming condition, suggesting that avoidant people's implicit PTSD vulnerability remained even in the presence of security primes.

Overall, Mikulincer et al.'s (2006) findings support the hypothesis that mobilizing external or internal forms of security during traumatic and posttraumatic periods reduces the intensity of PTSD symptoms. The studies also show that at least some traumatized individuals respond favorably to actual support offered by familiar others in their immediate environment and to the contextual manipulation of their sense of attachment security.

Does Persistent PTSD Erode Attachment Security?

Most studies that have examined associations between PTSD and attachment orientations have been cross-sectional and so cannot reveal the causal direction of the association. Moreover, the few published prospective longitudinal studies examined changes in PTSD over time as a function of attachment orientations (e.g., Fraley et al., 2006), but not the reverse. In these studies, attachment orientations were measured only once.

The first attempt to examine within-person variability in attachment orientations over time as a function of PTSD severity was conducted by Solomon, Dekel, and Mikulincer (2008). In this study, a sample of Israeli ex-prisoners of war from the 1973 Yom Kippur War (henceforth called the "ex-POWS") and a matched control group of non-imprisoned Israeli combat veterans from the same war reported on PTSD severity and attachment orientations twice: 18 and 30 years after the war. The findings indicated that, whereas attachment anxiety and avoidance remained stable over time among control veterans, these forms of insecurity increased from Time 1 to Time 2 among ex-POWs. Moreover, increases in attachment anxiety and avoidance were associated with increases in PTSD symptoms, and PTSD severity at Time 1 predicted increases in attachment insecurities better than attachment orientations at Time 1 predicted changes in PTSD severity. These results indicate that attachment security was eroded over time among traumatized victims and that this erosion was particularly strong in cases of more severe PTSD.

In a subsequent study, Mikulincer, Ein-Dor, Solomon, and Shaver (2011) recontacted the ex-POWs and control veterans (35 years after the war) and again assessed PTSD severity and attachment orientations. Findings from a latent growth curve analysis of the impact of war captivity and PTSD revealed that attachment anxiety and avoidance continued to increase from Time 2 to Time 3 among ex-POWs and that PTSD severity was associated with attachment insecurities at each of the three time points. Thus, prolonged PTSD can erode attachment security among trauma victims.

Additional research is needed, however, to determine whether this erosion is specific to the complex trauma of captivity or can be generalized to other types of traumatic events. In answering this question, one should consider that the trauma of captivity can be viewed as an attachment injury that has repercussions on the attachment system. According to Herman (1992), "...prolonged captivity disrupts all human relationships and amplifies the dialectic of trauma. The survivor oscillates between intense attachment and terrified withdrawal" (p. 93). Therefore, it is important to discover whether or not attachment-unrelated traumas also erode attachment security over time.

Does Persistent PTSD Disrupt Regulatory Functions of the Attachment System?

In an initial attempt to explore whether the recursive, amplifying cycle of PTSD and attachment insecurities disrupt regulatory functions of the attachment system, Mikulincer, Solomon, Shaver, and Ein-Dor (2014) selected a random subsample of ex-POWs and control veterans from the 1973 Yom Kippur war who had completed self-report measures of PTSD and attachment orientations 18, 30, and 35 years after the war. The authors assessed the activation and functioning of representations of attachment security in three computerized cognitive tasks. First, participants completed Mikulincer et al.'s (2002) Stroop color-naming procedure to assess the activation of the names of security-enhancing attachment figures following subliminal priming of trauma-related words. Second, participants completed Mikulincer et al.'s (2001) affective priming procedure to assess the ability of security-related representations to color previously neutral stimuli (Chinese ideographs) with positive affect. Third, participants completed Mikulincer et al.'s (2006) Stroop color-naming procedure to assess the ability of security priming (subliminal exposure to names of security-enhancing attachment figures) to reduce the accessibility of trauma-related words.

Using data from the three waves of measurement described above, Mikulincer et al. (2011) first identified three subgroups of ex-POWs showing different trajectories of PTSD: (a) a *stable PTSD trajectory* (ex-POWs with relatively high levels of PTSD symptoms at all three time points), (b) a *unstable PTSD trajectory* (ex-POWs who reported relatively low levels of PTSD symptoms in the first wave of measurement but reported increasing levels of symptoms in the second or third waves), and (c) a *stable resilience trajectory* (ex-POWs who reported relatively low levels of PTSD symptoms at all three points). These three ex-POW groups and a group of control veterans were then compared with respect to the activation and functioning of mental representations of security.

In the Stroop task assessing activation of security representations, no significant difference was found between the various ex-POW groups and the controls. In this task, all groups exhibited longer color-naming latencies for names of attachment figures following a trauma-related prime (as compared with a neutral prime)—a sign of attachment-system activation following implicit threat. In the affective priming task, controls and ex-POWs with a stable resilience trajectory or an unstable PTSD trajectory were more likely to have a positive reaction to Chinese ideographs following a security prime (the name of an attachment figure) than following a neutral prime—a sign that security representations infused the previously neutral stimuli with positive affect. However, among ex-POWs with a stable PTSD trajectory, the usual affective priming effect did not appear, and instead, priming the name of an attachment figure led to lower ratings of the ideographs (a sign of negative affect). Finally, findings for the Stroop task assessing the healing effects of security representations revealed that ex-POWs with an unstable PTSD trajectory, as compared to controls, showed heightened access to trauma-related words following a neutral prime (an implicit symptom of PTSD), and that this heightened access was dramatically reduced by a security prime (the name of an attachment figure). Ex-POWs with a stable PTSD trajectory also evinced greater accessibility to trauma-related words (relative to controls), but the security prime failed to reduce this heightened accessibility.

Overall, these findings indicate that persistent PTSD (e.g., a stable PTSD trajectory over 17 years) not only elevates attachment anxiety and avoidance but also disrupts the regulatory functioning of the attachment system. Among trauma victims with persistent PTSD, the priming of security representations (the name of security-enhancing attachment figures) failed to induce a positive mood or lower the mental availability of trauma-related thoughts (a typical PTSD symptom). Rather, these 'security' representations seemed to be associated, implicitly, with negative mood. However, these ex-POWS still showed increased mental access to the names of security providers following exposure to trauma-related words. That is, they still implicitly sought connections with a security provider, although this person's name failed to relieve their symptoms or inhibit their access to trauma-related thoughts. In other words, persistent PTSD does not block automatic activation of the attachment system in times of need, but it keeps a trauma victim submerged in a swamp of frustration, despair, and helplessness that is not remedied by contact with symbols of human comfort and support.

In contrast, among ex-POWs with an unstable PTSD trajectory, security representations were still effective in creating a positive mood and inhibiting access to trauma-related thoughts. Moreover, these ex-POWs showed increased accessibility of names of security providers following exposure to trauma-related words. These findings indicate that their attachment systems were working properly: Ex-POWs with an unstable PTSD trajectory activated representations of security providers in times of need and these representations created a more positive mood and reduced access to trauma-related thoughts. In these ex-POWs, heightened symptoms might have been only a temporary reflection of particular life events or developmental transitions, not a sign of persistent and pervasive personality disorder.

Conclusions and Future Directions

The empirical evidence reviewed in this chapter supports our theoretical analysis of the attachment-PTSD linkage. Overall, attachment insecurities are associated with PTSD severity, and the mobilization of external or internal sources of security during traumatic and posttraumatic periods reduces the likelihood and intensity of PTSD symptoms. This helps to explain why dispositionally secure people are less likely than their insecurely attached counterparts to develop PTSD. In addition, recent studies conducted with Israeli ex-POWs show that persistent PTSD can erode attachment security and disrupt the regulatory functions of the attachment system. This makes it seem that persistent PTSD can be crystallized by a recursive, amplifying cycle of PTSD and attachment insecurities by which attachment worries and doubts contribute to heightened PTSD symptoms, and heightened PTSD (involving repeated reactivation of a trauma) can further erode the sense of security.

This research has important clinical implications. In treating trauma victims who are suffering from PTSD, one cannot ignore the associated attachment worries and doubts. Increasing a sense of security in the client–therapist relationship or through the evocation of memories or images of security-enhancing attachment figures can have a soothing effect that facilitates a good therapeutic outcome. Therapists should recognize that PTSD victims may suffer not only from trauma itself but also from a sense of loneliness, isolation, rejection, and distrust. Therapists also need to recognize that even in cases of persistent and pervasive PTSD, trauma victims are implicitly searching for a security provider when they experience threats and face painful memories. It is possible that providing experiences of security within the therapeutic setting can counteract the regulatory deficits reviewed here and reestablish the healing role of attachment security. To this end, therapists should also identify and foster other sources of security in the client's life (e.g., family members, friends, a religious community) that can facilitate and support the healing process.

Although the research reviewed here is an important initial step in understanding links between the attachment system and traumatic and posttraumatic processes, more research is needed on the hypothesized connection between traumatic helplessness and feelings of isolation, rejection, and loneliness. It is important to determine whether such feelings actually arise during and after trauma, whether they intensify PTSD symptoms, and whether interventions aimed at enhancing a person's sense of connectedness, belongingness, and community can reduce or prevent PTSD. Research should also examine the extent to which attachment security contributes to reconstruction and strengthening of comforting, health-sustaining beliefs shattered by trauma—i.e., to posttraumatic growth (Tedeschi & Calhoun, 2004). In fact, attachment security has already been associated with cognitive openness and creative exploration of personal experiences (e.g., Mikulincer, 1997), which Tedeschi and Calhoun (2004) viewed as important ingredients of posttraumatic growth. Finally, future research should examine more thoroughly the process of security erosion produced by persistent PTSD and the ways in which this harmful outcome can be prevented or reversed.

Acknowledgment Preparation of this chapter was facilitated by a grant from the US–Israel Bi-national Science Foundation.

References

Ainsworth, M. D. S., Blehar, M. C., Waters, E., & Wall, S. (1978). *Patterns of attachment: Assessed in the Strange Situation and at home*. Hillsdale, NJ: Erlbaum.

Alexander, P. C., Anderson, C. L., Brand, B., Schaeffer, C. M., Grelling, B. Z., & Kretz, L. (1998). Adult attachment and long-term effects in survivors of incest. *Child Abuse and Neglect, 22*, 45–61.

American Psychiatric Association. (1994). *Diagnostic and statistical manual of mental disorders* (4th ed.). Washington, DC: Author.

Baldwin, M. W., & Fehr, B. (1995). On the instability of attachment style ratings. *Personal Relationships, 2*, 247–261.

Ball, T. M., & Stein, M. B. (2012). Classification of posttraumatic stress disorder. In J. G. Beck & D. M. Sloan (Eds.), *The Oxford handbook of traumatic stress disorders* (pp. 39–53). New York: Oxford University Press.

Benoit, M., Bouthillier, D., Moss, E., Rousseau, C., & Brunet, A. (2010). Emotion regulation strategies as mediators of the association between level of attachment security and PTSD symptoms following trauma in adulthood. *Anxiety, Stress, and Coping, 23*, 101–118.

Berant, E., Mikulincer, M., & Shaver, P. R. (2008). Mothers' attachment style, their mental health, and their children's emotional vulnerabilities: A seven-year study of children with congenital heart disease. *Journal of Personality, 76*, 31–66.

Besser, A., & Neria, Y. (2010). The effects of insecure attachment orientations and perceived social support on posttraumatic stress and depressive symptoms among civilians exposed to the 2009 Israel-Gaza war: A follow-up cross-lagged panel design study. *Journal of Research in Personality, 44*, 335–341.

Besser, A., & Neria, Y. (2012). When home isn't a safe haven: Insecure attachment orientations, perceived social support, and PTSD symptoms among Israeli evacuees under missile threat. *Psychological Trauma, 4*, 34–46.

Besser, A., Neria, Y., & Haynes, M. (2009). Adult attachment, perceived stress, and PTSD among civilians exposed to ongoing terrorist attacks in Southern Israel. *Personality and Individual Differences, 47*, 851–857.

Bogaerts, S., Daalder, A. L., Van Der Knaap, L. M., Kunst, M. J. J. M., & Buschman, J. (2008). Critical incident, adult attachment style, and posttraumatic stress disorder: A comparison of three groups of security workers. *Social Behavior and Personality, 36*, 1063–1072.

Bogaerts, S., Kunst, M. J. J., & Winkel, F. W. (2009). Dismissive attachment and posttraumatic stress disorder among securely and insecurely attached Belgium security workers. *Psychological Reports, 105*, 889–899.

Bowlby, J. (1973). *Attachment and loss: Vol. 2. Separation: Anxiety and anger*. New York: Basic Books.

Bowlby, J. (1980). *Attachment and loss: Vol. 3. Sadness and depression*. New York: Basic Books.

Bowlby, J. (1982). *Attachment and loss: Vol. 1. Attachment* (2nd ed.). New York: Basic Books.

Bowlby, J. (1988). *A secure base: Clinical applications of attachment theory*. London: Routledge.

Brennan, K. A., Clark, C. L., & Shaver, P. R. (1998). Self-report measurement of adult attachment: An integrative overview. In J. A. Simpson & W. S. Rholes (Eds.), *Attachment theory and close relationships* (pp. 46–76). New York: Guilford Press.

Cassidy, J., & Kobak, R. R. (1988). Avoidance and its relationship with other defensive processes. In J. Belsky & T. Nezworski (Eds.), *Clinical implications of attachment* (pp. 300–323). Hillsdale, NJ: Erlbaum.

Cassidy, J., & Shaver, P. R. (Eds.). (2008). *Handbook of attachment: Theory, research, and clinical applications* (2nd ed.). New York: Guilford Press.

Cohen, E., Dekel, R., & Solomon, Z. (2002). Long-term adjustment and the role of attachment among Holocaust child survivors. *Personality and Individual Differences, 33*, 299–310.

Davila, J., & Cobb, R. J. (2004). Predictors of changes in attachment security during adulthood. In W. S. Rholes & J. A. Simpson (Eds.), *Adult attachment: Theory, research, and clinical implications* (pp. 133–156). New York: Guilford Press.

Davis, D., Shaver, P. R., & Vernon, M. L. (2003). Physical, emotional, and behavioral reactions to breaking up: The roles of gender, age, emotional involvement, and attachment style. *Personality and Social Psychology Bulletin, 29*, 871–884.

Declercq, F., & Willemsen, J. (2006). Distress and post-traumatic stress disorders in high risk professionals: Adult attachment style and the dimensions of anxiety and avoidance. *Clinical Psychology and Psychotherapy, 13*, 256–263.

Dekel, R., Solomon, Z., Ginzburg, K., & Neria, Y. (2004). Long-term adjustment among Israeli war veterans: The role of attachment style. *Anxiety, Stress, and Coping, 17*, 141–152.

Dieperink, M., Leskela, J., Thuras, P., & Engdahl, B. (2001). Attachment style classification and posttraumatic stress disorder in former prisoners of war. *American Journal of Orthopsychiatry, 71*, 374–378.

Elwood, L. S., & Williams, N. L. (2007). PTSD-related cognitions and romantic attachment style as moderators of psychological symptoms in victims of interpersonal trauma. *Journal of Social and Clinical Psychology, 26*, 1189–1209.

Emilien, G., Penasse, C., Charles, G., Martin, D., Lasseaux, L., & Waltregny, A. (2000). Post-traumatic stress disorder: Hypotheses from clinical neuropsychology and psychopharmacology research. *International Journal of Psychiatry in Clinical Practice, 4*, 3–18.

Forbes, D., Parslow, R., Fletcher, S., McHugh, T., & Creamer, M. (2010). Attachment style in the prediction of recovery following group treatment of combat veterans with post-traumatic stress disorder. *Journal of Nervous and Mental Disease, 198*, 881–884.

Fraley, R. C., Fazzari, D. A., Bonanno, G. A., & Dekel, S. (2006). Attachment and psychological adaptation in high exposure survivors of the September 11th attack on the World Trade Center. *Personality and Social Psychology Bulletin, 32*, 538–551.

Fraley, R. C., & Shaver, P. R. (2000). Adult romantic attachment: Theoretical developments, emerging controversies, and unanswered questions. *Review of General Psychology, 4*, 132–154.

Fredrickson, B. L. (2001). The role of positive emotions in positive psychology: The broaden-and-build theory of positive emotions. *American Psychologist, 56*, 218–226.

George, C., & West, M. (2001). The development and preliminary validation of a new measure of adult attachment: The adult attachment projective. *Attachment and Human Development, 3*, 30–61.

Ghafoori, B., Hierholzer, R. W., Howsepian, B., & Boardman, A. (2008). The role of adult attachment, parental bonding, and spiritual love in the adjustment to military trauma. *Journal of Trauma and Dissociation, 9*, 85–106.

Harari, D., Bakermans-Kranenburg, M. J., de Kloet, C. S., Geuze, E., Vermetten, E., Westenberg, H. G. M., et al. (2009). Attachment representations in Dutch veterans with and without deployment-related PTSD. *Attachment and Human Development, 11*, 515–536.

Hazan, C., & Shaver, P. R. (1987). Romantic love conceptualized as an attachment process. *Journal of Personality and Social Psychology, 52*, 511–524.
Herman, J. L. (1992). *Trauma and recovery*. New York: Basic Books.
Horowitz, M. J. (1982). Psychological processes induced by illness, injury, and loss. In T. Millon, C. Green, & R. Meagher (Eds.), *Handbook of clinical health psychology* (pp. 53–68). New York: Plenum Press.
Horowitz, M. J., Wilner, N., & Alvarez, W. (1979). Impact of Event Scale: A measure of subjective stress. *Psychosomatic Medicine, 41*, 209–218.
Kanninen, K., Punamaki, R. L., & Qouta, S. (2003). Personality and trauma: Adult attachment and posttraumatic distress among former political prisoners. *Peace and Conflict: Journal of Peace Psychology, 9*, 97–126.
Main, M., Hesse, E., & Goldwyn, R. (2009). Studying differences in language usage in recounting attachment history: An introduction to the AAI. In H. Steele & M. Steele (Eds.), *Clinical applications of the adult attachment interview* (pp. 31–68). New York: Guilford Press.
McNally, R. J. (1998). Experimental approaches to cognitive abnormality in posttraumatic stress disorder. *Clinical Psychology Review, 18*, 971–982.
Mikulincer, M. (1997). Adult attachment style and information processing: Individual differences in curiosity and cognitive closure. *Journal of Personality and Social Psychology, 72*, 1217–1230.
Mikulincer, M., Ein-Dor, T., Solomon, Z., & Shaver, P. R. (2011). Trajectories of attachment insecurities over a 17-year period: A Latent Growth Curve analysis of the impact of war captivity and posttraumatic stress disorder. *Journal of Social and Clinical Psychology, 30*, 960–984.
Mikulincer, M., Florian, V., & Weller, A. (1993). Attachment styles, coping strategies, and posttraumatic psychological distress: The impact of the Gulf War in Israel. *Journal of Personality and Social Psychology, 64*, 817–826.
Mikulincer, M., Gillath, O., & Shaver, P. R. (2002). Activation of the attachment system in adulthood: Threat-related primes increase the accessibility of mental representations of attachment figures. *Journal of Personality and Social Psychology, 83*, 881–895.
Mikulincer, M., Hirschberger, G., Nachmias, O., & Gillath, O. (2001). The affective component of the secure base schema: Affective priming with representations of attachment security. *Journal of Personality and Social Psychology, 81*, 305–321.
Mikulincer, M., Horesh, N., Eilati, I., & Kotler, M. (1999). The association between adult attachment style and mental health in extreme life endangering conditions. *Personality and Individual Differences, 27*, 831–842.
Mikulincer, M., & Shaver, P. R. (2003). The attachment behavioral system in adulthood: Activation, psychodynamics, and interpersonal processes. In M. P. Zanna (Ed.), *Advances in experimental social psychology* (Vol. 35, pp. 53–152). San Diego, CA: Academic Press.
Mikulincer, M., & Shaver, P. R. (2007a). *Attachment in adulthood: Structure, dynamics, and change*. New York: Guilford Press.
Mikulincer, M., & Shaver, P. R. (2007b). Boosting attachment security to promote mental health, prosocial values, and inter-group tolerance. *Psychological Inquiry, 18*, 139–156.
Mikulincer, M., Shaver, P. R., Sapir-Lavid, Y., & Avihou-Kanza, N. (2009). What's inside the minds of securely and insecurely attached people? The secure-base script and its associations with attachment-style dimensions. *Journal of Personality and Social Psychology, 97*, 615–633.
Mikulincer, M., Shaver, P. R., & Horesh, N. (2006). Attachment bases of emotion regulation and posttraumatic adjustment. In D. K. Snyder, J. A. Simpson, & J. N. Hughes (Eds.), *Emotion regulation in families: Pathways to dysfunction and health* (pp. 77–99). Washington, DC: American Psychological Association.
Mikulincer, M., Solomon, Z., Shaver, P. R., & Ein-Dor, T. (2014). Attachment-related consequences of war captivity and trajectories of posttraumatic stress disorder: A 17-year longitudinal study. *Journal of Social and Clinical Psychology, 33*, 207–228.
Muller, R. T., & Lemieux, K. E. (2000). Social support, attachment, and psychopathology in high risk formerly maltreated adults. *Child Abuse and Neglect, 24*, 883–900.
Muller, R. T., & Rosenkranz, S. E. (2009). Attachment and treatment response among adults in inpatient treatment for posttraumatic stress disorder. *Psychotherapy, 46*, 82–96.

Muller, R. T., Sicoli, L. A., & Lemieux, K. E. (2000). Relationship between attachment style and posttraumatic stress symptomatology among adults who report the experience of childhood abuse. *Journal of Traumatic Stress, 13*, 321–332.

Neria, Y., Guttmann-Steinmetz, S., Koenen, K., Levinovsky, L., Zakin, G., & Dekel, R. (2001). Do attachment and hardiness relate to each other and to mental health in real-life stress? *Journal of Social and Personal Relationships, 18*, 844–858.

Nye, E. C., Katzman, J., Bell, J. B., Kilpatrick, J., Brainard, M., & Haaland, K. Y. (2008). Attachment organization in Vietnam combat veterans with posttraumatic stress disorder. *Attachment & Human Development, 10*, 41–57.

Renaud, E. F. (2008). The attachment characteristics of combat veterans with PTSD. *Traumatology, 14*, 1–12.

Roche, D. N., Runtz, M. G., & Hunter, M. A. (1999). Adult attachment: A mediator between child sexual abuse and later psychological adjustment. *Journal of Interpersonal Violence, 14*, 184–207.

Sandberg, D. A. (2010). Adult attachment as a predictor of posttraumatic stress and dissociation. *Journal of Trauma and Dissociation, 11*, 293–307.

Sandberg, D. A., Suess, E. A., & Heaton, J. L. (2010). Attachment anxiety as a mediator of the relationship between interpersonal trauma and posttraumatic symptomatology among college women. *Journal of Interpersonal Violence, 25*, 33–49.

Scott, S., & Babcock, J. C. (2010). Attachment as a moderator between intimate partner violence and PTSD symptoms. *Journal of Family Violence, 25*, 1–9.

Shapiro, D. L., & Levendosky, A. A. (1999). Adolescent survivors of childhood sexual abuse: The mediating role of attachment style and coping in psychological and interpersonal functioning. *Child Abuse and Neglect, 23*, 1175–1191.

Shaver, P. R., & Hazan, C. (1993). Adult romantic attachment: Theory and evidence. In D. Perlman & W. Jones (Eds.), *Advances in personal relationships* (Vol. 4, pp. 29–70). London: Jessica Kingsley.

Shaver, P. R., & Mikulincer, M. (2002). Attachment-related psychodynamics. *Attachment and Human Development, 4*, 133–161.

Shaver, P. R., & Mikulincer, M. (2008). Augmenting the sense of security in romantic, leader-follower, therapeutic, and group relationships: A relational model of psychological change. In J. P. Forgas & J. Fitness (Eds.), *Social relationships: Cognitive, affective, and motivational processes* (pp. 55–74). New York: Psychology Press.

Simpson, J. A., & Rholes, W. S. (2002). Fearful-avoidance, disorganization, and multiple working models: Some directions for future theory and research. *Attachment and Human Development, 4*, 223–229.

Solomon, Z., Dekel, R., & Mikulincer, M. (2008). Complex trauma of war captivity: A prospective study of attachment and posttraumatic stress disorder. *Psychological Medicine, 38*, 1427–1434.

Solomon, Z., Ginzburg, K., Mikulincer, M., Neria, Y., & Ohry, A. (1998). Coping with war captivity: The role of attachment style. *European Journal of Personality, 12*, 271–285.

Stroop, J. R. (1935). Studies of interference in serial verbal reactions. *Journal of Experimental Psychology, 18*, 643–662.

Tedeschi, R. G., & Calhoun, L. G. (2004). Posttraumatic growth: Conceptual foundations and empirical evidence. *Psychological Inquiry, 15*, 1–18.

Twaite, J. A., & Rodriguez-Srednicki, O. (2004). Childhood sexual and physical abuse and adult vulnerability to PTSD: The mediating effects of attachment and dissociation. *Journal of Child Sexual Abuse, 13*, 17–38.

Waters, H. S., & Waters, E. (2006). The attachment working models concept: Among other things, we build scriptlike representations of secure base experiences. *Attachment and Human Development, 8*, 185–198.

Zakin, G., Solomon, Z., & Neria, Y. (2003). Hardiness, attachment style, and long-term psychological distress among Israeli POWs and combat veterans. *Personality and Individual Differences, 34*, 819–829.

Chapter 5
Delayed-Onset PTSD in Israeli Combat Veterans: Correlates, Clinical Picture, and Controversy

Danny Horesh, Zahava Solomon, Giora Keinan, and Tsachi Ein-Dor

Introduction

Combat Stress and Its Psychological Toll

It is a well-established fact that combat experiences are often highly traumatic. Combat has both short-term (acute) and long-term (chronic) pathological implications. Combat stress reaction (CSR) is the most common acute reaction on the battlefield. It consists of polymorphic and labile psychiatric and somatic symptoms, and is diagnosed by trained clinicians based on impaired functioning. Among the symptoms that may characterize this condition are paralyzing fear of death, emotional and physical numbness, and impaired combat functioning (Kardiner & Spiegel, 1947). In some instances, the initial reaction to stress subsides after a period of time, while in other instances it crystallizes into a more chronic disorder (Solomon, 1993). The long-term consequences of exposure to stress may be expressed in several ways, the most common of which is posttraumatic stress disorder (PTSD).

D. Horesh, Ph.D. (✉)
Department of Psychology, Bar Ilan University, Ramat Gan 5290002, Israel

Department of Psychiatry, New York University, School of Medicine, New York, NY 10016, USA
e-mail: danny.horesh@biu.ac.il

Z. Solomon, Ph.D.
Bob Shapell School of Social Work, Tel Aviv University, Tel Aviv 69978, Israel
e-mail: Solomon@post.tau.ac.il

G. Keinan, Ph.D.
Department of Psychology, Tel Aviv University, Tel Aviv 69978, Israel
e-mail: giorak@post.tau.ac.il

T. Ein-Dor, Ph.D.
School of Psychology, Interdisciplinary Center (IDC), Herzliya 46150, Israel
e-mail: teindor@idc.ac.il

M.P. Safir et al. (eds.), *Future Directions in Post-Traumatic Stress Disorder*,
DOI 10.1007/978-1-4899-7522-5_5

In most cases, PTSD erupts after a relatively short period following the traumatic event. However, in some cases PTSD onset is delayed for months and even years. According to DSM-V (APA, 2013), when PTSD erupts at least 6 months post-trauma it is defined as delayed-onset PTSD (DPTSD). This phenomenon is yet to be fully understood. For many years, there has been considerable debate regarding its validity, prevalence, and etiology. Despite interest aroused among the trauma research community, a relatively small number of empirical investigations of DPTSD have been conducted. The following chapter will discuss the prevalence, correlates, and clinical picture of DPTSD among Israeli veterans who were longitudinally assessed following the 1982 Lebanon War.

Delayed-Onset PTSD: Controversy and Prevalence

Reports of DPTSD have appeared for at least 60 years (e.g., Krystal, 1968). Still, there has been a substantial medicolegal debate regarding the validity of this phenomenon. Some have argued that seemingly new cases of PTSD are actually manifestations of malingering (Smith & Frueh, 1996), while others (e.g., Pary, Turns, & Tobias, 1986) have claimed that in many cases it is not the disorder that is delayed, but rather its diagnosis, or seeking of treatment for posttraumatic symptoms.

Although some have questioned the validity of DPTSD, a growing body of literature has been published supporting the existence of this phenomenon (e.g., Smid, van der Velden, Gersons, & Kleber, 2012). In fact, DPTSD has been found among victims of various kinds of traumatic events, such as motor vehicle accidents (Mayou, Bryant, & Duthrie, 1993), natural disasters (Green et al., 1990), incest (Green, Coupe, Fernandez, & Stevens, 1995), and combat (Solomon, Mikulincer, Waysman, & Marlowe, 1991). In addition, a meta-analysis of prospective DPTSD studies (Smid, Mooren, Van der Mast, Gersons, & Kleber, 2009) has demonstrated convincing evidence supporting the validity of this phenomenon, as well as specific factors associated with it.

The first aim of our study was to assess the prevalence of DPTSD among a sample of both traumatized and non-traumatized war veterans. Throughout the years, epidemiological studies have shown great variance in the prevalence of DPTSD among trauma survivors (Andrews, Brewin, Philpott, & Stewart, 2007), with rates ranging from around zero (Frueh, Grubaugh, Yeager, & Magruder, 2009) to almost 20 % (McFarlane, 1988) of entire samples (participants both with and without PTSD) and from zero (Epstein, 1993) to 68 % (Op den Velde et al., 1993) of participants with PTSD. This extremely wide variance in prevalence may stem from various reasons, mainly differences in the definition of DPTSD, study design, and sample size. The type of trauma examined may also be associated with prevalence of DPTSD. For example, in recent years, there has been at least some evidence that the prevalence of DPTSD following combat is relatively high compared to other types of traumatic events (Prigerson, Maciejewski, & Rosenheck, 2001).

The Clinical Picture of DPTSD

A second aim of our study was to assess the clinical picture of DPTSD, and more specifically to examine whether it may be clinically differentiated from non-delayed PTSD. Previous studies have reported mixed results regarding the clinical picture of DPTSD, with some showing DPTSD to be associated with less severe psychopathology than non-delayed PTSD (Bryant & Harvey, 2002), and others failing to find any connection between the time of PTSD onset and the level of psychopathology (Andrews, Brewin, Stewart, Philpott, & Hejdenberg, 2009). Thus, a question still remains as to whether DPTSD should be considered a clinical subtype of PTSD, with its own unique characteristics.

Another question that remains regarding the nature of DPTSD is whether symptoms erupt after a purely non-symptomatic period, or rather that this phenomenon is a manifestation of a latent disorder that has existed "in the background" for some time. While case reports of DPTSD often give the impression of a very sudden PTSD onset, which occurred after a very long non-symptomatic period (e.g., Reich, 2006), these descriptions, for the most part, do not stand the test of empirical examination. Most studies reveal that DPTSD appears after the victim had already suffered from some previous level of symptoms (e.g., Smid, Lensvelt-Mulders, Knipscheer, Gersons, & Kleber, 2011).

Finally, another clinical issue that has yet to be clarified is the association between acute reactions to stress and DPTSD. Acute stress disorder has been shown to serve as a risk factor for various subsequent psychiatric problems and disorders (Bryant & Harvey, 1998). This was also found specifically regarding combat stress reaction (CSR), an acute reaction to combat trauma (Solomon & Mikulincer, 2006). To date, only one study that we know of reexamined the possible relation between acute stress disorder and the time of PTSD onset (Bryant & Harvey, 2002), and none have examined the association between CSR and DPTSD. Thus, in this study, we have attempted to bridge this gap by including CSR as a possible predictor for the time on PTSD onset.

The Underlying Mechanisms of DPTSD

DPTSD is still a poorly understood phenomenon. A few years after the Vietnam War, Horowitz and Solomon (1975) suggested that when soldiers return from the battlefield to the safe and comfortable environment of their homes, they gradually let go of the defense mechanisms which they employed on the battlefield. This, in turn, allows the eruption of posttraumatic symptoms that remained hidden for some time. Over the years, several cognitive (Ehlers & Clark, 2000), psychodynamic, (Shatan, 1973) and biological (Pitman, 1989) explanations for DPTSD have been proposed. However, evidence supporting these explanations remains scarce, and there is a need for empirical studies attempting to explain DPTSD.

The present study aimed to examine the role of several personal and social resources in DPTSD: Social support, locus of control, and both emotion- and problem-focused coping. Studies have consistently found that resources may shield against the effects of traumatic stress (e.g., Hyman, Gold, & Cott, 2003), including combat-related stress (King, King, Fairbank, Keane, & Adams, 1998). The role of resources in the realm of traumatic stress is perhaps best described by Hobfoll's (1988) Conservation of Resources (COR) theory. The theory's basic assumption is that people strive to retain, protect, and build resources, and that what is threatening to them is the potential or actual loss of these resources. The prominent role of resource loss in COR theory makes it a very useful theoretical framework for the study of trauma. Following a traumatic event, resource loss is often fast, extensive, and deep. An example of a loss spiral is the one created by the combat stress (Hobfoll, 1998). Traumatic experiences during combat often deplete the same resources the veteran will need in order to recover from his emotional wounds (Solomon et al., 1992).

Locus of Control, Social Support, and Ways of Coping

The present study examined the role of three resources in DPTSD: locus of control, social support, and ways of coping. These three variables have been traditionally known for their stress-buffering role following trauma.

Locus of control

The concept of perceived control has been known to have special importance in the study of stress. One of the best-known formulations of perceived control is the concept of locus of control, i.e., the patterned ways in which an individual perceives the sources of control over unforeseen stressors (Rotter, 1975). An internal locus of control refers to the belief that events are contingent upon one's own behavior, while external locus of control refers to the belief that events are not contingent upon one's actions but rather on luck, fate, chance, or powerful others. While many studies have found a positive connection between PTSD and external locus of control (e.g., Brown, Mulhern, & Joseph, 2002), some studies have failed to find such a connection (Barouk, 2005).

Social support

Social support has been consistently found to buffer adverse psychological consequences of traumatic events (e.g., Hyman et al., 2003). Cohen, Hettler, and Park (1997) have suggested several potential functions of social support, including emotional support, social integration or network support, esteem support, and informational support. Much of the research on the stress-moderating function of social support has been conducted on combat-related PTSD (e.g. Solomon, Mikulincer, & Waysman, 1991). However, it should be noted that while the negative association between combat-related PTSD and social support is well established (e.g., Koenen, Stellman, Stellman, & Sommer, 2003), the directionality of this association is often the subject of debate (King, Taft, King, Hammond, & Stone, 2006).

Ways of coping

Lazarus and Folkman (1984) have defined coping as constantly changing cognitive and behavioral efforts to manage specific external and/or internal demands that are appraised as taxing or exceeding the resources of the person. Studies on stress have identified several major categories of coping strategies, among them problem-focused coping, emotion-focused coping, seeking social support, and religious coping (Aldwin & Yancura, 2004). Of these, the most common distinction is between problem-focused, or "active" coping, and emotion-focused, or "palliative" coping. Problem-focused strategies are intended to manage the problem by removing or circumventing the stressor; Emotion-focused coping, on the other hand, is designed to regulate, reduce, or eliminate the emotional distress associated with the stressful situation (e.g., emotional avoidance, positive reappraisal of the threatening situation). Much of this research indicates that problem-focused coping with stress has positive psychological outcomes (e.g., Silver, Holman, McIntosh, Poulin, & Gil-Rivas, 2002). Emotion-focused coping, on the other hand, has often been found to be associated with higher levels of posttraumatic stress (Zeidner & Ben-Zur, 1994), anxiety, and depression (Compas, Worsham, Ey, & Howell, 1996). Nonetheless, findings about both emotion and problem-focused coping remain, for the most part, inconclusive.

Coping was also often found to mediate the effects of other resources on psychological well-being. Lazarus and Folkman (1984) defined personal and social resources as what an individual "draws on in order to cope", and argued that these resources "precede and influence coping" (p. 158). This definition strongly suggests the mediating role of coping, which has been confirmed by several studies (e.g. Brown et al., 2002; Holahan & Moos, 1994).

Psychological Resources and DPTSD

The role of psychological resources was also studied specifically in the context of DPTSD. However, these studies are few and far between. Studies examining the role of social support in DPTSD have yielded mixed results. Some studies have found an association between social support and DPTSD (e.g., McFarlane, 1988), including following war trauma (Nitto, 2001), while others have failed to find such a connection (e.g., Buckley, Blanchard, & Hickling, 1996). The locus of control and coping has been scarcely studied vis-à-vis DPTSD. In an earlier assessment conducted by members of our team, veterans with DPTSD did not differ from veterans with non-delayed PTSD in their locus of control. The former did, however, use more problem-focused coping than the latter (Solomon, 1989).

Mixed findings were also found regarding the role of other resources (e.g., self-esteem, positive perceptions) in relation to DPTSD (Boscarino & Adams, 2009; Gray, Bolton, & Litz, 2004). Reviewed together, studies that have examined the role of psychological resources in DPTSD have failed to reveal a clear picture. This may result from vast differences between these studies in design, sample size, type of trauma, and length of follow-up period.

The Present Study: Veterans of the 1982 Lebanon War

As may be seen, the literature regarding DPTSD does not present a clear picture regarding the prevalence, clinical characteristics, and correlates of this phenomenon. In many ways, delayed PTSD remains an enigma, and its underlying mechanisms have yet to be fully understood, as most of our knowledge regarding DPTSD comes from studies with significant methodological weaknesses. Many are case studies (e.g., Ramchandani, 1990) and/or studies with retrospective designs (e.g. Yule et al., 2000). While prospective studies of DPTSD do exist, they are relatively rare, and are often based on short-term follow-ups (e.g., Koren, Arnon, & Klein, 2001) that limit the ability to examine the true scope of this phenomenon. Finally, to the best of our knowledge, no study of delayed PTSD has empirically examined a multivariable model for this phenomenon. The vast majority of studies examined the role of various factors that may contribute to DPTSD, without exploring their complex interrelationships.

In light of these gaps, the present study presents a longitudinal prospective examination of DPTSD, across a 20-year period. The study also examined a multivariable model for the possible role of psychological resources in DPTSD. The study aimed to prospectively examine the prevalence, clinical picture, and correlates of DPTSD among a large sample of Israeli veterans of the 1982 Lebanon War. The study is part of a large scale longitudinal study, which was initiated 30 years ago by the Israel Defense Forces (IDF) mental health research branch. This data set has already yielded many reports concerning various aspects of posttraumatic distress among veterans (e.g., Solomon & Mikulincer, 2006; Zerach, Solomon, Horesh, & Ein-Dor, 2013), including several studies of delayed-onset PTSD (e.g. Horesh et al., 2011; Solomon, Mikulincer, & Waysman, 1991).

Research Hypotheses

This study examined the clinical picture and psychological correlates of DPTSD, among a sample of both combat stress reaction (CSR) casualties and comparable combatants. We examined a model of the role of three resources in DPTSD: locus of control, social support, and ways of coping. This model prospectively examined whether the levels of these resources 2 years following the war predicted the future course of PTSD. More specifically, the model attempted to uncover whether there is an association between the level of psychological resources 2 years following the war and the duration of delay in PTSD onset over the course of 20 years after the war.

The study examined the following hypotheses:

1. The duration of delay in PTSD onset (the time gap between exposure to trauma and first onset of PTSD) will be negatively associated with the severity of psychopathology: veterans with longer delays in PTSD onset will report lower levels of psychopathology.
2. Combat stress reaction (CSR) will be negatively associated with the duration of delay in PTSD onset: veterans with antecedent CSR will demonstrate a shorter delay in PTSD onset.
3. In most cases, DPTSD will appear after a symptomatic, rather than asymptomatic, period.
4. The duration of delay in PTSD onset will be positively associated with higher levels of psychological resources (i.e., more social support, internal locus of control, and problem-focused coping); Emotion-focused coping will be negatively associated with the duration of delay in PTSD onset.
5. Coping will mediate the associations between social support/locus of control and the duration of delay in PTSD onset.

Method

Participants

Six-hundred and seventy-five male veterans from the 1982 Lebanon War were assessed at three points in time after the war had ended: 1 year postwar (Time 1), 2 years postwar (Time 2), and 20 years postwar (Time 3). All 675 participants were divided into four study groups, according to the duration of delay in PTSD onset: (1) the "*1983 onset*" group consisted of veterans who already met PTSD symptom criteria at the first assessment. (2) The "*1984 onset*" group consisted of veterans who did not meet PTSD symptom criteria at the first assessment, but did meet the criteria at the second assessment. (3) The "*2002 onset*" group consisted of veterans who did not meet PTSD symptom criteria at the first and second assessments, but did meet criteria at the third assessment. (4) The "*no PTSD*" group consisted of veterans who did not meet PTSD symptom criteria at any of the three assessments.

These four groups represent different levels of delay in PTSD onset, with the 1983 onset group representing the shortest duration of delay, and the no PTSD group representing the longest duration of delay, as these veterans still have not suffered from any PTSD. Thus, DPTSD is not defined here according to the 6-month DSM threshold. Rather, we assess the *relative* delay in PTSD onset. The delay in PTSD is regarded as a continuum in time, on which a first PTSD onset 2 years after the war represents a longer delay in onset than a first PTSD onset 1 year postwar. No differences were found between the study groups in family status, military rank, socioeconomic status before the war, level of education, age, and number of children.

Of the 675 veterans participating in this study, 369 experienced psychic breakdown on the battlefield and were identified as suffering from Combat Stress Reaction (CSR). The remaining 306 veterans served in the same frontline combat units as the CSR group, but did not show symptoms of CSR. For each CSR casualty, a matched control participant was randomly selected from among eligible soldiers who had similar socio-demographic characteristics (age, education, military rank, and assignment).

Procedure

One and two years following the 1982 Lebanon War, participants were asked to report to the headquarters of the IDF Surgeon General to take part in this study. They filled out a battery of questionnaires in small groups. Data in the third wave (2002) were collected at the veterans' homes. The participants' consent was obtained, and they were informed that the data will remain confidential, and will in no way influence their status in military or civilian life.

Measures of psychopathology and physical health were administered at all 3 points of measurement. Battle exposure and socio-demographic variables were examined at time 1. The resources included in the research model were all measured at time 2 (1984), to ensure standardization in time.

Attrition and Handling of Missing Data

Six-hundred and seventy-five veterans participated in the study at 1983 (Time 1). Of those, 462 also participated at 1984 (Time 2), constituting a 68.4 % participation rate at follow-up. Of those 462 veterans, 296 participated in the third and final follow-up at 2002, constituting 64.1 % of those who participated in the first two assessments. Overall, these final 296 veterans constitute 43.9 % of the original sample that started at 1983. Missing data were handled using Multiple Imputation (MI; Rubin, 1987), a widely used and recommended method for handling missing data in longitudinal studies (e.g., Newman, 2003). In order to examine whether our data filled the basic requirements of MI, we employed Little's missing completely at random (MCAR) test ($\chi^2 = 2{,}865.160$, df = 5,829, Sig. = 1.000).

Measures

Posttraumatic Stress Disorder Inventory

The PTSD inventory (Solomon, Weisenberg, Schwarzwald, & Mikulincer, 1987) consists of 13 statements describing the DSM-III (APA, 1980) symptoms of PTSD, as adapted for combat trauma. DSM-III was the standard used when the study commenced, and was therefore employed to allow standardization across measurements. The 13 symptoms correspond to the three DSM criteria groups for the diagnosis of PTSD: (1) reexperiencing of the trauma (2) numbing of responsiveness to- or avoidance of the external world (3) additional symptoms, including hyper-alertness, sleep disturbance, and memory or concentration difficulties. Participants were asked to indicate whether or not they had suffered from each symptom during the month preceding the assessment. In line with DSM-III symptom criteria, participants were diagnosed with PTSD if they endorsed at least one reexperiencing symptom, one numbing/avoidance symptom, and two hyper-alertness symptoms. The PTSD inventory was previously found to have good psychometric qualities (see Solomon et al., 1993). In the present study, Cronbach's Alphas for this inventory ranged from 0.89 in 1983 and 1984 to 0.92 in 2002.

Impact of Event Scale (IES)

The IES (Horowitz, Wilner, & Avlarez, 1979) describes 16 emotional reactions tapping intrusion and avoidance symptoms. The respondent is asked to indicate (on a 4-point scale ranging from "not at all" to "very often") how frequently he/she experienced each reaction during the previous week. Two total scores—intrusion and avoidance—are then calculated by summing the items corresponding to each scale. The IES was translated into Hebrew and tailored to the specific stressor of combat. The Hebrew version was found to have high validity (Schwarzwald, Solomon, Weisenberg, & Mikulincer, 1987). In the present study, Cronbach's alphas across waves of measurement ranged from 0.91 to 0.95 for the entire scale, 0.78 to 0.87 for the avoidance subscale, and 0.93 to 0.95 for the intrusion subscale.

Symptoms Checklist-90-R (SCL-90-R)

The SCL-90-R (Derogatis, 1977) is composed of 90 self-report items, each referring to a specific psychiatric symptom. For each item, the respondent is asked to rate on a 5-point scale ranging from "not at all" to "very much" the degree to which he suffered from the symptom during the preceding 2 weeks. The scale includes nine symptom dimensions: somatization, obsessive–compulsive problems, interpersonal sensitivity, depression, anxiety, hostility, phobic anxiety, paranoid ideation, and psychoticism. In addition, the scale yields a global score—The Global Severity Index (GSI)—which represents the participant's mean score on all 90 symptoms. The SCL-90-R was found to have good validity (Peveler & Fairburn, 1990). In the present study, Cronbach's alphas ranged from 0.98 to 0.99 across the waves of measurement.

Problems in functioning

A self-report questionnaire assessing problems in functioning was constructed for the purpose of the present study. Participants were presented with a list of 33 problems from various areas of life, and asked to indicate whether or not each item describes a problem that arose since the Lebanon War (Yes/No). A factor analyses with Promax rotation yielded four factors, each comprising of problems in: (1) family functioning. (2) Inter-personal relationships. (3) Work and physical health. (4) Receiving help from others. A general score was calculated for the entire questionnaire, as well as separate scores for each subscale. Cronbach's alpha for the entire scale was 0.93 at all three measurements. Good reliabilities were also found for the following subscales across measurements: receiving help ($\alpha=0.81$–0.83), relationships ($\alpha=0.88$ at all waves), and work/physical health ($\alpha=0.81$–0.83). Adequate reliability was found for family functioning ($\alpha=0.60$–0.74).

Physical health

Physical health was assessed using two questions: (a) Perceived health status was assessed via the question: "How would you define your present physical health status?" (from 1—"very bad" to 5—"very good"). This question is commonly used in health surveys and was consistently found to have an independent contribution to the prediction of mortality and future health outcomes (Benyamini & Idler, 1999). (b) Veterans were also asked whether or not they began suffering from health problems in the following areas from the beginning of the Lebanon War (Yes/No): allergies, high blood pressure, ulcers and other digestion problems, heart disease, chest pains, diabetes, problems of the nervous system, back pain, and other pains or disease not otherwise specified. The number of problems for which the veterans answered "yes" was then summed to produce a total score.

Locus of control

Control expectancies were assessed by a shortened version of Rotter's Internal-External Locus of Control Scale (Rotter, 1966). In this study, a Hebrew version of the scale was used, consisting of the most reliable 15 items. Each item is comprised of two sentences—one presenting an attitude typical of an external locus of control and the other presenting an attitude typical of an internal locus of control. For each item, the participant is asked to select the one sentence with which he agrees more. The scale was found to have adequate reliability ($\alpha = 0.68$).

Social support

The social support questionnaire was based on Mueller's (1980) social network interview, and was revised for the purpose of this study. Participants were presented with seven questions regarding expressive and instrumental support that they received from their network's members. They were asked to indicate on a 4-point scale (1 = "not at all" to 4 = "very much") to what extent they received support from their social network. In the present study, the scale was found to have good reliability (Cronbach's $\alpha = 0.86$).

Ways of coping

Coping was assessed with a 44-item shortened version of Folkman and Lazarus (1980) Ways of Coping Checklist. The scale was translated into Hebrew, and pre-tested in a small sample of soldiers. Participants were asked to recall stressful episodes that had taken place in the previous 3 months. Next, they were asked to indicate on a 4-point scale (1 = "not used" to 4 = "used a great deal") the extent to which they tend to use each coping strategy when confronted with the stressful episodes that they encountered. This questionnaire was factor-analyzed many times in the past, yielding different categorizations of coping factors (e.g. Sørlie & Sexton, 2001). For the present study, an exploratory factor analysis with Varimax rotation was conducted yielding eight coping factors. Of those, problem-focused coping and emotion-focused coping were used in the present study. This checklist is known to have good validity (Vitaliano, Russo, Carr, Maiuro, & Becker, 1985). Cronbach's alphas in the present study were 0.90 for the entire scale, 0.86 for problem-focused coping, and 0.69 for emotion-focused coping.

Combat exposure

Combat exposure was assessed using questions that were composed specifically for the purpose of this study: (1) "what role did you serve during combat? (active fighting role/assisting role/service role)", and (2) "did you take part in war-related activities, such as evacuation of bodies or injured soldiers?"

Socio-demographic characteristics were assessed using a questionnaire developed especially for the present study, which includes questions regarding the veteran's family status, military rank, prewar financial status, level of education, age, and number of children.

Data Analyses

Between-group differences in psychopathology levels at time of PTSD onset (PTSD, SCL-90, IES, etc.) were examined using a series of two-way ANOVAs, with CSR and onset group as the independent variables and each measure of psychopathology as the dependent variable. Differences in CSR rates among the study groups were examined using Chi Square test. Structural Equation Modeling (SEM) was used to examine the role of psychological resources in DPTSD, and specifically the hypothesized mediating role of coping. Ordinal regression was used to examine the relative contribution of all independent variables to DPTSD.

Results

Group Differences in Battle Exposure

The four study groups (1983/1984/2002 onset, and no PTSD) did not differ in the two measures of battle exposure examined. No differences were found in the number of veterans from each group who participated in war-related activities such as evacuation of dead or injured soldiers, $\chi^2(3) = 6.61$, $p = 0.09$, nor in the number of veterans who served in active combat role, assisting role, or service role during the war, $\chi^2(6) = 7.01$, $p = 0.32$.

Delayed-Onset PTSD: Prevalence

As noted, the study compared four groups of veterans, according to the time of first reported PTSD onset (1983, 1984, 2002, and no PTSD). Two types of information regarding prevalence are presented. Figure 5.1 presents the number and percentage of veterans from each group compared to the entire sample. Figure 5.2 presents numbers and percentages compared only to those veterans who endorsed PTSD at any time.

It should be noted that the present study employed a continuum of delays across time, instead of a rigid division into "delayed/acute" PTSD cases. However, for the purpose of the prevalence analyses we shall treat the 1984 and 2002 groups as those representing DPTSD. Thus, veterans who did not endorse PTSD in the first assessment, but did experience first PTSD onset at either 1984 or 2002, are considered cases of delayed PTSD. This 1-year cutoff differs from the 6-month threshold presented by the DSM. However, it is in line with other studies of delayed PTSD (Andrews et al., 2007).

As can be seen, when using the entire sample as a point of reference, the largest group consisted of veterans who experienced their first PTSD onset 1 year after the war, followed by veterans who did not suffer from PTSD at any time of assessment during the study's 20-year period. Together, the two groups that represent relative delays in PTSD onset (2 years and 20 years delay) consisted of 16.5 % of the sample. Interestingly, the rate of veterans who experienced a 2-year delay was very similar to that of veterans experiencing a 20-year delay.

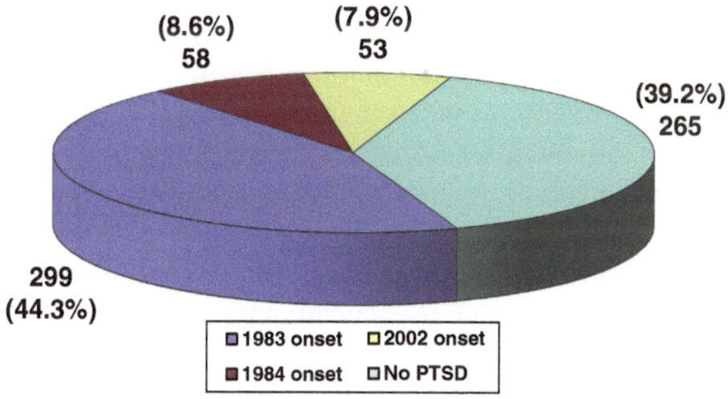

Fig. 5.1 Group rates compared to the entire sample

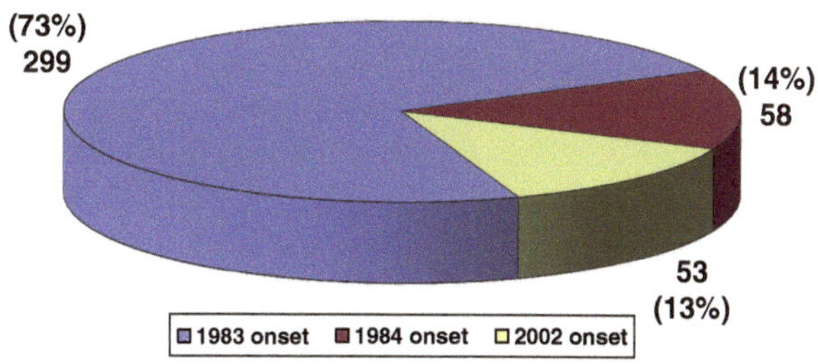

Fig. 5.2 Group rates compared to those who endorsed PTSD at any time

When examining only those veterans who endorsed PTSD, the 1983 onset group remains the largest. Veterans with relative delays in PTSD onset (2 and 20 years postwar) consist of 27 % of the entire PTSD population, again with the 1984 and 2002 showing quite similar rates.

Clinical Characteristics of DPTSD

Group Differences in Psychopathology

The four study groups were compared with regard to the following measures of psychopathology: number of PTSD symptoms, IES intrusion and avoidance symptoms, general psychiatric problems (GSI), problems in functioning, and number of physical health problems. A series of two-way ANOVAs was conducted, with each ANOVA comprising of two independent variables (onset group and CSR) and one dependent variable (psychopathology measure). The data entered into analysis for each group refers only to the year of first reported PTSD onset. For example, the 1983 onset group was assessed for psychiatric problems, functioning problems, etc. *only at 1983*, which was the year of its first PTSD onset. Data for the no PTSD group was collected at 2002, the last time point possible. Results are presented in Table 5.1.

As can be seen in Table 5.1, group had a main effect on all measures of psychopathology. LSD post hoc tests were conducted separately for each ANOVA. Taken together, the results regarding psychopathology supported our hypothesis predicting a negative association between the duration of delay (DOD) in PTSD onset and the severity of psychopathology. Thus, the shorter the delay in PTSD onset, the more severe the psychopathology was reported. The 1983 onset group reported significantly higher scores than the other three groups on the vast majority of psychopathology measures (excluding health problems, on which the 1983 and 1984 onset groups did not differ). Also, as expected, the no PTSD group reported lower levels of psychopathology than the 1983, 1984, and 2002 onset groups (excluding only IES avoidance, on which the 2002 onset and no PTSD groups did not differ). Interestingly, the 1984 and 2002 onset groups did not significantly differ with regard to most measures of psychopathology (excluding only health problems and IES intrusion, on which the 1984 onset group was more symptomatic).

CSR, DPTSD, and Psychopathology

The results of this study supported our hypothesis that CSR would be associated with shorter delays in PTSD. The four groups differed in the number of veterans who experienced antecedent CSR ($\chi^2(3)=151.72, p<0.001$). As expected, the highest rate of CSR was found among the 1983 onset group (79.3 %, $N=237$), followed by the 1984 onset (58.6 %, $N=34$), 2002 onset (45.3 %, $N=24$), and no PTSD (27.9 %, $N=74$) groups.

Table 5.1 Means, SDs, and F values for psychopathology measures according to CSR and study group

PTSD symptoms							GSI							Functioning problems						
		M	SD	F group (3,667)	F CSR (1,667)	F inter-action (3,667)			M	SD	F group (3,667)	F CSR (1,667)	F inter-action (3,667)			M	SD	F group (3,667)	F CSR (1,667)	F interac-tion (3,667)
CSR	1983	8.91	2.20	151.64***	38.57***	2.67*	CSR	1983	1.37	0.72	21.56***	7.82**	3.15*	CSR	1983	13.65	6.47	30.35***	7.63**	2.41 n.s.
	1984	7.00	1.91					1984	1.05	0.73					1984	9.74	5.85			
	2002	7.38	1.95					2002	0.98	0.41					2002	9.38	4.58			
	No PTSD	3.88	2.68					No PTSD	0.72	0.52					No PTSD	7.36	4.41			
Non-CSR	1983	6.98	2.08				Non-CSR	1983	0.97	0.67				Non-CSR	1983	10.37	6.26			
	1984	5.25	1.78					1984	0.85	0.60					1984	7.83	4.07			
	2002	6.07	2.37					2002	0.92	0.42					2002	8.90	3.05			
	No PTSD	3.12	1.91					No PTSD	0.66	0.41					No PTSD	6.72	3.80			

(continued)

Table 5.1 (continued)

IES intrusion							IES avoidance							Physical health problems						
		M	SD	F group (3,667)	F CSR (1,667)	F interaction (3,667)			M	SD	F group (3,667)	F CSR (1,667)	F interaction (3,667)			M	SD	F group (3,667)	F CSR (1,667)	F interaction (3,667)
CSR	1983	3.08	1.25	68.29***	35.64***	0.89 n.s.	CSR	1983	2.10	1.09	31.93***	5.15*	0.85 n.s.	CSR	1983	1.31	1.32	10.98***	0.97 n.s.	0.40 n.s.
	1984	2.38	1.28					1984	1.50	0.96					1984	1.71	1.36			
	2002	1.77	0.74					2002	1.23	0.85					2002	0.92	0.83			
	No PTSD	1.47	1.12					No PTSD	1.07	0.89					No PTSD	0.81	0.75			
Non-CSR	1983	2.26	1.10				Non-CSR	1983	1.68	1.14				Non-CSR	1983	1.35	1.31			
	1984	1.57	0.81					1984	1.21	0.76					1984	1.42	1.18			
	2002	1.21	0.87					2002	1.17	0.91					2002	0.97	0.94			
	No PTSD	0.96	0.71					No PTSD	0.91	0.70					No PTSD	0.86	0.71			

$^*p<0.05$, $^{**}p<0.01$, $^{***}p<0.001$

As indicated in Table 5.1, CSR and non-CSR veterans also significantly differed on the vast majority of psychopathology measures (excluding only number of health problems). Thus, overall, CSR veterans reported more severe psychopathology than non-CSR veterans.

This study was designed to examine interaction effects between CSR and study group, with regard to the various measures of psychopathology. As can be seen in Table 5.1, two significant interaction effects were found, one for PTSD symptoms and the other for GSI. Thus, group differences in PTSD symptoms and GSI were more accentuated among the CSR group compared to the non-CSR group.

Is DPTSD an "All-or-Nothing" Condition?

Another aim of this study was to examine whether DPTSD appears after a completely asymptomatic period. In order to answer that question, we examined whether veterans from the 1984 onset group suffered from PTSD symptoms in the previous measurement (1983), or if they had no symptoms at all. Two similar analyses were conducted for the 2002 onset group and the no PTSD group. For the 2002 onset group, we examined whether the veterans suffered from PTSD symptoms at any of the two previous assessments (i.e., 1983 and/or 1984). For the no PTSD group, we examined whether veterans were symptomatic at any of the three assessments. It should be noted that we adopted a dichotomous approach here, comparing those with no prior symptoms at all to those with at least one prior PTSD symptom. For further analyses based on a more continuous approach for measuring number of prior symptoms, see Horesh, Solomon, Keinan, & Ein-Dor, 2013).

When we assessed the number of veterans who had at least some level of PTSD symptoms at any of the previous assessments, the rate of previously symptomatic veterans from the 1984 onset, 2002 onset, and no PTSD groups were 86.2 % ($n = 50$), 98.11 % ($n = 52$), and 93.58 % ($n = 248$), respectively. Taken together, these results confirmed our hypothesis that among the majority of veterans with DPTSD, full-blown PTSD will appear following a symptomatic period. All groups were generally symptomatic prior to PTSD onset.

The Role of Personal and Social Resources in DPTSD

Our research model hypothesized associations between psychological resources (social support, locus of control, problem- and emotion-focused coping) and the duration of delay in PTSD onset. The aim of our model was to examine the prospective contribution of these resources to the delay in PTSD onset. Since all independent variables were measured at 1984, the model is based only on data collected at 1984 and 2002, and does not include data from 1983. This was done in order to avoid the violation of the prospective nature of this study, as well as the basic assumptions of any mediation model. In order to examine the model, a new ordinal variable was created, called "duration of delay" (DOD). The DOD variable is based on the previous categorization into study groups, with "1984 onset" representing the shortest duration of delay, followed by "2002 onset" and finally "no PTSD." This resulted in a three-point ordinal variable.

Social Support, Locus of Control and Coping: A Mediation Model

The mediation hypotheses were examined using the EQS 6.1 Structural Equation Models (SEM) software (Bentler & Wu, 1995). Model fit was estimated with the comparative fit index (CFI), the non-normed fit index (NNFI), and the root mean-square error of approximation (RMSEA). CSR was entered as a covariate, in order to test the model for the entire sample. Since DOD was entered as an ordinal variable, the SEM analysis was adjusted accordingly. Most importantly, the chi-square test used to assess model fit was the Satorra–Bentler (S-B) scaled chi-square (Satorra & Bentler, 2001), which incorporates a scaling correction for the chi-square statistic when distributional assumptions are violated.

Did Social Support and Locus of Control Predict DOD?

The structural model describing the pattern of relationships between the variables produced an excellent fit to the data: S-B χ^2 $(1, N=376)=0.0000$, $p=1.00$, CFI = 1, GFI = 1, 1-RMSEA = 1. Veterans' DOD was significantly predicted by both social support ($\beta=0.11$, $p<0.05$) and locus of control ($\beta=0.24$, $p<0.001$). In line with our hypothesis, the more social support a veteran had, the longer was the delay in PTSD onset; In line with another hypothesis, the more internal a veteran's locus of control was, the longer was the delay in his PTSD onset. The next step was to examine whether these two paths were mediated by coping.

Were the Mediation Paths Significant?

The structural model describing the pattern of relationships between the variables produced an excellent fit to the data: S-B χ^2 $(1, N=376)=0.0000$, $p=1.00$, CFI = 1, NNFI = 1, 1-RMSEA = 1. Veterans' social support significantly predicted both emotion-focused coping ($\beta=0.21$, $p<0.001$) and problem-focused coping ($\beta=0.43$, $p<0.001$). That is, the more social support a veteran had, the more he employed both problem- and emotion-focused coping. Moreover, a significant positive association was found between veterans' problem-focused coping and DOD ($\beta=0.23$, $p<0.001$), i.e., the more a veteran employed problem-focused coping, the longer was the delay in PTSD onset. A significant negative association was found between veterans' emotion-focused coping and DOD ($\beta=-0.20$, $p<0.001$). In line with our hypothesis, the more a veteran employed emotion-focused coping, the shorter was the delay in PTSD onset. Locus of control was not significantly associated with either problem-focused coping ($\beta=-0.06$, n.s.) nor emotion-focused coping ($\beta=-0.07$, n.s.). Thus, the mediation paths were found to be significant for social support, but not for locus of control.

Assuming that A represents predicting variables, B represents mediating variables, and C represents the outcome variable, in order to examine the mediation effect the overall fit of the A–B–C model was first calculated when the A–C paths were constrained to zero. The model produced excellent fit to the data under the constrained condition: S-B χ^2 (2, $N=376$)=0.0001, p=0.1.00, CFI=1, NNFI=1, 1-RMSEA=1). Next, the overall fit of the A–B–C model was calculated when the A–C paths were not constrained. The model produced an excellent fit to the data: S-B χ^2 (1, $N=376$)=0.0001, $p=0.99$, CFI=1, NNFI=1, 1-RMSEA=1). The results indicated that there was no significant improvement in fit on the basis of the difference between the two model chi-squares ($\Delta\chi^2=0$, Δdf=1, n.s.). This indicates that the association between social support and DOD is fully mediated by both problem- and emotion-focused coping.

It should be noted that the analysis showed that social support was positively related to DOD. However, when the mediation paths were examined more closely, it was found that social support was positively related to emotion-focused coping, which in turn was *negatively* related to DOD. Initially, this may seem as a peculiar finding, as it seemingly contradicts the overall positive relation between social support and DOD. This finding seems to represent what is known as "inconsistent mediation" (MacKinnon, Krull, & Lockwood, 2000; Shrout & Bolger, 2002), i.e., the mediation path produces an overall correlation opposite in sign (in this case, a minus sign) to that of the overall correlation (in this case, a positive correlation). On the other hand, the second mediation path, through problem-focused coping, was consistent with the overall association of social support and DOD.

To summarize, Fig. 5.3 presents a graphic illustration of the research model.

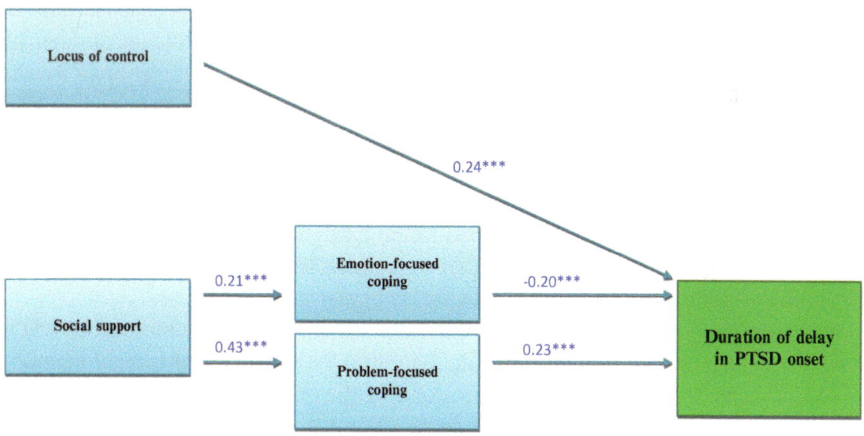

***p<.001
-Values on arrows represent standardized solution coefficients from SEM with ordinal data
-CSR was entered into the model as a covariant

Fig. 5.3 Research model describing the associations between Locus of control, social support, ways of coping, and DOD. ***$p<0.001$. *Values* on *arrows* represent standardized solution coefficients from SEM with ordinal data. CSR was entered into the model as a covariant

Table 5.2 Prediction of DOD according to psychological resources and CSR

	Estimate	Wald	Sig.
Social support	0.14	0.91	0.397
Locus of control	0.41	9.13**	0.004
P-F coping	0.43	8.39**	0.004
E-F coping	−0.47	10.04**	0.002
CSR	−1.10	21.01***	0.000

**$p<0.01$, ***$p<0.001$; df=1

To assess the relative contributions of the predictors included in this study to DOD, an ordinal regression was conducted, with social support, locus of control, both coping factors and CSR as the independent variables, and DOD as the ordinal dependent variable (Table 5.2).

As can be seen, when all predictors were examined together, only social support became nonsignificant. Of the remaining variables, CSR was the most powerful predictor of DOD, followed by emotion-focused coping, locus of control, and problem-focused coping.

Discussion

The Prevalence of DPTSD

The delay in PTSD is treated in this study as a continuum in time, where a PTSD onset 2 years after the war, for example, represents a longer delay in onset than a PTSD onset 1 year after the year. Our results indicate that a significant number of veterans reported a delay in PTSD onset. The two study groups that represent a relative delay in PTSD onset (the 1984 onset and 2002 onset groups) comprised 16.5 % of the entire sample and 27 % of those veterans who reported PTSD. The 16.5 % found here is higher than the rate found in most studies employing this method of calculation (e.g., Frueh et al., 2009). However, some studies have found similar rates (e.g., McFarlane, 1988). The 27 % found here seems to represent a midpoint between very low and very high rates that were previously found (Smid et al., 2009). Thus, the present study reveals a relatively high rate of DPTSD cases.

First and foremost, this finding empirically validates the existence of DPTSD, despite the turbulent medicolegal debate regarding the validity of this phenomenon. In recent years, the public discourse surrounding the military campaigns in Iraq and Afghanistan is increasingly becoming centered on the issue of "the hidden costs of war," from both a financial (Hartung, 2004) and psychological (Coleman, 2007) perspective. The results of the present study clearly support the notion of a delayed PTSD as a hidden cost of war.

The relatively high rate of DPTSD in the present study may be attributed to several factors. First, our results seem to support Prigerson et al.'s contention (2001)

that a delayed onset of PTSD symptoms is particularly common among survivors of war trauma. Combat is perhaps the most "masculine" trauma of all. Being tagged as "posttraumatic" following participation in combat often entails a social stigma. This may be especially true in a war-ridden country such as Israel, where the ability to endure the effects of battle is a desirable, even admirable, attribute. A second reason why war trauma may entail relatively high rates of DPTSD may be that during combat, soldiers enter a survival mode that is particularly insistent. The soldier cannot afford to experience psychological breakdown on the battlefield, as his life depends on his functioning. Thus, the psychological scars caused by the war may not manifest themselves on the battlefield or shortly thereafter, but rather remain unseen for a long period of time.

Another possible explanation for the relatively high rate of DPTSD in this study is that it was conducted in Israel, a country that may be viewed as a "stress lab," where citizens are exposed to ongoing war and terror. DPTSD is known to be associated with external triggers, i.e., events that somehow resemble the index trauma and therefore trigger its recollections (e.g., Green et al., 1995). Thus, the security situation in Israel may provide many opportunities for the early trauma of war to rise to the foreground, even after a long latency period.

Our finding that for some veterans in this study PTSD onset was delayed for 20 years after the war may be attributed to two major factors. First, the third assessment of this study was conducted in 2002, in the midst of the Al-Aqsa Intifada, the violent armed conflict between Israel and the Palestinians. At the time, the Israeli civilian population was under constant terrorist attacks. As expected, studies have shown that this violent atmosphere was also implicated in posttraumatic distress (e.g., Bleich, Gelkopf, & Solomon, 2003). Therefore, it is highly reasonable that the events of that period served as a trigger for DPTSD. The second explanation for DPTSD at 2002 is related to the fact that many of the veterans in this study were approaching midlife, and were already experiencing various aging processes. There is considerable evidence (e.g., Davison et al., 2006) regarding the role of aging processes in the onset of PTSD. Decreased activity during midlife and old age provides one with more opportunities to reminisce and review one's life, a process often accompanied by the recollection of early traumatic events. In addition, aging often entails many losses and exit events (e.g., retirement, death of loved ones) that may be particularly distressing for previously traumatized individuals (Christenson, Walker, Ross, & Maltbie, 1981).

The Clinical Picture of DPTSD

Previous studies have yielded mixed results regarding the severity of psychopathology in DPTSD (e.g., Bryant & Harvey, 2002; Solomon, Mikulincer, Waysman, & Marlowe, 1991; Watson, Kucala, Manifold, Vassar, & Juba, 1988). Our findings clearly indicate that the longer the delay in onset, the lower the symptom severity. The 1983 onset group was the most vulnerable, followed by the 1984 and 2002 onset groups, who did not differ from one another on most psychopathology measures, and finally the no PTSD group, which, as expected, endorsed the lowest psychopathology levels. Overall, these findings indicate that DPTSD may be considered a unique clinical subtype of PTSD, with an attenuated clinical picture. These findings also suggest that there may be a critical period, potentially a 1-year delay, during which the delay in PTSD onset is particularly related to the severity of psychopathology. However, once this temporal threshold is crossed, further delays in PTSD onset do not significantly affect the level of psychopathology. One possible explanation for our findings is that the initial impact of combat subsides with time, such that when it resurfaces, it takes a less severe form. A second possible explanation may be that veterans with DPTSD were initially more resilient to the effects of combat. This explanation was supported by earlier studies showing that casualties with DPTSD endorsed more psychological resources than those with immediate or chronic PTSD (e.g., Nitto, 2001).

We also found that veterans with antecedent CSR reported more severe psychopathology than non-CSR veterans. This finding falls in line with previous studies, indicating that both ASD (Bryant & Harvey, 1998) and CSR (Solomon et al., 2006) are risk factors for subsequent psychopathology. This is also congruent with the "vulnerability perspective," which postulates that an initial traumatic experience may weaken one's ability to effectively cope with subsequent stress (e.g., Danieli, 2007). In addition, we have found an interaction effect between CSR and study group (i.e., time of onset) regarding the number of PTSD symptoms and general psychiatric distress. Thus, the negative association between the DOD in PTSD onset and psychopathology was stronger among CSR veterans.

Our results also reveal that, in most cases, PTSD onset follows residual posttraumatic symptoms that already exist. This is consistent with other studies of DPTSD (Andrews et al., 2007). This finding may be attributed to the process of "fear incubation" (Eysenck, 1968), in which responses to fear-conditioned cues increase over time in the absence of further stress exposure. Recent studies have suggested fear incubation as an underlying mechanism in DPTSD (Pickens, Golden, Adams-Deutsch, Nair, & Shaham, 2009). Finally, a small number of veterans presented DPTSD following a completely asymptomatic period. While there are some researchers who see this pattern as unlikely (e.g., Blanchard & Hickling, 2004), this pattern has been previously reported by studies of DPTSD (e.g., Carty, O'Donnell, & Creamer, 2006), particularly case studies (e.g., Ramchandani, 1990).

The Role of Social and Personal Resources in DPTSD

Our findings suggest a model depicting the possible relationships between psychological resources and DPTSD. The model attempts to prospectively predict the duration of delay in PTSD onset. It does so by assessing all predicting variables at 1984, and examining their contribution to the course of PTSD from 1984 onwards.

Social Support, Coping, and DPTSD

In line with the research hypothesis, a positive association was found between social support and DOD. Thus, the higher one's perceived social support, the longer was the delay in PTSD onset. This finding is in line with a very large body of work, showing social support to be a protective factor in the face of traumatic stress (For a review see Kaniasty, 2005). It is also in line with previous studies of DPTSD, revealing an association between perceived social support and DPTSD (e.g., Nitto, 2001). However, it seems that social support plays a complex role vis-à-vis the delay in PTSD onset. Our results indicate that the association between social support and DOD was fully mediated by both emotion- and problem-focused coping. This finding is in line with the notion of social support as "coping assistance" (Kosciulek, 2007). However, the two mediation paths examined in the study deserve some elaboration. With regard to the first mediation path that included social support and problem-focused coping, our findings were in line with previous studies that have shown social support to be positively associated with problem-focused coping in the face of stress (e.g., Tan, 2007). Social support often bestows one with the sense of safety and confidence needed in order to try and directly confront the problems and tasks one is facing. As expected, we also found that problem-focused coping was positively associated with DOD. Problem-focused coping was often found to be negatively associated with PTSD (e.g., Dirkzwager, Bramsen, & Van der Ploeg, 2003).

The second mediation path included social support, emotion-focused coping, and DOD. Contrary to expectations, a positive association was found between social support and emotion-focused coping. Most previous studies have found a negative association between these two variables (e.g., Green & Pomeroy, 2007). Emotion-focused coping primarily includes intrapsychic coping strategies, and is therefore generally thought to be used in circumstances where social support is not readily available. However, in line with the present study, several studies have found a positive association between perceived social support and emotion-focused coping in stressful situations (e.g., Cayley, 2004). The finding that social support is positively related to emotion-focused coping may be explained by the fact that in order to confront the traumatic memories and losses associated with the war, veterans often must feel that they are safe, and that they are part of a solid social network that will support them if and when the processing of trauma-related emotions becomes unbearable. This notion corresponds with Winnicott's idea of a "holding environment" (1974), which facilitates one's encounter with his emotional self. In a similar vein, social support may facilitate the veteran's encounter with his traumatic memories and emotions.

Only one study, conducted by members of our team, had previously examined the role of emotion-focused coping in DPTSD (Solomon, 1989), but failed to find any difference in this type of coping between veterans with delayed PTSD and acute PTSD. Our finding that emotion-focused coping is associated with a shorter delay in PTSD onset may be attributed to the fact that the emotions associated with war and combat are often very negative. They may include rage, guilt, and helplessness (Herman, 1992).

The homecoming veteran employing emotion-focused coping is thus at risk of encountering these emotions, and subsequently experiencing great emotional pain. If PTSD is considered a manifestation of that pain, it may erupt at a relatively early stage.

The second mediation path (social support—emotion-focused coping—DOD), in its entirety, seems to be in line with Horowitz and Solomon's (1975) original theory of DPTSD, which postulated that some veterans return home from the battlefield, and continue to employ the psychological defenses of denial and emotional numbing that protected them from the horrors of war. However, when they return home to the safe environment of their friends and family, veterans may gradually let go of these rigid defense mechanisms, thus allowing themselves more direct contact with the emotional residues of their traumatic experiences. This process often results in the delayed surfacing of posttraumatic symptoms. The process described by Horowitz and Solomon is in some ways analogous to the mediation path found in this study: veterans who perceive themselves as having high levels of social support may consequently let go of their defenses more quickly and adapt a more emotion-focused coping style, in which trauma-related feelings and memories are faced rather than denied. This, in turn, may result in a faster emergence of posttraumatic symptoms.

Another possible explanation for this mediation effect is that while one's social network may promote emotion-focused coping, there is no guarantee that the social network's response to the emotionally coping individual will be positive. In other words, a supportive environment that initially encourages an emotional coping style on the veteran's part might later have difficulty containing the veteran's emotions and show little tolerance for this coping style. Subsequently, the veteran may experience mental distress, or in our case—an accelerated onset of PTSD. Many studies have reported the difficulties of the environment in accepting the veteran's emotional turmoil following the war (e.g., Figley & Leventman, 1980). In a similar vein, Hobfoll and London (1986) have argued that when social support increases rather than decreases emotional distress in the face of war, this may be the results of a "pressure cooker" effect. This refers to situations where the total amount of resources in one's environment is limited. Therefore, when one receives social support, one may deplete the environment of valuable resources that are essential for its functioning and well-being.

Overall, a close examination of the mediation paths found in this study reveals an interesting pattern. Social support was positively associated with problem-focused coping, which in turn was positively associated with DOD. However, social support was also positively associated with emotion-focused coping, which in turn was negatively associated with DOD. We have interpreted this interesting pattern of results as a case of "inconsistent mediation" (Shrout & Bolger, 2002). In other words—how can social support be positively associated with DOD of PTSD onset on one hand, but also associated with a factor that seems to exceed PTSD onset, on the other hand? The answer to this question seems to be that social support plays a twofold role with regard to DOD in PTSD onset. The total effect of this variable is indeed positive: higher levels of social support contribute to the delay in PTSD onset. However, a closer look reveals that social support contributes to two conflicting forces working in parallel. One is emotion-focused coping and the other is problem-focused coping; the former is associated with a shorter delay, while the latter is associated with a longer delay.

Locus of Control and DPTSD

Internal locus of control was found to be positively associated with DOD. Thus, veterans with a more internal locus of control experienced a longer delay in PTSD onset. However, the research hypotheses that this association will be mediated by both emotion- and problem-focused coping were not confirmed. The positive association between internal locus of control and DOD is in line with previous studies (e.g., Chung, Preveza, Papandreou, & Prevezas, 2007). Locus of control has been scarcely studied in the context of DPTSD. To the best of our knowledge, the present study is the first to find an association between locus of control and the delay in PTSD onset.

The finding that internal locus of control was associated with a longer delay in PTSD onset is to be expected. Control has been known to play a key role in the dynamics of trauma. Looked at from the conservation of resources perspective (Hobfoll, 1989), control may be one of the first resources depleted following exposure to a traumatic event. In the words of Judith Lewis Herman (1992): "Trauma robs the victim of a sense of power and control; the guiding principle of recovery is to restore power and control to the survivor" (p. 159).

The research hypothesis that the association between locus of control and the DOD in PTSD onset will be mediated by both emotion- and problem-focused coping was not confirmed. This may have several explanations. First, it is possible that a direct, rather than indirect, connection exists between locus of control and DOD. If this is indeed the case, than locus of control may play a primarily intrapsychic role in DPTSD. That is, one's sense of control does not affect one's ability to behave or cope in certain ways, but rather works through internal emotional mechanisms to change one's feeling and well-being. Another explanation for the lack of mediation effect in this study may be that the association between locus of control and DOD is mediated by other variables that were not examined in the study, such as treatment seeking (Page & Scalora, 2004).

The Relative Contribution of Study Variables to the Duration of Delay in PTSD Onset

This study also examined the relative contribution of each predictor to the DOD in PTSD onset. The findings demonstrated that CSR was the most powerful predictor, followed by emotion-focused coping, locus of control, and problem-focused coping. When all variables were examined together, no significant contribution was found for social support.

Previous PTSD studies have yielded mixed findings regarding the relative strength of various types of resources. While some have found social resources to play a more important role in PTSD than personal resources (e.g., Al-Turkait & Ohaeri, 2008; King et al., 1998), others showed personal resources to be more powerful predictors of PTSD (e.g., Williams, 2008). In the field of DPTSD, studies comparing the relative predictive power of different resources are quite rare, and the ones that do exist fail to present a clear picture (e.g., Adams & Boscarino, 2006; Nitto, 2001).

The fact that in the present study CSR made the most powerful contribution to the delay in PTSD onset is hardly surprising. CSR was previously found to be an early marker for future PTSD (Solomon, 1993; Solomon & Mikulincer, 2006). Of the psychological resources examined in this study, emotion-focused coping was found to be the strongest predictor of DOD in PTSD onset. The strength of emotion-focused coping as a predictor of DOD is to be expected when one considers Horowitz and Solomon's (1975) theory of delayed stress response. As already noted, this influential theory places a strong emphasis on veterans' ability to avoid emotional encounters with the memory of their trauma, and sees this process as the key factor in delayed stress responses. The powerful role of emotion-focused coping may also be taken to show the importance of the coping concept in general. It seems that in order to fully understand the reasons for the delay in PTSD onset, it is not sufficient to understand the veteran's personality and/or interpersonal interactions. Rather, it is crucial to move one step further and understand what types of behavioral, cognitive, and emotional strategies one employs in order to deal with stress.

Study Limitations

This study has several methodological limitations. First, it is based on self-report measures that, although very common in trauma studies, still entail the risk of biased reporting and/or biased memory. Another limitation is related to our definition and measurement of DPTSD. The first assessment occurred 1 year following the war, thereby exceeding the 6-month mark determined by the DSM for DPTSD. In addition, because of the time lag between assessments, we have no way of knowing if veterans suffered from PTSD in the time periods between our assessments. However, as has already been noted, due to significant measurement difficulties, studies of DPTSD traditionally show great variability in their threshold for defining delayed onset (e.g., Andrews et al., 2007). A final limitation is the diagnosis of PTSD according to DSM-III criteria. It may be expected that applying the more stringent criteria of DSM-IV or DSM-V would have resulted in lower rates of DPTSD (e.g., Solomon & Horesh, 2007).

Study Importance and Implications

The present study offers a unique opportunity for examining the under-studied phenomenon of DPTSD. First, this is one of the largest prospective studies ever conducted in the field of DPTSD. Also, much of the knowledge in this field has so far come from case reports, retrospective studies, or prospective studies with relatively short-term follow-ups. This study is based on a prospective, longitudinal design. This should be considered a major methodological advantage. Also, the present study covers a long follow-up period. Horowitz and Solomon (1975), in their early efforts of studying DPTSD, have predicted that as years will go by, time will unravel more and more delayed cases of PTSD. Thus, short-term follow-ups are not sufficient in order to understand the true scope and nature of this phenomenon. The present study also uses a large and unique sample, comprising of both a clinical and nonclinical group. Thus, it offers a rare look into the role of CSR in DPTSD.

This study imparts several theoretical implications. First, it offers further validation for the existence of DPTSD. The rates of delayed-onset cases found here clearly indicate that this is by no means a negligible phenomenon, but rather one which touches upon the lives of many war veterans. The second theoretical implication of this study is the conceptualization of delayed PTSD as a unique and separate clinical subtype of PTSD, with an attenuated clinical picture. Moreover, the fact the delayed PTSD was associated with lower levels of psychopathology stands in sharp contrast to some views of delayed psychopathology (e.g., delayed grief), which often consider the early (rather than delayed) manifestation of emotional distress as a predictor of better mental health. Third, our research model confirms that the delay in PTSD onset may be seen as a sign of psychological resilience, i.e., the veteran's ability to rely on his psychological resources for a significant period of time, without developing PTSD. Specifically, the study reveals that resilience may be defined not only in terms of the question: "*Did* the veteran suffer from PTSD?," but also the question: "*When* did the veterans suffer from PTSD?".

This study also has important clinical and other practical implications, some of which are tightly linked to the theoretical implications noted above. First, the identification of various resources associated with DPTSD may be of great importance for mental health professionals. Therapeutic interventions are encouraged to put emphasis on resources that were found to be most strongly associated with delayed PTSD, and to design interventions according to the "hierarchy of resources" found here. Second, our finding that delayed PTSD is not an "all-or-nothing" phenomenon, but rather one that appears after some PTSD symptoms were already present, should encourage professionals to closely follow the emergence of PTSD symptoms among their patients, even—and perhaps especially—if they have not reached the clinical or sub-clinical threshold of PTSD. These symptoms may serve as the platform upon which PTSD will later appear, sometimes many years later. Third, the fact that the severity of psychopathology varies across PTSD patients may be of great value to therapists. When a patient seeks treatment for PTSD, it is important to inquire as to the time in which the disorder first appeared, as this may affect treatment decisions.

Finally, since DPTSD seems to represent a unique clinical subtype of PTSD, mental health professionals are encouraged to design specific interventions for veterans suffering from this condition. One interesting example is the work of Charles Kaiman (2003), who has started a therapeutic group for aging war veterans suffering from delayed and exacerbated PTSD.

Our findings may also carry legal and financial implications. As already noted, DPTSD is often regarded with suspicion, and interpreted as an attempt to gain compensation. We believe that our findings provide significant support for the existence of DPTSD as a legitimate clinical entity. Therefore, the military, legal, and financial authorities are encouraged to consider lowering their sometimes-increased level of suspicion towards veterans who report delayed-onset PTSD. It seems that with the gradual proliferation of delayed PTSD studies, this point is already being taken into account in other war-ridden areas of the world (e.g., Šivert & Miloševic, 2004).

Suggestions for Future Research

Despite a recent growing interest in DPTSD, studies in this area are still relatively scarce. Also, there is a lack of variety in studies of DPTSD, with most studies employing similar methodologies and exploring a rather limited set of variables. To the best of our knowledge, the present study is the first to suggest a multivariable model of DPTSD, examining mediation effects, as well as intercorrelations between predictors. Future studies are encouraged to expand on this effort, and to develop other multivariable models of DPTSD. Future studies are also encouraged to develop specific measures for assessing DPTSD. If, as the results of this study suggest, DPTSD is indeed a unique subtype of PTSD, then it may be useful to employ more specific measurement tools that take into account its unique characteristics. A significant step in this direction may be seen in the development and validation of specific measures such as the LOSS questionnaire (King et al., 2007), assessing late-onset stress symptomatology. Finally, in the future, there may also be a need to draw a clearer line between two major types of delayed PTSD studies. Some studies, the present one included, place a stronger emphasis on factors contributing to the delay in PTSD onset. Thus, they explore variables that may inhibit symptom onset for significant periods of time. Other studies, however, focus on factors that may serve as triggers for PTSD onset. In the future, the trauma literature may greatly benefit from studies attempting to integrate these two lines of research.

References

Adams, R. E., & Boscarino, J. A. (2006). Predictors of PTSD and delayed PTSD after disaster: The impact of exposure and psychosocial resources. *Journal of Nervous and Mental Disease, 194*(7), 485–493.

Aldwin, C. M., & Yancura, L. A. (2004). Coping and health: A comparison of the stress and trauma literatures. In P. P. Schnurr & B. L. Green (Eds.), *Physical health consequences of exposure to extreme stress* (pp. 99–126). Washington, DC: American Psychological Association.

Al-Turkait, F. A., & Ohaeri, J. U. (2008). Post-traumatic stress disorder among wives of Kuwaiti veterans of the first Gulf War. *Journal of Anxiety Disorders, 22*, 18–31.

American Psychiatric Association. (1980). *Diagnostic and statistical manual of mental disorders* (3rd ed.). Washington, DC: Author.

American Psychiatric Association. (2013). *Diagnostic and statistical manual of mental disorders* (5th ed.). Washington, DC: Author.

Andrews, B., Brewin, C., Philpott, R., & Stewart, L. (2007). Delayed-onset posttraumatic stress disorder: A systematic review of the evidence. *American Journal of Psychiatry, 164*, 1319–1326.

Andrews, B., Brewin, C. R., Stewart, L., Philpott, R., & Hejdenberg, J. (2009). Comparison of immediate-onset and delayed onset posttraumatic stress disorder in military veterans. *Journal of Abnormal Psychology, 118*(4), 767–777.

Barouk, N. (2005). *The relationships between individual characteristics and long-term persistence of PTSD symptoms*. Doctoral dissertation, Fairleigh Dickinson University, USA.

Bentler, P. M., & Wu, E. J. C. (1995). *EQS for windows user's guide*. Encino, CA: Multivariate Software.

Benyamini, Y., & Idler, E. L. (1999). Community studies reporting association between self-rated health and mortality: Additional studies, 1995–1998. *Research on Aging, 21*(3), 392–401.

Blanchard, E. B., & Hickling, E. J. (2004). *After the crash: Psychological assessment and treatment of survivors of motor vehicle accidents*. Washington, DC: American Psychological Association.

Bleich, A., Gelkopf, M., & Solomon, Z. (2003). Exposure to terrorism, stress-related mental health symptoms, and coping behaviors among a nationally representative sample in Israel. *JAMA: The Journal of the American Medical Association, 290*(5), 612–620.

Boscarino, J. A., & Adams, R. E. (2009). PTSD onset and course following the World Trade Center disaster: Findings and implications for future research. *Social Psychiatry and Psychiatric Epidemiology, 44*(10), 887–898.

Brown, J., Mulhern, G., & Joseph, S. A. (2002). Incident-related stressors, locus of control, coping, and psychological distress among firefighters in Northern Ireland. *Journal of Traumatic Stress, 15*(2), 161–168.

Bryant, R. A., & Harvey, A. G. (1998). The relationship between acute stress disorder and post-traumatic stress disorder following mild traumatic brain injury. *American Journal of Psychiatry, 155*, 625–629.

Bryant, R. A., & Harvey, A. G. (2002). Delayed-onset posttraumatic stress disorder: A prospective evaluation. *Australian and New Zealand Journal of Psychiatry, 36*, 205–209.

Buckley, T. C., Blanchard, E. B., & Hickling, E. J. (1996). A prospective examination of Delayed onset PTSD secondary to motor vehicle accidents. *Journal of Abnormal Psychology, 103*(4), 617–625.

Carty, J., O'Donnell, M. L., & Creamer, M. (2006). Delayed-onset PTSD: A prospective study of injury survivors. *Journal of Affective Disorders, 90*(2–3), 257–261.

Cayley, C. (2004). *Coping with interpersonal sport stress in female adolescent soccer players: The role of perceived social support, cognitive appraisal, and trait social anxiety*. Master's Thesis, University of British Columbia.

Christenson, R. M., Walker, J. I., Ross, D. R., & Maltbie, A. A. (1981). Reactivation of traumatic conflicts. *American Journal of Psychiatry, 138*, 984–985.

Chung, M. C., Preveza, E., Papandreou, K., & Prevezas, N. (2007). Locus of control among spinal cord injury patients with different levels of posttraumatic stress disorder. *Psychiatry Research, 152*(2–3), 253–260.

Cohen, L. H., Hettler, T. R., & Park, C. L. (1997). Social support, personality, and life stress adjustment. In G. R. Pierce & B. Lakey (Eds.), *Sourcebook of social support and personality* (pp. 215–228). New York: Plenum Press.

Coleman, P. (2007, November 11). *Veterans' suicides: A hidden cost of Bush's wars*. Retrieved May 1, 2008, from http://www.Alternet.org

Compas, B. E., Worsham, N. L., Ey, S., & Howell, D. C. (1996). When mom or dad has cancer: II. Coping, cognitive appraisals and psychological distress in children of cancer patients. *Health Psychology, 15*(3), 167–175.

Danieli, Y. (2007). *International handbook of multigenerational legacies of trauma*. New York: Springer.

Davison, E. H., Pless, A. P., Gugliucci, M. R., King, L. A., King, D. W., Salgado, D. M., et al. (2006). Late-life emergence of early-life trauma: The phenomenon of late-onset stress symptomatology among aging combat veterans. *Research on Aging, 28*(1), 84–114.

Derogatis, L. R. (1977). *SCL-90-R: Administration, scoring and procedures manual, I, for the Revised version*. Baltimore: Johns Hopkins University, Clinical Psychometrics Research Unit.

Dirkzwager, A. J. E., Bramsen, I., & Van der Ploeg, H. M. (2003). Social support, coping, life events, and posttraumatic stress symptoms among former peacekeepers: A prospective study. *Personality and Individual Differences, 34*(8), 1545–1559.

Ehlers, A., & Clark, D. M. (2000). A cognitive model of posttraumatic stress disorder. *Behaviour Research and Therapy, 38*, 319–345.

Epstein, R. (1993). Avoidant symptoms cloaking the diagnosis of PTSD in patients with severe accidental injury. *Journal of Traumatic Stress, 6*, 451–458.

Eysenck, H. J. (1968). A theory of incubation of anxiety of fear responses. *Behaviour Research and Therapy, 6*, 309–322.

Figley, C. R., & Leventman, S. (1980). *Strangers at home: Vietnam veterans since the war*. New York: Praeger.

Folkman, S., & Lazarus, R. S. (1980). An analysis of coping in a middle-aged community sample. *Journal of Health and Social Behavior, 21*, 219–239.

Frueh, B. C., Grubaugh, A. L., Yeager, D. E., & Magruder, K. M. (2009). Delayed-onset posttraumatic stress disorder among war veterans in primary care clinics. *The British Journal of Psychiatry, 194*(6), 515–520.

Gray, M. J., Bolton, E. E., & Litz, B. T. (2004). A longitudinal analysis of PTSD symptom course: Delayed-onset PTSD in Somalia peacekeepers. *Journal of Consulting and Clinical Psychology, 72*(5), 909–913.

Green, A. H., Coupe, P., Fernandez, R., & Stevens, B. (1995). Incest revisited: Delayed posttraumatic stress disorder in mothers following the sexual abuse of their children. *Child Abuse & Neglect, 19*(10), 1275–1282.

Green, B. L., Lindy, J. D., Grace, M. C., Gleser, G. C., Leonard, A. C., Korol, M., et al. (1990). Buffalo creek survivors in the second decade: Stability of stress symptoms. *American Journal of Orthopsychiatry, 60*, 43–54.

Green, D. L., & Pomeroy, E. (2007). Crime victims: What is the role of social support? *Journal of Aggression, Maltreatment & Trauma, 15*(2), 97–113.

Hartung, W. D. (2004, March). Iraq and the costs of war. From http://www.fpif.org

Herman, J. L. (1992). *Trauma and recovery*. New York: Basic Books.

Hobfoll, S. E. (1988). *The ecology of stress*. Washington, DC: Hemisphere.

Hobfoll, S. E. (1989). Conservation of resources: A new attempt at conceptualizing stress. *American Psychologist, 44*(3), 513–524.

Hobfoll, S. E. (1998). *Stress, culture, and community: The psychology and philosophy of stress*. New York: Plenum Press.

Hobfoll, S. E., & London, P. (1986). The relationship of self-concept and social support to emotional distress among women during war. *Journal of Social and Clinical Psychology, 4*(2), 189–203.

Holahan, C. J., & Moos, R. H. (1994). Life stressors and mental health: Advances in conceptualizing stress resistance. In W. R. Avison & I. H. Gotlib (Eds.), *Stress and mental health: Contemporary issues and prospects for the future* (pp. 213–238). New York: Plenum Press.

Horesh, D., Solomon, Z., Zerach, G., & Ein-Dor, T. (2011). Delayed-onset PTSD among war veterans: the role of life events throughout the life cycle. *Social Psychiatry and Psychiatric Epidemiology, 46*(9), 863–870.

Horesh, D., Solomon, Z., Keinan, G., & Ein-Dor, T. (2013). The clinical picture of late-onset PTSD: A 20-year longitudinal study of Israeli war veterans. *Psychiatry Research, 208*(3), 265–273.

Horowitz, M. J., & Solomon, G. F. (1975). A prediction of delayed stress response syndromes in Vietnam veterans. *Journal of Social Issues, 31*(4), 67–80.
Horowitz, M. J., Wilner, N., & Avlarez, W. (1979). Impact of event scale: A measure of subjective stress. *Psychosomatic Medicine, 41*, 209–218.
Hyman, S. M., Gold, S. N., & Cott, M. A. (2003). Forms of social support that moderate PTSD in childhood sexual abuse survivors. *Journal of Family Violence, 18*(5), 295–300.
Kaiman, C. (2003). PTSD in the World War II Combat Veteran. *American Journal of Nursing, 103*(11), 32–41.
Kaniasty, K. (2005). Social support and traumatic stress. *PTSD Research Quarterly, 16*(2), 1–3.
Kardiner, A., & Spiegel, H. (1947). *War stress and neurotic illness*. New York: Hoeber.
King, L. A., King, D. W., Fairbank, J. A., Keane, T. M., & Adams, G. A. (1998). Resilience-recovery factors in post-traumatic stress disorder among female and male Vietnam veterans: Hardiness, postwar social support, and additional stressful life events. *Journal of Personality and Social Psychology, 74*(2), 420–434.
King, D. W., Taft, C., King, L. A., Hammond, C., & Stone, E. R. (2006). Directionality of the association between social support and posttraumatic stress disorder: A longitudinal investigation. *Journal of Applied Social Psychology, 36*(12), 2980–2992.
King, L. A., King, D. W., Vickers, K., Davison, E. H., & Spiro III, A. (2007). Assessing late-onset stress symptomatology among aging male combat veterans. *Aging & Mental Health, 11*(2), 175–191
Koenen, K., Stellman, J. M., Stellman, S. D., & Sommer, J. F. (2003). Risk factors for the course of posttraumatic stress disorder among Vietnam veterans: A 14-year follow-up of American legionnaires. *Journal of Consulting and Clinical Psychology, 71*, 980–986.
Koren, D., Arnon, I., & Klein, E. (2001). Long-term course of chronic post-traumatic stress disorder in traffic accident victims: A three-year prospective follow-up study. *Behaviour Research and Therapy, 39*, 1449–1458.
Kosciulek, J. F. (2007). The social context of coping. In E. Martz & H. Livneh (Eds.), *Coping with chronic illness and disability: Theoretical, empirical, and clinical aspects* (pp. 73–88). New York: Springer.
Krystal, H. (1968). *Massive psychic trauma*. New York: Little, Brown.
Lazarus, R. S., & Folkman, S. (1984). *Stress, appraisal, and coping*. New York: Springer.
MacKinnon, D. P., Krull, J. L., & Lockwood, C. M. (2000). Equivalence of the mediation, confounding and suppression effects. *Prevention Science, 1*, 173–181.
Mayou, R., Bryant, B., & Duthrie, R. (1993). Psychiatric consequences of road traffic accidents. *British Medical Journal, 307*, 647–651.
McFarlane, A. C. (1988). The longitudinal course of posttraumatic morbidity: The range of outcomes and their predictors. *Journal of Nervous and Mental Disease, 176*, 30–39.
Mueller, D. P. (1980). Social networks: A promising direction for research on the relationship of the social environment to psychiatric disorder. *Social Science Medicine, 14*, 147–161.
Newman, D. A. (2003). Longitudinal modeling with randomly and systematically missing data: A simulation of Ad Hoc, Maximum Likelihood, and Multiple Imputation techniques. *Organizational Research Methods, 6*, 328–362.
Nitto, M. M. (2001). *An investigation of factors contributing to delays in the onset of PTSD among Vietnam veterans*. Doctoral dissertation, University of Hartford, USA.
Op den Velde, W., Falger, P. R. J., Hovens, J. E., De Groen, J. H. M., Lasschuit, L. J., Van Dijn, H., et al. (1993). Posttraumatic stress disorder in Dutch resistance veterans from World War II. In J. P. Wilson & B. Raphael (Eds.), *International handbook of traumatic stress syndromes* (pp. 219–230). New York: Plenum.
Page, G. L., & Scalora, M. J. (2004). The utility of locus of control for assessing juvenile amenability to treatment. *Aggression and Violent Behavior, 9*(5), 523–534.
Pary, R., Turns, D. M., & Tobias, C. R. (1986). A case of delayed recognition of posttraumatic stress disorder. *American Journal of Psychiatry, 143*(7), 941.
Peveler, R. C., & Fairburn, C. G. (1990). Measurement of neurotic symptoms by self-report questionnaire: Validity of the SCL-90R. *Psychological Medicine, 20*(4), 873–879.

Pickens, C. L., Golden, S. A., Adams-Deutsch, T., Nair, S. G., & Shaham, Y. (2009). Long-lasting incubation of conditioned fear in rats. *Biological Psychiatry, 65*, 881–886.
Pitman, R. K. (1989). Post-traumatic stress disorder, hormones, and memory. *Biological Psychiatry, 26*, 221–223.
Prigerson, H. G., Maciejewski, P. K., & Rosenheck, R. A. (2001). Combat trauma: Trauma with highest risk of delayed onset and unresolved posttraumatic stress disorder symptoms, unemployment and abuse among men. *The Journal of Nervous and Mental Disease, 189*(2), 99–108.
Ramchandani, D. (1990). Distinguishing features of delayed-onset posttraumatic stress disorder. *Bulletin of the Menninger Clinic, 54*(2), 247–254.
Reich, H. (2006). *The first and final nightmare of Sonia Reich: A son's memoir*. New York: PublicAffairs.
Rotter, J. B. (1966). Generalized expectancies for internal versus external control of reinforcement. *Psychological Monographs: General and Applied, 80*(1), 1–28.
Rotter, J. B. (1975). Some problems and misconceptions related to the construct of internal versus external control of reinforcement. *Journal of Consulting and Clinical Psychology, 43*(1), 56–67.
Rubin, D. B. (1987). *Multiple imputation for nonresponse in surveys*. New York: Wiley.
Satorra, A., & Bentler, P. M. (2001). A scaled difference chi-square test statistic for moment structure analysis. *Psychometrika, 66*(4), 507–514.
Schwarzwald, J., Solomon, Z., Weisenberg, M., & Mikulincer, M. (1987). Validation of the Impact of Event Scale for the psychological sequelae of combat. *Journal of Consulting and Clinical Psychology, 55*, 251–256.
Shatan, C. F. (1973). The grief of soldiers: Vietnam combat veterans' self-help movement. *American Journal of Orthopsychiatry, 43*(4), 640–653.
Shrout, P. E., & Bolger, N. (2002). Mediation in experimental and nonexperimental studies: New procedures and recommendations. *Psychological Methods, 7*, 422–445.
Silver, R. C., Holman, E. A., McIntosh, D. N., Poulin, M., & Gil-Rivas, V. (2002). Nationwide longitudinal study of psychological responses to September 11. *Journal of the American Medical Association, 288*(10), 1235–1244.
Šivert, M., & Miloševic, V. (2004). Legal consequences of the delayed occurrence of posttraumatic stress disorder. In Z. Spiric, G. Knezevic, V. Jovic, & G. Opacic (Eds.), *Torture in war: Consequences and rehabilitation of victims – Yugoslav experience* (pp. 369–376). Belgrade: International Aid Network.
Smid, G. E., Lensvelt-Mulders, G. J., Knipscheer, J. W., Gersons, B. P., & Kleber, R. J. (2011). Late-onset PTSD in unaccompanied refugee minors: Exploring the predictive utility of depression and anxiety symptoms. *Journal of Clinical Child & Adolescent Psychology, 40*(5), 742–755.
Smid, G. E., Mooren, T. T. M., Van der Mast, R. C., Gersons, B. P. R., & Kleber, R. J. (2009). Delayed posttraumatic stress disorder: Systematic review, meta-analysis, and meta-regression analysis of prospective studies. *Journal of Clinical Psychiatry, 70*(11), 1572–1582.
Smid, G. E., van der Velden, P. G., Gersons, B. P. R., & Kleber, R. J. (2012). Late-onset posttraumatic stress disorder following a disaster: A longitudinal study. *Psychological Trauma: Theory, Research, Practice, and Policy, 4*(3), 312–322.
Smith, D. W., & Frueh, B. C. (1996). Compensation seeking, comorbidity, and apparent exaggeration of PTSD symptoms among Vietnam combat veterans. *Psychological Assessment, 8*(1), 3–6.
Solomon, Z. (1989). *Delayed PTSD: Course and correlates*. Tel Aviv: Medical Corps, Research Branch, Department of Mental Health, IDF.
Solomon, Z. (1993). *Combat stress reaction: The enduring toll of war*. New York: Plenum Press.
Solomon, Z., Benbenishty, R., Neria, Y., Abramowitz, M., Ginzburg, K., & Ohry, A. (1993). Assessment of PTSD: Validation of the revised PTSD Inventory. *Israel Journal of Psychiatry and Related Sciences, 30*(2), 110–115.
Solomon, Z., & Horesh, D. (2007). Changes in diagnostic criteria of PTSD: Implications from two prospective longitudinal studies. *American Journal of Orthopsychiatry, 77*(2), 182–188.

Solomon, Z., & Mikulincer, M. (2006). Trajectories of PTSD: A 20-year longitudinal study. *American Journal of Psychiatry, 163*, 659–666.

Solomon, Z., Shklar, R., Singer, Y., & Mikulincer, M. (2006). Reactions to combat stress in Israeli veterans twenty years after the 1982 Lebanon war. *The Journal of Nervous and Mental Disease, 194*(12), 935–939.

Solomon, Z., Mikulincer, M., & Waysman, M. (1991). Delayed and immediate posttraumatic stress disorder: The role of life events and social resources. *Journal of Community Psychology, 19*, 231–236.

Solomon, Z., Mikulincer, M., Waysman, M., & Marlowe, D. (1991). Delayed and immediate onset posttraumatic stress disorder: I. Differential clinical characteristics. *Social Psychiatry and Psychiatric Epidemiology, 26*, 1–7.

Solomon, Z., Waysman, M., Levy, G., Fried, B., Mikulincer, M., Benbenishty, R., et al. (1992). From front line to home front: A study of secondary traumatization. *Family Process, 31*(3), 289–302.

Solomon, Z., Weisenberg, M., Schwarzwald, J., & Mikulincer, M. (1987). Posttraumatic stress disorder among frontline soldiers with combat stress reaction: The 1982 Israeli experience. *American Journal of Psychiatry, 144*(4), 448–454.

Sørlie, T., & Sexton, H. C. (2001). The factor structure of "The Ways of Coping Questionnaire" and the process of coping in surgical patients. *Personality and Individual Differences, 30*(6), 961–975.

Tan, M. (2007). Social support and coping in Turkish patients with cancer. *Cancer Nursing, 30*(6), 498–504.

Vitaliano, P. P., Russo, J., Carr, J. E., Maiuro, R. D., & Becker, J. (1985). The ways of coping checklist: Revision and psychometric properties. *Multivariate Behavioral Research, 20*(1), 3–26.

Watson, C. G., Kucala, T., Manifold, V., Vassar, P., & Juba, M. (1988). Differences between posttraumatic stress disorder patients with Delayed and immediate onsets. *The Journal of Nervous and Mental Disease, 76*(9), 568–572.

Williams, L. F. (2008). *Psychosocial protection following exposure to sexual assault: Predictive value and malleability of multiple psychosocial protective factors.* Doctoral dissertation, University of Missouri – Saint Louis.

Winnicott, D. W. (1974). Fear of breakdown. *The International Review of Psycho-Analysis, 1*, 103–107.

Yule, W., Bolton, D., Udwin, O., Boyle, S., O'Ryan, D., & Nurrish, J. (2000). The long-term psychological effects of a disaster experienced in adolescence, I: The incidence and course of PTSD. *Journal of Child Psychology and Psychiatry, 41*, 503–511.

Zeidner, M., & Ben-Zur, H. (1994). Individual differences in anxiety, coping and post-traumatic stress in the aftermath of the Persian Gulf War. *Personality and Individual Difference, 16*(3), 459–476.

Zerach, G., Solomon, Z., Horesh, D., & Ein-Dor, T. (2013). Family cohesion and posttraumatic intrusion and avoidance among war veterans: a 20-year longitudinal study. *Social Psychiatry and Psychiatric Epidemiology, 48*(2), 205–214.

Part II
Preventing PTSD

Chapter 6
Cutting Edge Research on Prevention of PTSD

Megan C. Kearns, Alex O. Rothbaum, Cole G. Youngner, Mark S. Burton, Alexander McCarthy, and Barbara Olasov Rothbaum

Prevention of PTSD

Nearly 6 years ago, Hurricane Katrina devastated the gulf coast region of the United States, the city of New Orleans in particular. Beyond the physical destruction—lives lost, homes destroyed, entire city disfigured—the psychological damage was equally powerful. An amalgamation of various news reports and research surveys estimated that nearly three million individuals in the New Orleans area were exposed to the traumatic natural disaster (Dalton, Scheeringa, & Zeanah, 2008). By comparing diagnostic rates for Posttraumatic Stress Disorder (PTSD), with rates from relief effort studies in the wake of Hurricane Katrina, Dalton et al. (2008) approximated that 260,612 individuals likely had diagnosable PTSD after exposure to Katrina. Shockingly still, this was a conservative calculation, with the upper estimate being over 500,000 people (Dalton et al., 2008). These data underscore the catastrophic potential of PTSD to affect mass numbers of individuals.

Occurring after exposure to a perceived life-threatening event, PTSD is an anxiety disorder characterized by three core sets of symptoms: reexperiencing, avoidance, and hyperarousal. These symptoms are often ubiquitous in the aftermath of a trauma and fortunately tend to diminish over time for the majority of trauma-exposed individuals. For some individuals, however, their symptoms do not extinguish

M.C. Kearns, Ph.D. • C.G. Youngner, B.A. • M.S. Burton, B.A. • A. McCarthy
B.O. Rothbaum, Ph.D., ABPP (✉)
Emory University School of Medicine, 1256 Briarcliff Road, Atlanta, GA 30306, USA
e-mail: megan.kearns@emory.edu; cyoungn@emory.edu; Mark.burton@case.edu; aj.mccarthy17@gmail.com; brothba@emory.edu

A.O. Rothbaum
Virtually Better, Inc., 2440 Lawrenceville Hwy, Decatur, GA 30033, USA
e-mail: arothba@emory.edu

M.P. Safir et al. (eds.), *Future Directions in Post-Traumatic Stress Disorder*,
DOI 10.1007/978-1-4899-7522-5_6

and interfere with their functioning, leading to a diagnosis of PTSD. Despite the many large-scale disasters since Hurricane Katrina in 2006, not to mention war and individual traumatic events, little progress has been made in interventions to prevent trauma survivors from developing PTSD. While such estimates can aid in the assessment of damage and the targeting of mental health services, clinicians and relief workers still need a treatment strategy that can prevent the normal distress of the trauma from becoming full-blown, diagnosable PTSD, especially in more vulnerable individuals.

The lack of such an established early intervention produces negative consequences for both the individuals suffering from PTSD and greater society. A regrettably common experience, an estimated 37–92 % of all people will be exposed to a severe traumatic situation during their lifetime (Breslau et al., 1998). Kessler et al.'s (2005) work from the most recent National Comorbidity Survey-Replication suggested that 6.8 % of adult Americans (3.6 % of males and 9.7 % of females) currently have PTSD. The prevalence is significantly higher in military personnel as 13.8 % of veterans of the war in Iraq and Afghanistan met DSM-IV criteria for PTSD (Tanielian & Jaycox, 2008). Furthermore, the strong relationship between PTSD and suicide makes the disorder even more troubling. In a recent replication of the National Comorbidity Survey, Cougle, Keough, Riccardi, and Sachs-Ericsson (2009) showed that 18.8 % of individuals diagnosed with PTSD had attempted suicide while 40.3 % reported suicidal ideation. More specifically, PTSD uniquely predicted suicidal ideation among individuals with other anxiety disorders, being associated with increased suicide risk in men and uniquely predictive of suicide attempts in women (Cougle et al., 2009).

In addition, the economic impacts of PTSD expand far beyond the threat of suicide as people suffering from PTSD accrue costs from their symptoms and other related health problems. Such significant health conditions as hypertension, bronchial asthma, peptic ulcers, gastrointestinal problems, and increased rates of surgery occur more commonly in those with PTSD (Leserman et al., 1996), resulting in encumbering financial issues. More specifically, the ensuing work impairment, hospitalization, and health visits due to PTSD culminate in higher economic costs than the costs associated with any other anxiety disorder (Greenberg et al., 1999; Marciniak et al., 2005). Although putting the total costs into an accurate, quantifiable amount remains difficult, Miller, Brody, and Summerton (1988) suggested that mental healthcare costs, the majority being likely due to PTSD stemming from criminal violence, reached $166 billion. The total costs may be significantly higher as these data do not account for the financial costs due to other traumas such as motor vehicle accidents and natural disasters.

Because of these tremendous health risks and potential financial burdens that stem from PTSD, there is an unmistakable need for preventative approaches to this anxiety disorder. In this chapter, we present an overview of research on predictors of PTSD and a review of past along with cutting edge efforts to develop early detection of and interventions for PTSD. Further research and progress show promise in treating those likely to develop PTSD before the disorder has a chance to adversely alter their lives.

Predictors of PTSD

Due to the high rates of trauma exposure across the world and the emotional toll for individuals who develop chronic PTSD, finding preventative treatment is a worthwhile endeavor. Research in developing early intervention for PTSD can be a difficult task due to the nature of the disorder. As discussed above, 37–92 % of all people will be exposed to a severe traumatic situation during their lifetime (Breslau et al., 1998), yet only a small minority will develop chronic PTSD. Traumatic events are not predictable; it is not known who will develop chronic PTSD following trauma, which leaves no option but to treat all trauma-exposed individuals. This blanket approach hopes to prevent chronic PTSD from developing for a minority of individuals after a trauma while also providing some relief for individuals with acute stress symptoms but not at risk for developing chronic PTSD. The shortfalls of prevention research have urged the study of predictors for PTSD in order to identify those most at risk for developing PTSD and thereby pinpoint the individuals who would most likely benefit from an early intervention. Predictors of PTSD can be classified into pre-trauma variables, trauma characteristics, and post-trauma variables. A brief review of predictor types is necessary to understand the current body of PTSD prevention research.

Pre-trauma Variables

Variables that may leave a person susceptible to trauma before a trauma occurs may be physiological, biological, or environmental (i.e., previous trauma history). For example, heightened pre-trauma physiological responses to perceived danger cues have been linked to PTSD symptom severity. Pole et al. (2009) found that police cadets who exhibited higher pre-trauma fear potentiated startle and greater skin conductance to both high and low threat danger cues were more likely to develop PTSD and have greater PTSD symptom severity after a traumatic event. Monitoring pre-trauma physiological responses to aversive stimuli may help determine who may need immediate preventative treatment following a trauma. The prevalence of PTSD has also been linked to previous trauma history. This is found in patients who experience trauma in both adulthood and childhood (Binder et al., 2008). In a meta-analysis, Ozer, Best, Lipsey, and Weiss (2008) found that both child and adult trauma experiences significantly and equally increased the likelihood of developing PTSD after a current trauma.

Some genetic underpinnings have recently been discovered to correspond with the development of PTSD. Segman et al. (2005) showed that gene expression patterns in the immediate aftermath of a trauma were predictive of later development of PTSD. Koenen et al. (2005) was the first to show that FKBP5 gene alleles were associated with increased peritraumatic dissociation in children which has been linked to PTSD development (Saxe et al., 2005). Since then, a number of studies have looked at single nucleotide polymorphisms (SNPs) within the FKBPF gene and how they are related to symptoms of PTSD in children and adults. Binder et al. (2008)

studied 8 SNPs within this gene and found that while the SNPs did not directly predict PTSD outcome or correlate with non-child abuse trauma, 4 of the 8 SNPs interacted with history of child abuse to predict adult PTSD symptoms. It was shown that children with these particular alleles experienced greater amounts of peritraumatic dissociation, which was related to higher rates of PTSD in adulthood. Xie et al. (2010) found a relationship between childhood trauma experience and later PTSD development. In this study, SNPs of the FKBP5 genotype moderated the effect of childhood trauma experience on risk for PTSD but only for African American participants. Recently published data (Ressler et al., 2011) shows a sex-specific gene predictor of PTSD. These data reveal that a single SNP in a putative estrogen response element within the PACAP-PACI receptor pathway predicts PTSD diagnosis and symptoms in females. This latter finding may help explain why PTSD occurs about twice as frequently in females as in males.

Trauma Variables

In addition to pre-trauma factors, some predictors of PTSD occur during the trauma. These factors can include trauma severity and type, duration and amount of trauma, and emotions felt during the trauma. In regards to trauma type, certain life-threatening experiences are more likely to lead to PTSD. Using data from the National Comorbidity Survey, Kessler, Sonnega, Bromet, Hughes, and Nelson (1995) found that PTSD is most common after combat exposure among men and rape among women. In a prospective study of rape victims, Rothbaum, Foa, Riggs, Murdock, and Walsh (1992) showed that 94 % of rape victims experience PTSD symptoms within the first 2 weeks of trauma, with natural recovery leading to rates of 47 % after 3 months. Furthermore, the 13.8 % prevalence of PTSD in military veterans from the wars in Iraq and Afghanistan (Tanielian & Jaycox, 2008) is twice that of the civilian population, 6.8 %, according to data from the most recent National Comorbidity Survey (Kessler et al., 2005). Motor vehicle crashes have been shown to have a higher PTSD rate than other traumas such as robbery or tragic death (Norris, 1992). While past data suggest that certain types of traumatic experiences put individuals at a higher risk for PTSD, they do not fully account for the variance in PTSD diagnoses and symptom severity. Thus, additional factors related to the trauma ought to be considered in predicting PTSD.

Other characteristics of traumatic events have been examined to better predict PTSD. Indicators of trauma severity such as subjective assessment of life threat have been implicated as consistent predictors of PTSD. Resnick, Kilpatrick, Best, and Kramer (1992) showed that individuals who thought they would be seriously injured or killed were more likely to develop PTSD. Furthermore, in a meta-analysis of studies on PTSD predictors, Ozer et al. (2008) found that perceived life threat was a systematic and consistent predictor of both PTSD diagnosis and symptoms. Duration of trauma exposure may also be linked to PTSD. For example, some research indicates that more deployments to a combat zone can increase the risk of PTSD (Tanielian & Jaycox, 2008). The continued stress in the recovery phase following a traumatic event may also exacerbate PTSD. After the September 11th attacks, for example, Galea et al. (2002) found that having lost one's possessions during the course of the traumatic event was related to higher rates of PTSD. Finally, one's initial response to the traumatic event may influence their likelihood of developing PTSD. Such appraisals often manifest themselves in how the patient experiences trauma, with two common reactions being peritraumatic emotionality (i.e., high levels of emotions during or immediately after the trauma) and peritraumatic dissociation (i.e., dissociative experiences during or immediately after the trauma). In their meta-analysis of PTSD predictor studies, Ozer et al. (2008) concluded that both emotionality and dissociation during or immediately after the trauma correspond to greater PTSD symptoms and rates of PTSD. Peritraumatic dissociation in particular was the strongest of seven statistically significant predictors of PTSD found by the meta-analysis; thus, especially when including emotionality, the psychological response one has during and immediately following a trauma appears to have a very strong relationship to his or her risk for developing PTSD. Noting responses of high emotionality or dissociative feelings may help identify individuals at a greater risk for eventually being diagnosed with PTSD. Ultimately, however, the typical response after a trauma suggests that PTSD symptoms dissipate over time, leaving a minority of trauma survivors with chronic PTSD (Bryant, 2003). Merely having reactions like dissociation and emotionality that are highly related to PTSD does not necessitate that an individual with such peri-traumatic responses will in fact develop chronic PTSD.

Post-trauma Variables

In many cases, the consequences that occur in the aftermath of trauma can indicate whether someone will later develop PTSD. One important aspect in the immediate aftermath of trauma is one's perceived social support. From a meta-analysis of 11 studies, totaling 3,537 patients, Ozer et al. (2008) found an inverse relationship between social support and PTSD symptoms. Specifically, after the trauma had occurred, individuals who reported lower levels of social support tended to have either more PTSD symptoms or a higher rate of PTSD diagnosis. Furthermore, the strength of the relationship between social support and PTSD symptoms or diagnosis increased as the length of the study increased (Ozer et al., 2008). As more time elapses since the trauma occurred, social support appears to play a stronger role in abating the symptoms of PTSD. Similar results have been noted in studies of large-scale disasters such as the events on September 11th, as low social support was linked to a higher prevalence of PTSD (Galea et al., 2002). However, whether the passage of time allows for more people to provide social support to those with PTSD or whether social support is less important in the immediate aftermath of a trauma remains unclear.

Not only do external factors influence the course of PTSD, but one's own personal responses to the traumatic event play an important role as well. Cognitive appraisals in particular are key predictors as Bryant (2003) notes that exaggerated, catastrophic appraisals in particular have been linked both directly to PTSD and to acute stress disorder (ASD), which often subsequently leads to or predicts PTSD. In addition to psychological factors, physiological indicators immediately following a trauma, such as heart rate (Bryant, Harvey, Guthrie, & Moulds, 2000; Shalev et al., 1998) and cortisol levels (Delahanty, Raimonde, & Spoonster, 2000; Resnick, Yehuda, Pitman, & Foy, 1995), have been shown to be predictors of subsequent PTSD development. However, at this stage of our knowledge, there have been no prospective studies validating any predictor in the immediate aftermath of trauma as specific and sensitive enough to determine who requires intervention and who will recover on their own.

Prevention Approaches to PTSD

Psychological Debriefing

Psychological debriefing (PD) is a term which refers to a number of different methods of crisis intervention, the most common of which is Critical Incident Stress Debriefing (CISD-Mitchell, 1983; Mitchell & Everly, 1996). CISD was developed as a crisis intervention to be implemented within 48 h of a trauma event. CISD intervention involves 7 phases. Phase 1, *the introduction phase*, consists of a description of the CISD process. Phase 2, *the fact phase*, involves the participant explaining what happened. Phase 3, *the thought phase*, is when participants convey their thoughts from the incident. In phase 4, *the feeling phase*, participants share their emotional reactions to the incident. Phase 5, *the assessment phase*, examines physical and psychological symptoms. Phase 6, *the education phase*, explains stress reactions and management. Finally, Phase 7, *the reentry phase*, sums up the debriefing and offers referrals for the participant. CISD is designed to be completed in 3–4 h and can be given individually or in a group session. The term CISD is often used interchangeably with PD in the literature. It should be noted that CISD is one form of PD and can be implemented in a number of different ways. CISD was created for emergency service personnel and offers an alternative to more time consuming psychotherapy. However, this model, as well as PD in general, has been heavily scrutinized in the literature for lacking sufficient support for its claim to be a prevention method for the development of PTSD. As a whole, debriefing literature reviews have determined the practice to be equivocal at best and harmful at worst (Litz, Gray, Bryant, & Adler, 2002; Rose, Bisson, Churchill, & Wessely, 2002). One randomized, controlled trial provided PD for individuals admitted to the hospital after a motor vehicle crash (MVC) (Mayou, Ehlers, & Hobbs, 2000). This method of PD included a review of the accident, addressed initial cognitive appraisals of the trauma, and discussed appropriate emotional expressions. Participant's trauma intrusion and avoidance symptoms were measured using the impact of event scale (IES) at both a 4-month and 3-year follow-up. Results indicate that individuals who had high initial scores on the IES remained symptomatic if they received the intervention and recovered if they did not receive the intervention at follow-up.

The authors suggest that PD may interfere with the natural recovery process and that individuals more likely to develop chronic PTSD may be harmed by a 1-h debriefing intervention. Due to these adverse findings and negative reviews, emphasis has been placed on conducting more methodologically rigorous studies of early intervention for PTSD.

The unpredictability of trauma events makes randomized-controlled trials of debriefing a difficult task. The developers of CISD have used this fact to maintain the credibility of debriefing based mainly on anecdotal accounts of the method (Everly, Flannery, & Mitchell, 2000). Multiple reviewers have condemned the methodology of research cited by CISD supporters (Devilly, Gist, & Cotton, 2006). A number of RCTs have been conducted which show a lack of support for the implementation of debriefing immediately following a trauma event. These studies are critiqued in depth in the Cochrane Review (Rose et al., 2002) which concludes that single session individual psychological debriefing is not useful as a preventative treatment for PTSD and in some cases (Bisson, Jenkins, Alexander, & Bannister, 1997) may lead to increased long-term PTSD symptoms. The Cochrane Review went as far as to suggest that "compulsory debriefing of victims of trauma should cease". These negative reviews have led to a transformation of PD into a more encompassing model which utilizes group CISD as the main treatment model but also includes aspects of trauma support such as pre-incident planning, crisis assessment, and individual crisis intervention. This integrated model is known as Critical Incident Stress Management (CISM) and is described by its authors not as psychotherapy, but as a collection of support services for trauma victims (Everly et al., 2000). Supporters suggest that CISD provided within the CISM model is a more efficacious approach to PD. However, Devilly et al. (2006) determined that there is not enough empirical study to warrant this claim.

PD research has lacked specificity in terms of defined components of the treatment. Generally the term PD refers to an overarching crisis intervention strategy and it is necessary to parse out the specific aspects of the treatment in order to implement the treatment properly. In a randomized, controlled trial, Sijbrandij, Olff, Reitsma, Carlier, and Gersons (2006) analyzed two key aspects of PD based on the CISD protocol, psychoeducation, and emotional ventilation. In this study participants received the CISD treatment with the education phase excluded or with the emotional reaction phase excluded or they received no intervention. Results indicate that PTSD symptoms significantly reduced for all treatment groups with no differences between the two debriefing methods or no debriefing. In addition, individuals with early hyperarousal symptoms experienced an adverse effect of emotional debriefing in that these individuals had higher rates of PTSD at 6-month follow-up than the no debriefing group, further acknowledging that debriefing may be harmful for some people.

More recent reviews acknowledge that the lack of empirically supported research of PD is problematic and may be harmful to the emergency worker groups that utilize the practice most frequently (Suveg, 2007; Tuckey, 2007). These reviews suggest that it is necessary for groups which utilize PD to invest in the necessary scientifically sound research to prove the utility of PD or abandon the practice all together in favor of alternative evidence-based approaches.

Pharmacological Treatments

In recent years, more attention has been given to pharmacological approaches in preventing PTSD. However, there are no currently recommended pharmacological treatments for early prevention of PTSD. A conceptual model of the pathogenesis of PTSD developed by Pitman and Delahanty (2005) suggests that the body's release of stress hormones in response to traumatic events leads to over-consolidation of the traumatic memory and fear conditioning. Thus, pharmacological treatments that inhibit this stress response may prevent the subsequent development of PTSD. Research examining the use of medications such as benzodiazepines, however, has suggested that early administration of these drugs can actually worsen outcomes in recently traumatized individuals, as demonstrated by higher rates of PTSD compared to control conditions (Gelpin, Bonne, Peri, & Brandes, 1996; Mellman, Bustamante, David, & Fins, 2002).

Other medications such as morphine, ketamine, and propranolol are being explored for their impact on subsequent PTSD. Propranolol, for instance, is a beta-adrenergic antagonist that blocks the reuptake of norepinephrine and is often used to treat hypertension (Fletcher, Creamer, & Forbes, 2010). A recent study showed that administration of propranolol reduces neural reactivity in the amygdala, which supports the idea that propranolol may inhibit anxiety responses in trauma-exposed individuals (Hurlemann et al., 2010). In clinical studies, Pitman et al. (2002) conducted a double-blind, placebo-controlled pilot study examining the effectiveness of propranolol at preventing the development of PTSD. Results indicated that administering propranolol within 6 h of the traumatic event and continuing a 10-day course of propranolol led to a reduction in one measure of physiological reactions to trauma-related stimuli 3 months later (Pitman et al., 2002). Similar results were documented by Vaiva et al. (2003) in a nonrandomized study of trauma-exposed individuals, with early administration of propranolol leading to lower rates of PTSD 2 months later. However, another double-blind, randomized-controlled trial of propranolol administered within 48 h of trauma exposure failed to produce significant differences in PTSD rates compared to placebo (Stein, Kerridge, Dimsdale, & Hoyt, 2007). A recent randomized-controlled trial that administered a 19-day trial of up to 240 mg a day of propranolol found no differences in PTSD severity, diagnostic outcome, or physiological reactivity at 4 and 12 weeks post-trauma between propranolol and placebo (Hoge et al., 2012). Thus, results on propranolol as a preventative strategy have been inconsistent and are likely to be abandoned, especially in light of these recent Hoge et al. (2012) data.

Morphine use following traumatic injury has been examined for its potential in preventing PTSD, presumably due to its inhibiting effect of norepinephrine, although the mechanism of action of the PTSD reduction remains speculation (Fletcher et al., 2010). Bryant, Creamer, O'Donnell, Silove, and McFarlane (2009) conducted a naturalistic study of acute morphine administration following traumatic injury and found that patients with greater morphine doses reported less PTSD symptoms 3 months after the initial trauma. A review of medical records of military personnel who experienced combat injury in Iraq indicated that early morphine administration, regardless of dose, were associated with decreased rates of PTSD (Holbrook, Galarneau, Dye, Quinn, & Dougherty, 2010). Similar findings have been found in child trauma populations (Nixon et al., 2010; Saxe et al., 2001). While these studies point to the potential of morphine to prevent subsequent PTSD symptomatology, randomized-controlled trials are needed to further investigate the efficacy of morphine as a preventative strategy and to elucidate the mechanism of action. It is unlikely that physicians will adopt widespread administration of morphine to trauma survivors in the absence of severe physical injury.

Another pharmacological treatment that has been examined for its relationship to PTSD development is ketamine. Ketamine is an *N*-methyl-D-aspartate receptor antagonist that is often used in emergency settings as an anesthetic or sedative (Schonenberg, Reichwald, Domes, Badke, & Hautzinger, 2005). Schonenberg et al. (2005) found that ketamine use in accident victims was actually associated with elevated rates of PTSD. However, a study of military service members with burn injuries found that ketamine administration during surgery was associated with lower rates of PTSD (McGhee, Maani, Garza, Gaylord, & Black, 2008). These contradictory findings are perplexing and point to the need for further research.

In summary, the use of pharmacotherapy to prevent the development of PTSD in trauma-exposed individuals is an important area to explore, but research on potential medications such as morphine and ketamine is in the preliminary stages. Inconsistent results have been documented and few randomized-controlled trials have been conducted. The recent negative RCT with propranolol has effectively eliminated it as a preventative strategy (Hoge et al., 2012). Thus, more work is needed in this area to determine the efficacy of these or other pharmacological treatments as preventive strategies.

Brief Psychosocial Interventions

Besides debriefing approaches such as CISD, there are other brief interventions that have been developed and tested for their ability to reduce distress associated with traumatic events and to prevent the development of PTSD. For example, another intervention that utilizes a group-based debriefing model specifically with military populations is a program called Battlemind Psychological Debriefing. Three different versions of Battlemind Debriefing exist, including a version at postdeployment, event-driven debriefing (e.g., following a specific traumatic event), and time-driven debriefing that occurs in theater at regularly scheduled intervals (Adler, Bliese, et al. 2009; Adler, Castro, & McGurk, 2009). The intervention consists of five phases, including introducing the program, identifying specific events that may be causing difficulties for unit members, normalizing reactions to the event, identifying common problems to look for in themselves and their buddies (e.g., anger, sleep problems), and finally reinforcing certain training principles (Adler, Bliese, et al. 2009; Adler, Castro, & McGurk, 2009). Battlemind Psychological Debriefing is said to diverge from other forms of PD in its lack of emphasis on recounting the traumatic event, its focus on specific deployment-related issues, and its group application and delivery at regularly scheduled intervals during deployment (Adler, Bliese, et al. 2009; Adler, Castro, & McGurk, 2009). A recent study documented some preliminary support for this program compared to a stress education condition, with results suggesting that Battlemind Debriefing led to fewer PTSD and depression symptoms, especially among groups with high combat exposure (Adler, Bliese, et al. 2009; Adler, Castro, & McGurk, 2009). However, more research is needed to establish the efficacy of this intervention.

Other interventions have been developed as well. Gidron et al. (2001) created a memory-structuring intervention based on the theory that memories of traumatic events tend to be fragmented and that creating a more organized, chronological memory of the event can prevent the development of PTSD. The intervention consisted of phone contact with a therapist who would listen to the patient's recounting of the traumatic memory and clarify details. The therapist would then read back a more organized and structured version of the traumatic memory, which would be repeated and practiced by the patient to facilitate processing. In a small pilot study utilizing a randomized-controlled design, results indicated that patients who received the memory-structuring intervention had lower PTSD symptoms 3 months later. However, a follow-up study found no overall group differences, although the intervention did appear effective at reducing PTSD symptoms specifically among women (Gidron et al., 2007). Given the small sample size utilized in both of these studies, these results should be considered preliminary with more research needed to interpret the results.

Another intervention developed specifically for survivors of sexual assault is a video-based treatment designed to precede a forensic rape exam. This brief 17-min video first provides information about the exam itself to prepare survivors for the procedure. Following this segment, the video goes on to provide psychoeducation about common reactions to rape and strategies to help limit avoidance and reduce anxiety (Resnick, Acierno, Holmes, Kilpatrick, & Jager, 1999). Results of a randomized study indicated preliminary support for reduced distress and marijuana abuse among women who watched the video compared to women who received standard care, with women with prior assaults appearing to benefit the most from the intervention (Resnick, Acierno, Kilpatrick, & Holmes, 2005). A more recent report on this intervention not only continued to identify significant benefits for women with a prior assault history but also documented a small increase in PTSD and anxiety at the 6-week follow-up among women with no prior assault history (Resnick et al., 2007). Further research on this video-based treatment is needed, but the potential of such a brief and easily disseminated intervention could be significant for trauma survivors and PTSD prevention.

Psychoeducation about common trauma reactions has also been tested in other formats, specifically in the form of self-help booklets provided to patients who have presented to emergency departments for injuries related to trauma exposure. Turpin, Downs, and Mason (2005) tested the efficacy of a brief self-help booklet that reviewed common physical and emotional reactions to trauma and that provided advice on seeking emotional support and preventing avoidance behavior. Results indicated that those who received the self-help booklet did not have greater improvements in PTSD and depression compared to individuals who did not receive the same information (Turpin et al., 2005). In a second examination of this approach that targeted high-risk patients with greater levels of acute stress, results again showed no advantage to receiving the self-help information in regards to subsequent PTSD and depression symptoms (Scholes, Turpin, & Mason, 2007). Thus, research evaluating the utility of self-help information that provides psychoeducation to recent trauma survivors suggests that these approaches are not useful prevention strategies for PTSD.

Exposure Therapy

Exposure therapy (ET) is a therapeutic approach to treating PTSD that utilizes cognitive-behavioral treatment strategies (CBT) and for PTSD, typically includes asking the patient to remember and recount a narrative of their traumatic experience, known as imaginal exposure. This account is often tape-recorded and given to the patient to listen to for homework. In vivo exposure involves helping the patient to encounter situations that are realistically safe, yet have been avoided because they trigger memories of the traumatic event. Prolonged Exposure (PE) is a specific program with specific components of ET (Foa, Hembree, & Rothbaum, 2007). First disseminated in the early 1990s by Foa, Rothbaum, Riggs, and Murdock (1991), PE has continually shown itself as a very effective method of treating PTSD in many different populations (Powers, Halpern, Ferenschak, Gillihan, & Foa, 2010). PE traditionally consists of 9–12 therapy sessions that are anywhere from 90 to 120 min each with the addition of homework to be done by the patient in between therapy sessions (Foa et al., 2007). The therapist personalizes the sessions and homework assignments for each individual patient in order for the patient to be exposed repeatedly to the traumatic memory and to reduce anxiety and PTSD symptoms over time via extinction and modify their maladaptive thoughts about the event (Foa et al., 2007). According to a meta-analysis by Powers and colleagues in 2010, using a sample size of 658 participants, 86 % of participants suffering from PTSD who received ET as opposed to control conditions did not meet PTSD diagnostic criteria at posttreatment. The data in support of ET in and of itself is overwhelming for chronic PTSD and suggests it may be an effective option for the prevention of PTSD in people exposed to traumatic situations (Bryant, Sackville, Dang, Moulds, & Guthrie, 1999).

ET adds to the CBT approach of anxiety management by activating the traumatic memory to aid in emotional processing of the trauma in addition to the reduction of anxiety (Foa et al., 2007). ET also aims to reduce avoidance of the traumatic memory or triggering situations. Several studies support the use of ET with participants who have been exposed to traumatic events (Bryant et al., 1999, 2008; Bryant, Moulds, Guthrie, Dang, & Nixon, 2003; Foa et al., 2005; Hembree, Rauch, & Foa, 2003; Rothbaum, Astin, & Marsteller, 2005). With the exception of one study conducted by Bryant et al. in 2003, which left out the in-vivo exposure element of ET (though still finding ET effective), studies have shown the key factor to be exposure even when paired with other treatments, such as cognitive restructuring (CR) and anxiety management (Bryant et al., 1999, 2003; Foa et al., 2005). In addition, though some treatments have shown benefit to PTSD sufferers, PE seems to work more quickly (Hembree et al., 2003).

Recent research has found that a percentage of people exposed to a traumatic event tend to develop what is known as Acute Stress Disorder (ASD), and a large percentage of these people go on to develop full-blown PTSD (Bryant et al., 1999). As an example, in participants who had experienced a motor vehicle crash and subsequently enrolled in a study conducted by Bryant and colleagues in 1999, 78–82 % of participants with ASD had PTSD 6 months following the accident. ASD occurs within a period of 2 days to 4 weeks following a traumatic event; however, not everyone who eventually develops PTSD after a traumatic event develops ASD, (Bryant et al., 1999, 2008) indicating that it is clearly not a perfect predictor of PTSD.

Along with studies investigating ASD, researchers have tried therapeutic methods used in treating full-blown PTSD to test whether or not they can also prevent the development of chronic PTSD. Various studies have shown ET to be an effective option in the prevention of PTSD development when administered to patients exhibiting symptoms of ASD soon after a nonsexual or combat-related traumatic event (Bryant et al., 1999, 2008). Bryant et al. (1999, 2008) administered only five ET sessions in their trials, thereby condensing the normal timeline of ET treatment. One study paired ET and anxiety management training (AMT) against both ET alone and supportive counseling (SC) and found that both groups that included ET had positive results (Bryant et al., 1999). Even more interesting is that ET with AMT was not significantly different from ET alone (Bryant et al., 1999). Foa, Zoellner, and Feeny (2006) had similar results in an early CBT intervention based on PE for female assault survivors. Results from this study indicated that the brief PE intervention produced lower rates of PTSD severity and general anxiety at post-intervention and a 3-month follow-up compared to SC, although later assessments identified equivalent outcomes between the two groups. Bryant et al. (2008) used ET in an early intervention trial against CR alone and a wait-list condition and found that ET's results were significantly better. At follow-up, 12 % of participants who had received ET exhibited symptoms of PTSD whereas 47 % of those in the CR group exhibited symptoms of PTSD. This suggests that exposure may be a key element for preventing and treating PTSD (Bryant et al., 2008).

ET has been shown to be an effective therapy for treating chronic PTSD and now shows promise as a possibly effective method for the prevention of chronic PTSD. Hembree and colleagues have found that PE can be effectively and efficiently disseminated using nonexpert therapists in very little time (Hembree et al., 2003). The Department of Veterans Affairs (VA) and the Substance Abuse and Mental Health Services Administration (SAMHSA) have begun efforts to internally disseminate PE protocols within their mental health services. Despite all of the promising data to date, there is still much unknown. Many studies exclude combat and sexual assault-related trauma victims (Bryant et al., 1999, 2008). There has also not been in-depth assessment in regards to the development of long-term psychopathology often associated with exposure to trauma and PTSD, such as depression and substance abuse (Bryant et al., 1999). As far as the actual ET delivered, there is no set or widely accepted formula for ET delivery for prevention of PTSD, as protocols have been altered in studies in order to further differentiate the ET treatment with the other experimental groups (Bryant et al., 2008). Investigations using combat and sexual assault trauma victims as well as a more clearly defined ET prevention protocol are needed. With further research, an ET protocol for acute trauma response can hopefully be developed and disseminated in order to prevent the suffering associated with chronic PTSD.

PTSD as a Disorder of Extinction: Extinction and Habituation

We view PTSD partly as a disorder of extinction. The symptoms of PTSD can be considered as part of the normal response to trauma but in the majority of trauma-exposed individuals, will decrease over time. Extinction is a widely documented and empirically validated phenomenon which involves a decrease in conditioned response when the conditioned stimulus (e.g., trauma-related cues that are not dangerous) is introduced repeatedly without the presence of the unconditioned stimulus (e.g., the trauma itself; Myers & Davis, 2002). Recent findings suggest that habituation may play an important role in moderating extinction (McSweeney & Swindell, 2002). Habituation, the decrease in responsiveness to a stimulus, occurs as a result of repeated and prolonged exposure to the stimulus (McSweeney & Swindell, 2002). Since habituation and extinction seem to share common processes, it would seem plausible to assume that deficits in habituation would retard the process of extinction and that together these deficits could maintain PTSD symptomatology and severity.

Indeed, research tends to support this assumption. Rothbaum, Kozak, Foa, and Whitaker (2001) found that rape victims with PTSD required more trials to habituate to auditory stimuli than non-PTSD controls. There was also a higher percentage of non-habituators to the auditory stimuli in the PTSD group than in the non-PTSD group. Similar findings were documented in a study with Vietnam veterans with PTSD, which found that current PTSD severity influenced the patients' ability to inhibit the fear response to safety cues in an experimental paradigm (Jovanovic et al., 2009). Specifically, patients with greater PTSD symptomatology had more difficulty inhibiting the fear response. Other research has documented impaired fear inhibition in civilian populations and found that this impairment appears specific to PTSD, versus other disorders such as major depression (Jovanovic et al., 2010). There is some indication that there may be specific PTSD symptom subclusters that are more strongly associated with difficulty inhibiting the fear response. Norrholm et al. (2011) found that in a civilian population, individuals with higher levels of reexperiencing symptoms exhibit greater startle responses than individuals with lower levels of reexperiencing symptoms during both the fear acquisition phase and the extinction phase.

Consistent with this conceptualization of PTSD as a failure of extinction are the findings that exposure therapy, which utilizes extinction mechanisms in which patients are helped to recall the traumatic memory through imagery and to confront safe but feared reminders, is an efficacious treatment for PTSD (Foa & Rothbaum, 1998). Animal research has indicated that the length of time that passes between the original acquisition of fear and subsequent extinction training influences the extinction process, with shorter delays producing more lasting fear extinction (Myers, Ressler, & Davis, 2006). Thus, extinction training done very shortly after fear conditioning may prevent consolidation of the original fear memory (Myers et al., 2006). In a translational study that utilized human subjects, participants were fear conditioned and extinguished at either 10 min or 72 h after conditioning. Participants who were immediately put through the extinction training had significantly lower levels of fear potentiated startle than those participants who underwent extinction training at a later time (Norrholm et al., 2008). Thus, earlier application of extinction training appears more effective than delayed training, which points to the potential need for more immediate intervention with trauma-exposed individuals.

Early Intervention for Trauma-Exposed Individuals in the Emergency Department

Based on these scientific findings, prevention approaches that utilize the early application of exposure therapy, a form of extinction training, may be effective at preventing the subsequent development of PTSD. The effectiveness of PE as both a treatment for chronic PTSD and acute stress disorder has already been documented. However, given the greater efficacy of early versus delayed extinction training in basic and preclinical studies (Myers et al., 2006; Norrholm et al., 2008), the application of prolonged imaginal exposure in the immediate aftermath of the trauma may have great potential as a preventative approach.

Thus, Rothbaum et al. (2008) have initiated pilot testing of an early exposure-based intervention delivered in the emergency department within hours of the initial trauma exposure. An initial study designed to assess feasibility of conducting this type of intervention in an emergency setting identified that a majority of patients would agree to participate in an intervention for PTSD (Rothbaum et al., 2008). This pilot study also tested an abbreviated intervention involving one session of prolonged imaginal exposure versus an assessment only condition. Although participants were nonrandomized, results suggested that individuals who received the intervention reported slightly lower levels of depression and clinician-rated global ratings of distress 1 week after the initial trauma (Rothbaum et al., 2008).

A randomized clinical trial was then conducted at a Level I trauma center located in a large metropolitan area in the Southeast (Rothbaum et al., 2012). All patients who had experienced a criterion A traumatic event were approached and screened within hours of arriving in the emergency department. Interested individuals who consented to participate were randomly assigned to an assessment only condition or to the intervention condition. In this research trial, the intervention consisted of 3 h-long sessions of an adaptation of prolonged imaginal exposure, with the first session being conducted in the emergency department before patients were discharged. The remaining two sessions were conducted 1 and 2 weeks post-trauma. The first session consisted of a brief overview of the treatment rationale, followed by 30–45 min of imaginal exposure to the traumatic memory. This was followed by briefly processing the exposure with the therapist, identifying maladaptive cognitions, discussing self-care, and assigning therapeutic homework. Homework consisted of identifying and practicing in vivo exposures to combat avoidance, identifying and correcting unhelpful cognitions, and promoting self-care strategies. Finally, participants were taught a brief breathing retraining exercise. Subsequent sessions consisted of homework review, further imaginal exposure (30–45 min) and processing, and assignment of new in vivo exposures and self-care strategies for homework. At 4 and 12-weeks post-trauma, participants returned for follow-up with an assessor who was blind to their assigned condition. Clinician ratings of PTSD were collected, as well as self-report measures of depression and past trauma symptoms.

Results of this clinical trial indicated that emergency room patients receiving the early intervention experienced lower posttraumatic stress reactions at 4 and 12 weeks post-injury compared to patients receiving assessment only (Rothbaum et al., 2012). Intervention participants also endorsed lower depressive symptoms at 4 weeks post-injury. When examining intervention impact across different types of traumas, results suggested that the intervention was most effective at reducing PTSD in rape victims (Rothbaum et al., 2012). In addition, genetic biomarkers of PTSD were shown to predict higher posttraumatic stress reactions in patients who did not receive the intervention (Rothbaum et al., in press). However, among patients receiving the intervention, there was no relationship between genetic risk for PTSD and posttraumatic stress symptoms at 12 weeks post-injury. Thus, early exposure-based intervention delivered immediately post-trauma appeared in this study to mitigate potential genetic risk for PTSD (Rothbaum et al., in press). Although additional research is needed, we believe that early provision of exposure-based treatment in the immediate aftermath of trauma exposure may represent an effective strategy for preventing the development of PTSD.

Summary and Conclusions

Exposure to potentially traumatic events is a relatively common experience with most trauma-exposed individuals experiencing acute stress reactions immediately following the trauma that subside over time. Identifying who is most at risk for subsequent development of PTSD can help aid prevention efforts by focusing resources and intervention on those who are most likely to suffer long-term consequences as a result of trauma exposure as opposed to a blanket approach (Ehlers et al., 2003). Although more work is needed, the above research suggests that progress has been made in understanding risk factors for PTSD and that, in the future, we may have a better understanding of how to effectively and efficiently intervene with those most vulnerable to developing PTSD. However, at this stage of our knowledge, there have been no prospective studies validating any predictor in the immediate aftermath of trauma as specific and sensitive enough to determine who requires intervention and who will recover on their own.

Unfortunately, past efforts to prevent PTSD intervene indiscriminately, primarily relying on PD (psychological debriefing) and CISD (critical incident stress debriefing), and lack empirical support. By attempting to intervene with every person exposed to a traumatic event, the natural healing process is interrupted in addition to wasting precious resources (Ehlers et al., 2003). The results of debriefing research are equivocal at best with some cases of individuals subjectively reporting improvement in PTSD symptoms, while other studies show rates of increased PTSD in individuals who receive PD (Bisson et al., 1997; Mayou et al., 2000). Despite empirical evidence suggesting single-session interventions early on are not effective, they are still widely practiced and their use should be reconsidered (Ehlers et al., 2003).

The shortcomings of debriefing highlight the need for a truly effective early intervention that can prevent PTSD. Both psychosocial and pharmacological approaches have been developed, but most remain in the preliminary stages and require further testing and replication before they can be recommended as effective prevention strategies in trauma-exposed individuals. Prolonged exposure represents one empirically supported treatment for PTSD that has also shown promise as an early intervention designed to prevent chronic PTSD. However, it has typically been provided only to individuals with more severe symptoms who meet criteria for Acute Stress Disorder. Even so, the application methods of PE as an intervention mechanism widely differ, as the traditional delivery model of PE is dropped in favor of variations that are less cumbersome (Bryant et al., 1999). Pharmacological approaches that seem viable have quirks as well, many of which are still unknown due to the lack of clinical trials.

While there are many possibilities that seem promising for the prevention of chronic PTSD, the reality is that it is still extremely difficult to predict who will heal naturally and who needs help doing so following traumatic exposure. More research is needed in all areas, from predictors to actual intervention techniques, whether they are pharmacological or psychological. What is known, however, is that PTSD can be detected early on and educating both survivors of traumatic events as well as their social support networks in which warning signs to look for in the weeks and months following traumatic exposure is important (Ehlers et al., 2003; Roberts et al. 2009). Intervening for PTSD early on will save money, lives, and help many people understand that they are not alone in their suffering.

References

Adler, A. B., Bliese, P. D., McGurk, D., Hoge, C. W., & Castro, C. A. (2009). Battlemind debriefing and Battlemind training as early interventions with soldiers returning from Iraq: Randomization by platoon. *Journal of Consulting and Clinical Psychology, 77*, 928–940.

Adler, A. B., Castro, C. A., & McGurk, D. (2009). Time-driven Battlemind Psychological Debriefing: A group-level early intervention in combat. *Military Medicine, 174*, 21–28.

Binder, E., Bradley, R., Liu, W., Epstein, M., Deveau, T., Binder, E., et al. (2008). FKBP5 polymorphisms moderate effects of child abuse on risk for PTSD in adults. *Journal of the American Medical Association, 299*(11), 1291–1305.

Bisson, J. I., Jenkins, P. L., Alexander, J., & Bannister, C. (1997). Randomised controlled trial of psychological debriefing for victims of acute burn trauma. *British Journal of Psychiatry, 171*, 78–81.

Breslau, N., Kessler, R. C., Chilcoat, H. D., Schultz, L. R., Davis, G. C., & Andreski, P. (1998). Trauma and posttraumatic stress disorder in the community: the 1996 Detroit Area Survey of Trauma. *Archives of General Psychiatry, 55*, 626–632.

Bryant, R. (2003). Early predictors of posttraumatic stress disorder. *Society of Biological Psychiatry, 53*, 789–795.

Bryant, R. A., Creamer, M., O'Donnell, M., Silove, D., & McFarlane, A. C. (2009). A study of protective function of acute morphine administration on subsequent posttraumatic stress disorder. *Biological Psychiatry, 65*, 438–440.

Bryant, R. A., Harvey, A. G., Guthrie, R. M., & Moulds, M. L. (2000). A prospective study of psychophysiological arousal, acute stress disorder, and posttraumatic stress disorder. *Journal of Abnormal Psychology, 109*(2), 341–344.

Bryant, R. A., Mastrodomenico, J., Felmingham, K. L., Hopwood, S., Kenny, L., Kandris, E., et al. (2008). Treatment of acute stress disorder: A randomized controlled trial. *Archives of General Psychiatry, 65*(6), 659–667. doi:10.1001/archpsyc.65.6.659.

Bryant, R. A., Moulds, M. L., Guthrie, R. M., Dang, S. T., & Nixon, R. D. V. (2003). Imaginal exposure alone and imaginal exposure with cognitive restructuring in treatment of posttraumatic stress disorder. *Journal of Consulting and Clinical Psychology, 71*, 706–712.

Bryant, R. A., Sackville, T., Dang, S., Moulds, M., & Guthrie, R. (1999). Treating acute stress disorder: An evaluation of cognitive behavior therapy and supportive counseling techniques. *American Journal of Psychiatry, 156*(11), 1780–1786.

Cougle, J. R., Keough, M. E., Riccardi, C. J., & Sachs-Ericsson, N. (2009). Anxiety disorders and suicidality in the National Comorbidity Survey-Replication. *Journal of Psychiatric Research, 43*(9), 825–829.

Dalton, R., Scheeringa, M. S., & Zeanah, C. H. (2008). Did the prevalence of PTSD following Hurricane Katrina match a rapid needs assessment prediction? A template for future public planning after large-scale disasters. *Psychiatric Annals, 38*(2), 134–141.

Delahanty, D. L., Raimonde, A., & Spoonster, E. (2000). Initial posttraumatic urinary cortisol levels predict subsequent PTSD symptoms in motor vehicle accident victims. *Biological Psychiatry, 48*(9), 940–947.

Devilly, G. J., Gist, R., & Cotton, P. (2006). Ready! Fire! Aim! The status of psychological debriefing and therapeutic interventions: In the work place and after disasters. *Review of General Psychology, 10*(4), 318–345.

Ehler, A., & Clark, D. (2003). Early psychological interventions for adult survivors of trauma: A review. *Biological Psychiatry, 53*, 817–826.

Everly, G. R., Flannery, R. R., & Mitchell, J. T. (2000). Critical incident stress management (CISM): A review of the literature. *Aggression and Violent Behavior, 5*(1), 23–40.

Fletcher, S., Creamer, M., & Forbes, D. (2010). Preventing posttraumatic stress disorder: Are drugs the answer? *Australian and New Zealand Journal of Psychiatry, 44*, 1064–1071.

Foa, E. B., Hembree, E. A., Cahill, S. P., Rauch, S. A. M., Riggs, D. S., Feeny, N. C., et al. (2005). Randomized trial of prolonged exposure for posttraumatic stress disorder with and without cognitive restructuring: Outcome at academic and community clinics. *Journal of Consulting and Clinical Psychology, 73*(5), 953–964. doi:10.1037/0022-006x.73.5.953.

Foa, E. B., Hembree, E. A., & Rothbaum, B. (2007). *Prolonged exposure therapy for PTSD: Emotional processing of traumatic experiences: Therapist guide*. New York, NY: Oxford University Press.

Foa, E. B., & Rothbaum, B. O. (1998). *Treating the trauma of rape: Cognitive-behavioral therapy for PTSD*. New York, NY: The Guilford Press.

Foa, E. B., Rothbaum, R. O., Riggs, D. S., & Murdock, T. B. (1991). Treatment of posttraumatic stress disorder in rape victims: A comparison between cognitive-behavioral procedures and counseling. *Journal of Consulting and Clinical Psychology, 59*, 715–723.

Foa, E. B., Zoellner, L. A., & Feeny, N. C. (2006). An evaluation of three brief programs for facilitating recovery after assault. *Journal of Traumatic Stress, 19*, 29–43.

Galea, S., Ahern, J., Resnick, H., Kilpatrick, D., Bucuvalas, M., Gold, J., et al. (2002). Psychological sequelae of the September 11 terrorist attacks in New York city. *New England Journal of Medicine, 346*(13), 982–987.

Gelpin, E., Bonne, O., Peri, T., & Brandes, D. (1996). Treatment of recent trama survivors with benzodiazepines: A prospective study. *Journal of Clinical Psychiatry, 57*, 390–394.

Gidron, Y., Gal, R., Freedman, S., Twiser, I., Lauden, A., Snir, Y., et al. (2001). Translating research findings to PTSD prevention: Results of a randomized-controlled pilot study. *Journal of Traumatic Stress, 14*(4), 773–780.

Gidron, Y., Gal, R., Givati, G., Lauden, A., Snir, Y., & Benjamin, J. (2007). Interactive effects of memory structuring and gender in preventing posttraumatic stress symptoms. *Journal of Nervous and Mental Disease, 195*, 179–182.

Greenberg, P. E., Sistsky, T., Kessler, R. C., Finkelstein, S. N., Berndt, E. R., Davidson, J. R., et al. (1999). The economic burden of anxiety disorder in the 1990's. *Journal of Clinical Psychiatry, 60*, 427–435.

Hembree, E. A., Rauch, S. A. M., & Foa, E. B. (2003). Beyond the manual: The insider's guide to prolonged exposure therapy for PTSD. *Cognitive and Behavioral Practice, 10*(1), 22–30. doi:10.1016/s1077-7229(03)80005-6.

Hoge, E. A., Worthington, J. J., Nagurney, J. T., Chang, Y., Kay, E. B., Feterowski, C. M., et al. (2012). Effect of acute posttrauma propranolol on PTSD outcome and physiological responses during script-driven imagery. *CNS Neuroscience and Therapeutics, 18*, 21–27. doi:10.1111/j.1755-5949.2010.00227.x.

Holbrook, T. L., Galarneau, M. R., Dye, J. L., Quinn, K., & Dougherty, A. L. (2010). Morphine use after combat injury in Iraq and posttraumatic stress disorder. *New England Journal of Medicine, 362*, 110–117.

Hurlemann, R., Walter, H., Rehme, A. K., Kukolja, J., Santoro, S. C., Schmidt, C., et al. (2010). Human amygdale reactivity is diminished by the β-noradrenergic antagonist propranolol. *Psychological Medicine, 40*, 1839–1848.

Jovanovic, T., Norrholm, S. D., Blanding, N. Q., Davis, M., Duncan, E., Bradley, B., et al. (2010). Impaired fear inhibition is a biomarker of PTSD but not depression. *Depression and Anxiety, 27*, 244–251.

Jovanovic, T., Norrholm, S. D., Fennell, J. E., Keyes, M., Fiallos, A., Meyers, K. M., et al. (2009). Posttraumatic stress disorder may be associated with impaired fear inhibition: Relation to symptom severity. *Psychiatry Review, 167*, 151–160.

Kessler, R. C., Berglund, P., Delmer, O., Jin, R., Merikangas, K. R., & Walters, E. E. (2005). Lifetime prevalence and age-of-onset distributions of DSM-IV disorders in the National Comorbidity Survey Replication. *Archives of General Psychiatry, 62*(6), 593–602.

Kessler, R. C., Sonnega, A., Bromet, E., Hughes, M., & Nelson, C. B. (1995). Posttraumatic stress disorder in the National Comorbidity Survey. *Archives of General Psychiatry, 52*(12), 1048–1060.

Koenen, K. C., Saxe, G. G., Purcell, S. S., Smoller, J. W., Bartholomew, D. D., Miller, A. A., et al. (2005). Polymorphisms in FKBP5 are associated with peritraumatic dissociation in medically injured children. *Molecular Psychiatry, 10*(12), 1058–1059.

Leserman, J., Drossman, D. A., Zhiming, L., Toomey, T. C., Nacman, G., & Glogau, L. (1996). Sexual and physical abuse history in gastroenterology practice: How types of abuse impact health status. *Psychosomatic Medicine, 58*, 4–15.

Litz, B., Gray, M., Bryant, R., & Adler, A. (2002). Early intervention for trauma: Current status and future directions. *Clinical Psychology: Science and Practice, 9*(2), 112–134.

Marciniak, M. D., Lage, M. J., Dunayevich, E., Russell, J. M., Bowman, L., Landbloom, R. P., et al. (2005). The cost of treating anxiety: The medical and demographic correlates that impact total medical costs. *Depression and Anxiety, 21*, 178–184.

Mayou, R. A., Ehlers, A. A., & Hobbs, M. M. (2000). Psychological debriefing for road traffic accident victims: Three-year follow-up of a randomised controlled trial. *British Journal of Psychiatry, 176*, 589–593.

McGhee, L. L., Maani, C. V., Garza, T. H., Gaylord, K. M., & Black, I. H. (2008). The correlation between ketamine and posttraumatic stress disorder in burned service members. *Journal of Trauma-Injury Infection and Critical Care, 64*(2 Suppl), S195–S199.

McSweeney, F. K., & Swindell, S. (2002). Common processes may contribute to extinction and habituation. *The Journal of General Psychology, 129*(4), 364–400.

Mellman, T. A., Bustamante, V., David, D., & Fins, A. I. (2002). Hypnotic medication in the aftermath of trauma. *Journal of Clinical Psychiatry, 63*, 1183–1184.

Miller, S. M., Brody, D. S., & Summerton, J. (1988). Styles of coping with threat: Implications for health. *Journal of Personality and Social Psychology, 54*, 142–148.

Mitchell, J. T. (1983). When disaster strikes. The critical incident stress debriefing process. *Journal of Emergency Medical Service, 8*, 36–39.

Mitchell, J. T., & Everly, G. S., Jr. (1996). *Critical incident stress debriefing: An operations manual for the prevention of traumatic stress among emergency services and disaster workers* (2nd ed.). Ellicott City, MD: Chevron Publishing Corporation.

Myers, K. M., & Davis, M. (2002). Behavioral and neural analysis of extinction. *Neuron, 36*, 567–584.

Myers, K. M., Ressler, K. J., & Davis, M. (2006). Different mechanisms of fear extinction dependent on length of time since fear acquisition. *Learning and Memory, 13*, 216–223.

Nixon, R. D. V., Nehmy, T. J., Ellis, A. A., Ball, S. A., Menne, A., & McKinnon, A. C. (2010). Predictors of posttraumatic stress in children following injury: The influence of appraisals, heart rate, and morphine use. *Behaviour Research and Therapy, 48*(8), 810–815.

Norrholm, S. D., Jovanovic, T., Olin, I. W., Sands, L. A., Karapanou, I., Bradley, B., et al. (2011). Fear extinction in traumatized civilians with posttraumatic stress disorder: Relation to symptom severity. *Biological Psychiatry, 69*, 556–563.

Norrholm, S. D., Jovanovic, T., Vervliet, B., Boshoven, W., Myers, K. M., Davis, M., et al. (2008). Timing of extinction relative to acquisition: A parametric analysis of fear extinction in humans. *Behavioral Neuroscience, 122*, 1016–1030.

Norris, F. H. (1992). Epidemiology of trauma: Frequency and impact of different potentially traumatic events on different demographic groups. *Journal of Consulting and Clinical Psychology, 60*(3), 409–418.

Ozer, E. J., Best, S. R., Lipsey, T. L., & Weiss, D. S. (2008). Predictors of posttraumatic stress disorder and symptoms in adults: A meta-analysis. *Psychological Trauma: Theory, Research, Practice, and Policy, S*(1), 3–36.

Pitman, R. K., & Delahanty, D. L. (2005). Conceptually driven pharmacologic approaches to acute trauma. *CNS Spectrums, 10*, 99–106.

Pitman, R., Sanders, K., Zusman, R., Healy, A., Cheema, F., & Lasko, N. (2002). Pilot study of secondary prevention of posttraumatic stress disorder with propranolol. *Biological Psychiatry, 51*(2), 189–192.

Pole, N., Neylan, T. C., Otte, C., Henn-Hasse, C., Metzler, T. J., & Marmar, C. R. (2009). Prospective prediction of posttraumatic stress disorder symptoms using fear potentiated auditory startle responses. *Biological Psychiatry, 65*(3), 235–240.

Powers, M. B., Halpern, J. M., Ferenschak, M. P., Gillihan, S. J., & Foa, E. B. (2010). A meta-analytic review of prolonged exposure for posttraumatic stress disorder. *Clinical Psychology Review, 30*, 635–641. doi:10.1016/j.cpr.2010.04.007.

Resnick, H., Acierno, R., Holmes, M., Kilpatrick, D. G., & Jager, N. (1999). Prevention of post-rape psychopathology: Preliminary findings of controlled acute rape treatment study. *Journal of Anxiety Disorders, 13*, 359–370.

Resnick, H., Acierno, R., Kilpatrick, D. G., & Holmes, M. (2005). Description of an early intervention to prevent substance abuse and psychopathology in recent rape victims. *Behavior Modification, 29*, 156–188.

Resnick, H., Acierno, R., Waldrop, A. E., King, L., King, D., Danielson, C., et al. (2007). Randomized controlled evaluation of an early intervention to prevent post-rape psychopathology. *Behaviour Research and Therapy, 45*, 2432–2447.

Resnick, H. S., Kilpatrick, D. G., Best, C. L., & Kramer, T. L. (1992). Vulnerability-stress factors in development of posttraumatic stress disorder. *Journal of Nervous and Mental Disease, 180*(7), 424–430.

Resnick, H. S., Yehuda, R., Pitman, R. K., & Foy, D. W. (1995). Effect of previous trauma on acute plasma cortisol level following rape. *The American Journal of Psychiatry, 152*(11), 1675–1677.

Ressler, K. J., Mercer, K. B., Bradley, B., Jovanovic, T., Mahan, A., Kerley, K., et al. (2011). Posttraumatic stress disorder is associated with PACAP and the PAC1 receptor. *Nature, 470*, 492–497.

Roberts, N. P., Kitchiner, N. J., Kenardy, J., & Bisson, J. I. (2009). Systematic review and meta-analysis of multiple-session early interventions following traumatic events. *American Journal of Psychiatry, 166*, 293–301.

Rose, S., Bisson, J., Churchill, R., Wessely, S. (2002). Psychological debriefing for preventing post traumatic stress disorder (PTSD). The Cochrane Database of Systematic Review, (2), CD000560.

Rothbaum, B. O., Astin, M. C., & Marsteller, F. (2005). Prolonged exposure vs. EMDR for PTSD rape victims. *Journal of Traumatic Stress, 18*, 607–616.

Rothbaum, B. O., Foa, E. B., Riggs, D. S., Murdock, T., & Walsh, W. (1992). A prospective examination of posttraumatic stress disorder in rape victims. *Journal of Traumatic Stress, 5*, 455–475.

Rothbaum, B. O., Houry, D., Heekin, M., Leiner, A. S., Daugherty, J., Smith, L. S., et al. (2008). A pilot study of an exposure-based intervention in the ED designed to prevent posttraumatic stress disorder. *American Journal of Emergency Medicine, 26*, 326–330.

Rothbaum, B. O., Kearns, M. C., Price, M., Malcoun, E., Davis, M., Ressler, K. J., et al. (2012). Early intervention may prevent the development of posttraumatic stress disorder: A randomized pilot civilian study with modified prolonged exposure. *Biological Psychiatry, 72*(11), 957–963.

Rothbaum, B.O., Kearns, M.C., Reiser, E., Davis, J.S., Kerley, K.A., Rothbaum, A.O., et al. (in press). Early intervention following trauma may mitigate genetic risk for PTSD in civilians: A pilot prospective emergency department study. *Journal of Clinical Psychiatry, 75*.

Rothbaum, B. O., Kozak, M. J., Foa, E. B., & Whitaker, D. J. (2001). Posttraumatic stress disorder in rape victims: Autonomic habituation to auditory stimuli. *Journal of Traumatic Stress, 14*, 283–293.

Saxe, G., Stoddard, F., Courtney, D., Cunningham, K., Chawla, N., Sheridan, R., et al. (2001). Relationship between acute morphine and the course of PTSD in children with burns. *Journal of American Academy of Child Adolescent Psychiatry, 40*(8), 915–921.

Saxe, G. N., Stoddard, F., Hall, E., Chawla, N., Lopez, C., Sheridan, R., et al. (2005). Pathways to PTSD, Part I: Children with burns. *The American Journal of Psychiatry, 162*(7), 1299–1304.

Scholes, C., Turpin, G., & Mason, S. (2007). A randomised controlled trial to assess the effectiveness of providing self-help information to people with symptoms of acute stress disorder following a traumatic injury. *Behaviour Research and Therapy, 45*, 2527–2536.

Schonenberg, M., Reichwald, U., Domes, G., Badke, A., & Hautzinger, M. (2005). Effects of peritraumatic ketamine medication on early and sustained posttraumatic stress symptoms in moderately injured accident victims. *Psychopharmacology, 182*, 420–425.

Segman, R. H., Shefi, N. N., Goltser-Dubner, T. T., Friedman, N. N., Kaminski, N. N., & Shalev, A. Y. (2005). Peripheral blood mononuclear cell gene expression profiles identify emergent post-traumatic stress disorder among trauma survivors. *Molecular Psychiatry, 10*(5), 500–513.

Shalev, A. Y., Sahar, T., Freedman, S., Peri, T., Glick, N., Brandes, D., et al. (1998). A prospective study of heart rate response following trauma and the subsequent development of posttraumatic stress disorder. *Archives of General Psychiatry, 55*, 553–559.

Sijbrandij, M., Olff, M., Reitsma, J. B., Carlier, I. E., & Gersons, B. R. (2006). Emotional or educational debriefing after psychological trauma: Randomised controlled trial. *British Journal of Psychiatry, 189*(2), 150–155.

Stein, M. B., Kerridge, C., Dimsdale, J. E., & Hoyt, D. B. (2007). Pharmacotherapy to prevent PTSD: Results from a randomized controlled proof-of-concept trial in physically injured patients. *Journal of Traumatic Stress, 20*, 923–932.

Suveg, C. (2007). Implications of the debriefing debate for research and clinical practice. *Clinical Psychology: Science and Practice, 14*(2), 117–120.

Tanielian, T., & Jaycox, L. H. (Eds.). (2008). *Invisible wounds of war: Psychological and cognitive injuries, their consequences, and serves to assist recovery*. Santa Monica, CA: RAND Corporation.

Tuckey, M. R. (2007). Issues in the debriefing debate for the emergency services: Moving research outcomes forward. *Clinical Psychology: Science and Practice, 14*(2), 106–116.

Turpin, G., Downs, M., & Mason, S. (2005). Effectiveness of providing self-help information following acute traumatic injury: Randomised controlled trial. *British Journal of Psychiatry, 187*, 76–82.

Vaiva, G., Ducrocq, F., Jezequel, K., Averland, B., Lestavel, P., Brunet, A., et al. (2003). Immediate treatment with propranolol decreases posttraumatic stress disorder two months after trauma. *Biological Psychiatry, 54*, 947–949.

Xie, P., Kranzler, H. R., Poling, J., Stein, M. B., Anton, R. F., Farrer, L. A., et al. (2010). Interaction of FKBP5 with childhood adversity on risk for post-traumatic stress disorder. *Neuropsychopharmacology, 35*(8), 1684–1692.

Chapter 7
Systems of Care for Traumatized Children: The Example of a School-Based Intervention Model

Danny Brom, Naomi L. Baum, and Ruth Pat-Horenczyk

Introduction

Terrorism and war threaten not only law enforcement and the military but also, and, in the case of terrorism, mainly the civilian population. The same is true for natural disasters and domestic violence. When disaster strikes, the immediate response is characterized by activities that have to ensure survival. Only when initial safety has been reached, there is room for emotional and cognitive processing of what happened. In a society, such as Israel, where war and terrorism are continuous, the threat to functioning, well-being, and mental health of both adults and children is a pressing public health issue.

Public health, social welfare, and mental healthcare systems tend to work as separate entities. The contact and collaboration between these systems is both a natural need for systems that partly overlap, have common interests and often serve the same population. At the same time these collaborations, and certainly the integration of the services, remain ongoing challenges.

Community wide traumatic experiences in Israel have created an opportunity to reach out to communities and populations and design cross-system services (Laor, Wiener, Spirman, & Wolmer, 2005).

In this chapter we will describe the development of a system of care for children through educational systems. Providing a continuum of trauma services for Israeli school children during long periods of exposure to trauma focuses on an array of services ranging from prevention to intervention. The school-based intervention model incorporates principles of both community and clinical psychology. Traditionally, services have focused on those who have been identified as suffering

D. Brom (✉) • N.L. Baum • R. Pat-Horenczyk
The Israel Center for the Treatment of Psychotrauma, Herzog Hospital, Jerusalem, Israel
e-mail: dbrom@herzoghospital.org; Naomi.baum@gmail.com; rpat@herzoghospital.org

M.P. Safir et al. (eds.), *Future Directions in Post-Traumatic Stress Disorder*,
DOI 10.1007/978-1-4899-7522-5_7

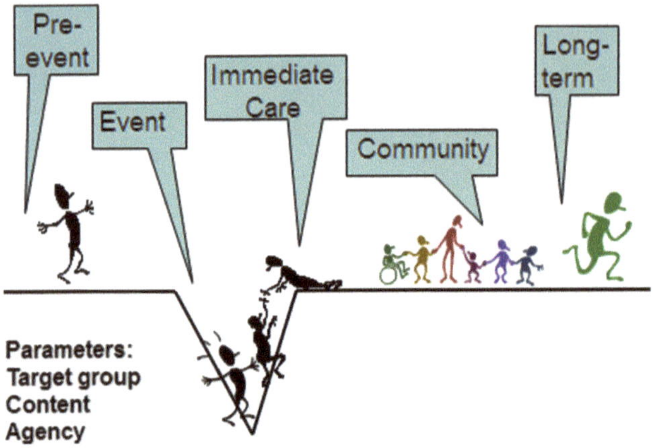

Chart 7.1 The continuum of services

from posttraumatic stress disorders or other clinical diagnoses. The continuum of trauma services model recognizes the importance of treating those who are suffering, while not overlooking the large, silent majority of the population who cope reasonably well through other trajectories (Layneet al., 2009).The provision of a range of services, from community interventions to clinical interventions within one system of care, form one of the touchstones of this model.

An overall model for developing trauma-related services can be seen in Chart 7.1.

The chart shows the need to think in multiple dimensions in the development of services. The first dimension is the time in relationship to traumatic events. Ideally, resilience-building interventions should be done before people are exposed to traumatic events so that they can cope better. The services during, immediately after, and long-term after will differ from each other in goals and techniques used. A second dimension is the target group for intervention. Are we talking about general population, high-risk groups, highly exposed groups, clinical populations, young children, adolescents, adults, elderly? A third dimension is the content and aims of the intervention. Some interventions might aim at strengthening the sense of community, others aim at showing victims that society cares, and yet others aim at speeding the coping process. The last dimension is the decision about who can and should execute the chosen intervention. Emergency and trauma-related interventions attract a large amount of volunteer and NGO work and philanthropy is often easy to recruit for this kind of work. NGOs are often also much more flexible and can respond to emergencies quicker than established systems of care that are not designed for emergency interventions. Strategically, however, it is important to make sure that trauma care will not be isolated and will not compete with the existing system of care.

Traumatized Children in Society: A Model of Care

We present a comprehensive model for building resilience in school communities that have been exposed to the trauma of terrorism and war. We will describe the various levels of intervention beginning with the principal and the leading teams in the school, and then highlight our resilience-building workshops for teachers. The guidelines for school-based screening for identifying posttraumatic distress will be clarified followed by three different modules of school-based treatment interventions. We conclude with challenges for implementation and future directions based on our experience.

Children Exposed to Mass Trauma

In the aftermath of war and terrorism, children may downplay or deny their symptoms for fear of overtaxing their already overburdened parents, and adolescents may avoid, ignore, or numb their symptoms either to assert their independence or simply to move on (Hoven, Duarte, & Mandell, 2003). After the Oklahoma bombing in 1995, Pfefferbaum et al. (2003) found that only 5 % of 2,720 children surveyed after the Oklahoma bombing in 1995 received counseling. Further, after 9/11, a large school-based screening conducted by the NYC Board of Education 6 months after the attacks, reported that 2/3 of children identified with posttraumatic distress were not referred to any type of treatment (Hoven et al., 2003). Such findings highlight the need to actively reach out and provide screening and treatment resources for children and adolescents suffering in silence from war- and terrorism-related traumas.

Increasing evidence suggests that when students are directly asked to report their own reactions and behaviors, they tend to express their posttraumatic distress (Pat-Horenczyk, Abramovitz, et al., 2007). Similarly, adolescents clearly indicate when they feel they need help, and these reports have a strong correlation with their answers on questionnaires about symptoms (Schiff et al., 2010). This underscores the importance of simply asking the proper questions to elicit responses that can help *identify* child and adolescent postwar and post-terrorism syndromes.

Most individuals exposed to traumatic experiences seem to cope well or even thrive in the aftermath of traumatic events. There are various ways to conceptualize what constitutes resilience and what constitutes a "resilience factor." Such factors could include a combination of protective *characteristics*, such as competence or self-efficacy (Garmezy, 1991; Masten & Coatsworth, 1998), or the underlying *processes* of coping that an individual adopts in the face of adversity (Luthar, Cicchetti, & Becker, 2000). Discussions abound regarding what constitutes a resilient response to trauma. Most agree that resilient individuals can still experience some difficulty or distress in the course of coping with traumatic events, but they also must be able to draw on their resources to resume normal functioning.

Bonanno (2004) claims that resilient individuals maintain a degree of equilibrium *during* their traumatic experiences and "generally exhibit a stable trajectory of healthy functioning across time" (p. 21), which separates them from individuals who "recover" from psychopathological episodes consequent to adversity. Our working definition of resilience is based on the formulation suggested by Masten (2001), which regards resilience as "ordinary magic," in contrast to extraordinary behavior in the face of adversity.

School-Based Intervention Model

Schools are natural venues for intervention following trauma, where the goal is to strengthen resilience and assess and treat posttraumatic distress, functional impairment, and related distress. Children spend most of their active daytime hours in school, making it a natural venue for developing mental-health initiatives. It has been argued that providing mental-health services in schools can minimize the stigma surrounding psychological care, and thus encourage students to seek care and incorporate therapeutic techniques in their lives (Kataoka et al., 2003). Situating mental-health programs in schools also makes health care more physically accessible and immediately available, which is an important factor, when one considers how many diagnosed cases of trauma-related symptoms remain untreated. On a practical level as well, schools are an excellent venue for intervention because they are already structured in a way conducive to program development and maintenance. Resources already embedded in the school systems, many of which are underutilized, can be used to create an effective and financially feasible mental-health response.

Not all school interventions target the same groups or aim for similar outcome measures. The Institute of Medicine (1994) delineated three different models of intervention that aim to improve the mental health of students: universal, selective, and indicated. In each of these categories, students with different profiles are slated for intervention. *Universal interventions* focus resources for all students; *selective interventions* are addressed only towards high-risk students; and *indicated interventions* address the needs of students on the brink of risk, when signs of problem behavior begin to emerge (Power, 2003). Inherent in these three models is the desire to promote health and resilience, on one hand, and the necessity to intervene and possibly offer treatment in the case of risk or psychopathology, on the other. The distinction between preventative and curative interventions for child mental health necessitates the assessment of the differential needs of students.

Often, in work with trauma, selective interventions in schools aim to identify children with PTSD, acute stress disorder, or depression, and then initiate group or individual treatment to alleviate these symptoms (Amaya-Jackson et al., 2003; Caplan, 1974; Cohen & Mannarino, 2004; Stein et al., 2003). Selective interventions usually borrow heavily from cognitive-behavioral models, where identified students are given a mixture of counseling, psycho-education, and techniques to alleviate stress, identify maladaptive cognitions, and process traumatic experiences

(Amaya-Jackson et al., 2003; Caplan, 1974; Cohen & Mannarino, 2004; Stein et al., 2003). In contrast, universal interventions target entire student bodies indiscriminately, focusing less on psychopathology or at-risk children, and more on creating individual and community resources so that all students can become more resilient. Universal interventions often involve multiple levels of school and community contributions to the program, such as parental involvement and teacher training (Berger, Pat-Horenczyk, & Gelkopf, 2007).

There is evidence to support the benefits of both selective and universal school interventions following a variety of traumatic experiences, including natural disasters and hurricanes (Chemtob, Nakashima, & Hamada, 2002; La Greca, Silverman, Vernberg, & Prinstein, 1996; Norris, Friedman, Watson, & Byrne, 2002), war (Laor et al., 1997; Saltzman, Pynoos, Layne, Steinberg, & Aisenberg, 2001; Saltzman, Steinberg, Layne, Aisenberg, & Pynoos, 2001), terrorism (Baum, 2005; Berger et al., 2007; Hoven et al., 2003; Koplewicz et al., 2002; Pat-Horenczyk, 2004; Pfefferbaum, 2001) and violence in communities and schools (Stein et al., 2003). However, while studies indicate that school-based screenings and interventions can be used to mitigate the effects of exposure to trauma (or potential exposure, in the case of resilience-building), many questions remain. A particular concern is the long-term validity of intervention programs and their ability to ensure long-term benefits to students. Additionally, at this early stage of development, there are still uncertainties regarding which critical ingredients of intervention are central to a program's success. Intervention must thus remain in constant dialogue with the theoretical and evidence-based currents in the field, and the strengths and weaknesses of its current programs must be assessed so as to create better practices (Power, 2003).

There are many practical constraints inherent in school-based work. School systems are vast and complex, involving multiple layers of organization and players. Thus, often even the best of programs can falter in the realm of implementation. It has been argued that mental-health objectives in schools often do not succeed, or at least are not sustainable, because there is a disconnect between the education and mental-health orientations, where educators focus on competence and achievement and mental-health practitioners focus on psychopathology and social and emotional growth (Masten, 2003). Political, economic, and cultural barriers can also be expected when intervention takes place in any real-life setting, and there will be particular demands at each research site that require additional resources (Kratochwill & Shernoff, 2004). Such concerns are of primary importance for programs where teachers and administrators, rather than researchers, become the key conduits of conveying mental-health programs.

The Building Resilience Project, in fact, pairs these two factors into a holistic model, bringing both selective and universal elements into one integrative process in schools. The resilience workshop is the first element of the model, which helps administrators, teachers, and other school personnel to acquire a basic understanding and practice of resilience, including trauma awareness education and building coping strategies. The trained personnel are guided to apply this experience and conduct resilience training in the classroom, teaching students through modeling and hands-on activities how to develop strengths that can buffer trauma. Parents also are involved in this program and attend informational seminars and workshops.

The second element is a comprehensive school screening program to identify those students who require individual and group treatment for trauma-related symptoms. Students identified through the screening ideally receive treatment from practitioners who work within the school setting, transforming schools into centers of immediate mental health care. Both elements work together; the nuance is not so much the bridging of two different models, but rather the unique character the program acquires as the two models work together in synergy.

Furthermore, while many interventions introduce outside protocols and procedures and "intervene" in the organic school environment, our model works to embed the solution, skills, and procedures of resilience development into the school system itself. This is the second unique feature of the program—namely, its sensitive approach to effecting change on a systems level. The first order of change involves structural concerns, such as including the Ministry of Education and local boards of education, reviewing program protocol, mapping an organizational framework, and identifying key players who can help make the program a success. Furthermore, since each school is a complex system in its own right, cultural concerns about school ideals and priorities must be addressed. Through the combination of teacher-training workshops, screening, and treatment, we aim to educate school personnel and bring mental-health concerns to the forefront of the educational discourse. In so doing, the program encourages educators to begin thinking in terms of students' social and emotional development, and thus inspires a reorientation of school culture and a redirecting of educational priorities. Training school-based mental health professionals furthers the empowerment of the local system, and builds capacity for professional trauma treatment and intervention in local schools.

In our experience, this model changes the way educators view their personal role in supporting the mental-health needs of their students, and empowers them to become the agents of this change. Staff training workshops focus on the teacher's experience and provide tools for intervention, thus challenging school personnel to take part in developing their own school-wide mental health program. By involving school personnel in the long-term goals of the program, and also ensuring that the school infrastructure can support the program, we help secure the long-term sustainability of mental health interventions in schools.

There are six major components of the model:

Preparing the School System

In order to ensure proper implementation of the program, including its sustainability after the initial intervention and implementation, strong working relationships need to be established with municipalities, supervisors of boards of education, and principals in individual schools. Creating a core of committed professionals ensures the continuation of the resilience-building work in the school setting long after the completion of the initial intervention. In this first component of the model, the goal is empowering the local school communities. Working from the top down, after meeting and gaining commitment from municipal education leaders and policy makers in the Ministry of Education, we involve all levels of school administration, staff, and parents in training about trauma and stress and the role of resilience. Their commitment to the program is critical in effecting change on all levels of the school community.

First we identify the key players in the school system. We ask: Which teachers are most excited about this project? Which administrators will oversee its proper implementation? Who will be the internal school contact who can help coordinate concerns from the field? During this initial phase, we also meet with the principal and leading school team (which may consist of the guidance counselor, psychologist, head teachers, or division heads) to assess the school's trauma history, including how both national and local traumatic events have affected the school atmosphere and the students' health. Such questions may include: Has the school sustained any losses (students, teachers, parents)? Were any of the students' family members wounded or killed in war? Did any students or faculty lose their houses during recent events? Has a student or teacher ever died in a car accident or of cancer? All of this information is necessary to tailor the program to the specific needs of the school. After a working relationship with the principal and the leading team has been established, the program is then explained and a timeline set up, with expectations and responsibilities for both sides. This element is critical, as it ensures that both external and internal parties are involved, as well as coordinated in their efforts to construct the school mental-health intervention.

Training Mental-Health Professionals

School mental-health professionals often lack the confidence and the specific tools needed to provide appropriate interventions in the wake of trauma. In addition, the system is often eager to show that everything is "back to normal" and so encourages professionals to go about their daily work. By helping the mental-health professionals acknowledge existing needs as well as empowering them to implement interventions, we aim to strengthen the mental-health system in the schools.

In the Israeli system, school psychologists and school guidance counselors address different mental-health needs. Psychologists play the dual role of consultant to school personnel including the principal and teachers, as well as treating children with a variety of psychological disorders. As such, the model trains psychologists to facilitate teacher resilience workshops, as well as provides training for the specialized treatment of severe manifestations of trauma exposure and posttraumatic stress disorder in a school-based group setting.

Guidance counselors are also key players, acting as the mental health advocates in school, helping direct school resources and energies in the changing environment that trauma creates. Guidance counselors can be trained to conduct post-screening interviews and refer children for individual or group therapy. They are also trained in the six-session protocolized program for reducing anxiety and posttraumatic symptoms that we will describe later.

Building Resilience with Teachers

Teachers are natural partners in developing resilience within the student body. Rather than relying on sporadic visits of outside experts, our program works with teachers to develop their skills so as to embed mental-health objectives in each classroom. The in-service workshop enhances the teachers' ability to cope with stress and trauma, and increases their resilience by expanding their understanding of trauma, self-awareness, and skill base for dealing with emotions in the classroom. By becoming aware of how they are coping on a personal level, teachers can more effectively communicate with their students about traumatic events and develop the confidence to work with children normatively after exposure to trauma. Furthermore, they learn to identify overt and subtle symptoms of posttraumatic stress disorder, and learn what referral services are available for them and their students, thus enhancing their ability to identify students who need these services and increasing the students' treatment prospects. Developing the teachers' repertoire of classroom activities, involving emotions and resilience-building activities, round out the intervention.

The workshop consists of four 3-h in-service meetings, led by trained resilience facilitators who have a community mental health background and familiarity with trauma studies and group work. While the immediate objective is to work on the teachers' strengths and coping strategies, the ultimate goal is to encourage them to apply their skills and tools in their classrooms, where children can then learn through example and exercises how to utilize their own internal resources. In so doing, teachers can change the classroom environment into one that encourages communication about the range of emotions and a center of social support and care.

While workshop facilitators can vary their particular programs to the needs of each teacher cohort, four underlying objectives of the workshop, known as the four "**S**"s, are presented throughout the sessions: **S**elf-awareness and regulation, **S**trengths and personal resources for coping, social **S**upport from colleagues, family and friends, and finding **S**ignificance, meaning, and hope. These "**S**"s were culled from the resilience literature. In addition to being evidence based, they are variables that we can effect, form the cornerstone of the teacher training, and inform the ideas and hands-on activities that the teachers subsequently implement in their classrooms. The workshop is divided into four sections, with correlating sub-themes, activities, and skills to apply in the classroom (Table 7.1).

Teachers' manuals (Baum, Bamberger, & Kerem, 2004) are distributed to all participants, containing information pages as well as guides for facilitating sharing of emotions and exercises in leading group conversations on emotional topics in the classroom. Different activities, ranging from meditation techniques to expressive art therapy, are explained further in the manual, and presented in an easily accessible

Table 7.1 Resilience workshop session content

Sessions	Psycho-education themes	Activities	Skills	Comments
One: Self-awareness and self-regulation	(a) Developing a common language (b) Resilience, stress, and trauma (c) Trauma and children	• Breathing • Minute meditation • Where am I? Where do I want to be? Drawings	• Trauma vocabulary • Understanding the normal trajectory of healing from trauma • Self-expression • Self-regulation • Mindfulness	*Trauma creates deregulation in both physiological and psychological responses. Understanding this and understanding ourselves is the first step to resilience*
Two: Feelings	(a) Empathic communication (b) Accessing feelings (c) Expressing feelings (d) Eliciting feelings in others (e) Childhood fears	• Clay molding activity involving feelings • Breathing exercises	• Self-regulation • Self-awareness	*Developing empathy, initially to oneself, paves the way to listening to others, especially students. Creating a listening environment aids healthy emotional development*
Three: Strengths and coping strategies	(a) Models of coping (b) BASIC-Ph model (Ayalon and Lahad, 2000)	• Coping: What works? What doesn't? (worksheets)	• Identifying successful coping • Initiating new coping activities	*This model allows participants to analyze their coping styles discussing whether they are predominantly based on belief, affect, social, imagination, cognitive, or physical*
Four: Creating meaning and hope	Understanding posttraumatic growth	• Meaningful moments: exercise • Writing a prayer	• Activities for bringing meaning into the classroom	*Creating meaning can take many forms, ranging from creating narrative to developing action plans to help others*

format for classroom implementation. Teachers are encouraged to choose activities from the manual and adapt or develop new exercises based on the four themes of the workshops.

Parental Involvement

Even though parent involvement is a crucial part of resilience programs for children, it is often the most challenging. Changing communication between teachers and children in school is just one step in creating a resilient environment.

Bringing parents into the picture adds a critical aspect. We have been most successful at recruiting parental involvement in the preschool setting, running many four-session parent groups entitled "Resilient Parent–Resilient Child." In contrast, parental participation at the elementary and high school level has proven more difficult. Due to difficulties in recruiting ongoing parental participation, we have adjusted the parent program, allowing schools to choose from a menu of possibilities in addition to the workshop series. The most popular choice has been a single-event "Parents' Night." This one-time session includes a lecture to parents on the subject of how adults and children cope during prolonged periods of stress and exposure to trauma, as well as teaching parents how to communicate with children about these topics. The importance of regulating media exposure is discussed, as well as activities and behaviors that can help develop the parents' own personal and family resilience. In addition, the components of the school project are presented. Often a workshop exercise is performed with the parents as well. Parents' night is an ideal time to present information about the screening program and to obtain signed consent from parents for screening as well.

Screening and Identification of Students with PTSD

The aim of school-based screening is to identify students who have developed symptoms on a clinical level, through direct or indirect exposure to terrorism or war, in order to be able to provide them with treatment. Specifically, the program screens students for posttraumatic symptoms, functional impairment and related distress, as well as protective factors. Using self-report screening questionnaires within the school has become the consensus method for identifying and triaging students for school-based interventions, as evidenced by the screening studies conducted after Hurricane Andrew in Hawaii (Chemtob et al., 2002), the war in Bosnia (Saltzman, Pynoos et al., 2001), the Oklahoma City bombing (Pfefferbaum et al., 2001), the terrorist attacks in Kenya and Tanzania (Pfefferbaum et al., 2003), the first bombing of the Twin Towers (Koplewicz et al., 2002), and in Palestinian and Israeli children (Solomon & Lavi, 2005).

In Israel, we have been conducting school-based screening and interventions since the outbreak of the Second Intifada in September 2000. We have shown, based on a sample of nearly 7,000 students that more than 32 % reported personal exposure to terrorist attacks, and an additional 22 % reported near-miss experiences (Pat-Horenczyk, Abramovitz et al., 2007). Although more than 2/3 of the youth reported extreme fear and helplessness, only 7.6 % reported posttraumatic symptoms that met the DSM criteria for PTSD. Children and adolescents may sometimes develop posttraumatic distress without being directly exposed to the traumatic event. For example, media coverage and indirect exposure (such as the death of a close relative or friend, even if not directly witnessed) may be enough to prompt the onset of PTSD (Pfefferbaum, Pfefferbaum, North, & Neas, 2002).

Screening Measures

Our screening procedures are aimed at identifying both risk and protective factors that are relevant to one's ability to cope in the aftermath of traumatic events (Pat-Horenczyk, Rabinowitz, Rice, & Tucker-Levin, 2009). We adapted screening inventories from an array of evidence-based settings, and translated (and cross-translated) all measures into Hebrew.

In our screening project during the ongoing terrorism of the Second Intifada, we asked children and adolescents to report on their rate of exposure to terrorism and war, and evaluated their reports of distress factors, including posttraumatic symptoms, functional impairment, somatic complaints, and symptoms of depression and anxiety. We further assessed the ability of children and adolescents to maintain their daily routine despite their ongoing exposure to terrorism and looked at the protective measures that help students achieve resilient outcomes. Such measures include coping strategies, students' ability to request assistance, school support, the ability to generate hope and meaning, and ego protection (see Benbenishty, Khoury-Kassabri, & Astor, 2005; Block & Block, 1980; Carver, 1997; Seidman et al., 1995; Snyder et al., 1997). In addition, the association between posttraumatic distress and increased risk-taking behavior was demonstrated in youth exposed to ongoing terrorism (Pat-Horenczyk, Abramovitz et al., 2007). This increase in risk-taking behavior among symptomatic adolescents is alarming in that it may make them more vulnerable to future trauma. Adolescents may be stimulated by psychological trauma to seek revenge, engage in defiant or even violent behaviors, or seek an escape from traumatic stress symptoms through social withdrawal, substance abuse, and self-harm (Pat-Horenczyk, Peled, Miron, Brom, Villa & Chemtob, 2007).

The combined clinical picture of both risk and protective factors gives educators and clinicians a richer understanding of each student's profile, as well as directing the intervention and decision-making procedures. The screening battery for each school is constructed according to the specific needs of the school and the context of the traumatic events.

School-Based Treatment of Children

Children who have been identified with high levels of stress-related symptoms are referred to one of two group interventions in the school. Because of the high number of children that were detected, we have developed two group treatment protocols for work with children who suffer from either a high level of symptoms or fully developed symptoms of posttraumatic stress disorder. Both group interventions are designed to prevent stigmatization, are delivered within the school, and are presented as "additional lessons" for special groups.

A 6-week school-based group intervention led by guidance counselors, entitled "Journey to Resilience" is geared to students who have been screened with the protocol described above, and have been found to have moderate to high levels of posttraumatic distress, but do not fulfill the full criteria for PTSD (Pat-Horenczyk, R., Berger, R., Kaplinsky, N. & Baum. N. (2004). The journey to resilience: Coping with ongoing stressful situations. Protocol for guidance counsellors (adolescents version) Unpublished Manuscript). This intervention is comprised of sessions of psycho-education about the normal reactions to trauma and stress, stress management techniques, including increased awareness, training in strengthening and utilizing personal resources, self-care, peer group support, and cognitive restructuring techniques.

An additional group protocol that we have more limited experience with is a 12-session school-based group intervention geared to students who have been found to be suffering from posttraumatic stress disorder at clinical levels (Pat-Horenczyk, R., & Kaplinsky, N. (2003). School-based treatment protocol for posttraumatic-related distress (adolescent version). Unpublished manuscript). This group is run by psychologists specially trained in trauma treatment. Cognitive-behavioral treatment techniques to process the traumatic event, including the building of a consistent narrative of the traumatic circumstances in the frame of the life narrative, are employed in this group setting, along with units on psycho-education, relaxation, and relapse prevention.

Concluding Comments

In this chapter we have outlined an integrative approach that reaches out actively to children and delivers non-stigmatizing services. The combination of a community approach that aims at increasing resilience and a clinical approach that reaches out to the most vulnerable children and offers treatment serves all parts of the school community. Group participation in school-based therapy groups was associated with improvement in posttraumatic stress, grief symptoms, and academic performance (Jaycox, 2004; Saltzman, Pynoos et al., 2001).

A major challenge in implementing these school-based community mental health programs is to make them sustainable within the local community. In order to do so we have partnered with the Israeli Ministry of Education and municipal authorities, and this has led to the establishment of city-wide programs in several cities in Israel. In the city wide model, all schools in a given municipality participate in the entire intervention, creating an impact throughout entire community. The city wide approach is also important in the light of our experience in the first years of the project that showed that when schools are offered these kinds of interventions, the organizationally and economically stronger schools tend to get involved. When the local authorities are involved, there is a good chance to also engage schools that are the most needy.

In order to take care of the children that are detected through screening, local school psychologists and group facilitators are trained who then facilitate teacher workshops. Guidance counselors and school psychologists are trained to treat traumatized children. In this way we increase the capacity of communities to take care of their own needs and create a sustainable foundation of mental health services that enrich the system and will continue to exist once the "official project" has concluded.

In the course of the past few years, the Israeli school-based intervention program has been applied in hundreds of schools, and over 20,000 children and adolescents have participated in screening procedures. An additional issue that creates a challenge for our approach is the active parental consent that is required by the authorities. When parents are asked to sign a form, it is often the more educated parents that respond and a systematic bias may result. The consent issue to screen for health problems is part of a discussion on ethical practice.

The future challenge is to evaluate and provide an evidence base for the effects of resilience-building interventions. Initial data show promising results Programs for building resilience are relatively new and tend to be funded only after major disaster strikes. The ideal way of strengthening resilience in children is to make this standard practice, certainly in high risk areas, such as the Middle East.

The school-based Intervention program is an example of an integrative way of service delivery, taking care of a wide range of needs in the face of mass trauma. A similar model has been developed for the care of young children (1–6 years old). We maintain that responses to mass trauma should include differential responses to people and communities that are at risk for varying levels of posttraumatic or other stress-related symptoms. This is true for soldiers after combat, for first responders who are highly exposed to traumatic sights and for civilian populations living in war zones or areas that are exposed to natural disaster.

References

Amaya-Jackson, L., Reynolds, V., Murray, M. C., McCarthy, G., Nelson, A., Cherney, M. S., et al. (2003). Cognitive-behavioral treatment for pediatric posttraumatic stress disorder: Protocol and application in school and community settings. *Cognitive and Behavioral Practice, 10*, 204–213.

Ayalon, O. and Lahad, M. (2000). *Living on the border*. Haifa: Nord Publishers.

Baum, N. (2005). Post-traumatic distress in adolescents exposed to ongoing terror: Findings from a school-based screening project in the Jerusalem Area. In Y. Daniely, D. Brom, J. Sills, & M. I. Holland (Eds.), *The trauma of terrorism: Sharing knowledge and shared care, an international handbook* (pp. 335–348). Binghamton, NY: Haworth Press.

Baum, N., Bamberger, E., & Kerem, R. (2004). *Building resilience in the classroom: Teacher's Manual. Unpublished manual. Israel Center for the Treatment of.* Jerusalem: Psychotrauma.

Baum, N. L., Lopes-Cardozo, B., Pat-Horenczyk, R., Ziv, Y., Blanton, C., Reza, A., Weltman, A., & Brom, D. (2013). Training teachers to build resilience in children in the aftermath of war: A cluster randomized trial. *Child & Youth Care Forum*, 42, 339–350.

Benbenishty, R., Khoury-Kassabri, R., & Astor, R. A. (2005). *Violence in the school system 2005*. Jerusalem: Hebrew University School of Social Work.

Berger, R., Pat-Horenczyk, R., & Gelkopf, M. (2007). School-based intervention for prevention and treatment of elementary-students' terror-related distress in Israel: A quasi-randomized controlled trial. *J Trauma Stress, 20*(4), 541–551.

Block, J. H., & Block, J. (1980). The role of ego control and ego resiliency in the organization of behavior. In W. A. Collins (Ed.), *The Minnesota symposia on child psychology* (Vol. 13, pp. 39–101). Hillsdale, NJ: Erlbaum.

Bonanno, G. (2004). Loss, trauma, and human resilience. *Am Psychol, 59*(1), 20–28.
Caplan, G. (1974). *Support system and community mental health*. New York: Behavioral Publications.
Carver, C. S. (1997). You want to measure coping but your protocol's too long: Consider the Brief COPE. *International Journal of Behavioral Medicine, 4*, 92–100.
Chemtob, C., Nakashima, J., & Hamada, R. (2002). Psychosocial intervention for postdisaster trauma symptoms in elementary school children (reprinted). *Archive of Pediatric Adolescent Medicine, 156*, 211–216.
Cohen, J. A., & Mannarino, A. P. (2004). Treating childhood traumatic grief. *Journal of Clinical Child and Adolescent Psychology, 33*, 819–831.
Garmezy, N. (1991). Resilience in children's adaptation to negative life events and stressed environments. *Pediatr Ann, 20*(9), 459-60–460. 463–466.
Hoven, C., Duarte, C., & Mandell, D. (2003). Children's mental health after disasters: The impact of the World Trade Center attack. *Current Psychiatry Reports, 5*(2), 101–107.
Institute of Medicine. (1994). *Reducing risks for mental disorders: Frontiers for preventive intervention research*. Washington, DC: National Academy Press.
Jaycox, L. (2004). *Cognitive-behavioral intervention for trauma in schools*. Longmont, CO: Sopris West Educational Services.
Kataoka, S., Stein, B., Jaycox, L., Wong, M., Escudero, P., Tu, W., et al. (2003). A school-based mental health program for traumatized Latino immigrant children. *American Academy of Child and Adolescent Psychiatry, 42*(3), 311–318.
Koplewicz, H. S., Vogel, J. M., Solanto, M. V., Morrissey, R. F., Alonso, C. M., Abikoff, H., et al. (2002). Child and parents response to the 1993 World Trade Center bombing. *J Trauma Stress, 15*, 77–85.
Kratochwill, T., & Shernoff, E. (2004). Evidence based practice: Promoting evidence-based interventions in school psychology. *Sch Psychol Rev, 33*(1), 34–48.
La Greca, A., Silverman, W. K., Vernberg, E. M., & Prinstein, M. J. (1996). Symptoms of posttraumatic stress in children after Hurricane Andrew: A prospective study. *J Consult Clin Psychol, 64*(4), 712–723.
Laor, N., Wiener, Z., Spirman, S., & Wolmer, L. (2005). Community mental health in emergencies and mass disasters: The Tel Aviv model. In Y. Danieli, D. Brom, & J. Sills (Eds.), *The trauma of terrorism: sharing knowledge and shared care. An international handbook*. New York: Haworth.
Laor, N., Wolmer, L., Mayes, L. C., Gershon, A., Weizman, R., & Cohen, D. J. (1997). Israeli preschool children under Scuds: A 30-month follow-up. *Journal of the American Academy of Adolescent Psychiatry, 36*(3), 349–356.
Layne, C. M., Beck, C. J., Rimmasch, H., Southwick, J. S., Moreno, M. A., & Hobfoll, S. E. (2009). Promoting "resilient" posttraumatic adjustment in childhood and beyond: "Unpacking" life events, adjustment trajectories, resources, and interventions. In: D. Brom, R. Pat-Horenczyk and J. Ford (Eds.) Treating Traumatized Children: Risk, Resilience and Recovery, Routledge, pp. 51–71.
Luthar, S., Cicchetti, D., & Becker, B. (2000). The construct of resilience: A critical evaluation and guidelines for future work. *Child Dev, 71*, 543–562.
Masten, A. (2001). Ordinary magic: Resilience processes in development. *Am Psychol, 56*(3), 227–238.
Masten, A. (2003). Commentary: developmental psychopathology as a unifying context for mental health and education models, research, and practice in schools. *Sch Psychol Rev, 32*(2), 169–173.
Masten, A., & Coatsworth, D. J. (1998). The development of competence in favorable and unfavorable environments: Lessons from research on successful children. *Am Psychol, 53*(2), 205–220.
Norris, F. H., Friedman, M. J., Watson, P. J., & Byrne, C. M. (2002). 60,000 disaster victims speak: Part I. An empirical review of the empirical literature, 1981-2001. *Psychiatry, 65*, 207–239.
Pat-Horenczyk, R. (2004). Post-traumatic distress in adolescents exposed to ongoing terror: Findings from a school-based screening project in the Jerusalem Area. *Journal of Aggression, Maltreatment and Trauma, 9*(3/4), 335–347.

Pat-Horenczyk, R., Abramovitz, R., Peled, O., Brom, D., Daie, A., & Chemtob, C. (2007). Adolescent exposure to recurrent terrorism in Israel: Posttraumatic distress and functional impairment. *Am J Orthopsychiatry, 77*(1), 76–85.
Pat-Horenczyk, R., Dopplet, O., Miron, T., Villa, Y., Brom, D., & Chemtob, C. M. (2007). Risk taking behaviors among Israeli Adolescents exposed to recurrent terrorism. *Am J Psychiatr, 164*(1), 66–72.
Pat-Horenczyk, R., Peled, O., Miron, T., Villa, Y., Brom, D. &Chemtob, C.M. (2007). Risk-Taking Behaviors among Israeli Adolescents Exposed to Recurrent Terrorism, *American Journal of Psychiatry, 164*(1), 66–72.
Pat-Horenczyk, R., Rabinowitz, R., Rice, A., & Tucker-Levin, A. (2009). The search for risk and protective factors in childhood PTSD: From variables to processes. In D. Brom, R. Pat-Horenczyk, & J. Ford (Eds.), *Treating traumatized children: Risk, resilience and recovery*. London: Routledge.
Pfefferbaum, B. (2001). Special report: Lessons from the 1995 bombing of the Alfred P Murrah Federal Building in Oklahoma City. *Lancet, 358*, 940.
Pfefferbaum, B., Nixon, S. J., Tivis, R. D., Doughty, D. E., Pynoos, R. S., Gurwitch, R. H., & Foy, D. W. (2001). Television exposure in children after a terrorist incident. *Psychiatry: Interpersonal and Biological Processes, 64*, 202–211.
Pfefferbaum, B., Pfefferbaum, R., Gurwitch, R., Nagumalli, S., Brandt, E., Robertson, M., et al. (2003). Children's response to terrorism: A critical review of the literature. *Current Psychiatry Report, 5*, 95–100.
Pfefferbaum, B., Pfefferbaum, R. L., North, C. S., & Neas, B. R. (2002). Does television viewing satisfy criteria for exposure in posttraumatic stress disorder? *Psychiatry, 65*(4), 306–309.
Power, T. (2003). Promoting children's mental health: Reform through interdisciplinary and community partnerships. *Sch Psychol Rev, 32*(1), 3–16.
Saltzman, W. R., Pynoos, R. S., Layne, C. M., Steinberg, A. M., & Aisenberg, E. (2001). Trauma and grief-focused intervention for adolescents exposed to community violence: Results of a school based screening and group treatment protocol. *Group Dynamics, 5*(4), 291–303.
Saltzman, W. R., Steinberg, A. M., Layne, C. M., Aisenberg, E., & Pynoos, R. S. (2001). A developmental approach to school-based treatment of adolescents exposed to trauma and traumatic loss. *Journal of Children and Adolescent Group Therapy, 11*, 43–51.
Schiff, M., Pat-Horenczyk, R., Benbenishty, R., Brom, D., Baum, N., & Astor, R. A. (2010). Seeking help: Do adolescents know when they need help? Jewish and Arab youths report on their posttraumatic distress in the aftermath of war. *J Trauma Stress, 23*(5), 657–660.
Seidman, E., Allen, L., Aber, J. L., Mitchell, C., Feinman, J., Yoshikawa, H., et al. (1995). Development and validation of adolescent perceived microsystem scales: Social support, daily hassles, and involvement. *Am J Community Psychol, 23*, 355–388.
Snyder, C. R., Hoza, B., Pelham, W. E., Rapoff, M., Ware, L., Danovsky, M., et al. (1997). The development and validation of the Children's Hope Scale. *J Pediatr Psychol, 22*(3), 399–421.
Solomon, Z., & Lavi, T. (2005). Israeli youth in the second Intifada: PTSD and future orientation. *Journal of the American Academy of Child and Adolescents Psychiatry, 44*, 1167–1175.
Stein, B. D., Jaycox, L. H., Kataoka, S. H., Wong, M., Tu, W., Elliott, M. N., et al. (2003). A mental health intervention for school children exposed to violence. *J Am Med Assoc, 290*, 603–611.

Chapter 8
Is Prevention Better than Cure? How Early Interventions Can Prevent PTSD

Sara A. Freedman and Arieh Y. Shalev

"…speaking as a mental health professional, why do we need to do anything at all?…" (Wessely, 2007).

In reference to the necessity of providing early interventions following mass disasters such as 9/11, the author suggested that the focus on the need for immediate intervention for those psychologically affected by traumatic events might be misplaced. In the debate regarding provision of interventions in the aftermath of a trauma, opinions range from mandatory provision of such services (e.g., Hokanson & Wirth, 2000) to the recommendation of wait, reevaluate, and delay treatment until necessary (e.g., Brewin et al., 2008).

The concept that it is preferable to prevent a problem from occurring rather than to treat it once it occurs is not novel, and has been applied to many areas of medicine, including dentistry (Grant, Roberts, Brown, & Quinoñez, 2007), heart disease (Lin et al., 2010), and vaccination programs (Elliman, Sengupta, El Bashir, & Bedford, 2007). Within psychiatry, the concept is perhaps less widely recognized, perhaps because most psychiatric illnesses have insidious onset, and unclear etiology, thus making prevention appear illusive. However, recent studies have shown that prevention also has potential with psychiatric problems. Posttraumatic stress disorder (PTSD) is unusual within psychiatric diagnoses in that its definition includes a clear etiology, along with well-documented paths of development

S.A. Freedman, Ph.D. (✉)
Department of Psychiatry, Center for Traumatic Stress, Hadassah University Hospital, Jerusalem, Israel

School of Social Work, Bar Ilan University, Ramat Gan, Israel
e-mail: sarafreedman@gmail.com

A.Y. Shalev, M.D.
Department of Psychiatry, Center for Traumatic Stress, Hadassah University Hospital, Jerusalem, Israel
e-mail: Arieh.Shalev@nyumc.org

M.P. Safir et al. (eds.), *Future Directions in Post-Traumatic Stress Disorder*,
DOI 10.1007/978-1-4899-7522-5_8

(e.g., Sveen, Ekselius, Gerdin, & Willebrand, 2011). This enables potential opportunity for speedy intervention before the disorder takes hold.

In this chapter, we will review the rationale for preventing posttraumatic stress disorder (PTSD), and review the studies examining early interventions for PTSD. In addition, the results of a large effectiveness and efficacy study of early PTSD treatment will be discussed. Lastly, the implications of these studies will be evaluated in terms of service planning and provision.

Background

Following exposure to a potentially traumatic event, a significant percentage of individuals will exhibit psychological symptoms, and many will subsequently develop PTSD. Studies have shown that most people will exhibit initial symptoms, and lifetime prevalence for chronic PTSD is 7.8 % (e.g., Kessler, Sonnega, Bromet, Hughes et al., 1995). The levels of chronic PTSD are related to the severity of the initial trauma (Shalev & Freedman, 2005), and trauma type (Kessler et al., 1995), such that exposure to a terrorist attack results in approximately 35 % chronic PTSD, and exposure to a straightforward traffic accident around 17 % (Shalev & Freedman, 2005).

PTSD is defined in DSM-IV-TR as including at least one symptom of reexperiencing, three of avoidance, and two of arousal. Symptoms must be present for at least 1 month, and result in significant impairment in functioning. PTSD is defined as acute when the duration of symptoms is under 3 months and chronic when the duration is over 3 months (APA, 2000).

PTSD is related to a host of other problems. For instance, PTSD is related to other comorbid psychiatric disorders, including a higher risk of suicide. In addition, PTSD sufferers are more likely to fail in higher education, become teenage parents, and have marital difficulties. Individuals with PTSD have 150 % increased odds of unemployment (Kessler, 2000). Patients with PTSD following traffic accidents use medical services eight times more frequently than non-PTSD patients with similar injuries (e.g., O'Donnell, Creamer, Elliott, & Atkin, 2005). Thus, in addition to the significant effects on sufferers, PTSD results in a significant burden to society (Kessler, 2000), and its early treatment is a public health necessity (e.g., Kartha et al., 2008).

The development of PTSD, regardless of traumatic event or PTSD severity, follows a path of initial symptoms which gradually decline over time. Most of this natural recovery takes place within the first 6 months following the traumatic event with significantly less recovery occurring after the first year (McFarlane, 2000). According to DSM-IV-TR, these initial symptoms can been classified as acute stress disorder (ASD) when they take place within the first 2 weeks following a traumatic event, including symptoms of: reexperiencing, avoidance, arousal, and dissociation, and cause significant impairment in various areas of functioning (APA, 2000).

Treatment of PTSD

Over the past 20 years, there have been significant advances in the successful treatment of chronic PTSD. Far from the refractory disorder it was once considered, a significant number of PTSD sufferers now benefit from effective treatment. According to the treatment guidelines of the ISTSS (Foa, Hembree et al., 2005; Foa, Keane et al. 2005), cognitive behavior therapy (CBT) is identified as an effective therapy (Cukor, Olden, Lee, & Difede, 2010; Foa, 2006). Specifically, several studies have shown that Prolonged Exposure (PE), a behavior treatment developed by Foa and colleagues, is an extremely effective intervention (Powers, Halpern, Ferenschak, Gillihan, & Foa, 2010). In addition, cognitive therapy (CT) and cognitive processing therapy (CPT) have also been shown to be effective (Cukor et al., 2010). Studies that have compared different types of CBT have concluded that all appear equally effective (although the largest number of studies have examined PE). Furthermore, addition of more than one component (e.g., PE plus CT) yields no added benefit (Mendes, Mello, Ventura, Passarela, & Mari, 2008, Foa, 2006).

Despite this success of these treatments, there remain several questions regarding treatment for chronic PTSD. Firstly, most of these studies show a relatively high level of dropouts from therapy (e.g., 21 %, Foa et al., 1999; 46 %, Foa, Hembree et al., 2005; Foa, Keane et al. 2005; 22–23 %, Rizvi, Vogt, & Resick, 2009; 24 %, Bryant et al., 2008). Although dropout from research protocols may not reflect dropout rates in clinical settings, this still reflects a barrier to treatment that must be overcome, if more people are to benefit from treatment.

Second, although CBT is significantly more effective than waitlist or control groups, following such treatments a significant percentage of patients remain with a diagnosis of PTSD. Foa et al. (1999) found a range of 40–60 % persistent PTSD after the completion of various treatment modalities. More recently, Bryant et al. (2008) found similar rates (35–65 %). Thus, despite successful therapies available to date, a significant percentage of patients do not respond sufficiently.

Early Interventions for PTSD

As previously stated, most individuals normally exhibit posttraumatic symptoms following exposure to a traumatic event that decrease over time. Even amongst those who develop PTSD, around 50 % will recover within 6 months (Freedman, Brandes, Peri, & Shalev, 1999). This pattern of spontaneous recovery suggests that following a traumatic event, there may be a critical time period within which symptoms of PTSD are not yet permanent, and recovery is more likely to take place. This may also serve as a therapeutic window of opportunity in which early interventions may prevent the consolidation of intrusive memories into chronic PTSD.

This notion is supported by studies that have examined conditioned responses to loud noises (e.g., Shalev et al., 2000; Griffin, 2008). Shalev et al. (2000) showed that individuals with chronic PTSD show no habituation when presented with unexpected loud noises: they display the startle response which is a hallmark symptom of PTSD. In contrast, individuals exposed to traumatic events, but who do not develop PTSD, habituate quickly. This significant difference is apparent 4 months post-trauma, but not before this time, suggesting that there still exist plasticity until this time (Shalev et al., 2000). Griffin (2008) showed that startle differences between PTSD and non-PTSD assault victims is apparent at 6 months post-trauma, but not at 1 month. Additional evidence comes from studies examining very early responses to traumatic events, demonstrating that memories are initially stored in short term memory, and over 6–8 h become consolidated in long term memory (e.g., Cohen et al., 2012). This process has been described in terms of its neurochemistry, and some recent studies have shown that memory consolidation, both in rats and humans, can be interrupted with the use of anisomycin (Cohen et al., 2006), propanolol (Pitman et al., 2002), and morphine (Holbrook, Galarneau, Dye, Quinn, & Dougherty, 2010). These studies suggest that the critical time period occurs immediately following a traumatic event, and before the person has had an opportunity to sleep (e.g., Wagner, Hallschmid, Rasch, & Born, 2006; Hu, Stylos-Allan, & Walker, 2006; Cohen et al., 2012).

Early interventions to prevent PTSD have a long history (e.g., Sokol, 1989), although randomized controlled trials are relatively more recent (e.g., Bisson, Jenkins, Alexander, & Bannister, 1997). These interventions will be divided into two groups, those based on the debriefing model and those based on CBT.

Debriefing

The concept of debriefing has its origins in Critical Incident Stress Management (CISM, Everly, Flannery, & Mitchell, 2000). CISM includes several components, from interventions prior to the traumatic event, through immediate post-event and follow-up. Based on initial work with preexisting, high risk teams, such as firefighters, CISM takes place in group format. CISM includes seven integrated elements: (1) precrisis preparation; (2) large scale demobilization procedures for use after disasters; (3) individual acute crisis counseling; (4) brief small group discussions, called defusings, designed to assist in acute symptom reduction; (5) Critical Incident Stress Debriefing (CISD): longer small group discussions designed to assist in achieving a sense of psychological closure postcrisis and/or facilitate the referral process; (6) family crisis intervention techniques; and (7) follow-up procedures, and/or referral for psychological assessment or treatment (Mitchell, 1983; Everly et al., 2000). Research shows that group participants are generally satisfied with CISM, although there is a paucity of research examining the long term effects of this intervention in randomized controlled trials.

Other studies have taken the concept of debriefing from critical incident stress management, and provided immediate debriefing, as a stand-alone intervention.

These interventions have included individual treatment, group treatments for convenience groups, and have included some, rather than all, the elements of the original model (Mitchell, 1983). Randomized controlled trials that have examined debriefing are summarized in Table 8.1. As can be seen, most studies conclude that debriefing is ineffective in preventing PTSD. Two studies show that providing debriefing to individuals as a stand-alone treatment immediately following a traumatic event may actually increase the development of PTSD (Bisson et al., 1997). Thus, recommendations from ISTSS treatment guidelines are that single session individual debriefing should not be offered, and that although there may be elements of group debriefing that are helpful, there is not sufficient evidence to warrant its recommendation (Foa, Hembree et al., 2005; Foa, Keane et al. 2005).

Cognitive Behavior Therapy: Early Intervention

Cognitive behavior therapy (CBT) is a well-established effective treatment for anxiety disorders in general (Olatunji, Cisler, & Deacon, 2010), and PTSD in particular (Kar, 2011). It has also been used as an early intervention for PTSD (Table 8.2). These studies show that brief early CBT both decreases initial symptoms levels, as well as prevents the long term development of PTSD. However, results are not entirely consistent. For example: in one study that compared CBT versus an assessment only control group, the CBT groups showed significantly lower PTSD symptoms at 1 week posttreatment, but by 4 months, this significant difference had disappeared (Sijbrandij et al., 2007).

Remaining Questions Regarding Early Interventions

Although the studies we have reviewed suggest that CBT offered close in time to a traumatic event may be effective at preventing PTSD, there remain several important questions:

First, optimal timing of early interventions remains unclear. These studies include interventions timed between several hours (Rothbaum, Meuli & Landolt 2012) or days (Zehnder et al., 2010) to a few months (Wagner et al., 2007) after the event. Knowledge of natural decline in symptoms indicates that interventions offered at 4 days and 10 weeks are dealing with different patient sets and needs.

Second, the interventions, while all falling under the umbrella of CBT, vary widely in the specific interventions included. Therefore, it is unclear which components are essential, and which may be less necessary.

Third, many of these studies have focused on patients with diagnoses of Acute Stress Disorder (ASD). A significant percentage of individuals with ASD subsequently develop PTSD, and therefore this is a vulnerable group. However, research shows that only between 30 (Creamer, O'Donnell, & Pattison, 2004) and 84 %

Table 8.1 Early intervention for PTSD: randomized studies of psychological debriefing

Authors	Study population	Study design	*N*	Timing of treatment post trauma	Treatment/s	Outcome
Adler et al. (2008)	Peacekeepers	RCT	952	Not timed to a specific event	Groups CISD vs. Survey only vs. Stress management	No overall effects
Bisson, Shepherd, Joy, Probert, & Newcombe (2004)	Burns victims	RCT	133	2–19 days	Debriefing vs. no treatment control	Debriefing groups had higher levels of PTSD at follow-up
Lee, Slade, & Lygo (1996)	Miscarriage	RCT	60	14 days	Individual counseling vs. treatment as usual	No overall effects
Marchand et al. (2006)	Armed robbery victims	RCT	75	2–22 days (first session); 1 week after that (second session)	Debriefing vs. no treatment control	No overall effects
Mayou, Ehlers, & Hobbs (2000) [3 year follow-up of Hobbs et al. (1996)]	Road traffic accident victims	RCT	160	24–48 h	Debriefing vs. no treatment control	At 3 months post-intervention: no difference between groups; at 3 years: intervention group had higher symptom levels
Rose, Brewin, Andrews, & Kirk (1999)	Violent crime	RCT	157	<1 month	Debriefing vs. education vs. assessment	No overall effects
Sijbrandij, Olff, Reitsma, Carlier, & Gersons (2006)	Adult civilian trauma	RCT	236	11–19 days	Emotional debriefing vs. educational debriefing vs. no treatment control	All groups showed similar results
Stallard et al. (2006)	Children aged 7–18, following road traffic accident	RCT	158	Within 1 month	Debriefing vs. no treatment control	Groups showed similar results
Wu et al. (2012)	Military rescuers	RCT	1,267	1 month	Cohesion debriefing vs. Debriefing vs. no treatment	Cohesion debriefing resulted in lower PTSD at follow-up

Table 8.2 Early intervention for PTSD: randomized studies of CBT

Authors	Study population	*N*	Timing of treatment post trauma	Treatment/s	Outcome
Bisson et al. (2004)	Physically injured trauma survivors	152	5–10 weeks	CBT vs. TAU	CBT led to significantly lower PTSD symptoms at follow-up
Bryant, Moulds, Guthrie, & Nixon (2005)	Adult civilian trauma with ASD	87	Within 1 month	CBT, CBT+hypnosis, Supportive e counseling	CBT & CBT-hypnosis lead to greater treatment effects than supportive counseling; CBT-hypnosis reduced reexperiencing symptoms
Bryant (2008)	Adult civilian trauma with ASD	90	Within 1 month	Exposure vs. cognitive restructuring vs. waitlist control	Exposure based therapy leads to more significant changes than cognitive restructuring
Bryant, Sackville, Dang, Moulds, & Guthrie (1999)	Adult civilian trauma with ASD	45	Within 2 weeks	PE vs. PE+AM vs. Supportive counseling	Less chronic PTSD in PE and PE+AM groups
Bryant, Harvey, Dang, Sackville, & Basten (1998)	Adult civilian trauma with ASD	24	Within 2 weeks	CBT vs. supportive counseling	CBT leads to significantly lower PTSD at posttreatment and follow-up
Bugg, Turpin, Mason, & Scholes (2009)	Adult civilian trauma	36	Within 6 weeks	Structured writing vs. information only	No significant difference between groups at follow-up.
Cox, Kenardy, & Hendrikz (2010)	Children, accidental injury	85	2 weeks	Web based CBT vs. waitlist control	Decrease in anxiety in treatment group
Ehlers et al. (2003)	Motor vehicle accident	96	Within 6 months	Cognitive therapy vs. self-help booklet vs. repeated assessments	Cognitive therapy resulted in fewer symptoms of PTSD and depression. Self help not useful
Freyth, Elsesser, Lohrmann, & Sartory (2010)	Civilian trauma with ASD	40	1 month	PE vs. supportive counseling (three sessions)	No difference between groups at follow-up
Foa, Hembree et al. (2005), Foa, Keane et al. (2005)	Adult female sexual assault victims	90	Within 4 weeks	4 2-h sessions CBT vs. assessment vs. supportive counseling	Less anxiety at 3 months follow-up for CBT; no significant differences at 9 months follow-up

(continued)

Table 8.2 (continued)

Authors	Study population	*N*	Timing of treatment post trauma	Treatment/s	Outcome
Nixon (2012)	Physical and sexual assault victims	30	Not stated	PT vs. supportive counseling	No difference between groups at follow-up
Rothbaum et al. (2012)	Civilian trauma survivors	137	During emergency room visit	Modified prolonged exposure in ER	Less PTSD at 4 and 12 weeks follow-up
Sijbrandij (2007)	Civilian trauma survivors	143	Within 3 months	Brief CBT vs. waitlist control	Accelerated recovery in the CBT group; no difference in long term outcome
Wagner, Zatzick, Ghesquiere, & Jurkovich (2007)	Injured trauma survivors	8	Between 1 and 3 months	TAU vs. behavioral activation	Behavioral activation resulted in fewer symptoms of PTSD, but not in depression
Zehnder, Meuli, & Landolt (2010)	Children, RTA	101	7–10 days	30 min intervention vs. treatment as usual	Reduced depression and beh problems in treatment group, who were preadolescent; no effect in older children

(Bryant & Harvey, 1998) of individuals with ASD will develop PTSD, whereas between 10 (Schnyder, Moergeli, Klaghofer, & Buddeberg, 2001) and 72 % (Harvey & Bryant, 2000) of individuals with PTSD suffered from ASD. Therefore offering intervention only to those patients with ASD potentially neglects a large number of people who are at risk for PTSD.

Fourth, although it seems clear to clinicians that early interventions are important and essential, clients seem less accepting. Studies have shown that even when early interventions are readily available, a significant percentage of patients are reluctant to accept treatment (e.g., Hoge et al., 2004). Several explanations for this have been suggested, including stigma (Kim, Thomas, Wilk, Castro, & Hoge, 2010). However, a better understanding of these barriers to treatment is essential in planning acceptable, and not just effective, treatments.

The Jerusalem Trauma Outreach and Prevention Study

The Jerusalem Trauma Outreach and Prevention Study (J-TOPS) project was designed in an attempt to answer some of the questions outlined above. It will be briefly described here (Shalev, Ankri, Peleg, Israeli-Shalev, & Freedman, 2011, gives more detailed information regarding its design), and the major results presented (Shalev et al., 2012).

J-TOPS consisted of two overlapping research methodologies: first, a longitudinal prospective outreach study and second, an embedded randomized controlled trial. Tracking all admissions to the Emergency Room of a large hospital in Israel, the outreach program identified, via computer, patients as suitable for the study (aged between 18 and 65, lived within the greater Jerusalem area, came to the ER as a result of a potentially traumatic event). These individuals were phoned within 2 weeks of their ER visit. This telephone interview (Telephone Interview I, or TI-1) identified whether the person had experienced a traumatic event, as per DSM (i.e., both objectively experienced an event as well as subjective responded to that event), as well as suffering from symptom levels of PTSD and depression. Figure 8.1 details the design of the study.

A second telephone interview was conducted 7 months post-trauma. At this point in time all subjects who had experienced a traumatic event were reinterviewed. In addition, 10 % of those subjects deemed not to have had experienced a traumatic event were randomly chosen and reinterviewed.

In the first telephone interview, 5,286 individuals were called, and 5,053 (94 %) agreed to participate. A large proportion of these people had not actually experienced a traumatic event, as defined in Criteria A1 and A2 of DSM IV. Of the 1996 that had experienced an event, 1,502 were considered to be sufficiently symptomatic as to warrant further investigation, and were invited to a clinical interview. Only 50 % actually attended. Of the 756 people interviewed at this stage, 397 exhibited PTSD symptoms, and were eligible for the randomized control trial. Of these, 296 (75 %) started treatment.

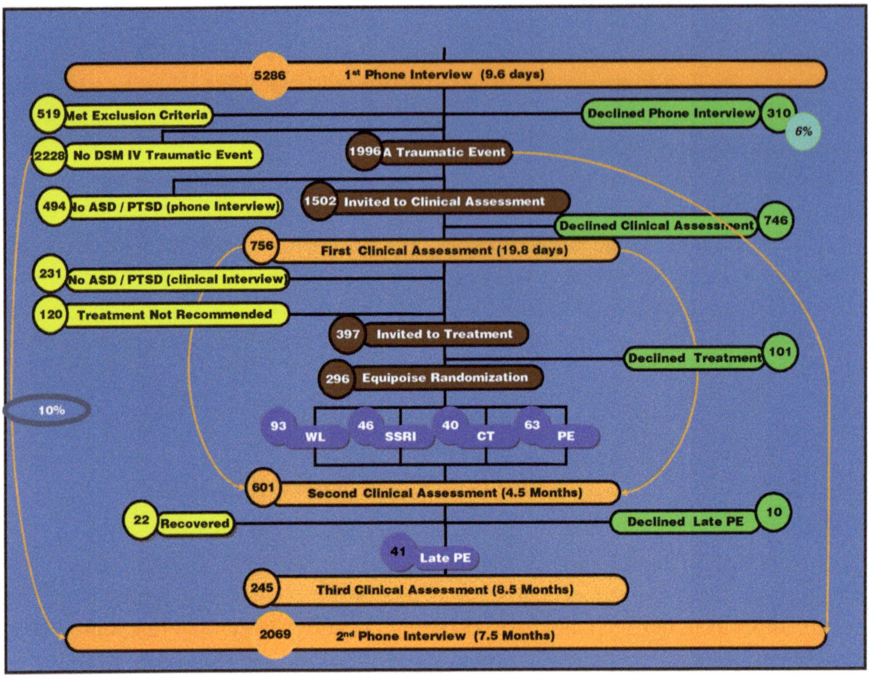

Fig. 8.1 J-TOPS study design

Participants who were invited to either the clinical interview, or to participate in the treatment trial, but did not attend, showed less symptom reduction over time. This difference between attendees and non-attendees remained significant, even when initial symptoms levels were taken into account. Thus, this study revealed that even when approached by a treatment team dedicated to outreach, the majority of recently traumatized individuals preferred not to meet with a mental health professional. However, acceptance of telephone contact was extremely high. As refusing an interview, or treatment, is clearly associated with poorer outcome, this represents a significant barrier to successful treatment.

The randomized controlled trial (Shalev et al., 2012) assessed effectiveness of three different treatment modalities. The first treatment, Prolonged Exposure (PE, Foa & Rothbaum, 1998), is a behavior based treatment that includes psychoeducation, breathing retraining, in vivo exposure, and imaginal exposure to the trauma narrative. Many studies, as described above, have demonstrated the effectiveness of PE as a treatment for both chronic PTSD as well as an early intervention. The latter, however, usually consisted of 4–5 sessions. In this study, the full protocol of 12 sessions was offered. The second treatment, cognitive therapy (CT, Marks, Lovell, Noshirvani, Livanou, & Thrasher, 1998), focuses on the negative interpretations that patients make about their trauma, themselves, and their reactions. It includes no elements of exposure, and therefore, can be compared with PE. CT been shown to be effective in treating chronic PTSD (Marks et al., 1998), although results as an early intervention were less positive (Bryant et al., 2008). In the third treatment group, patients received an SSRI in a double blind comparison with placebo. A fourth group of patients were a waitlist control. If they were symptomatic at the end of the waitlist condition, they received Prolonged Exposure. Thus, early and late interventions could be compared.

The results indicated that both PE and CT were successful in treating early symptoms. There were no significant differences between PE and CT in treatment acceptance, drop out from treatment, or its effectiveness. There were no significant difference between SSRI, placebo, and waitlist control, and all were significantly less effective than PE and CT.

This study allowed patients to refuse up to two treatment conditions within the randomization process: thus a patient could refuse PE, and then be re-randomized to one of the other conditions. This type of randomization better reflects real world clinical settings, where patients are able to choose their treatment. This study found that relatively few patients refused psychological treatments (CT: 8, 3.1 %; PE: 3, 1.2 %). However, a significantly higher number refused medication (103, 42.6 %).

The study found that early and late PE resulted in similar recovery rates.

While the majority of patients who entered the RCT presented with full PTSD or ASD symptoms, others met two out of the three necessary criteria and therefore could be said to have "partial PTSD." When these patients with partial PTSD who received CT or PE were compared with waitlist control, no significant differences were found. This indicates that the effectiveness of PE and CT over natural recovery is only apparent in those presenting with all the symptoms of PTSD.

Service Planning

At the beginning of this chapter, we raised the question as to whether early interventions are necessary. The assumption has usually been not only are they needed, but that in the event of a mass disaster existing service provision will not be sufficient to cope with demand. Indeed, following 9/11, immediate government funding of 40 million dollars was allocated to provide additional services that arose as a result of the terror attacks (Emergency Supplemental Appropriations Act for Recovery from and Response to Terrorist Attacks on the United States, 2001).

In the present study, potential patients' reception of early interventions was examined. For every 100 patients who attended the Emergency Room, six received early treatment; for every 100 patients who experienced a traumatic event as identified by initial telephone interviews, only 15 accepted early treatment (Shalev et al., 2011). These figures indicate that even with systematic outreach, by a highly experienced and dedicated team, few individuals actually accept early treatment. Outreach rarely exists in real life settings, given its cost. This data is novel and extremely salient in treatment planning. As relatively few individuals are interested in early treatment, most clinical settings would be able to accommodate the extra patients needing interventions following a traumatic event, without the addition of extra resources. Since this study also demonstrated that delaying treatment did not result in reduced treatment effectiveness, service planning can also reliably employ a "wait and see" approach, when resources are stretched. Finally, this study showed that providing early treatment to individuals, who did not have all symptoms of PTSD, was no more effective than the waitlist control. This indicates that resources should not be provided for this population: natural recovery is best with this group.

Conclusions

In answer to the question posed by Wessely: "why do we need to do anything at all?"—the answer appears to be "we don't always need to." The studies reviewed here have shown that while one-off interventions are rarely helpful, cognitive behavioral interventions can help prevent the development of PTSD. These interventions seem most effective with more severely symptomatic individuals, as natural recovery results in the same rate of symptom reduction as psychological interventions with patients who do not have full PTSD. When mental health resources are unable to cope with a surge in demand, interventions carried out at a later stage are as effective as more immediate ones.

An important task for us as mental health professionals is to uncover why many people who require psychological intervention do not receive it (Kazdin & Blasé, 2011). It is important to identify barriers to treatment, and to employ strategies to overcome them, in order to successfully treat a larger proportion of individuals who need treatment. This may include systematic outreach, employing novel treatment modalities, and psycho-education regarding the benefits of treatment.

References

Adler, A. B., Litz, B. T., Castro, C. A., Suvak, M. T., Jeffrey, L., Burrell, L., et al. (2008). A group randomized trial of critical incident stress debriefing provided to U.S. peacekeepers. *Journal of Traumatic Stress, 21*(3), 253–263.

American Psychiatric Association. (2000). *Diagnostic and statistical manual of mental disorders*. (4th ed. text revision). Washington, DC.

Bisson, J. L., Jenkins, P. L., Alexander, J., & Bannister, C. (1997). Randomised controlled trial of psychological debriefing for victims of acute burn trauma. *British Journal of Psychiatry, 171*, 78–81.

Bisson, J. I., Shepherd, J. P., Joy, D., Probert, R., & Newcombe, R. G. (2004). Early cognitive-behavioral therapy for post-traumatic stress symptoms after physical injury. *British Journal of Psychiatry, 184*, 63–9.

Brewin, C. R., Scragg, P., Robertson, M., Thompson, M., d'Ardenne, P., & Ehlers, A. (2008). Promoting mental health following the London bombings: A screen and treat approach. *Journal of Traumatic Stress, 21*(1), 3–8.

Bryant, R. A., & Harvey, A. G. (1998). Relationship of acute stress disorder and posttraumatic stress disorder following mild traumatic brain injury. *American Journal of Psychiatry, 155*, 625–629.

Bryant, R. A., Harvey, A. G., Dang, S. T., Sackville, T., & Basten, C. (1998). Treatment of acute stress disorder: A comparison of cognitive-behavioral therapy and supportive counseling. *Journal of Consulting and Clinical Psychology, 66*(5), 862–866.

Bryant, R. A., Mastrodomenico, J., Felmingham, K. L., Hopwood, S., Kenny, L., Kandris, E., et al. (2008). Treatment of acute stress disorder: A randomized controlled trial. *Archives of General Psychiatry, 65*(6), 659–667.

Bryant, R. A., Moulds, M., Guthrie, R., & Nixon, R. D. V. (2003). Treating acute stress disorder following mild traumatic brain injury. *American Journal of Psychiatry, 160*, 585–7.

Bryant, R. A., Moulds, M. L., Guthrie, R. M., & Nixon, R. D. V. (2005). The additive benefits of hypnosis and cognitive-behavioral therapy in treating acute stress disorder. *Journal of Consulting and Clinical Psychology, 73*(2), 334–40.

Bryant, R. A., Sackville, T., Dang, S. T., Moulds, M., & Guthrie, R. (1999). Treating acute stress disorder: An evaluation of cognitive behavior therapy and supporting counseling techniques. *American Journal of Psychiatry, 156*(11), 1780–1786.

Bugg, A., Turpin, G., Mason, S., & Scholes, C. (2009). A randomised controlled trial of the effectiveness of writing as a self-help intervention for traumatic injury patients at risk of developing post-traumatic stress disorder. *Behaviour Research and Therapy, 47*, 6–12.

Cohen, H., Kaplan, Z., Matar, M. A., Loewenthal, U., Kozlovsky, N., & Zohar, J. (2006). Anisomycin, a protein synthesis inhibitor, disrupts traumatic memory consolidation and attenuates posttraumatic stress response in rats. *Biological Psychiatry, 60*(7), 767–76.

Cohen, S., Kozlovsky, N., Matar, M. A., Kaplan, Z., Zohar, J., & Cohen, H. (2012). Post-exposure sleep deprivation facilitates correctly timed interactions between glucocorticoid and adrenergic systems, which attenuate traumatic stress responses. *Neuropsychopharmacology, 37*(11), 2388–2404.

Cox, C. M., Kenardy, J. A., & Hendrikz, J. K. (2010). A randomized controlled trial of a web-based early intervention for children and their parents following unintentional injury. *Journal of Pediatric Psychology, 35*(6), 581–592.

Creamer, M. C., O'Donnell, M. L., & Pattison, P. (2004). The relation-ship between acute stress disorder and posttraumatic stress disorder in severely injured trauma survivors. *Behaviour Research and Therapy, 42*(3), 315–328.

Cukor, J., Olden, M., Lee, F., & Difede, J. (2010). Evidence-based treatments for PTSD, new directions, and special challenges. *Annals of New York Academy of Sciences, 1208*, 82–9.

Ehlers, A., Clark, D. M., Hackmann, A., McManus, F., Fennell, M., Herbert, C., et al. (2003). A randomized controlled trial of cognitive therapy, a self help booklet, and repeated assessments as early interventions for posttraumatic stress disorder. *Archives of General Psychiatry, 60*(10), 1024–1032.

Elliman, D., Sengupta, N., El Bashir, H., & Bedford, H. (2007). Measles, mumps, and rubella: prevention. *Clinical Evidence, pii*, 0316.

Emergency Supplemental Appropriations Act for Recovery from and Response to Terrorist Attacks on the United States of 2001, Pub. L.107–38.

Everly, G. S., Flannery, R. B., & Mitchell, J. T. (2000). Critical incident stress management (CISM): A review of the literature. *Aggression and Violent Behavior, 5*, 23–40.

Foa, E. B. (2006). Psychosocial therapy for posttraumatic stress disorder. *Journal of Clinical Psychiatry, 67*(Suppl. 2), 40–5.

Foa, E. B., Dancu, C. V., Hembree, E. A., Jaycox, L. H., Meadows, E. A., & Street, G. P. (1999). A comparison of exposure therapy, stress innoculation training, and their combination for reducing posttraumatic stress disorder in female assault victims. *Journal of Consulting and Clinical Psychology, 67*(2), 194–200.

Foa, E. B., Hembree, E. A., Cahill, S. P., Rauch, S. A., Riggs, D. S., Feeny, N. C., et al. (2005). Randomized trial of prolonged exposure for posttraumatic stress disorder with and without cognitive restructuring: Outcome at academic and community clinics. *Journal of Consulting and Clinical Psychology, 73*(5), 953–964.

Foa, E. B., Keane, T. M., Friedman, M., & Cohen, J. A. (Eds.). (2005). *Effective Treatments for PTSD: Practice guidelines from the International Society for Traumatic Stress Studies (ISTSS)* (2nd ed.). New York, NY: Guilford Press.

Foa, E. B., & Rothbaum, B. O. (1998). *Treating the trauma of rape: Cognitive-behavioral therapy for PTSD*. New York, NY: Guilford Press.

Foa, E. B., Zoellner, L. A., & Feeny, N. C. (2006). An evaluation of three brief programs for facilitating recovery after assault. *Journal of Traumatic Stress, 19*(1), 29–43.

Freedman, S. A., Brandes, D., Peri, T., & Shalev, A. Y. (1999). Predic-tors of chronic post-traumatic stress disorder: A prospective study. *British Journal of Psychiatry, 174*, 353–359.

Freyth, C., Elsesser, K., Lohrmann, T., & Sartory, G. (2010). Effects of additional prolonged exposure to psychoeducation and relaxation in acute stress disorder. *Journal of Anxiety Disorders, 24*(8), 909–917.

Grant, J. S., Roberts, M. W., Brown, W. D., & Quinoñez, R. B. (2007). Integrating dental screening and fluoride varnish application into a pediatric residency outpatient program: Clinical and financial implications. *Clinical Pediatric Dentistry, 31*(3), 175–8.

Griffin, M. G. (2008). A prospective assessment of auditory startle alterations in rape and physical assault survivors. *Journal of Traumatic Stress, 21*(1), 91–99.

Harvey, A. G., & Bryant, R. A. (2000). A two-year prospective evaluation of the relationship between acute stress disorder and post-traumatic stress disorder following mild traumatic brain injury. *American Journal of Psychiatry, 157*, 626–628.

Hobbs M1, Mayou R, Harrison B, Worlock P. (1996). A randomised controlled trial of psychological debriefing for victims of road traffic accidents. BMJ. Dec 7;313(7070):1438-9.

Hoge, C. W., Castro, C. A., Messer, S. C., McGurk, D., Cotting, D. I., & Koffman, R. L. (2004). Combat duty in Iraq and Afghanistan, mental health problems, and barriers to care. *New England Journal of Medicine, 351*(1), 13–22.

Hokanson, M., & Wirth, B. (2000). The critical incident stress debriefing process for the Los Angeles county fire department: Automatic and effective. *International Journal of Emergency Mental Health, 2*(4), 249–257.

Holbrook, T. L., Galarneau, M. R., Dye, J. L., Quinn, K., & Dougherty, A. L. (2010). Morphine use after combat injury in Iraq and post-traumatic stress disorder. *New England Journal of Medicine, 362*(2), 110–7.

Hu, P., Stylos-Allan, M., & Walker, M. P. (2006). Sleep facilitates consolidation of emotional declarative memory. *Psychological Science, 17*(10), 891–8.

Kar, N. (2011). Cognitive behavioral therapy for the treatment of post-traumatic stress disorder: A review. *Neuropsychiatric Disease and Treatment, 7*, 167–81.

Kartha, A., Brower, V., Saitz, R., Samet, J. H., Keane, T. M., & Liebschutz, J. (2008). The impact of trauma exposure and post-traumatic stress disorder on healthcare utilization among primary care patients. *Medical Care, 46*(4), 388–393.

Kazdin, A. E., & Blasé, S. L. (2011). Rebooting psychotherapy research and practice to reduce the burden of mental illness. *Perspectives on Psychological Science, 6*, 21.

Kessler, R. C. (2000). Posttraumatic stress disorder: The burden to the individual and to society. *Journal of Clinical Psychiatry, 61*(Suppl 5), 4–12.

Kessler, R. C., Sonnega, A., Bromet, E., Hughes, M., et al. (1995). Posttraumatic stress disorder in the National Comorbidity Survey. *Archives of General Psychiatry, 52*(12), 1048–1060.

Kim, P. Y., Thomas, J. L., Wilk, J. E., Castro, C. A., & Hoge, C. W. (2010). Stigma, barriers to care, and use of mental health services among active duty and National Guard soldiers after combat. *Psychiatric Services, 61*(6), 582–8.

Lee, C., Slade, P., & Lygo, V. (1996). The influence of psychological debriefing on emotional adaption in women following early miscarriage: A preliminary study. *British Journal of Medical Psychology, 69*(1), 47–58.

Lin, J. S., O'Connor, E., Whitlock, E. P., Beil, T. L., Zuber, S. P., Per-due, L. A., Plaut, D., Lutz, K. (2010). *Behavioral counseling to promote physical activity and a healthful diet to prevent cardiovascular disease in adults: Update of the evidence for the U.S. Preventive Services Task Force* [Internet]. Rockville, MD: Agency for Healthcare Research and Quality (US); Report No.: 11-05149-EF-1.

Marchand, A., Guay, S., Boyer, R., lucci, S., Martin, A., & St Hilaire, M. (2006). A randomized controlled trial of an adapted form of individual critical incident stress debriefing for victims of an armed robbery. *Brief Treatment and Crisis Intervention, 6*(2), 122–129.
Marks, I., Lovell, K., Noshirvani, H., Livanou, M., & Thrasher, S. (1998). Treatment of posttraumatic stress disorder by exposure and/or cognitive restructuring: a controlled study. *Archives of General Psychiatry, 55*(4), 317–25.
Mayou, R. A., Ehlers, A., & Hobbs, M. (2000). Psychological debriefing for road traffic accident victims: Three-year follow-up of a randomised controlled trial. *British Journal of Psychiatry, 176*, 589–593.
McFarlane, A. C. (2000). Posttraumatic stress disorder: A model of the longitudinal course and the role of the risk factors. *Journal of Clinical Psychiatry, 61*(Suppl. 5), 15–23.
Mendes, D. D., Mello, M. F., Ventura, P., Passarela, C. M., & Mari, J. J. (2008). A systematic review on the effectiveness of cognitive behavioral therapy for posttraumatic stress disorder. *International Journal of Psychiatry in Medicine, 38*(3), 241–59.
Mitchell, J. T. (1983). When disaster strikes: The critical incident stress debriefing process. *Journal of Emergency Services, 8*, 36–39.
Nixon, R. D. V. (2012). Cognitive processing therapy versus supportive counseling for acute stress disorder following assault: A randomized pilot trial. *Behavior Therapy, 43*(4), 825–836.
O'Donnell, M. L., Creamer, M., Elliott, P., & Atkin, C. (2005). Health costs following motor vehicle accidents: The role of posttraumatic stress disorder. *Journal of Traumatic Stress, 18*(5), 557–61.
Olatunji, B. O., Cisler, J. M., & Deacon, B. J. (2010). Efficacy of cognitive behavioral therapy for anxiety disorders: a review of meta-analytic findings. *The Psychiatric Clinics of North America, 33*(3), 557–77.
Pitman, R. K., Sanders, K. M., Zusman, R. M., Healy, A. R., Cheema, F., Lasko, N. B., et al. (2002). Pilot study of secondary prevention of posttraumatic stress disorder with propranolol. *Biological Psychiatry, 51*(2), 189–92.
Powers, M. B., Halpern, J. M., Ferenschak, M. P., Gillihan, S. J., & Foa, E. B. (2010). A meta-analytic review of prolonged exposure for posttraumatic stress disorder. *Clinical Psychology Review, 30*(6), 635–41.
Rizvi, S. L., Vogt, D. S., & Resick, P. A. (2009). Cognitive and affective predictors of treatment outcome in Cognitive Processing Therapy and Prolonged Exposure for posttraumatic stress disorder. *Behaviour Research and Therapy, 9*, 737–43.
Rose, S., Brewin, C. R., Andrews, B., & Kirk, M. (1999). A randomized controlled trial of individual psychological debriefing for victims of violent crime. *Psychological Medicine: A Journal of Research in Psychiatry and the Allied Sciences, 29*(4), 793–799.
Rothbaum, B. O., Kearns, M. C., Price, M., Malcoun, E., Davis, M., Ressler, K. J., et al. (2012). Early intervention may prevent the development of posttraumatic stress disorder: A randomized pilot civilian study with modified prolonged exposure. *Biological Psychiatry, 72*(11), 957–63.
Schnyder, U., Moergeli, H., Klaghofer, R., & Buddeberg, C. (2001). Incidence and prediction of posttraumatic stress disorder symptoms in severely injured accident victims. *American Journal of Psychiatry, 158*, 594–599.
Shalev, A. Y., Ankri, Y., Peleg, T., Israeli-Shalev, Y., Adessky, R., & Freedman, S. A. (2012). Early treatment for PTSD: Results from the Jerusalem Trauma Outreach and Prevention Study (J-TOPS). *Archives of General Psychiatry, 69*, 166–176.
Shalev, A. Y., Ankri, Y. L., Peleg, T., Israeli-Shalev, Y., & Freedman, S. (2011). Barriers to receiving early care for PTSD: Results from the Jerusalem trauma outreach and prevention study. *Psychiatric Services, 62*(7), 765–73.
Shalev, A. Y., & Freedman, S. A. (2005). PTSD following terrorist attacks: A prospective evaluation. *American Journal of Psychiatry, 162*, 1188–1191.
Shalev, A. Y., Peri, T., Brandes, D., Freedman, S., Orr, S. P., & Pitman, R. K. (2000). Auditory startle response in trauma survivors with posttraumatic stress disorder: A prospective study. *American Journal of Psychiatry, 157*(2), 255–261.

Sijbrandij, M., Olff, M., Reitsma, J. B., Carlier, I. V. E., De Vries, M. H., & Gersons, B. P. R. (2007). Treatment of acute posttraumatic stress disorder with brief cognitive behavioural therapy: A randomised controlled trial. *American Journal of Psychiatry, 164*, 82–90.

Sijbrandij, M., Olff, M., Reitsma, J. B., Carlier, I. V. E., & Gersons, B. P. R. (2006). Emotional or educational debriefing after psychological trauma: Randomised controlled trial. *British Journal of Psychiatry, 189*(2), 150–155.

Sokol, R. J. (1989). Early mental health intervention in combat situations: The USS Stark. *Military Medicine, 154*(8), 407–409.

Stallard, P., Velleman, R., Salter, E., Howse, I., Yule, W., & Taylor, G. (2006). A randomised controlled trial to determine the effectiveness of an early psychological intervention with children involved in road traffic accidents. *Journal of Child Psychology and Psychiatry, 47*(2), 127–134.

Sveen, J., Ekselius, L., Gerdin, B., & Willebrand, M. (2011). A prospective longitudinal study of posttraumatic stress disorder symptom trajectories after burn injury. *Journal of Trauma, 71*(6), 1808–15.

Wagner, U., Hallschmid, M., Rasch, B., & Born, J. (2006). Brief sleep after learning keeps emotional memories alive for years. *Biological Psychiatry, 60*(7), 788–90.

Wagner, A. W., Zatzick, D. F., Ghesquiere, A., & Jurkovich, G. J. (2007). Behavioral activation as an early intervention for posttraumatic stress disorder and depression among physically injured trauma survivors. *Cognitive and Behavioral Practice, 14*(4), 341–349.

Wessely, S. (2007). When being upset is not a mental health problem. *Psychiatry, 67*(2), 153–157.

Wu, S., Zhu, X., Zhang, Y., Liang, J., Liu, X., Yang, Y., et al. (2012). A new psychological intervention: "512 Psychological Intervention Model" used for military rescuers in Wenchuan Earthquake in China. *Social Psychiatry and Psychiatric Epidemiology, 47*(7), 1111–9.

Zehnder, D., Meuli, M., & Landolt, M. A. (2010). Effectiveness of a single-session early psychological intervention for children after road traffic accidents: A randomised controlled trial. *Child and Adolescent Psychiatry and Mental Health, 4*.

Part III
Diagnosing PTSD

Chapter 9
Evolution of PTSD Diagnosis in the *DSM*

Lennis G. Echterling, Thomas A. Field, and Anne L. Stewart

Evolution of PTSD Diagnosis in the *DSM*

Although the American Psychiatric Association's (APA) *Diagnostic and Statistical Manual of Mental Disorders* (*DSM*) introduced the diagnosis of posttraumatic stress disorder (PTSD) only a little over three decades ago, psychological trauma is as old as human history. Timeless Homeric epics gave eloquent voice to the psychic scars of war (Shay, 1991). In this chapter, we focus on the origins and rapid evolution of the syndrome's diagnosis in the *DSM*. We also address several of the controversies related to the conceptualization of PTSD. Finally, we provide an overview of the changes that have taken place in the *DSM-5*.

Origins

The origins of the PTSD diagnosis stem from two distinct movements that presented dramatically different conceptualizations of the syndrome's origins, features, process, prognosis, and treatment, viz., the psychological and the somatic movements. The psychological movement began in the 1790s, and considered the syndrome as primarily a mental one involving altered consciousness and amnesia, which later became known as "dissociation." During subsequent wars, psychological conceptualizations of the condition included "nostalgia" in the U.S. Civil War, "war neuroses" in WWI, and "combat fatigue" in WWII.

L.G. Echterling (✉) • T.A. Field • A.L. Stewart
James Madison University, Harrisonburg, VA 22807, USA
e-mail: echterlg@jmu.edu; tfield@cityu.edu; stewaral@jmu.edu

M.P. Safir et al. (eds.), *Future Directions in Post-Traumatic Stress Disorder*,
DOI 10.1007/978-1-4899-7522-5_9

The somatic movement, conceptualizing a physiological basis for the syndrome, began in England during the 1860s, when researchers described "railway spine" as a consequence of the physical traumas of railroad accidents (Trimble, 1981). At the same time in the United States, physicians proposed that traumatized Civil War combat veterans were suffering from a cardiac injury, labeling it "soldier's heart" or "irritable heart" (O'Brien, 1998). Later terms from the somatic perspective included "Da Costa's syndrome" and "neurocirculatory asthenia" in WWI.

These two movements were merged in the 1890s under the diagnosis of "hysteria," which later evolved into what is now known as PTSD (van der Kolk, 2007). In his conceptualization of hysteria, Freud (1892) rejected the notion that the traumatic event directly induced the disorder. Instead, he believed that it was actually the persistent memory of the incident that caused the onset of symptoms. Thus, the role of memory in traumatization was conceptualized early on, and the causation for posttraumatic reactions was chiefly attributed to the individual's dysfunctional response, rather than the severity of the stressor itself.

World War I

By 1914, physicians in Europe and the United States were becoming familiar with the concept of "traumatic memory" (Young, 1995). However, widespread traumatization on an epidemic level was not documented until WWI. By 1918, the British Royal Army Medical Corps (RAMC) had treated 80,000 cases of "shell shock" (Stone, 1988). Shell shock was considered to be the physiological reaction to the intense shock waves that emanated from an artillery explosion, producing some form of brain injury, such as a concussion (Mott, 1917). Although there is growing recognition that primary blast waves have caused serious and permanent traumatic brain injuries (TBI) among veterans of the Iraq and Afghanistan wars (Warden, 2006), the original diagnosis of shell shock was mired in complications from its genesis. It was found that some soldiers did not develop the condition until weeks or months following an incident, and many cases had no history of experiencing blast waves (Myers, 1940).

During WWI, the work of British psychiatrist W. H. R. Rivers pioneered the acceptance of posttraumatic reactions within the psychiatric field (Herman, 1997). Like Freud, Rivers believed that exposure to trauma only resulted in a disorder when the person had a neurotic predisposition, a conceptualization that represented a swing toward the internal causality model. A formal inquiry in 1922 by the Report of the War Office Committee of Enquiry on Shell Shock lent support for Rivers' opinion (Hargreaves, Wittkower, & Wilson, 1940), and the term "shell shock" was dropped after the end of the war (O'Brien, 1998). The acceptance of war neurosis in psychiatric circles eventually led to Freud's brief account of war neurosis in *Beyond the Pleasure Principle* (1920), which was largely based on the reports of his colleagues who had treated traumatized Austrian and German soldiers during WWI.

World War II

During the decades of peacetime immediately following WWI, practitioners and researchers largely neglected the lessons they had learned regarding the profound impact of trauma on military troops. However, with the beginning of WWII, many service members once again experienced posttraumatic reactions from exposure to the horrors of combat. Initially, those who developed war neuroses during WWII were discharged (Boone, 2011). However, the need for military personnel led to psychiatrists in North Africa to use a new diagnosis of "combat stress," also known as "combat fatigue" (Boone, 2011).

Grinker and Spiegel (1945) studied factors that prevented the development of combat fatigue, and proposed that the degree of relatedness in the military unit was a protective factor. These findings led to the development of treatment strategies during WWII that reduced the amount of separation from the military unit. With support and encouragement, these affected combatants could be returned rapidly to active duty. The dysfunction resulting from combat fatigue was understood to be fleeting and not the manifestation of psychopathology. The profound impact of these contrasting conceptualizations on both treatment approaches and military personnel policies continues today.

Kardiner (1941) and Rado (1941) published separate reports of "traumatic neurosis" in WWII soldiers. Many of the symptoms they described were similar to those formally identified in editions of the *DSM*. These symptoms included hypersensitivity, arousal, sleep disturbances, and vivid nightmares. In a study that was also significant in the genesis of the PTSD diagnosis, Appel and Beebe (1946) concluded that any soldier would become symptomatic after experiencing 200–240 combat days. Hence, combat stress was considered to be a normal reaction to prolonged exposure.

Again, interest in traumatic neuroses faded once WWII came to an end. Nevertheless, the first use of the diagnostic term "posttraumatic" occurred in 1955, when the Veterans Administration conducted a follow-up study on veterans who had been diagnosed with some form of war neurosis (Brill & Beeb, 1955). Kardiner (1959) later noted that the diagnosis of war neurosis remained "anarchic" (p. 245) and without structure or clarity. Attempts to systematically define war neurosis were initially fraught with problems, stemming from the use of psychoanalytic terminology to identify core symptoms (Young, 1995).

Early DSM Conceptualizations of PTSD

It was not until 1980 that the American Psychiatric Association formally accepted PTSD as a legitimate diagnostic category in the *DSM-III.* However, even in the *DSM-I* (APA, 1952), the Committee on Nomenclature and Statistics recognized the then current and disturbing findings on the prevalence of psychiatric casualties of World War II. Therefore, it introduced "gross stress reaction" under the category of "transient situational personality disorders." This syndrome was presented as a short-lived and fleeting reaction to a major stressor such as a "combat or a civilian catastrophe" (p. 40) that was resolved within a few weeks.

Although this reaction was not labeled as a formal psychiatric disorder and did not include diagnostic criteria, its inclusion in *DSM-I* was significant for several reasons. First, it acknowledged that the syndrome was a risk not only for veterans of war, but also for survivors of natural disasters, fires, and other calamitous events. Second, the *DSM-I* asserted that "this diagnosis applies to previously more or less 'normal' persons who experience intolerable stress" (APA, 1952, p. 40), disagreeing with the then dominant psychodynamic assumption that the psychiatric casualties of extreme stress were vulnerable individuals with predisposing neurotic conditions (Saigh & Bremner, 1999). Third, it stimulated more research on combat veterans, including those in the heat of battle in the Korean War, which was ongoing during the publication of the *DSM-I.*

The inclusion of the "normal personality" descriptor suggested that the pendulum had swung away from attributing the development of dysfunction to an individual's character flaws (i.e., "neuropathic personality") after exposure to a stressor. From WWII onward, the external event was given greater weight in its contribution to dysfunction. Attributing causation to the external stressor as reason for dysfunction would later be reflected in the first formal diagnostic classification of PTSD in *DSM-III* (APA, 1980). Andraesen (2010) hypothesized that this change in causation attribution occurred due to concerns that diagnosing WWI military personnel with a form of war neurosis had been stigmatizing. The later research into combat fatigue during WWII further strengthened the argument for the normality of experiencing transient distress following exposure to a major stressor.

In the next edition of the *DSM-II* (1968), APA dropped the term "gross stress reaction" and substituted in its place the classification of "transient situation disturbances." While reasons for its absence are unknown, some experts have hypothesized that the 1950s and 1960s, like the decades between WWI and WWII, were a period of relative peace following wartime, and thus the diagnosis was conveniently forgotten (Andraesen, 2010). These syndromes were characterized as disturbances "that occur in individuals without any underlying mental disorders and that represent an acute reaction to overwhelming environmental stress" (APA, 1968, p. 48). Therefore, what was initially conceptualized as a "reaction" in 1952 was now labeled with the more clearly negative term, "disturbance." Although identifying the syndrome as an adverse consequence, the *DSM-II*, like its predecessor, did not specify any diagnostic criteria for transient situation disturbances.

As the title suggested, any psychological disturbance was considered to be fleeting, and if "symptoms persist after the stress is removed, another mental disorder is indicated" (p. 48). Thus, the *DSM-II* diagnosis of transient situational disturbance was somewhat comparable to gross stress reaction in *DSM-I*, since both involved short-lived responses to situational stressors.

Vietnam War

It was not until the Vietnam War that the demand for a combat-related trauma diagnosis reached a tipping point. In the early 1970s, many returning U.S. veterans exhibited problematic and potentially life-threatening behaviors, such as suicide attempts, antisocial behavior, and drug abuse (Dean, 1992). At first, these behaviors were attributed to non-combat-related neurosis or psychosis (Scott, 1990). However, with public war protests and disaffection growing, veterans began to advocate for a new disorder called "Post-Vietnam Syndrome" (Andraesen, 2010).

Proponents of an as-yet unidentified disorder began to publish books and newspaper columns on the psychiatric problems found in Vietnam veterans. Robert Lifton and Chaim Shatan, two of the most well-known writers on the topic, began holding "rap groups" with Vietnam veterans about their experiences and led panel discussions at psychiatric conferences (van der Kolk, 2007). By 1975, these two men approached the head of the *DSM-III* taskforce, Elliot Spitzer, to request the formation of a subcommittee on "post-Vietnam syndrome" (Scott, 1990). Spitzer's initial rejection on the grounds of nonexistent research support had a proviso attached; he would reconsider if evidence could be found that supported their claims. In response, Shatan organized the Committee on Reactive Disorders to gather and review findings. Significantly, although lacking formal training, one of the six Committee members was a Vietnam War veteran who had been active in advocacy efforts. Thus, some degree of political motivation was present within the Committee.

The initial diagnosis proposed was renamed "catastrophic stress disorder," with "post-combat stress reaction" included as a subcategory (Scott, 1990). Evidence was gathered from Veteran's Affairs (VA) hospitals, where it was found that many veterans were already being diagnosed with "traumatic war neurosis" in place of a formal *DSM-II* disorder.

PTSD Comes of Age: The *DSM-III*

It was not until 1980 that the APA formally accepted PTSD as a legitimate diagnostic category in the *DSM-III*. PTSD can be considered a "disease of time" (Young, 1995, p. 7), in that a past event is re-experienced in the present moment through memory, thought, consciousness, and physiological response. Whereas many other forms of anxiety (e.g., panic disorder, phobias) are not defined by temporal causation, PTSD must contain a specific past event that causes dysfunction in the present. PTSD became the first and only disorder that included a diagnostic criterion—a traumatic event—that is entirely external to the individual. The *DSM-III* specified that the traumatic event must be a catastrophic stressor. Examples in the *DSM-III* of these traumatic events included rape, assault, torture, military combat, natural disasters, industrial or vehicular accidents, and exposure to violence. Therefore, if the event was a "normal" one, such as a sports injury, loss of a job, or divorce, then the person's reaction may be diagnosed as an adjustment disorder.

According to the *DSM-III*, the diagnosis of PTSD included a traumatic event and three symptom clusters. Criterion A required exposure to a catastrophic stressor. Criterion B involved the re-experiencing constellation, which included intrusive thoughts, nightmares, and "flashbacks." Criterion C, the avoidance and numbing cluster, included feeling detached from others, lacking interest in activities, and having constricted affect. Criterion D, the arousal cluster, included such symptoms as exaggerated startle response, sleep disturbance, guilt, memory impairment or trouble concentrating, and heightened reactivity to traumatic stimuli. The *DSM-III* definition even made reference to initial conceptualizations of trauma from the nineteenth century. The text stipulated that trauma often results from "direct damage to the central nervous system" (p. 236), such as head injury. This is consistent with early studies into the effects of nervous system damage in survivors of railway accidents.

Perhaps most importantly, the *DSM-III* stipulated that the stressor "would evoke significant symptoms of distress in almost anyone" (APA, 1980, p. 238). This clarified that dysfunction was caused by exposure to the traumatic event itself, and further consolidated the conceptualization that distress responses were normative. This criterion has its heritage in WWII, where combat fatigue was considered to be a normative reaction to prolonged combat exposure, and in the *DSM-I*, when any "normal" person could be expected to develop distress after exposure to the stressor (APA, 1952, p. 40). The stressor was also defined as "outside the range of usual human experience" (APA, 1980, p. 236). By requiring that the stressor must be outside normal human experience, and so severe that any normal person could be affected, causation was more exclusively placed upon the stressor/trauma in the development of individual psychopathology. In short, the *DSM-III* definition of PTSD reflected the farthest reach of the pendulum's swing toward onus for dysfunction being attributed to the stressor/traumatic event, rather than the individual's own response.

The inclusion of PTSD was not without controversy. Given its emphasis on combat-related trauma, there was concern that the Vietnam War had politicized the decision with its emphasis on the hidden wounds of combat veterans. Writing during the year the *DSM-III* was published, the leader of the PTSD workgroup mentioned the timeliness of PTSD's inclusion as a valid mental disorder: "The Vietnam War…provided convincing evidence for such a need" (Andraesen, 1980, p. 1518). It was the experiences of Vietnam veterans that also fueled additional research into PTSD, which continued well into the mid-1990s when the next edition of the *DSM* was published (van der Kolk, 2007).

The addition of this diagnosis had far-reaching implications in the treatment of returning U.S. veterans. PTSD clearly identified that this dysfunction resulted directly from a "recognizable stressor," such as combat traumatization. Furthermore, exposure to this stressor "would evoke significant symptoms of distress in almost anyone" (APA, 1980, p. 238). Because their dysfunction was directly tied to military service and not to personality flaws, the VA system was required to offer services to these affected soldiers. In addition, the VA recognized PTSD as a disorder that merited disability status (Atkinson, Henderson, Sparr, & Deale, 1982). Consequently, the VA requested more government funding to meet the increased need for psychological services (Friedman & Fuller, 1985). By 1990, The National Vietnam Veterans Readjustment Study found a 15.2 % incidence of PTSD in male Vietnam veterans, with an additional 11.1 % suffering from subthreshold symptoms of PTSD (Kulka et al., 1990).

One major trend in practice was that professionals began to diagnose PTSD in populations that had not been involved in combat. These included survivors of rape, abuse, natural disasters, and torture (van der Kolk, 2007). Since the entry of PTSD into the official psychiatric literature, organizations for the prevention and treatment of PTSD have been established. In the United States, these include the National Institutes of Health's Violence and Traumatic Stress branch, the VA's National Center for PTSD, and the National Child Traumatic Stress Network created by the U.S. Department of Health and Human Services (van der Kolk, 2007).

Further progress was made toward refining the diagnostic category in the revised version of the third edition, entitled *DSM-III-R* (APA, 1987). One serious limitation of the first three editions of the *DSM* was the lack of consideration of any potential developmental differences in reactions to extreme stress. Therefore, a major contribution of the *DSM-III-R* (1987) was to identify, for the first time, age-specific features that children and adolescents exhibit. For example, the *DSM-III-R* noted that young children were more likely to relive the trauma "in action, through repetitive play" (APA, 1987, p. 249). Researchers and clinicians working with children and youth have continued to revise, expand, and challenge the relative utility of the diagnosis in subsequent editions of the *DSM*.

The other refinements in PTSD diagnostic criteria in the *DSM-III-R* were minor revisions involving operationalizing and expanding the symptom clusters. In 1980, the four PTSD criteria were (A) traumatic event, (B) re-experiencing the event, (C) numbing phenomena, and (D) miscellaneous symptoms. By 1987, the third and fourth PTSD categories were changed to (C) attempts to avoid situations that might trigger re-experiences or distress/generalized numbing, and (D) autonomic arousal.

The first two categories remained unchanged. This change unified the diagnostic category by defining (C) avoidance and numbing and (D) forms of arousal as side effects of (B) painful re-experiencing. Prior to this, Criterion A and B did not seem to dynamically interact with C and D. A few other changes were included. The text "outside the range of usual human experience" was added to Criterion A (p. 247). This had previously been included in the main body of text pertaining to PTSD in the *DSM-III*. A change also was made to the nomenclature of the event that preceded symptom development: "recognizable stressor" was replaced with "traumatic event" (Criterion A).

The Pendulum Swings Back: The *DSM-IV*

PTSD continued to evolve in the *DSM-IV* (APA, 1994) based on studies into the relevance of each diagnostic criterion (van der Kolk, Roth, Pelcovitz, Sunday, & Spinazzola, 2005). The *DSM-III* diagnosis suggested that anyone exposed to such events listed above had been traumatized, though new evidence indicated that the majority of people did not develop PTSD after exposure to traumatic events. For example, the majority of individuals experience some form of trauma in their lives (Breslau & Kessler, 2001), but only 8 % of individuals in the United States will develop PTSD during their lifetime (APA, 2000). Thus, the etiology of individual dysfunction was changed in the *DSM-IV* (APA, 1994). Previously, dysfunction resulted directly from exposure to a traumatic event. In the *DSM-IV*, dysfunction was understood to result from both exposure to an event *and* an individual's emotional response to those events; "intense fear, helplessness, or horror" (p. 428) must be present for the event to be considered traumatizing. In other words, the event itself was no longer considered to solely cause PTSD.

In the *DSM-IV*, the pendulum appeared to swing back toward the interaction between internal and external causation for traumatization. The reader may recall that the diagnosis of *hysteria* (a form of war neurosis) was stigmatizing during WWI because it was commonly associated with a "neuropathic personality." In other words, the individual was solely responsible for the manifestation of the disorder. In the *DSM-III*, the pendulum swung in the other direction, attributing causation to the external traumatic event as the main culprit for psychological dysfunction, since it could "evoke significant symptoms of distress in most people" (p. 238). In the *DSM-IV*, a more balanced approach was sought, whereby the dynamic interaction between the traumatic event and the individual's response to the event caused distress. Thus, in the *DSM-IV*, both internal and external factors were considered equally important causative agents. Nevertheless, the text revision (*DSM-IV-TR*; APA, 2000) indicated: "this disorder can develop in individuals without any predisposing conditions, particularly if the stressor is especially extreme" (p. 466).

Two significant changes in *DSM-IV* included eliminating the requirement that the precipitating stressor must be outside the range of normal human experience, and broadening the definition of a traumatic event. Criterion A1 stated that a trauma had occurred when "the person experienced, witnessed, or been confronted with an event or events that involved actual or threatened death or serious injury, or a threat to the physical integrity to oneself or others" (APA, 1994, pp. 427–428). In other words, this criterion included not only direct victims, but also those indirectly affected, such as observers and loved ones. The broadening of the definition of a traumatic event and the inclusion of language about witnessing actual harm or the threat of harm had important implications for the relevance and utility of the diagnosis for children and youth experiencing or viewing interpersonal violence, and for children and youth living with the threat of violence to themselves or others. As mentioned, Criterion A2 was added to require that the person also experienced an intense emotional reaction—fear, helplessness, or horror—to the traumatic event. *DSM-IV* also attempted to address PTSD presentation in children with a change to Criterion A2 noting disorganized or agitated behavior.

The *DSM-IV* also made one small adjustment in the organization of the symptom clusters. Criterion B now included physiological reactivity to traumatic stimuli as one of five symptoms of re-experiencing. In the *DSM-III*, this symptom was part of Criterion D, the arousal cluster. Another change involved adding Criterion E, specifying a time period of at least 1-month duration of symptoms. Finally, Criterion F required that the disturbance must cause "clinically significant distress or impairments in social, occupational, or other important areas of functioning" (APA, 1994, p. 429).

Critics had noted that the *DSM* criteria did not capture the full range of symptoms among children exposed to traumatic events, particularly for children chronically exposed to traumatic experiences. A field trial conducted for a classification, termed Disorders of Extreme Stress (DES), for the *DSM-IV* helped indicate differential impact of a traumatic event on mature adults, compared with adults who were exposed to chronic interpersonal violence as children (van der Kolk et al., 2005). The DES symptoms were included in *DSM-IV* as associated features of PTSD, but the discussion of the proposed disorder and evidence helped increase awareness of the limits of PTSD diagnosis for children and youth.

This expansion of the traumatic event definition (i.e., to include vicarious traumatization) also broadened the criteria for meeting the diagnostic threshold of PTSD, such that the total number of combinations in which an individual could meet the diagnostic threshold changed from 135 (*DSM-III*) to 10,500 (*DSM-IV*). Between 1980 and 1994, the number of qualifying events for "traumatic event" increased by 59 % (Breslau & Kessler, 2001). No other diagnosis in the *DSM*'s history has experienced such a drastic expansion (known as "conceptual bracket creep"; McNally, 2009) from one volume to another (Rosen, Lilienfeld, Frueh, McHugh, & Spitzer, 2010). Table 9.1 depicts the changes and additions made to the PTSD diagnosis in the *DSM* nosology.

Table 9.1 Major changes in the evolution of PTSD in the DSM

DSM	Term	Event	Diagnostic criteria					
			B	C	D	E	F	G
I	Gross stress reaction	Catastrophe						
II	Transient situational disturbance	Overwhelming stress						
III	Posttraumatic stress disorder	Catastrophic stressor	Re-experience	Numbing	Misc.			
III-R	Posttraumatic stress disorder	Traumatic event	Re-experience	Avoidance/ numbing	Arousal			
IV	Posttraumatic stress disorder	Extreme, life-threatening, and intense reaction	Re-experience	Avoidance/ numbing	Arousal	>I month	Distress/ impairment	
5	Posttraumatic stress disorder	Actual or threatened death, serious injury, sexual violence	Re-experience	Avoidance	Alterations in cognitions or mood	Arousal	> 1 month	Distress/ impairment

Classification of PTSD

According to the *DSM-IV-TR*, in order to meet the criteria for a PTSD diagnosis, the traumatic event must have been "extreme" and "life-threatening" (APA, 2000, p. 467). The text specified that if symptoms develop as a result of exposure to a stressor that is not considered extreme (with examples given for "spouse leaving, being fired", p. 467), then an adjustment disorder was indicated rather than PTSD. The diagnosis of PTSD involved three major symptom clusters that stemmed from an exposure to a traumatic event: re-experiencing the traumatic event, avoidance/numbing, and hyperarousal (APA, 2000). The first cluster involved re-experiencing the event through intrusive thoughts and memories of the event, flashbacks of the event, nightmares of the event, psychological distress pertaining to the event, and physiological reactions to the event (e.g., shakiness). The second cluster involved avoidance of thinking about the event, feeling numb and having a restricted affective range, avoiding activities, people, and places related to the event, having an amnestic memory of the event, and feeling detached from others. The blunting of emotional response (called *psychic numbing* or *emotional anesthesia* in the *DSM-III*; APA, 1980) affected not only reactions to the traumatic event, but was pervasive and included the reduction of emotional responsiveness to others in that individual's life, such as romantic partners and family members. The third cluster of hyperarousal included sleep disturbance and insomnia, irritability, difficulty concentrating, hypervigilance or awareness of the external environment, and an exaggerated startle response.

Diagnostic specifiers included both "Acute" (experiencing PTSD for less than 3 months) and "Chronic" (experiencing PTSD for longer than 3 months) specifications. The development of PTSD symptoms could begin immediately following the event, or in some cases, delayed onset could occur whereby the individual did not exhibit symptoms until at least 6 months after the traumatic event (APA, 2000). Delayed onset was typically triggered by another event that mimicked or resembled the original event (p. 466). When PTSD symptoms appeared, sufferers could experience the disorder episodically (i.e., periods of remission punctuated with relapses) or chronically, over the course of a lifetime. In recent years, delayed onset has been better conceptualized as delayed help-seeking, and if PTSD was indicated, symptoms rarely developed in a delayed fashion. This has led some to call for the elimination of "delayed onset" as a specifier (Spitzer, First, & Wakefield, 2007). PTSD is treatable, and in some cases, sufferers experience full remission. However, longitudinal studies with WWII veterans and survivors of the Holocaust have found that the diagnosis can persist for more than 50 years (Schnurr, 1991). Other longitudinal studies have found that the disorder is typically chronic, persisting throughout a person's lifetime (Perkonigg et al., 2005).

Acute Stress Disorder and Combat Operational Stress Reaction

In *DSM-IV*, a PTSD diagnosis required that an individual must experience symptoms related to trauma for at least a month in order to meet the diagnostic threshold. Prior to this month, individuals could develop acute stress disorder (ASD) if they experienced similar symptoms to PTSD from 2 days to 4 weeks immediately following the traumatic event. This has been known as "combat operational stress reaction" (COSR) in military circles. The ASD/COSR diagnoses consist of similar symptomatology to PTSD, with some salient differences. Whereas in PTSD, no dissociative symptoms were necessary to meet diagnostic criteria, in ASD, an individual must have displayed three dissociative symptoms (APA, 2000). Examples included a reduced awareness, such as being in a daze or daydream (Criterion B2), derealization or feeling that the external world is strange or somehow unfamiliar (Criterion B3), depersonalization or feeling detached from oneself as if in a dream or an out-of-body experience (Criterion B4), and dissociative amnesia or unable to remember important information about the traumatic event (Criterion B5). In ASD, symptoms must only be present for the first month. If these symptoms persisted for longer than 1 month, an individual qualified for a diagnosis of PTSD.

Significantly, 70–80 % of individuals with ASD/COSR eventually developed PTSD, yet 60 % of individuals with a PTSD diagnosis did not meet the diagnostic criteria for ASD (Classen, Koopman, Hales, & Spiegel, 1998). This lack of consistency between PTSD and ASD has led for calls to abandon the ASD diagnosis, and replace it instead with a V-code entitled "acute stress reaction" (Spitzer et al., 2007). This would be harmonious with empirical knowledge that fully functioning (i.e., "normal") individuals often seek professional help after exposure to a stressor/trauma, though do not exhibit psychopathology (McHugh & Treisman, 2007). Changing ASD/COSR to a V-code could be considered a step toward reducing the stigma of help-seeking behavior following exposure to a stressor or traumatic event, but the change would also have implications for reimbursement for treatment.

The *DSM-5*

Approved by the American Psychiatric Association in December 2012, the DSM-5 was released in May 2013 (American Psychiatric Association, 2013). During the revision process, numerous comments had been published on the many proposed changes to the PTSD diagnosis. Ever since PTSD entered into the official psychiatric nosology in 1980, "no other psychiatric diagnosis, with the exception of Dissociative Identity Disorder (a related disorder), has generated so much controversy in the field as to the boundaries of the disorder, diagnostic criteria, central assumptions, clinical utility, and prevalence in various populations" (Spitzer et al., 2007, p. 233). Many practitioners have been concerned that broadening PTSD diagnostic criteria has had the unintended consequence of pathologizing natural human reactions to highly disturbing incidents (McNally, 2009). In other words, there is a danger of overdiagnosis in which expressions of personal distress may be characterized as symptoms of psychiatric disorder. Underdiagnosis can also be a serious problem when financial, medical, social, and other benefits may be involved. Currently, U.S. Army psychiatrists are under investigation for reversing PTSD diagnoses of soldiers in order to reduce treatment and benefit expenses (APA, 2012).

The following section reviews changes to the *DSM-5* classification of PTSD, summarizes the new diagnostic criteria for PTSD, and highlights related discourse in the professional literature.

Classification

During the planning phase for the *DSM-5*, many argued that PTSD should be considered a part of another diagnostic category (Miller, Resick, & Keane, 2009), rather than classified as an anxiety disorder. Proponents maintained that a separate category was warranted because the dysphoric symptoms of PTSD appeared to be more consistent with non-anxiety disorders, such a major depressive disorder and dysthymia, rather than fearful anxieties, such as phobias (Resick & Miller, 2009). Furthermore, PTSD could be conceptualized as a unique diagnostic condition, due to the necessary presence of an identifiable cause (i.e., "traumatic event") in order for a diagnosis to be made. Miller et al. (2009) proposed a distinct category for these types of disorders, which included PTSD, acute stress reaction, adjustment disorder, traumatic grief, and possibly complex PTSD. Yet another proposed change was to delineate heterogeneous classifications of posttraumatic disorders, such as "posttraumatic dental care anxiety," "posttraumatic grief disorder," "posttraumatic abortion syndrome," and "posttraumatic embitterment syndrome" (Coyne & Thompson, 2007; Rosen & Taylor, 2007). Research into the relationship between mild traumatic brain injury and PTSD resulting from military combat in the recent U.S.-Iraq war led to the proposed category of "combat-related mild-traumatic brain injury" (Hoge et al., 2008). In response to these arguments, the APA decided to include PTSD in a new chapter in the *DSM-5* on Trauma- and Stressor-Related Disorders, which also includes reactive attachment disorder, disinhibited social engagement disorder, acute stress disorder, and adjustment disorders.

Revision of Diagnostic Criteria

All primary diagnostic criteria identified by the *DSM-IV* for PTSD were examined for possible revisions, and the approved DSM-5 diagnostic criteria (APA, 2012, 2013) for PTSD included a number of significant restrictions to Criterion A1 that tightened the operational definition of exposure to a traumatic stressor. First, witnessing an event no longer qualified, unless the person was physically present.

Observing an event through the media (e.g., television, radio, Internet) was excluded, unless such mediated exposure was related to work (e.g., law enforcement), and involved repeated or extreme exposure. The second restriction was that learning about a loved one's trauma only qualified as exposure if the incident had involved an actual or threatened death by violence or accident. These revisions were in response to a vigorous debate among various scholars (e.g., Brewin, Lanius, Novac, Schnyder, & Galea, 2009; Friedman, Resick, Bryant, & Brewin, 2011; Long & Elhai, 2009; Spitzer et al., 2007).

Another major change in the *DSM-5* was the elimination of Criterion A2, which required an intense emotional reaction to the event, because it had been demonstrated that it lacked predictive utility (Bovin & Marx, 2011). Moreover, as McNally (2009) argued, this elimination brought greater conceptual clarity to Criterion A by focusing only on the external stimulus, rather than including the person's internal responses, which were covered more precisely in the other symptom clusters.

Minor revisions have been made in Criterion B specifying that nightmare content must be trauma-related, and clarifying that flashback episodes were dissociative reactions. The most prominent change in the symptom clusters involved highlighting the distinctions between avoidance and emotional numbing. Since the *DSM-III*, these symptoms have been combined in Criterion C. However, the new revision divided these into two separate symptom clusters because research had demonstrated that avoidance and numbing are distinct and separate factors (Asmundson, Stapleton, & Taylor, 2004; Elhai & Palmieri, 2011). The new Criterion C included two avoidance symptoms involving internal and external reminders of the traumatic event. Research in different countries had suggested that avoidance/numbing symptoms (Criterion C) have more predictive validity for a PTSD diagnosis than persistent re-experiencing of an event (Criteria B) or hyperarousal (Criterion D; North, Suris, Davis, & Smith, 2009). In addition to including psychic numbing, Criterion D of the *DSM-5* added new depressive symptoms. These included self-blame, pervasive negative emotions, and persistent negative perceptions of oneself, others, or the world (Contractor et al., 2013). Criterion E is an elaboration of the arousal symptom cluster that appeared in previous editions of the *DSM*. In addition to sleep disturbances, hypervigilance, and exaggerated startle response, it added reckless or self-destructive behavior, irritability, and aggressive behavior. Finally, *DSM-5* enabled specification of delayed expression of PTSD, even if some of the symptoms occurred up to 6 months after the event. As noted earlier, some studies have indicated that delayed onset of PTSD occurs very rarely (Andrews, Brewin, Philpott, & Stewart, 2007; Frueh, Grubaugh, Yeager, & Magruder, 2009).

These changes in PTSD in the *DSM-5* are considered by some to be minor improvements over the *DSM-IV* criteria (Frueh, Elhai, & Acierno, 2010). Although they may contribute to conceptual clarity, the changes are not likely to affect the prevalence of PTSD diagnoses (Elhai et al., 2012). Recent studies, using these PTSD criteria, have found that 89 % of veterans meeting the *DSM-IV* diagnostic threshold for PTSD also met the new *DSM-5* diagnostic threshold for PTSD (Miller, Chard, Schumm, & O'Brien, 2011). However, given the increase in the number of diagnostic criteria for PTSD in the *DSM-5*, Galatzer-Levy and Bryant (2013) calculated that

636,120 different combinations of symptoms could fulfill the diagnosis. They argued that such heterogeneity is a consequence of the *DSM's* checklist approach and threatens to sabotage the reliability and validity of the diagnosis of PTSD.

In an attempt to be more developmentally sensitive, a separate list of diagnostic criteria for children 6 years or younger is provided in the *DSM-5*. The major difference from the criteria for those older than 6 years, other than minor changes in wording, is that negative alterations in cognitions are not separated into a new major category. A proposal to include a new diagnosis, Developmental Trauma Disorder (DTD), was forwarded for inclusion in *DSM-5* (Moran, 2007; van der Kolk & Pynoos, 2009). This diagnosis was proposed based upon findings from developmental psychopathology, clinical presentations of children and youth exposed to chronic interpersonal violence, and emerging evidence from the field of neurobiology regarding the impact of trauma on brain development. Proponents noted that the *DSM*'s PTSD criteria did not capture clinically relevant symptoms for children living in chronically unsafe conditions. The supporters of DTD acknowledged the relevance of the PTSD diagnosis for a child experiencing a single incident trauma and living in a secure caregiving relationship. However, they argued, the practical impact of the PTSD criteria for *DSM-5* is harmful for children who undergo multiple and complex traumas, especially for children exposed to harmful caregiving. The supporters contended that the criteria may result in no diagnoses, inadequate diagnoses, or inaccurate diagnoses for these children (van der Kolk & Pynoos, 2009). The proposal for DTD was not accepted for inclusion in *DSM-5*, but the discussion of the merits of an alternative classification system for children experiencing complex trauma is continuing.

Importantly, DSM-5 includes the first developmental subtype of a disorder: Posttraumatic Stress Disorder in Preschool children. Studies that compared the use of developmentally sensitive criteria resulted in approximately three to eight times more children qualifying for diagnosis compared to the use of DSM-IV (Scheeringa, Myers, Putnam, & Zeanah, 2012; Scheeringa, Zeanah, & Cohen, 2011). These findings support need for age-related criteria, given the cognitive and verbal capacities of preschool age children. Some symptoms were deleted and the wording was modified on others to be more behaviorally based, for example, "Diminished interest in significant activities may manifest as constriction of play." Preliminary evidence supports the criterion, discriminant, and predictive validities of the preschool PTSD criteria (Scheeringa et al., 2011).

Current Issues of PTSD Diagnosis in the Military

Within the past decade, the PTSD diagnosis has garnered increased attention within the U.S. military, in part because the number of veterans diagnosed with PTSD has been increasing. The incidence of PTSD in Iraq and Afghanistan War veterans is estimated at 15 % (Tanielian, Jaycox, & Rand Corporation, 2008). This is nearly twice the estimated lifetime prevalence rate for civilians (5–10 %; Wittchen &

Jacobi, 2005), and comparable with longitudinal data for the incidence of PTSD in Vietnam veterans (Kulka et al., 1990). As of 2011, the VA estimated that 177,000 returning troops from Iraq and Afghanistan have PTSD, which did not include currently serving soldiers or those served in the VA system prior to the Iraq and Afghanistan conflicts (Boone, 2011). Several reasons may be postulated for this phenomenon. First, today's military personnel are far more likely to survive when injured than in previous wars, due to improvements in medical care and war zone evacuation. In the Iraq and Afghanistan wars of the past decade, only 10 % of military personnel died as a result of their injuries, compared to 25 % in prior wars (Gawande, 2004). Other possible reasons for the increased incidence of PTSD in the U.S. military include multiple and longer deployments, the difficulties of counterterrorism, and the use of National Guard members who may not have expected to engage in overseas military combat (Andraesen, 2010).

The armed forces have also developed more comprehensive procedures for identifying PTSD (Friedman, 2005). For example, every veteran who uses VA services is asked screening questions for PTSD, at least once per year, for the initial 5 years of service, and then every 5 years following (Katz & Karlin, 2009). The screening contains the following items:

In your life, have you ever had any experience that was so frightening, horrible, or upsetting that, in the past month, you:

1. Have had nightmares about it or thought about it when you did not want to?
2. Tried hard to not think about it or went out of your way to avoid situations that reminded you of it?
3. Were constantly on guard, watchful, or easily startled?
4. Felt numb or detached from others, activities, or your surroundings? (p. 121).

A positive response to three of the four items results in referral for clinical evaluation.

In 2010, the U.S. Army diagnosed 10,756 military personnel with PTSD, more than double the number (n=4,967) diagnosed in 2005 (New York Times, 2012). Current events at the time of writing powerfully demonstrate that PTSD remains a critical issue regarding the impact of war. In March 2012, U.S. Army Staff Sgt. Robert Bales, diagnosed with a Traumatic Brain Injury in 2010, is alleged to have killed 16 Afghan civilians. According to former General Peter Chiarelli, Staff Sgt. Bales, on his fourth deployment, would likely have been screened for behavioral health issues before, during, and after every deployment. The process is flawed, and Chiarelli reported his frustration at the inability to detect problems during screening. Chiarelli advocates eliminating the term "disorder" when referring to PTSD, stating: "one of the reasons I've dropped the 'D' is no soldier likes to be told that he has a 'disorder'" (National Public Radio, 2012). The military is now initiating programs, such as Comprehensive Soldier Fitness, aiming to increase resilience and posttraumatic growth (PTG) following deployment.

The increased incidence of PTSD in the veteran population has resulted in an overburdening of the VA health system. A recent study into validity of the PTSD diagnosis among war veterans was conducted by the Institute of Medicine.

Despite fears that PTSD is being overdiagnosed, the study's findings suggest that PTSD *is* being accurately diagnosed, and therefore increased services are needed to treat U.S. war veterans (Institute of Medicine, 2006, 2007). In May 2011, the U.S. Court of Appeals for the Ninth Circuit demanded that the VA overhaul its mental health services, since delayed and inadequate services were being provided to returning U.S. veterans with PTSD (Boone, 2011).

The Future: Will the Pendulum Swing Again?

The classification of PTSD is entwined in the controversy about whether the severity of the traumatic event is diagnostically relevant. As mentioned above, other voices in the field (e.g., Rosen, Spitzer, & McHugh, 2008) have suggested that Criterion A's presence of an "extreme" and "life-threatening" traumatic event should be removed entirely, which would extricate the focus of external causation in the disorder and thus also silence proponents of a new diagnostic category. This proposal represents the pendulum once again swinging back to the days of Freud, when distress was solely attributed to the individual and not the external stressor or traumatic event (see Fig. 9.1). Despite the *DSM-IV-TR*'s specification that the traumatic event must be "of an extreme (i.e., life threatening) nature" (APA, 2000, p. 467), evidence exists that PTSD is being diagnosed in routine situations, such as the dental extraction of wisdom teeth, giving birth to a healthy baby, and being exposed to sexually offensive jokes in the workplace (McNally, 2009). The broadening of the PTSD category is controversial on these grounds; critics have balked at the "patent absurdity" of PTSD being applied to both Auschwitz survivors and recipients of sexually offensive jokes (Shephard, 2004, p. 57). As McNally (2009) presciently

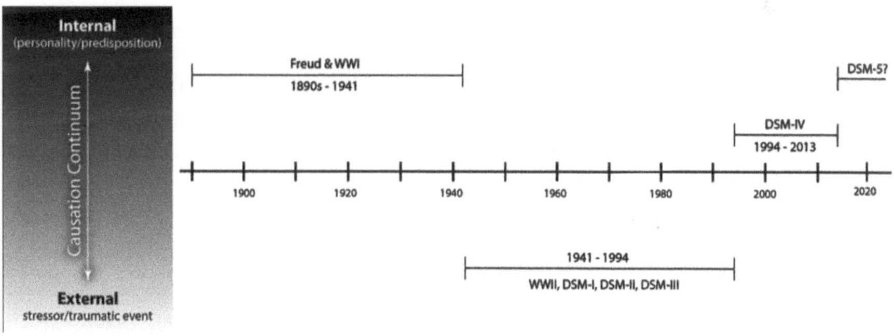

Fig. 9.1 The historical pendulum effect of causation attribution for the PTSD diagnosis. *Note.* The four pendulums on the timeline represent the four distinct changes in causation attribution regarding traumatization (what is now known as PTSD) over the course of the nineteenth, twentieth, and twenty-first centuries. The fourth pendulum represents the proposed removal of Criterion A in the *DSM-5*, which has been retained

wrote, "shifting the causal emphasis away from the stressor undermines the very rationale of having a diagnosis of PTSD in the first place" (p. 598). McNally advocated for Criterion A to be kept despite evidence that the traumatic event does not need to be "extreme" or "life-threatening" (APA, 2000, p. 467).

Evidence for the "dose–response" association between level of exposure and severity of the traumatic event suggests that the elimination of Criterion A may be hasty and reactive. In the United States, lifetime exposure to traumatic events is between 50 and 60 %, compared to 92 % in Algeria (De Jong et al., 2001; Kessler, Sonnega, Bromet, Hughes, & Nelson, 1995). As one might imagine, the prevalence of PTSD is much greater in Algeria (37.4 %) than in the United States (7.8 %). If exposure to a traumatic event were not a necessary criterion for PTSD diagnosis, then why are higher PTSD rates found in countries with higher rates of traumatic exposure? Differences in prevalence rates between nations may be derived from differences in cultural presentations and treatment availability. In addition, the incidence of PTSD is far greater among more severely traumatized populations. For example, the incidence of PTSD among female accident survivors is 8.8 %, compared to 45.6 % of female rape survivors (Kessler et al., 1995; Resnick, Kilpatrick, Dansky, Saunders, & Best, 1993). Thus, the level of exposure and severity of the traumatic event does appear to influence PTSD prevalence rates, suggesting that exposure to a traumatic event (Criterion A) is a crucial part of the current diagnostic criteria. Of course, it is important to also consider other potential mediating factors, such as culture and gender, in understanding prevalence rates.

Several leading figures in the field (e.g., McNally, 2009; Spitzer et al., 2007) have also advocated for Criterion A1 to require the *direct* presence of the individual at the trauma scene. This suggestion appears to ignore evidence that traumatization does not require physical presence. For example, 6 % of Manhattan residents without direct exposure to the World Trade Center's collapse during 9/11 reported traumatic reactions (Galea et al., 2002), and reactions were found in individuals as far away as Texas and California resulting from television viewing of the World Trade Center collapse (Schlenger et al., 2002; Silver, Holman, McIntosh, Poulin, & Gil-Rivas, 2002). These controversies have led some in the field to caution against eliminating the PTSD diagnosis, yet acknowledge that "PTSD in its current form should not be reified to the status of a distinct disorder in nature" (Rosen et al., 2010, p. 344).

It could be argued that the future of PTSD research should examine the possible predictive power of individual variables in the development of the disorder. As not all individuals who are exposed to a traumatic event develop PTSD, it would be beneficial to know why some develop the disorder and others do not. Answers to this question would enable institutions such as the military to select troops for front-line combat based on their level of resilience (or ability to withstand traumatic events and not develop PTSD), and find better-fitting duties for individuals with high predisposition for PTSD. Current risk factors include female gender, younger age, the severity of the stressor, and lack of social supports (Wittchen et al., 2009). Further research is needed into the relationship between genetic predisposition and PTSD development (Yehuda & Brier, 2009). Considering the vast cost and typical lifetime prevalence of the disorder (Perkonigg et al., 2005), a preventative approach would be more humane and cost-saving than merely attempting to remediate symptoms after they develop.

In addition to the controversies regarding the definition and criteria of PTSD and the lowering of diagnostic thresholds, it is clear that the changes have important implications for the availability and appropriateness of support services for veterans and other vulnerable populations. Discussions focusing on the weak empirical grounding for changes and the relative emphasis of sociocultural and biological influences have been prominent in the literature (American Counseling Association, 2011). Moreover, concerns have continued to emerge regarding the transparency, representation, and integrity of the process. Critics have cited the secrecy of the *DSM-5* development, and the apparent lingering presence of pharmaceutical company influence on *DSM* taskforce members, as factors affecting the process. Currently, 69 % of *DSM-5* taskforce members have ties to the pharmaceutical industry, a 21 % increase over the *DSM-IV* taskforce (Cosgrove & Krimsky, 2012). As to the taskforce responsible specifically for the PTSD diagnosis (under "anxiety, obsessive–compulsive spectrum, posttraumatic, and dissociative disorders"), 57 % have received financial support from the pharmaceutical industry, representing an ethical conflict of interest (Cosgrove & Krimsky, 2012). To its credit, the APA has instituted a mandatory disclosure policy for each workgroup and panel member regarding financial conflicts of interest (APA, 2007). However, critics have warned that this transparency cannot fully eliminate the potential for bias that may affect the integrity of the entire process.

Summary

This chapter reviewed the historical development of the PTSD diagnosis through the major U.S. conflicts of the twentieth and twenty-first centuries, leading up to current issues regarding the diagnostic criteria for *DSM-5*. Over the past few centuries, the attribution of causation for reactions resulting from exposure to a traumatic event has swung back and forth. In the time of Freud and WWI, causation was attributed largely to the individual's character deficits. During WWII, transient distress was understood to be a normal reaction to persistent conflict exposure. Thus, the pendulum began swinging back toward the stressor itself as the chief culprit of dysfunction. This was reflected in *DSM-I* (APA, 1952, p. 40), when any "normal" individual would develop symptoms after exposure to the stressor. As traumatized veterans returned from the Vietnam War, special interest groups began advocating for the inclusion of a combat-related diagnosis. Eventually, "posttraumatic stress disorder" was first introduced as a psychiatric diagnosis in the *DSM-III* (APA, 1980). Examples included war, torture, automobile accidents, and abuse/neglect. The *DSM-IV* (APA, 1994) represented the pendulum's swing back toward the middle, as the individual's emotional reaction to the traumatic event was judged to be just as crucial as the event itself in the development of psychopathology. This chapter concluded with a summary of changes to PTSD in the *DSM-5*, a review of current issues regarding the *DSM* diagnosis in military circles, and a discussion of future possibilities. Some leading figures have suggested that Criterion A should be removed entirely, a move that would resemble a return to Freud's conception of dysfunction being attributed solely to the individual and not the external event. In the current environment, PTSD remains a controversial diagnosis (Rosen et al., 2010) and in need of further conceptualization from a developmental perspective.

References

American Counseling Association. (2011). *An open letter to the American Psychiatric Association and DSM-5 Task Force*. Retrieved from http://www.counseling.org/

American Psychiatric Association. (1952). *Diagnostic and statistical manual of mental disorders*. Washington, DC: Author.

American Psychiatric Association. (1968). *Diagnostic and statistical manual of mental disorders* (2nd ed.). Washington, DC: Author.

American Psychiatric Association. (1980). *Diagnostic and statistical manual of mental disorders* (3rd ed.). Washington, DC: Author.

American Psychiatric Association. (1987). *Diagnostic and statistical manual of mental disorders* (3rd ed., rev.). Washington, DC: Author.

American Psychiatric Association. (1994). *Diagnostic and statistical manual of mental disorders* (4th ed.). Washington, DC: Author.

American Psychiatric Association. (2000). *Diagnostic and statistical manual of mental disorders* (4th ed., text rev.). Washington, DC: Author.

American Psychiatric Association. (2007). *APA names DSM-5 task force members: Leading experts to revise handbook for diagnosing mental disorders*. Retrieved from http://www.dsm5.org

American Psychiatric Association. (2012). *Army in midst of PTSD diagnosis controversy*. Retrieved from http://alert.psychiatricnews.org/2012/02/army-in-midst-of-ptsd-diagnosis.html

American Psychiatric Association. (2013). *Diagnostic and statistical manual of mental disorders* (5th ed.). Washington, DC: Author.

Andraesen, N. C. (1980). Post-traumatic stress disorder. In H. Kaplan, A. Freedman, & B. Sadock (Eds.), *Comprehensive textbook of psychiatry* (3rd ed., pp. 1517–1525). Baltimore, MD: Williams & Wilkins.

Andraesen, N. C. (2010). Posttraumatic stress disorder: A history and a critique. *Annals of the New York Academy of Sciences, 1208*, 67–71. doi:10.1111/j.1749-6632.2010.05699.x.

Andrews, B., Brewin, C. R., Philpott, R., & Stewart, L. (2007). Delayed-onset posttraumatic stress disorder: A systematic review of the evidence. *American Journal of Psychiatry, 164*, 1319–1326. doi:10.1176/appi.ajp.2007.06091491.

Appel, J. W., & Beebe, G. W. (1946). Preventive psychiatry: An epidemiological approach. *Journal of the American Medical Association, 131*, 1468–1471.

Asmundson, G. J. G., Stapleton, J. A., & Taylor, S. (2004). Are avoidance and numbing distinct PTSD symptom clusters? *Journal of Traumatic Stress, 17*, 467–475. doi:10.1007/s10960-004-5795-7.

Atkinson, R. M., Henderson, R. G., Sparr, L. F., & Deale, S. (1982). Assessment of Vietnam veterans for post-traumatic stress disorder in Veterans Administration disability claims. *American Journal of Psychiatry, 139*, 1118–1121.

Boone, K. N. (2011). The paradox of PTSD. *Wilson Quarterly, 35*(4), 18–22.

Bovin, M. J., & Marx, B. P. (2011). The importance of the peritraumatic experience in defining traumatic stress. *Psychological Bulletin, 137*, 47–67. doi:10.1037/a0021353.

Breslau, N., & Kessler, R. C. (2001). The stressor criterion in DSM-IV posttraumatic stress disorder: An empirical investigation. *Biological Psychiatry, 50*(9), 699–704.

Brewin, C. R., Lanius, R. A., Novac, A., Schnyder, U., & Galea, S. (2009). Reformulating PTSD for DSM-5: Life after Criterion A. *Journal of Traumatic Stress, 22*, 366–373. doi:10.1002/jts.20443.

Brill, N. Q., & Beeb, G. (1955). *A follow-up study of war neuroses*. Washington, DC: Government Printing Office.

Classen, C., Koopman, C., Hales, R., & Spiegel, D. (1998). Acute stress disorder as a predictor of posttraumatic stress symptoms. *American Journal of Psychiatry, 155*(5), 620–624.

Contractor, A. A., Durham, T. A., Brennan, J. A., Armour, C., Wutrick, H. R., Frueh, B. C., et al. (2013). DSM-5 PTSD's symptom dimensions and relations with major depression's symptom dimensions in a primary care sample. *Psychiatry Research, 215*(1), 146–153. Retrieved from http://dx.doi.org/10.1016/j.psychres.2013.10.015.

Cosgrove, L., & Krimsky, S. (2012). A comparison of DSM-IV and DSM-5 panel members' financial associations with industry: A pernicious problem exists. *PLoS Medicine, 9*(3), 1–4.

Coyne, J. C., & Thompson, R. (2007). Posttraumatic stress syndromes: Useful or negative heuristics? *Journal of Anxiety Disorders, 21*(2), 223–229. doi:10.1016/j.janxdis.2006.09.008.

De Jong, J. T., Komproe, I. H., Van Ommeren, M., El Masri, M., Araya, M., et al. (2001). Lifetime events and posttraumatic stress disorder in 4 postconflict settings. *Journal of the American Medical Association, 286*(5), 555–562. doi:10.1001/jama.286.5.555.

Dean, E. T. (1992). The myth of the troubled and scorned Vietnam veteran. *Journal of American Studies, 26*, 59–74.

Elhai, J. D., Miller, M. E., Ford, J. D., Biehn, T. L., Palmieri, P. A., & Frueh, B. C. (2012). Posttraumatic stress disorder in DSM-5: Estimates of prevalence and symptom structure in a nonclinical sample of college students. *Journal of Anxiety Disorders, 26*, 58–64.

Elhai, J. D., & Palmieri, P. A. (2011). The factor structure of posttraumatic stress disorder: A literature update, critique of methodology, and agenda for future research. *Journal of Anxiety Disorders, 25*, 849–854. doi:10.1016/j.janxdis.2011.04.007.

Freud, S. (1892). On the theory of hysterical attacks. In J. Strachey (Ed. & Trans.), *The standard edition of the complete psychological works of Sigmund Freud* (Vol. 1., pp. 151–154). London: Hogarth Press.

Freud, S. (1920). Beyond the pleasure principle. In J. Strachey (Ed. & Trans.), *The standard edition of the complete psychological works of Sigmund Freud* (Vol. 18, pp. 7–64). London: Hogarth Press.

Friedman, M. J. (2005). Veterans' mental health in the wake of war. *New England Journal of Medicine, 352*(13), 1287–1290. doi:10.111/j.1525-1497.2006.00367.x.

Friedman, M. J., & Fuller, R. B. (1985). War veterans' post-traumatic stress disorder and the U.S. congress. In W. Kelley (Ed.), *Post-traumatic stress disorder and the war veteran patient* (pp. 3–11). New York, NY: Brunner/Mazel.

Friedman, M. J., Resick, P. A., Bryant, R. A., & Brewin, C. R. (2011). Considering PTSD for DSM-5. *Depression and Anxiety, 28*, 750–769. doi:10.1002/da. 20767.

Frueh, B. C., Elhai, J. D., & Acierno, R. (2010). The future of posttraumatic stress disorder in the DSM. *Psychological Injury and Law, 3*, 260–270. doi:10.1007/s12207-010-9088-6.

Frueh, B. C., Grubaugh, A. L., Yeager, D. E., & Magruder, K. M. (2009). Delayed-onset posttraumatic stress disorder among war veterans in primary care clinics. *British Journal of Psychiatry, 194*, 515–520. doi:10.1192/bjp.bp.108.054700.

Galatzer-Levy, I. R., & Bryant, R. A. (2013). 636,120 ways to have posttraumatic stress disorder. *Perspectives on Psychological Science, 8*(6), 651–662. doi:10.1177/1745691613504115.

Galea, S., Ahern, J., Resnick, H., Kilpatrick, D., Bucuvalis, M., Gold, J., et al. (2002). Psychological sequelae of the Sept 11 terrorist attacks in New York City. *New England Journal of Medicine, 346*, 982–987.

Gawande, A. (2004). Casualties of war—military care for the wounded from Iraq and Afghanistan. *New England Journal of Medicine, 351*, 2471–2475.

Grinker, R. R., & Spiegel, J. P. (1945). *Men under stress*. Philadelphia, PA: Blakiston.

Hargreaves, G., Wittkower, E., & Wilson, A. T. M. (1940). Psychiatric organisation in the services. In E. Miller (Ed.), *The neurosis of war* (pp. 163–179). London: Macmillan.

Herman, J. L. (1997). *Trauma and recovery*. New York, NY: Basic.
Hoge, C. W., McGurk, D., Thomas, J. L., Cox, A. L., Engel, C. C., & Castro, C. A. (2008). Mild traumatic brain injury in U.S. soldiers returning from Iraq. *New England Journal of Medicine, 358*, 453–463.
Institute of Medicine. (2006). *Posttraumatic stress disorder: Diagnosis and assessment*. Washington, DC: Author.
Institute of Medicine. (2007). *PTSD compensation and military service*. Washington, DC: Author.
Kardiner, A. (1941). *The traumatic neuroses of war*. Washington, DC: National Research Council.
Kardiner, A. (1959). Traumatic neuroses of war. In S. Arieti (Ed.), *American handbook of psychiatry* (pp. 245–257). New York, NY: Basic.
Katz, I. R., & Karlin, B. (2009). A veteran's guide to mental health services in the VA. In P. P. Driscoll & C. Straus (Eds.), *Hidden battles on unseen fronts: Stories of American soldiers with traumatic brain injury and PTSD*. Drexel Hill, PA: CASEMATE.
Kessler, R. C., Sonnega, A., Bromet, E., Hughes, M., & Nelson, C. B. (1995). Posttraumatic stress disorder in the National Comorbidity Survey. *Archives of General Psychiatry, 52*, 1048–1060.
Kulka, R. A., Schlenger, W. E., Fairbank, J. A., Hough, R. L., Jordan, B. K., Marmar, C. R., et al. (1990). *Trauma and the Vietnam War generation: Report of findings from the National Vietnam Veterans Readjustment Study*. New York, NY: Brunner/Mazel.
Long, M. E., & Elhai, J. D. (2009). Posttraumatic stress disorder's traumatic stress or criterion: History, controversy, clinical and legal implications. *Psychological Injury and Law, 2*, 167–178. doi:10.1007/s12207-009-9043-6.
McHugh, P. R., & Treisman, G. (2007). PTSD: A problematic diagnostic category. *Journal of Anxiety Disorders, 21*, 211–222. doi:10.1016/j.janxdis.2006.09.003.
McNally, R. J. (2009). Can we fix PTSD in DSM-5? *Depression and Anxiety, 26*, 597–600. doi:10.1002/da.20586.
Miller, L. N., Chard, K. M., Schumm, J. A., & O'Brien, C. (2011). The impact of endorsing Spitzer's proposed criteria for PTSD in the forthcoming DSM-5 on male and female veterans. *Journal of Anxiety Disorders, 25*(5), 639–644. doi:10.1016/j.janxdis.2011.02.004.
Miller, M. W., Resick, P. A., & Keane, T. M. (2009). DSM-5: Should PTSD be in a class of its own? *British Journal of Psychiatry, 194*(1), 90. doi:10.1192/bjp.194.1.90.
Moran, M. (2007). Developmental trauma mertis DSM diagnosis, experts say. *Psychiatry News, 42*(3), 20.
Mott, F. W. (1917). The microscopic examination of the brains of two men dead of commotion cerebri (shell shock) without visible injury. *British Medical Journal, 2*, 612–615.
Myers, C. S. (1940). *Shellshock in France 1914-18: Based on a war diary*. Cambridge: Cambridge University Press.
National Public Radio. (2012, March 18). Troops' mental health: How much is unknown? Retrieved from http://www.npr.org
New York Times. (2012, March 22). Post-traumatic stress's surprisingly positive flip side. Retrieved from http://www.nytimes.com
North, C. S., Suris, A. M., Davis, M., & Smith, R. P. (2009). Toward validation of the diagnosis of posttraumatic stress disorder. *American Journal of Psychiatry, 166*, 34–41. doi:10.1176/appi.ajp.2008.08050644.
O'Brien, L. S. (1998). *Traumatic events and mental health*. Cambridge: Cambridge University Press.
Perkonigg, A., Pfister, H., Stein, M. B., Hofler, M., Lieb, R., et al. (2005). Longitudinal course of posttraumatic stress disorder and post-traumatic stress disorder symptoms in a community sample of adolescents and young adults. *American Journal of Psychiatry, 162*(7), 1320–1327. doi:10.11776/appi.ajp.162.7.1320.
Rado, S. (1941). Pathodynamics and treatment of traumatic war neurosis (traumatophobia). *Psychosomatic Medicine, 4*, 362–368.
Resick, P. A., & Miller, M. W. (2009). Posttraumatic stress disorder: Anxiety of traumatic stress disorder? *Journal of Traumatic Stress, 22*(5), 384–390. doi:10.1002/jts.20437.

Resnick, H. S., Kilpatrick, D. G., Dansky, B. S., Saunders, B. E., & Best, C. L. (1993). Prevalence of civilian trauma and posttraumatic stress disorder in a representative national sample of women. *Journal of Consulting and Clinical Psychology, 61*(6), 984–991.

Rosen, G. M., Lilienfeld, S. O., Frueh, B. C., McHugh, P. R., & Spitzer, R. L. (2010). Reflections on PTSD's future in DSM-5. *British Journal of Psychiatry, 197*, 343–344. doi:10.1192/bjp.bp.110.079699.

Rosen, G. M., Spitzer, R. L., & McHugh, P. R. (2008). Problems with the post-traumatic stress disorder diagnosis and its future in DSM-5. *British Journal of Psychiatry, 192*, 3–4. doi:10.1192/bjp.bp.107.043083.

Rosen, G. M., & Taylor, S. (2007). Pseudo-PTSD. *Journal of Anxiety Disorders, 21*(2), 201–210. doi:10.1016/j.anxdis.2006.09.011.

Saigh, P. A., & Bremner, D. (1999). *Posttraumatic stress disorder: A comprehensive text*. Boston, MA: Allyn & Bacon.

Scheeringa, M. S., Myers, L., Putnam, F. W., & Zeanah, C. H. (2012). Diagnosing PTSD in early childhood: an empirical assessment of four approaches. *Journal of Traumatic Stress, 25*(4), 359–367.

Scheeringa, M. S., Zeanah, C. H., & Cohen, J. A. (2011). PTSD in children and adolescents: Towards an empirically based algorithm. *Depression and Anxiety, 28*(9), 770–782. doi:10.1002/da.20736.

Schlenger, W. E., Caddell, J. M., Ebert, L., Jordan, B. K., Rourke, K. M., et al. (2002). Psychological reactions to terrorist attacks: Findings from the national study of Americans' reactions to Sept 11. *Journal of the American Medical Association, 288*(5), 581–588. doi:10.1001/jama.288.5.581.

Scott, W. (1990). PTSD in DSM-III: A case in the politics of diagnosis and disease. *Social Problems, 37*(3), 294–310.

Schnurr, P. P. (1991). PTSD and combat-related psychiatric symptoms in older veterans. *PTSD Research Quarterly, 2*, 1–6.

Shephard, B. (2004). Risk factors and PTSD. In G. M. Rosen (Ed.) *Posttraumatic Stress Disorder* (pp. 39–61). Chichester: Wiley.

Shay, J. (1991). Learning about combat stress from Homer's *Illiad. Journal of Traumatic Stress, 4*, 561–579.

Silver, R. C., Holman, E. A., McIntosh, D. N., Poulin, M., & Gil-Rivas, V. (2002). Nationwide longitudinal study of psychological responses to Sept 11. *Journal of the American Medical Association, 288*(10), 1235–1244. doi:10.1001/jama.288.10.1235.

Spitzer, R. L., First, M. B., & Wakefield, J. C. (2007). Saving PTSD from itself in DSM-5. *Journal of Anxiety Disorders, 21*, 233–241. doi:10.1016/j.janxdis.2006.09.006.

Stone, M. (1988). Shellshock and the psychologists. In W. F. Bynum, R. Porter, & M. Shepherd (Eds.), *The anatomy of madness: Essays in the history of psychiatry*. London: Tavistock.

Tanielian, T. L., Jaycox, L., & Rand Corporation (Eds.). (2008). *Invisible wounds of war: Psychological and cognitive injuries, their consequences, and services to assist recovery*. Santa Monica, CA: RAND.

Trimble, M. R. (1981). *Post-traumatic neurosis: From railway spine to the whiplash*. Chichester: Wiley.

van der Kolk, B. A. (2007). The history of trauma in psychiatry. In M. J. Friedman, T. M. Keane, & P. A. Resick (Eds.), *Handbook of PTSD: Science and practice* (pp. 19–36). New York, NY: Guilford.

van der Kolk, B. A., & Pynoos, R. (2009). Proposal to include a developmental trauma disorder diagnosis for children and adolescents in DSM-5. Retrieved from http://www.traumacenter.org/announcements/DTD_papers_Oct_09.pdf

van der Kolk, B. A., Roth, S., Pelcovitz, D., Sunday, S., & Spinazzola, J. (2005). Disorders of extreme stress: The empirical foundation of a complex adaptation to trauma. *Journal of Traumatic Stress, 18*(5), 389–399. doi:10.1002/jts.20047.

Warden, D. (2006). Military TBI during the Iraq and Afghanistan Wars. *Journal of Head Trauma Rehabilitation, 5*, 398–402.

Wittchen, H. U., & Jacobi, F. (2005). Size and burden of mental disorders in European Union. *European Neuropsychopharmacology, 15*, 357–376.

Wittchen H. U., Gloster A., Beesdo K., Schoenfeld S., & Perkonigg, A. (2009). Posttraumatic stress disorder: Diagnostic and epidemiological perspectives. *CNS Spectrums, 14*(1), 5–12.

Yehuda, R., & Bierer, L. M. (2009). The relevance of epigenetics to PTSD: Implications for the DSM-V. *Journal of Traumatic Stress, 22*(5), 427–434. doi:10.1002/jts.20448

Young, A. (1995). *The harmony of illusions: Inventing post-traumatic stress disorder*. Princeton, NJ: Princeton University Press.

Chapter 10
Functional Neuroanatomy of PTSD: Developmental Cytoarchitectonic Trends, Memory Systems, and Control Processes

Asaf Gilboa

Introduction

Posttraumatic Stress disorder's (PTSDs) three symptom clusters in the DSM IV (1994) have close correspondences with different cognitive-behavioral domains and their underlying neurocognitive substrates. The symptom clusters that may be most relevant to neurocognitive systems are re-experiencing and hyperarousal. Intrusive memories and realistic re-experiencing of the trauma (including flashbacks and nightmares) are hallmarks of PTSD and may be considered as reflecting dysfunctional memory systems. Persistent symptoms of increased physiological arousal, characterized by hypervigilance to any signs of threat in the environment, and an exaggerated startle response, may signify aberrations of fundamental attentional control systems, which in turn may lead to impairments in other cognitive domains (e.g., memory and executive functions) that depend on attention.

Within the memory domain, the primary candidate dysfunctional systems include the non-declarative fear-conditioning memory system (Kim & Jung, 2006; Maren, 2001), the declarative memory system (Squire, 1992, 1998), and the interaction between them. Fear conditioning and fear processing have been a primary focus of much of the neurocognitive research in PTSD (Grillon, Southwick, & Charney, 1996; Liberzon & Sripada, 2008; Rauch, Shin, & Phelps, 2006; Shin & Handwerger, 2009). Indeed, PTSD has been defined as a disorder characterized by pathological

A. Gilboa (✉)
The Rotman Research Institute at Baycrest, 3560 Bathurst Street, Toronto, ON, Canada M6A 2E1

Heart and Stroke Foundation Canadian Partnership for Stroke Recovery, 3560 Bathurst Street, Toronto, ON, Canada M6A 2E1

Department of Psychology, University of Toronto, 3560 Bathurst Street, Toronto, ON, Canada M6A 2E1
e-mail: agilboa@research.baycrest.org

M.P. Safir et al. (eds.), *Future Directions in Post-Traumatic Stress Disorder*,
DOI 10.1007/978-1-4899-7522-5_10

acquisition, expression, and persistence of leaned fear. This view of PTSD highlights the role of the medial prefrontal cortex, and the amygdala, in the evolution of the disorder. The amygdala mediates the assessment of threat-related stimuli and has a central role in acquisition and retention of fear conditioning (Grillon et al., 1996; Kim & Jung, 2006; Pare, 2002; Sehlmeyer et al., 2009). The medial prefrontal cortex and, in particular, the sub-callosal gyrus are involved in the process of extinction of fear conditioning, and retention of extinction learning in animals (Milad et al., 2009; Milad, Rauch, Pitman, & Quirk, 2006; Quirk & Beer, 2006; Rauch et al., 2006; Shin, Rauch, & Pitman, 2006). By focusing on these two regions, many have argued that PTSD is the result of failed medial prefrontal control over a hyperresponsive amygdala.

With regard to the declarative memory system, PTSD is associated with a somewhat confusing pattern of memory phenomena. On the one hand, patients experience highly vivid and detailed memories of aspects of the traumatic events that are reflected in flashbacks and nightmares. By contrast, when questioned or specifically probed, patients appear to have significant deficits in their recollection of the traumatic episode and the events surrounding it. They have difficulty constructing a coherent narrative that consists of both spatial and temporal continuities. They are often missing many central details in their accounts of the events surrounding their traumas. In addition to poor memory for the traumatic episode itself, patients often complain about impoverished memory in everyday situations. This suggests the possibility that PTSD involves a breakdown in the process of combining individual sensory features and placing them in the correct spatiotemporal context to form cohesive, stable memory representations (Brewin, 2007). The hippocampus is the epicenter of the neural substrate that enables such binding processes, which in humans serves the episodic memory system, as well as other reconstructive process (e.g., Hassabis & Maguire, 2007).

There is ample evidence of hippocampal deformity in PTSD. Reduced hippocampal volume has been frequently reported, likely associated with more chronic, severe forms of the disorder. There is some evidence that this may also be a risk factor in developing PTSD, rather than an acquired trait (Rauch et al., 2006; Shin et al., 2006). The functional consequence of the anomaly has been more elusive. It is often assumed that these hippocampal abnormalities lead to memory deficits in PTSD. However, hippocampal abnormalities are only rarely reported in functional neuroimaging studies. Instead, most functional neuroimaging reports have tended to emphasize the findings of hyperactive amygdala and a hypoactive medial prefrontal cortex, in line with the fear-conditioning and extinction hypothesis mentioned above (Charney, 2003; Gilboa et al., 2004; Rauch et al., 2006). For example, in a functional connectivity neuroimaging study, we provided partial support of this model, demonstrating abnormally increased direct influences of the amygdala on both medial prefrontal and posterior imagery-related regions. Others have provided support for the failed inhibition hypothesis. By contrast memory-related networks, including the hippocampus, appear to be co-activated equally in PTSD and non-PTSD trauma-exposed controls (Gilboa et al., 2004). Some neuroimaging studies have reported abnormal activations in the hippocampus. However there are mixed reports of increases, decreases, or no abnormal hippocampal activation (Shin et al., 2006). Irrespective of the indeterminate evidence, prevailing models of PTSD suggest important features of the disorder involve deficits in episodic memory and abnormal (hippocampal) contextual fear-conditioning acquisition (Rauch et al., 2006; Shin et al., 2006).

Current models of PTSD almost invariably feature both deficits in fear conditioning and extinction (mediated by abnormal vmPFC–amygdala interactions) and deficits in contextual fear and declarative memory (mediated by hippocampal dysfunction). Despite its appeal, empirical support for this canonical model of PTSD is equivocal. Although the fear-conditioning and extinction model of PTSD has been supported by a wealth of research, PTSD is characterized by emotion dysregulation that goes well beyond fear. In addition to fear recent models of the disorder have emphasized dysregulation of other affective states such as anger, guilt, and shame as well as the centrality of dissociation and numbing (Lanius et al., 2010; Resick & Miller, 2009). Moreover, the interchangeable use of the terms "fear memory" and "fear conditioning" in the literature reflects a reductionist, if not a misleading, view of the variety of mnemonic phenomena associated with the disorder. Although the fear-conditioning model is useful for cross-species investigations, it only captures one memory system that is dysfunctional in PTSD. Finally, the memory complaints and deficits, which are reported in many studies, often reflect actual attentional and working memory deficits and consequent poor encoding, rather than memory impairment per se (Brandes et al., 2002; Isaac, Cushway, & Jones, 2006; Vasterling, Brailey, Constans, & Sutker, 1998). In light of these complexities, neurofunctional models that focus on specific regions are likely to have limited success in explaining the full range of neurocognitive phenomena and underlying mechanisms of PTSD. In the present chapter I have attempted to examine the evidence for the neurobiological basis of PTSD from a developmental systems point of view. In what follows, I briefly present a framework, which I believe may be instructive in providing a broader perspective of this psychiatric disorder, and provide a brief review of the evidence within this framework.

Cytoarchitectonic Trends: A Framework for Understanding PTSD as a Neuropsychiatric Disorder

In the early twentieth century, Dart [1934; as cited by Sanides (1970)] observed a duality in the architecture and function of cortical structures in the reptilian brain and was the first to describe parapiriform and parahippocampal subdivisions. Abbie, in 1940 and 1942 [cited by Sanides (1970)], confirmed the dual origin of neocortical structures in Echidna and Platypus and later in the marsupial brain. His findings were the first to suggest that the same principle of duality also exists in the mammalian neocortex. These studies indicated that different cytoarchitectonic fields represent successive evolutionary waves of circumferential differentiation, commencing either from the hippocampus or from the piriform cortex and amygdala, respectively.

Sanides (1962) proposed a similar dual origin of the human neocortex based on cytoarchitectonic and myeloarchitectonic data of the human frontal lobe, and later confirmed the same principles in primates, carnivores, rodents, and other species (Sanides, 1970).

Increasing successions of cytoarchitectonic complexity and lamination are characteristic of both developmental trends. These begin with 3-layered allocortex in the limbic core through paralimbic periallocortical and proisocortical structures, culminating in six-layered isocortical regions (Mega, Cummings, Salloway, & Malloy, 1997; Pandya, Seltzer, & Barbas, 1988; Sanides, 1970). Based on an illustration by Giaccio (2006), we used Pandya and Petrides's cytoarchitectonic division (Petrides & Pandya, 1994) to denote the two developmental streams and the different cortical types of which they are comprised, and as depicted in Figs. 10.1 and 10.2 (Shalev, Gilboa, & Rasmusson, 2011).

The *archicortical trend* originates from the hippocampus. It then passes along the medial aspect of the temporal lobes with periallocortical, and proisocortical, parahippocampal cortices. This then gives rise to structures in the mediodorsal aspects of the parietal and frontal cortex, including proisocortical posterior cingulate cortex (Brodmann areas 31 and 23 posteriorly and 24, 25, and 32 anteriorly). Finally, this trend forms isocortical areas in the dorsomedial and dorsolateral prefrontal cortex (BA 9, 10, 46, and 8) (Pandya et al., 1988).

The *paleocortical trend* is differentiated from its limbic piriform/amygdala core, and journeys posteriorly along the entire temporal cortex from the proisocortical temporal pole, and progressively differentiates, as it extends caudally all the way to the caudalmost section of the temporal gyri. Anteriorly, the paleocortical trend differentiates into the proisocortical regions of the orbital and insular cortices, and the isocortical regions of the ventrolateral and lateral orbitofrontal cortex including Brodmann areas 10, 12, 46, 14, 8, and 11 (Pandya et al., 1988).

The functional significance of these two developmental trends for PTSD is discussed extensively below. Broadly, the two systems may be considered as serving distinctive roles in shaping and controlling behavior. The dorsal archicortical system, arising from the hippocampal area, is particularly suited for processing of spatial–temporal and contextual elements in the environment. The hippocampus best epitomizes this role as it specializes in binding items together to create novel arbitrary associations, and in spatial navigation. The ventral paleocortical system, arising from the olfactory cortex and amygdala, mediates the processing of object identity and the allocation of incentive significance to stimuli and supports motivational components of behavior. The centrality of neural systems that mediate motivational and reinforcement aspects of behavior, such as the amygdala and orbitofrontal cortex, exemplifies this role. Thus, evolutionary brain organization provides the basic architecture that supports independent processing of objects, and of contextual and spatial information, while maintaining synchronous representations of these processes. This structural design is reflected in two separate cortical systems that are also highly interconnected, allowing for efficient coordination. Both archicortical and paleocortical evolutionary trends have access to perimotor cortical structures at multiple levels, allowing them to control behavior through frontal

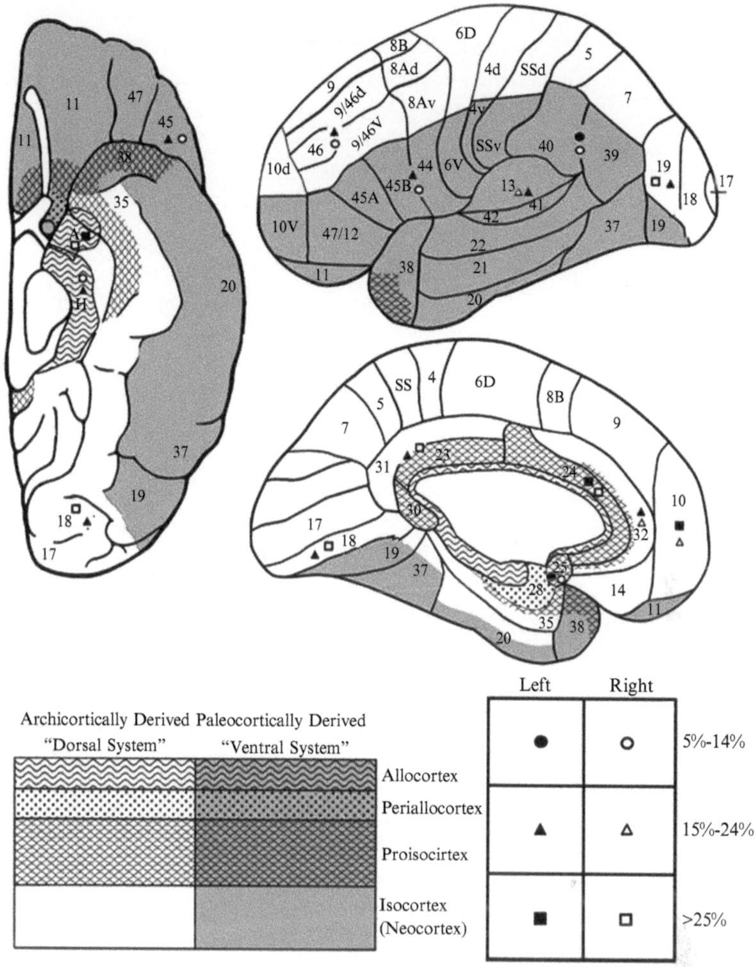

Fig. 10.1 Cartoon representation of ventral (*left*), lateral (*top right*), and medial (*bottom right*) of the human brain with Petrides and Pandya (1994) cytoarchitectonic delineation [adapted from Stuss et al. (2002)] and the evolutionary developmental trends with coding for the archicortical (*white*) and paleocortical (*gray*) cortical moieties and the cortical types within each trend [adapted after Giaccio (2006)]. Geometrical designs represent the percent of neuroimaging studies reporting activation differences between PTSD and controls on emotional/traumatic tasks and stimuli. *Black geometric designs* represent *left-sided* differences and *white designs* represent *right-sided* differences. The inferior parietal lobule is marked with an * because it is considered a transitional cortex belonging to both developmental trends (Pandya et al., 1988)

executive neural networks. For example, the dorsal prefrontal cortex, which is part of the archicortical dorsal route, has extensive connections with supplementary motor/premotor areas and may guide complex behaviors that require temporal structuring and cognitive planning. The ventrolateral motor system, with its paleocortical limbic base, may mediate an affective influence over behavior through

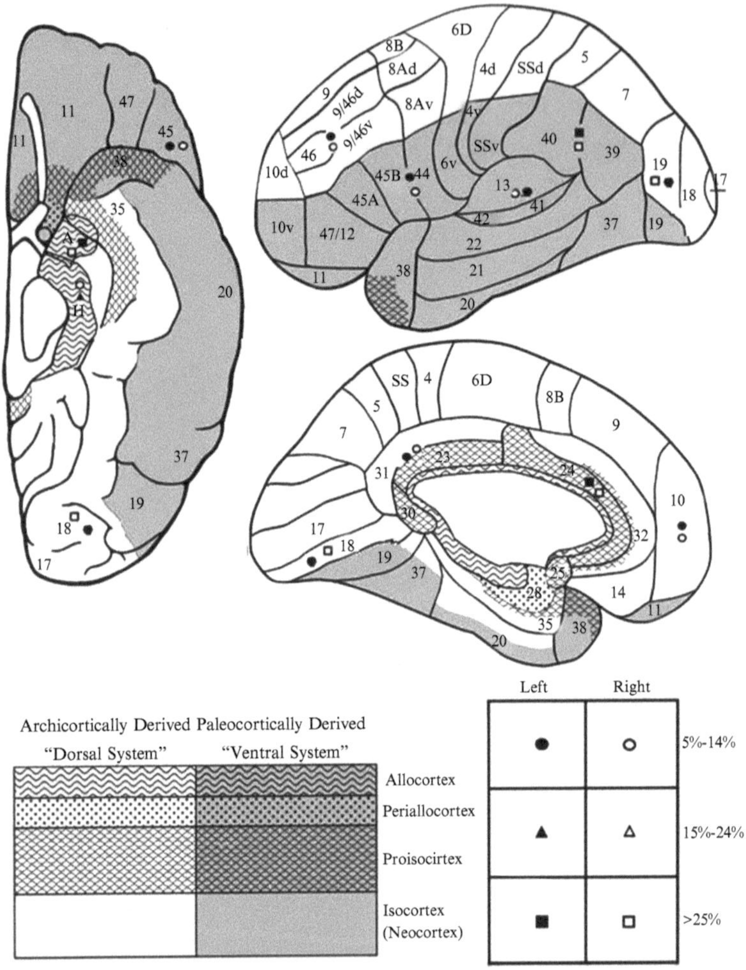

Fig. 10.2 Cartoon representation of ventral (*left*), lateral (*top right*), and medial (*bottom right*). Color and geometrical coding are identical to Fig. 10.1 except that *geometrical designs* represent the percent of neuroimaging studies reporting activation differences between PTSD and controls on neutral tasks and stimuli. *Black geometric designs* represent *left-sided* differences and *white designs* represent *right-sided* differences. The inferior parietal lobule is marked with * because it is considered a transitional cortex belonging to both developmental trends (Pandya et al., 1988)

extensive connections with the amygdala and insular and temporal pole cortices. Moreover, the intensive connectivity of this ventral system with the insula may be important for linking visceroautonomic associations to perceptual events and to the organization of action plans.

The dual cytoarchitectonic trends framework can be instructive for understanding the functional neuroanatomy of psychiatric disorders. Most advanced neuropsychiatric models emphasize aberrations at the level of large network interactions, and imbalances among remote brain regions, rather than deficits associated with particular brain regions. The phylogenetic and ontogenetic neurodevelopmental model presented here has recently begun to filter into the psychiatric literature, primarily as a model for understanding Schizophrenia, but also as a more general model of understanding psychiatric disorders (Antonova, Sharma, Morris, & Kumari, 2004; Christensen & Bilder, 2000; Giaccio, 2006).

Next, I briefly review current findings from structural and functional neuroimaging involving patients suffering from PTSD. I will then present these findings within the conceptual framework of the dual developmental trends. It is important to note that despite theoretical advancement, many functional and structural neuroimaging studies do not possess the methodological complexity that could directly support system-level theories. Therefore, analyses are still conducted in a voxel-wise manner, or focusing on regions of interest. Thus I will separately discuss findings from functional and effective connectivity, studies that may hold particular promise for our understanding of the neural basis of PTSD.

Structural Findings in PTSD

The first report of PTSD-related neural structural abnormalities revealed reduced MRI-derived left hippocampal volume in Vietnam veterans with PTSD, compared with non-PTSD controls (Bremner et al., 1995). These findings had been interpreted as reflecting the vulnerability of this structure to the effects of stress hormones, within the framework of Gluccocorticoid Cascade Hypothesis (Sapolsky, Krey, & McEwen, 1986). Thus, it has been suggested that smaller hippocampal volumes reflect an acquired trait. The rationale behind this claim is that PTSD involves a prolonged state of stress, which leads to loss of hippocampal neurons. As described above, the hippocampus is the core of the archicortical (dorsomedial) developmental trend that mediates the processing of spatiotemporal aspects of behavior. It has been described as "projectional," in that it mediates action derived from internal probabilistic models of the future, based on previous experiences.

The pioneering report by Bremner et al. (1995) has prompted a surge of studies investigating structural abnormalities in PTSD, with particular focus on the hippocampus. Many of these studies have reported either left, right, or bilateral hippocampal volume reduction ranging from approximately 5 % to an incredible 26 % (Bonne et al., 2008; Bossini et al., 2008; Bremner et al., 1997, 2003; Emdad et al., 2006; Felmingham et al., 2009; Gurvits et al., 1996; Hedges et al., 2003; Lindauer et al., 2004; Shin et al., 2004; Stein, Koverola, Hanna, Torchia, & McClarty, 1997; Vermetten, Vythilingam, Southwick, Charney, & Bremner, 2003; Villarreal et al., 2002; Vythilingam et al., 2005; Wang et al., 2010; Woon & Hedges, 2008). For comparison, a volume reduction of 40 % is thought to reflect a nearly complete loss of hippocampal neurons in acquired amnesia in adults (Gold & Squire, 2005). Or, if we consider hippocampal volume reduction to be a vulnerability factor (see below) developmental amnesia resulting from anoxia-induced hippocampal atrophy involves volume loss of 20–30 % (Isaacs et al., 2003). Given that amnesia (acquired or developmental) involves a severe inability to acquire new declarative memories, one might wonder why in PTSD neuropsychological deficits in the realm of memory are only found in some studies, and why even these effects are rather modest.

Volumetric studies of hippocampal structural changes in PTSD have often reported significantly reduced volumes. However, this is by no means a universal finding. There are several reports that found no hippocampal volume difference (Bonne et al., 2001; Carrion et al., 2001; De Bellis, Hall, Boring, Frustaci, & Moritz, 2001; De Bellis et al., 2002; Golier et al., 2005; Jatzko et al., 2006). In addition, we consider the possibility that additional unpublished null result studies also exist. That said, recent meta-analyses further support the verity of reduced hippocampal volume in PTSD (Karl et al., 2006; Woon & Hedges, 2008). The inconsistencies across studies with regard to the existence, laterality, and the extent of hippocampal structural abnormalities, suggest that mediating or moderating factors must be taken into account. For example, smaller hippocampal volumes may be related to comorbid conditions such as depression or alcohol abuse, which are known to independently affect hippocampal integrity (Hedges & Woon, 2010; Videbech & Ravnkilde, 2004). In addition, hippocampal atrophy may be characteristic of only a subgroup of PTSD patients with particularly chronic and severe conditions. This latter possibility receives some support from a study of hippocampal volume in monozygotic twins discordant for PTSD diagnosis (Gilbertson et al., 2002). In that study, twins who had been to Vietnam and developed PTSD were found to have significantly smaller hippocampal volumes, but only when 5 of the 17 PTSD patients with the lowest CAPS score were removed from the analysis. Thus, even in this very chronic sample, significant hippocampal atrophy as measured by MRI could only be verified in the most affected individuals.

Gilbertson et al. landmark study was designed to address the etiology of reduced hippocampal volumes in PTSD. One possibility mentioned above is that smaller hippocampal volumes are an acquired trait mediated by elevated levels of glucocorticoids, either during trauma or later during the posttraumatic response. Another possibility is that smaller hippocampus is a vulnerability factor, and may be part of what determines the development of the disorder. Indeed why some individuals develop PTSD following traumatic experiences while others do not remains unresolved. Gilbertson and colleagues' findings strongly support the latter possibility in that there were no differences between hippocampal volumes of PTSD patients and their non-traumatized twins, suggesting no disease-related atrophic processes. Moreover, there was a significant correlation between the hippocampal volumes of the unaffected siblings and the PTSD symptom severity of the affected twins. These findings strongly suggest smaller hippocampal volumes constitute a vulnerability factor, and point to the possibility that premorbid archicortical abnormalities lead to susceptibility to develop PTSD as a result of exposure to traumatic stress.

Structural abnormalities of the hippocampus in PTSD were the first to be reported and have received the most attention by far. However, more recent volumetric studies have also reported other morphometric differences associated with PTSD. These reports became more abundant with the advent of automatic methods for measuring brain volumes and atrophy. The primary gray matter regions reported in these studies as having reduced volumes in PTSD are the amygdala and regions within the anterior cingulate and the insula. There are also reports originating from pediatric PTSD investigations of white matter volume reductions primarily in the corpus callosum (De Bellis & Keshavan, 2003; De Bellis et al., 2002; Jackowski et al., 2008; Kitayama et al., 2007; Villarreal et al., 2004).

The amygdalae have been a target for structural investigations of PTSD from the outset, because of its role in emotional dysregulation in general, and particularly in fear conditioning. Most neurobiological models of PTSD have emphasized the role of the amygdala in the disorder's pathophysiology and both functional and structural studies have attempted to uncover PTSD-related abnormalities in this structure. The evidence for amygdalar structural alterations associated with PTSD are quite weak (Bonne et al., 2001; Bremner et al., 1997; Carrion et al., 2001; Cohen et al., 2006; De Bellis et al., 2001; Fennema-Notestine, Stein, Kennedy, Archibald, & Jernigan, 2002; Gurvits et al., 1996; Hara et al., 2008; Karl et al., 2006; Lindauer et al., 2004; Matsuoka, Yamawaki, Inagaki, Akechi, & Uchitomi, 2003; Rauch et al., 2003; Rogers et al., 2009; Wignall et al., 2004; Woodward et al., 2006; Woon & Hedges, 2008, 2009) possibly because this structure is more difficult to reliably measure than the hippocampus. Accordingly, two recent meta-analyses reached somewhat different conclusions. One found that there is overall evidence for smaller left amygdala volumes in adults with PTSD compared with controls, but not in pediatric PTSD (Karl et al., 2006). The other study, on the other hand, found no significant volumetric differences in either population (Woon & Hedges, 2008), emphasizing the great inconsistencies and variability across studies.

The anterior cingulate cortex (ACC) has also been a target of structural investigation in PTSD. Its established role in extinction learning (Milad et al., 2006; Quirk & Beer, 2006) has led to several theories suggesting failed inhibition of amygdala activity is a central contributor to the pathophysiology of the disorder (Bremner, 2006b; Liberzon & Sripada, 2008; Rauch et al., 2006; Shin & Handwerger, 2009). Several studies have pointed to abnormal structural characteristics associated with PTSD in the anterior cingulate cortex (ACC). Patients with PTSD have been shown to have reduced ACC gray matter volumes compared with controls (Abe et al., 2006; Corbo, Clement, Armony, Pruessner, & Brunet, 2005; Kitayama, Quinn, & Bremner, 2006; Woodward et al., 2006; Yamasue et al., 2003) as well as white matter abnormalities of the cingulum bundle (Abe et al., 2006). These reduced volumes may be particularly characteristic of the rostral (~Brodmann area 32) and subcallosal (~Brodmann area 25) portions of the ACC, rather than the dorsal ACC (Rauch et al., 2003). Rostral ACC volumes derived using VBM have also been found to predict response to cognitive-behavioral interventions such that larger volumes were associated with greater symptom reduction (Bryant et al., 2008). Finally a study of pregenual ACC volumes in monozygotic twins discordant for PTSD suggested reduced volumes may reflect an acquired trait of PTSD rather than a vulnerability factor (Kasai et al., 2008), in contrast with the findings of hippocampal volumes cited above.

One last cortical region that has been implicated in structural studies of PTSD is the insula. Reduced insular gray matter has been reported by several studies (Chen, Li, Xu, & Liu, 2009; Chen et al., 2006; Corbo et al., 2005; Kasai et al., 2008). However despite the proliferation of the use of whole-brain voxel-based morphometry in anatomical studies of PTSD, the evidence for insular structural deformities in PTSD appears to be very limited and awaits further research.

To conclude, more than 15 years of structural imaging in PTSD appear to indicate that the hippocampi, and less consistently the ACC, show abnormal morphology in the disorder. By contrast, abnormal structural findings in the amygdala and insular cortex have been inconsistently reported. Thus, of the two primordial core structures within the limbic ring, there seems to be better evidence for a structural abnormality associated with the dorsal-archicortical (hippocampus) than the ventral-paleocortical (amygdala) stream. Further down the archicortical stream, isocortical regions that belong to that system (i.e., the anterior ACC) also seem to be affected. Moreover, the structural deficit affecting the limbic core of the archicortical system appears to constitute a risk factor for developing the disorder, whereas further downstream, gray matter reduction in the ACC may represent an acquired sign of PTSD consistent with stress-induced loss.

Functional Imaging Findings

Current models of the neural basis of PTSD have greatly relied on evidence from human functional neuroimaging explorations of possible PTSD-related alterations in brain function. Functional neuroimaging studies include either studies of brain function at rest or studies of brain function during performance of tasks. The most prevalent task used in PTSD research is symptom provocation in response to processing of either individualized or generic trauma-related stimuli. However, many studies have also investigated possible neural alterations in processing and memory of generic emotional stimuli, as well as processing and memory of neutral stimuli. Several detailed reviews of these neuroimaging studies have been published in recent years (Bremner, 2006a, 2007; Cannistraro & Rauch, 2003; Deckersbach, Dougherty, & Rauch, 2006; Francati, Vermetten, & Bremner, 2007; Lanius, Bluhm, Lanius, & Pain, 2006; Liberzon & Sripada, 2008; Shin et al., 2006). Among others, these reviews have pointed to important heterogeneities in findings associated with factors such as subject characteristics, type of stimulus, type of imaging modality, and so forth. An extensive review is beyond the scope of the present chapter, but I attempt to sketch a fundamental picture of the functional neural systems that appear to be abnormally involved in the disorder. We (Shalev et al., 2011) have recently reviewed over 30 neuroimaging studies that have used emotional stimuli (Table 10.1; Fig. 10.1), and 15 studies that have used neutral stimuli and tasks (Table 10.2, Fig. 10.2).

Table 10.1 Emotion-related contrasts within studies used for Fig. 10.1

Contrasts	Imaging modality	Study
Combat-related slides and sounds vs. neutral slides and sounds.	PET	Bremner et al. (1999)
Script-driven imagery of autobiographical events: traumatic vs. neutral	PET	Bremner et al. (1999b)
Retrieval of deeply encoded emotional words vs. neutral deeply encoded words	PET	Bremner et al. (2003b)
Emotional stroop vs. neutral stroop	PET	Bremner et al. (2004)
Script-driven imagery of autobiographical events: traumatic vs. neutral	PET	Britton et al. (2005)
Visuo-verbal target detection: varying vs. fixed target conditions	PET	Clarck et al. (2003)
Cued recollection of autobiographical events: traumatic vs. negative (nontraumatic)	fMRI	Driessen et al. (2004)
Benign temperature vs. painful temperatures	fMRI	Geuze et al. (2007)
Audiotaped script-driven autobiographical imagery: traumatic vs. Neutral	PET	Gilboa et al. (2004)
Backward-masked images of combat vs. noncombat content	fMRI	Hendler et al. (2003)
Traumatic vs. neutral pictures	fMRI	Hou et al. (2007)
Fearful vs. neutral faces	fMRI	Kemp et al. (2009)
Script-driven imagery of autobiographical traumatic event vs. rest	fMRI	Lanius et al. (2001)
Script-driven imagery of autobiographical traumatic event vs. rest	fMRI	Lanius et al. (2002)
1. Script-driven imagery of autobiographical traumatic event vs. rest 2. Script-driven imagery of autobiographical sad event vs. rest 3. Script-driven imagery of autobiographical anxious event vs. rest	fMRI	Lanius et al. (2003)
Script-driven imagery of autobiographical traumatic event vs. rest	fMRI	Lanius et al. (2004)
Connectivity: script-driven imagery of autobiographical traumatic event vs. rest	fMRI	Lanius et al. (2005)
Trauma-related stimuli (combat sounds) vs. nonspecific arousing stimuli (white noise)	SPECT	Liberzon et al. (1999)
Script-driven imagery of autobiographical events: traumatic vs. neutral	PET	Liberzon et al. (2003)
Audiotaped script-driven imagery of autobiographical events: traumatic vs. neutral	SPECT	Lindauer et al. (2004)
Script-driven imagery of autobiographical events: fearful vs. neutral	PET	Pardo et al. (2009)
Trauma-related negative words vs. neutral words	fMRI	Protopopescu et al. (2005)
Masked fearful faces vs. masked happy faces	fMRI	Rauch et al. (2000)

(continued)

Table 10.1 (continued)

Contrasts	Imaging modality	Study
Visual mental images of pictures: combat vs. neutral	PET	Shin et al. (1997)
Audiotaped script-driven autobiographical imagery: traumatic vs. neutral	PET	Shin et al. (1999)
Counting stroop: combat-related vs. neutral	fMRI	Shin et al. (2001)
Audiotaped script-driven imagery of autobiographical events: traumatic vs. neutral	PET	Shin et al. (2004)
Fearful vs. happy facial expressions	fMRI	Shin et al. (2005)
Recognition: false alarms negative vs. baseline	fMRI	Thomaes et al. (2009)
	PET	Vermetten et al. (2007)
Emotional vs. neutral hits	fMRI	Whalley et al. (2009)
Combat sounds vs. white noise	SPECT	Zubieta et al. (1999)

Table 10.2 Neutral contrasts within studies used for Fig. 10.2

Contrasts	Imaging modality	Study
Virtual Morris Water Task: cued navigation to a hidden ball vs. navigation to a visible ball	fMRI	Astur et al. (2006)
Encoding of auditory paragraph vs. control condition (counting 'd's in the paragraph)	PET	Bremner et al. (2003)
Neutral stroop vs. control stimulus	PET	Bremner et al. (2004)
Target tones vs. standard tones	fMRI	Bryant et al. (2005)
Rest	SPECT	Chung et al. (2006)
Script-driven imagery of autobiographical neutral event vs. rest	fMRI	Lanius et al. (2004)
Script-driven imagery of autobiographical neutral event vs. rest.	fMRI	Lanius et al. (2005)
Rest	fMRI	Qingling et al. (2009)
Rest	SPECT	Sachinvala et al. (2000)
Auditory continuous performance task (tone volume discrimination) vs. rest	PET	Semple et al. (1996)
Rest vs. auditory continuous performance task	PET	Semple et al. (2000)
Neutral target words detection: varying vs. fixed target conditions	PET	Shaw et al. (2002)
Recollection of neutral deeply vs. neutral shallowly encoded words	PET	Shin et al. (2004b)
1. Encoding face-profession pairs (target stimuli) vs. watching face stimuli (control stimuli) 2. Retrieval of the matching-face profession vs. control task	fMRI	Werner et al. (2009)
Old vs. new items recognition	fMRI	Whalley et al. (2009)

Frequencies of regions that are consistently reported as abnormally activated in PTSD compared with controls (regardless of whether this involves hypo- or hyperactivation) were plotted on brain cartoons that depict the two developmental trends. Although very general, this representation allows an overall appreciation of the relationship between functional disorders and cytoarchitectonic principles of brain structure.

Functional differences between PTSD and controls are often reported for the amygdala, but less so for the hippocampus. Thus, in structures that constitute the limbic core of the developmental trends, it appears that the functional aberrations in the paleocortical stream are more characteristic of PTSD pathology. Interestingly this pattern is similar for both emotional tasks where one might expect greater differences in amygdala activation, but also for the neutral contrasts (Fig. 10.2). Interestingly this pattern is the reverse of what was described for structural abnormalities. Importantly, however, outside the limbic core the picture is more consistent with the anatomical reports. The vast majority of reported differences in activation between PTSD and controls do not occur in the paleocortical stream, but rather in proisocortical and isocortical territories of the dorsal, archicortical, stream. These include regions in the posterior, dorsal and anterior cingulate, occipital and medial prefrontal cortices, as well as dorsolateral prefrontal cortex. By contrast, relatively few reports exist of differences in activation in ventral paleocortical regions outside the amygdala itself. The only other regions that seem to be relatively consistently implicated are the bilateral insula and left ventrolateral prefrontal cortex.

When stimuli and tasks are neutral (Table 10.2, Fig. 10.2) it is possible to observe several differences in the patterns of abnormal activations associated with a diagnosis of PTSD. First, there is even less overall consistency across studies than there is for emotional studies. This, however, is likely a function of the more varied tasks and conditions. It should be noted that there are many fewer studies that have used neutral stimuli than those that use emotional ones. With respect to patterns of abnormal activations, the rostral ACC and sub-callosal ACC do not show unique patterns of activity in response to neutral conditions. Only the dorsal ACC still appears to be recruited differently in PTSD when compared with controls. However, despite these specific differences between neutral and emotional stimuli, the same overall pattern can be detected, in that the majority of abnormal activations in PTSD appear to occur in the dorsal protogradation, and primarily in proisocortical and isocortical territories.

The overall pattern that arises from both types of functional neuroimaging studies nicely converges with the reports of structural abnormalities discussed above. Neuroimaging investigations appear to point to a primary abnormality of the dorsal archicortical stream, both structurally and functionally. The neurobiological basis of PTSD involves both core and later developed cortical territories of the archicortical protogradation. By contrast, the ventral paleocortical protogradation appears to display aberrant functional activity (but less structural alterations) of only the core structures (amygdala and to an extent insula).

Hypothetical Functional Significance

The observed patterns of functional irregularity may illuminate and help clarify the unique configurations of pathology and cognitive disruption associated with PTSD. Archicortical neocortical structures are broadly associated with the critical and complex task of multimodal integration of information. As such these structures support the representation and maintenance over time of the spatiotemporal context, in which events occur and behavior is executed. To facilitate such complex representations, dorsal systems perform functions such as (1) online processing of spatial cues and the location of objects in space; (2) allocation of spatial attention; (3) mnemonic functions that allow the flexible coding and retrieval of all forms of relationships among objects and events in both working memory and long-term memory. Accordingly, behavior mediated by the archicortical system can be characterized as "projectional"; that is, actions are derived from probabilistic models of the future based on previous experiences (Goldberg, 1985). These behaviors are controlled through the dorsal systems' connection with dorsal sectors of the premotor cortex (see Figs. 10.1 and 10.2). Thus, the archicortical trend is responsible for coherence of both internal representations and motor behaviors, allowing for the creation and control of temporally and contextually bound and internally driven patterns of behavior and thought. They allow directed behavior to be organized over time, through support of working memory and extended planning processes. It is relatively straightforward to understand the characteristics of the re-experiencing and hyperarousal symptom clusters of PTSD in terms of dysfunction of archicortical neural structures. Contextually nonspecific "fight or flight" reactions, as well as difficulty maintaining attention, which are characteristic of hyperarousal, can result from aberrations from functional networks involving archicortical stream structures. Similarly, deficits in contextual fear conditioning leading to generalized nonspecific fear responses are known to result from damage to the hippocampus, the core structure of the archicortical stream. Finally, the fragmented, insulated nature of memory representations of traumatic memory can be a result of a dysfunction in systems whose role is to allow for coherent representations of time and space either at encoding or during retrieval and re-encoding.

On the other hand, paleocortical structures in the ventral stream code and respond to the motivational significance and the identity of external objects and stimuli. One of their most important functions is to support the integration of internally generated appetitive drives, with aversion, or attraction to external stimuli. The ventral system, through its extensive connections with and reliance on the amygdala and insular and temporal pole cortices, is well suited for integrating sensory information with viscera-autonomic responses. Thus it may serve an evaluative role in the processing of stimuli vis-à-vis their motivational significance in relation to internal states. One function the amygdala might carry out is parsing events or episodes out of the ongoing flow of ongoing experience. In doing so it instills visceroautonomic information into specific events, imbuing them with motivational significance, as part of the amygdala's role in mediation of the fear response (Pribram, 1991). As such it may link motor sequences to stimuli in the environment in a responsive, segmented way (Goldberg, 1985), irrespective of the larger spatiotemporal context in which these events or stimuli occur. It is tempting to speculate that disruptions to these processes are at the heart of PTSD, because such characteristics appear to dominate the behavior of patients with PTSD. However, as noted above, aberrations of the ventral system both functionally and structurally are less consistently reported than those associated with the dorsal system. Moreover, there are indications that dorsal system abnormalities may constitute a risk factor for developing the disorder both structurally, as reflected by hippocampal volume (Gilbertson et al., 2002), and functionally as reflected by processing of spatial information (Gilbertson et al., 2007). Neurocognitive risk factors of PTSD also appear to point to greater involvement of dorsal system structures as reflected in deficits in visuo-spatial memory (Marx, Doron-Lamarca, Proctor, & Vasterling, 2009), working memory, attention, short-term memory, and even vocabulary achievement (Parslow & Jorm, 2007). Thus, one may cautiously hypothesize that if a primary deficit exists in PTSD it may be related to decreased ability to organize information and process it in a coherent and contextually bound manner. Observations of hyperactive amygdala may represent the normal function of this structure under conditions in which the archicortical moiety fails to perform its function, either during acute stress or chronically, but does not constitute a risk factor for developing the disorder (Milad et al., 2008).

Current models of PTSD emphasize abnormal hyperactivity of the amygdala on the one hand, but also hypoactivity of the medial prefrontal cortex. These canonical models highlight the role of medial aspects of the prefrontal cortex in extinction of conditioned fear, suggesting a combination of failed extinction and increased processing of fear stimuli are the definitive features of the disorder. This idea receives apparent support from elegant lesion and electrophysiological studies on rats that have demonstrated the infralimbic cortex in the rat is critical for extinction learning (Lebron, Milad, & Quirk, 2004; Milad & Quirk, 2002). Thus, studies that have found medial prefrontal cortex hypoactivation in patients with PTSD have asserted that it may reflect failed extinction processes in PTSD akin to the findings in the rat (Bremner, 2007; Liberzon & Sripada, 2008; Milad et al., 2006; Rauch et al., 2006; Shin et al., 2006).

While supported in fear conditioning studies of rodents, there is little direct evidence to support this model in humans. As described below, there are at least four reasons to treat such direct parallels between the animal and human research with caution. (1) The first reason is the uncertain homology between rodent and primate cortical cytoarchitectonic and functional organization, and the even more dubious relationship between functional imaging data in PTSD and the rat infralimbic cortex. With respect to rodent–primate cortical parallels, it has been argued by some that both sub-callosal ACC (BA 25) and rostral ACC (BA 32) in the primate, and by extension in humans, are homologous to the rat infralimbic cortex (Milad et al., 2006). However others have taken a more conservative approach and argued, just as convincingly, that the homology is restricted to sub-callosal (BA 25) and more ventral and caudal orbitofrontal parts of the primate brain (Barbas, 1995; Vertes, 2004) which include caudal BA 11 and 14 but not anterior ACC. Even if one accepts the former interpretation, and includes both areas 25 and 32, there is still a question with respect to the degree of correspondence between findings from neuroimaging studies of PTSD and the infralimbic cortex in the rat. In fact, fewer than 40 % of studies show abnormal activity in these regions, and some of these studies show hyper rather than hypo activations. (2) A second issue is the specificity of aberrant prefrontal activations associated with PTSD. This pertains to the question as to the extent to which presumed failed extinction is a core, fundamental deficit resulting in PTSD or just one of many dysfunctional processes, which might even be epiphenomenal to other core deficits. As can be seen in the current brief review, as well as in other more systematic meta-analyses (Etkin & Wager, 2007), Abnormal activations in areas that are considered homologous to the prelimbic region in rats (dorsal mPFC and DLPFC) are just as common, if not more frequent than those reported for areas 32 and 25. Moreover, even when medial prefrontal hypoactivations are observed, the center of activation is more rostral and dorsal, extending well beyond the proisocortical territory of the archicortical stream and into isocortical regions in Brodmann areas 9 and 10 (see Fig. 10.1 and cf. Fig. 5 in Milad et al., 2006). Opposite effects are reported in the rat with regard to prelimbic–amygdala interactions and their effect on extinction. These dorsal structures are likely more associated with higher-level processes of emotion regulation than with the biologically more basic process of extinction, although they might play a modulatory role in fear conditioning and extinction (see #4 below). (3) Thus the relationship between activation in PET and fMRI human neuroimaging studies and electrophysiological findings in animals is less than straightforward. It should be noted that the two types of studies have very different timescale: millisecond temporal resolution in the latter, and seconds to minutes in the former. Moreover, the relationship between cellular inhibition and excitation and hyper- or hypoactivation in neuroimaging is unknown. For example, both inhibitory and excitatory activity at the cellular level might appear as an increase in activity in neuroimaging, and hypoactivation in medial prefrontal cortex in PTSD could be interpreted either as lack of inhibition or as lack of excitatory input into other regions. (4) Finally, human neuroimaging studies have demonstrated extinction-related activity in area 25 (Phelps, Delgado, Nearing, & LeDoux, 2004), which appears to support the extinction failure model of PTSD. However, studies with healthy individuals have also demonstrated that more complex processes associated with emotion regulation critically mediate the contribution of these lower-level mechanisms (Delgado, Nearing, LeDoux, & Phelps, 2008; Schiller & Delgado, 2010). These high-level cognitive control processes are mediated by dorsal Medial and dorsolateral aspects of the PFC. As noted above abnormalities in activation of these regions are highly characteristic of PTSD and may reflect failure of emotion regulation processes, associated with deficient dorsal stream connectivity. These might be as critical a component in the evolution and persistence of PTSD as failed extinction and may in fact precede it.

Connectivity

The most conspicuous aspect of the patterns of activation described above is that there is little consistency across studies with regard to the regions abnormally activated by PTSD and controls. The most consistently reported regions that reflect differential activity in PTSD vs. controls only appear in 25–40 % of studies. Moreover, the above review of neuroimaging reports did not distinguish between reports of abnormal hyperactivations from those of abnormal hypoactivations, so consistency across studies is even lower. One potentially useful way of understanding such inconsistent and sometimes contradictory results is to think of the neuroanatomical sites involved in this complex disorder, as a dynamic system comprised of a network of regions that when out of balance can lead to abnormal behaviors. Although the word "network" is often used in the course of describing the results of neuroimaging studies, most studies use univariate voxel-based statistics. In this context, the word network is misleading. What is often actually reported is a collection or an assembly of regions activated during a particular task compared with a baseline task, each analyzed independently of the other regions. Some univariate studies may add a correlational analysis focusing on few regions of interest. However, this is also quite limited compared with the rich complexity of abnormal neural networks that lead to the complex cognitive-emotional dysfunction in PTSD. In recent years, several studies have investigated the neural correlates of PTSD by considering the interactions among the different brain regions involved, in light of their intrinsic anatomical connections. This handful of studies uses more sophisticated multivariate analyses methods that are more appropriate for describing system-level functional and effective connectivity.

Based on the framework of dual evolutionary neural trends, one may think of three types of interactions between regions: within each of the neurodevelopmental moieties ([i] archicortical–archicortical and [ii] paleocortical–paleocortical) or interactions between them ([iii] paleocortical–archicortical). Figures 10.3 and 10.4 depict reported differences in functional or effective connectivity between PTSD and controls reported by different studies. Note that because of the very small number of studies, arrows in the figures represent any reported abnormality from any of the studies (rather than reflect some sort of summary data). This also means that some studies may have "contributed" more arrows to the figures than others, and in that sense may have biased the visual depiction. This is balanced by the text below which attempts to describe the patterns of interaction reported by different studies more specifically, and so the figures and text should complement and help balance each other.

[i] Despite the relatively small number of connectivity studies, there are many reports of differences in both functional and effective connectivity within the archicortical dorsal stream. Specifically, significantly weaker interactions have been reported between the rostral ACC (BA 32) and posterior dorsal cortices including retrosplenial cortex (BA 29/30), lateral parietal cortices (BA40 and BA7), and occipital cortex, as well as anterior dorsolateral prefrontal cortex (BA9) (Lanius

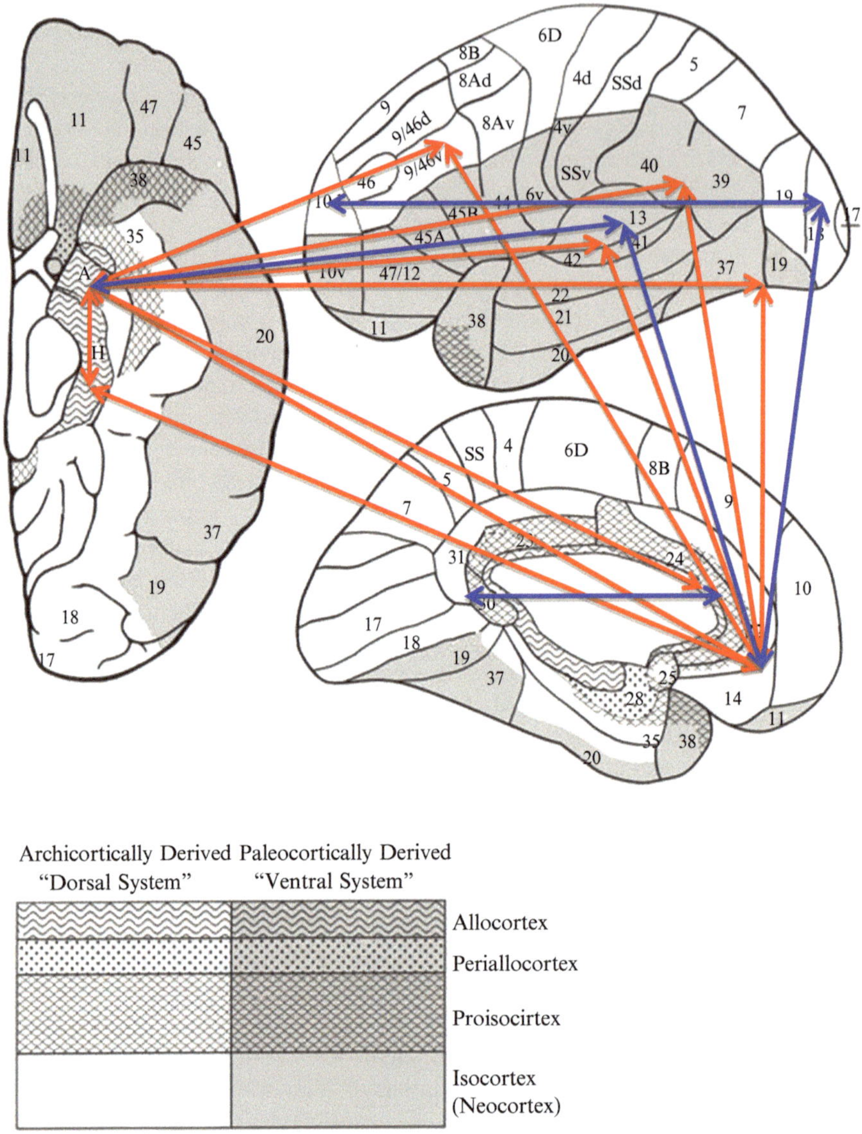

Fig. 10.3 Cartoon representation of ventral (*left*), lateral (*top right*), and medial (*bottom right*). Grayscale coding is identical to Fig. 10.1. *Arrows* represent significant difference in connectivity reported between PTSD and controls during emotional processing. *Red arrows* represent increased connectivity in PTSD, while *blue arrows* represent reduced connectivity in PTSD

et al., 2004). Similarly, reduced connectivity in PTSD has been reported between dorsal/polar prefrontal (BA10) and occipital cortex (BA19) during symptom provocation (Gilboa et al., 2004), and retrosplenial (BA31) and occipital (BA19) cortices at rest (Bluhm et al., 2009). Conversely, stronger interactions in PTSD within the

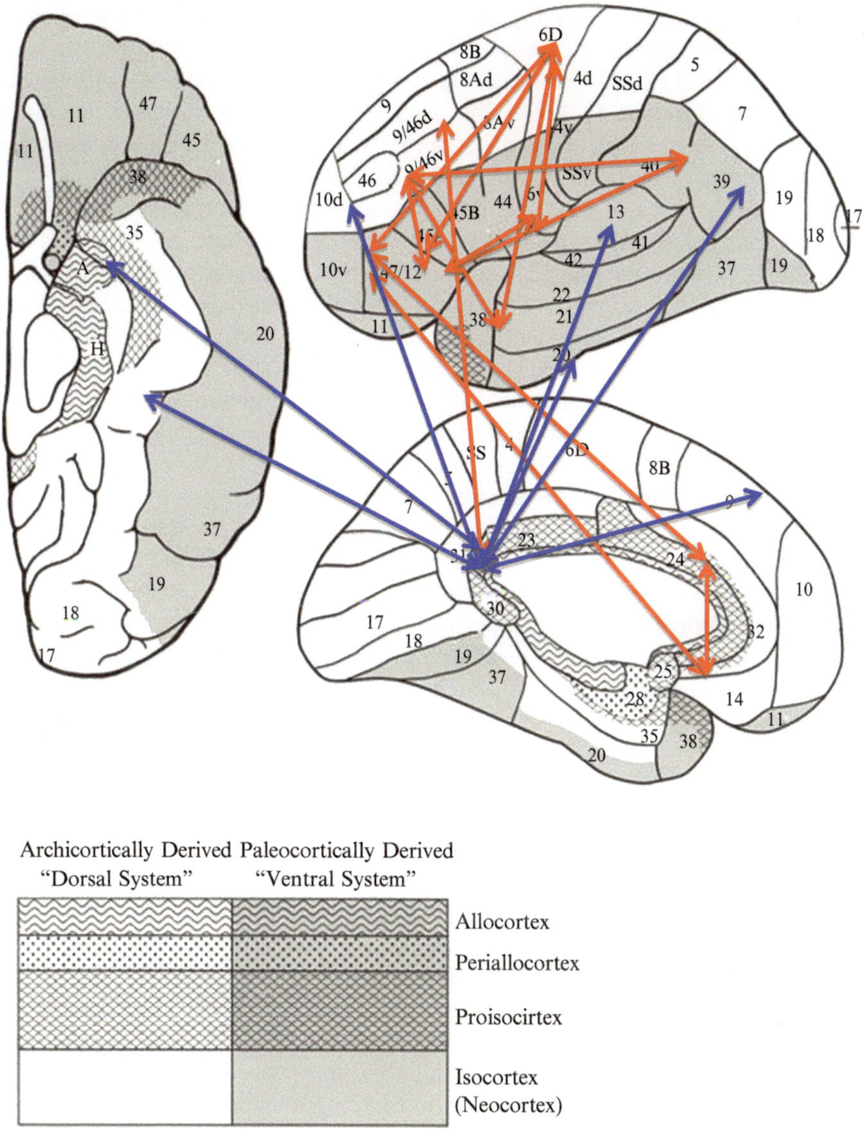

Fig. 10.4 Cartoon representation of ventral (*left*), lateral (*top right*), and medial (*bottom right*). Grayscale coding is identical to Fig. 10.1. *Arrows* represent significant difference in connectivity reported between PTSD and controls during neutral processing. *Red arrows* represent increased connectivity in PTSD. There were no reports of decreased connectivity in PTSD compared with controls

archicortical stream have also been reported. These include connections between the rostral ACC (BA32) with dorsolateral and medial PFC (BA9 and BA10) and with parietal cortex (BA40) (Lanius et al., 2004) as well as with the hippocampus (Shin et al., 2004).

[ii] By contrast, only very few differences in connectivity have been reported within the ventral moiety, all associated with the interactions of the amygdala with the fusiform gyrus (BA37) (Gilboa et al., 2004; Shin et al., 2004), and ventrolateral PFC (BA45) (Gilboa et al., 2004; Shin et al., 2004). Reports of amygdala–insula connectivity include both increases (Osuch, Willis, Bluhm, Ursano, & Drevets, 2008) and decreases (Simmons et al., 2008) in PTSD compared with controls.

[iii] The other type of connectivity abnormalities extensively reported in PTSD involves interactions across neurodevelopmental trends. These primarily involve interactions between the amygdala and archicortical structures ranging from allocortical to isocortical structures. Specifically, several studies have reported abnormal interactions between the amygdala and medial prefrontal cortices (BA 10/32) (Shin, Orr et al., 2004; Shin et al., 2005), BA24 (Gilboa et al., 2004; Osuch et al., 2008), BA 25 (Gilboa et al., 2004), dorsolateral PFC (BA9/10) (Gilboa et al., 2004), as well as with posterior regions including the precuneus (BA18/19) and posterior cingulate (BA31) (Gilboa et al., 2004). Stronger connectivity in PTSD between the amygdala and hippocampus has also been reported (Osuch et al., 2008).

Two primary patterns are evident from the above review of connectivity reports and from Figs. 10.3 and 10.4. One is that connectivity aberrations in PTSD are most commonly observed within the dorsal, archicortical, stream, and across paleocortical and archicortical streams, but are relatively infrequent within the ventral stream. The other is that there is great variability in reports, including reports of reverse patterns of stronger or weaker connectivity in different studies.

Conclusions

The current predominant view of PTSD as failed extinction of excessive fear processing cannot account for the variable profile of brain anatomy, brain activation, and system-level network interaction. The current canonical view of PTSD argues that the core and principal dysfunctional process in PTSD involves failed extinction learning, coupled with enhanced fear conditioning, and enhanced processing of fear-related stimuli. In animal models of fear conditioning and extinction this pattern is mediated by the amygdala and infralimbic prefrontal cortex. Thus, one would expect to see more consistent involvement of amygdala and sub-callosal ACC in PTSD, and consistent reports of abnormal interactions between them. Instead, it appears PTSD involves much more extensive abnormalities in widespread networks of neural structures, and variability appears to be a major characteristic of this involvement. Considering this variability from a systems perspective might however help better understand the complex interactions among neurocognitive structures in PTSD, particularly if one considers the different regions not only as foci of primary dysfunction but also as possibly sites for adaptive and maladaptive compensatory processes (Ressler & Mayberg, 2007).

Archicortical system vulnerability may mediate, among other processes, failed extinction and deficient contextual conditioning in PTSD. However it may also mediate other more complex adjustment and modulatory deficits. For example, some patients, or even some cohorts of patients, might exercise (or attempt to exercise) higher-level cognitive structuring and mood regulation strategies. Research with healthy controls has demonstrated such processing might considerably alter the conditioning-extinction network. This may account for the extensive differences in dorsal–dorsal connectivity alterations observed in PTSD, including among dorsolateral and medial prefrontal cortices. Such interactions have been shown to be modulatory during extinction in healthy controls (Delgado et al., 2008). Moreover, even the imaging data that appear to be supportive of the failed extinction hypothesis are not completely compatible with its predictions. A failed extinction mechanism of sub-callosal or rostral ACC cortex over the amygdala implies that such a process exists for controls, but not for patients. That is, if controls successfully extinguish fear conditioning, this should be reflected in enhanced connectivity between medial prefrontal cortex and amygdala. Instead the data reflect a reverse pattern, in which, when significant connectivity patterns are observed, they are observed only or primarily in the patient group—which may reflect compensatory processes rather than the absence of a process. Compensatory responses may include over-recruitment, failed attempted recruitment, or no attempt to recruit a particular process. Each of these profiles might induce different patterns of brain hypo- and hyperactivity as well as different patterns of connectivity. Extensive differences in activation and connectivity patterns, even at rest, or during processing of neutral stimuli in PTSD, further support the idea that brain alterations in the disorder are not limited to the processing of fear stimuli. Deficits in the efficient processing of contextual aspects of the environment may serve as a basis for enhanced processing of fear information. For full characterization of these complex interactions, more research is needed which would expand beyond a simple conditioning model of PTSD.

References

Abe, O., Yamasue, H., Kasai, K., Yamada, H., Aoki, S., Iwanami, A., et al. (2006). Voxel-based diffusion tensor analysis reveals aberrant anterior cingulum integrity in posttraumatic stress disorder due to terrorism. *Psychiatry Research, 146*(3), 231–242.

Antonova, E., Sharma, T., Morris, R., & Kumari, V. (2004). The relationship between brain structure and neurocognition in schizophrenia: A selective review. *Schizophrenia Research, 70*(2–3), 117–145.

Association, A. P. (1994). *DSM-IV: Diagnostic and statistical manual of mental disorders*. Washington, DC: American Psychiatric Association.

Astur, R. S., St. Germain, S. A., Tolin, D., et al. (2006). Hippocampus function predicts severity of post-traumatic stress disorder. *Cyberpsychology & Behavior, 9*(2), 234–240.

Barbas, H. (1995). Anatomic basis of cognitive-emotional interactions in the primate prefrontal cortex. *Neuroscience and Biobehavioral Reviews, 19*(3), 499–510.

Bluhm, R. L., Williamson, P. C., Osuch, E. A., Frewen, P. A., Stevens, T. K., Boksman, K., et al. (2009). Alterations in default network connectivity in posttraumatic stress disorder related to early-life trauma. *Journal of Psychiatry and Neuroscience, 34*(3), 187–194.

Bonne, O., Brandes, D., Gilboa, A., Gomori, J. M., Shenton, M. E., Pitman, R. K., et al. (2001). Longitudinal MRI study of hippocampal volume in trauma survivors with PTSD. *The American Journal of Psychiatry, 158*(8), 1248–1251.

Bonne, O., Vythilingam, M., Inagaki, M., Wood, S., Neumeister, A., Nugent, A. C., et al. (2008). Reduced posterior hippocampal volume in posttraumatic stress disorder. *The Journal of Clinical Psychiatry, 69*(7), 1087–1091.

Bossini, L., Tavanti, M., Calossi, S., Lombardelli, A., Polizzotto, N. R., Galli, R., et al. (2008). Magnetic resonance imaging volumes of the hippocampus in drug-naive patients with post-traumatic stress disorder without comorbidity conditions. *Journal of Psychiatric Research, 42*(9), 752–762.

Brandes, D., Ben-Schachar, G., Gilboa, A., Bonne, O., Freedman, S., & Shalev, A. Y. (2002). PTSD symptoms and cognitive performance in recent trauma survivors. *Psychiatry Research, 110*(3), 231–238.

Bremner, J. D. (2006a). The relationship between cognitive and brain changes in posttraumatic stress disorder. *Annals of the New York Academy of Sciences, 1071*, 80–86.

Bremner, J. D. (2006b). Stress and brain atrophy. *CNS & Neurological Disorders Drug Targets, 5*(5), 503–512.

Bremner, J. D., Randall, P., Scott, T. M., Bronen, R. A., Seibyl, J. P., Southwick, S. M., et al. (1995). MRI-based measurement of hippocampal volume in patients with combat-related post-traumatic stress disorder. *The American Journal of Psychiatry, 152*(7), 973–981.

Bremner, J. D., Randall, P., Vermetten, E., Staib, L., Bronen, R. A., Mazure, C., et al. (1997). Magnetic resonance imaging-based measurement of hippocampal volume in posttraumatic stress disorder related to childhood physical and sexual abuse–a preliminary report. *Biological Psychiatry, 41*(1), 23–32.

Bremner, J. D., Narayan, M., Staib, L. H., et al. (1999). Neural correlates of memories of childhood sexual abuse in women with and without posttraumatic stress disorder. *American Journal of Psychiatry, 156*(11), 1787–1795.

Bremner, J. D., Staib, L. H., Kaloupek, D., et al. (1999b). Neural correlates of exposure to traumatic pictures and sound in Vietnam combat veterans with and without posttraumatic stress disorder: A positron emission tomography study. *Biological Psychiatry, 45*(7), 806–816.

Bremner, J. D., Vythilingam, M., Vermetten, E., Southwick, S. M., McGlashan, T., Nazeer, A., et al. (2003). MRI and PET study of deficits in hippocampal structure and function in women with childhood sexual abuse and posttraumatic stress disorder. *The American Journal of Psychiatry, 160*(5), 924–932.

Bremner, J. D., Vermetten, E., Vythilingam, M., et al. (2004). Neural correlates of the classic color and emotional stroop in women with abuse-related posttraumatic stress disorder. *Biological Psychiatry, 55*(6), 612–620.

Bremner, J. D. (2007). Neuroimaging in posttraumatic stress disorder and other stress-related disorders. *Neuroimaging Clinics of North America, 17*(4), 523–538.

Brewin, C. R. (2007). Autobiographical memory for trauma: Update on four controversies. *Memory, 15*(3), 227–248.

Britton, J. C., Phan, K. L., Taylor, S. F., et al. (2005). Corticolimbic blood flow in posttraumatic stress disorder during script-driven imagery. *Biological Psychiatry, 57*(8), 832–840.

Bryant, R. A., Felmingham, K. L., Kemp, A. H., et al. (2005). Neural networks of information processing in posttraumatic stress disorder: A functional magnetic resonance imaging study. *Biological Psychiatry, 58*(2), 111–118.

Bryant, R. A., Felmingham, K., Whitford, T. J., Kemp, A., Hughes, G., Peduto, A., et al. (2008). Rostral anterior cingulate volume predicts treatment response to cognitive-behavioural therapy for posttraumatic stress disorder. *Journal of Psychiatry and Neuroscience, 33*(2), 142–146.

Cannistraro, P. A., & Rauch, S. L. (2003). Neural circuitry of anxiety: Evidence from structural and functional neuroimaging studies. *Psychopharmacology Bulletin, 37*(4), 8–25.

Carrion, V. G., Weems, C. F., Eliez, S., Patwardhan, A., Brown, W., Ray, R. D., et al. (2001). Attenuation of frontal asymmetry in pediatric posttraumatic stress disorder. *Biological Psychiatry, 50*(12), 943–951.

Charney, D. S. (2003). Neuroanatomical circuits modulating fear and anxiety behaviors. *Acta Psychiatrica Scandinavica Supplementum, 417*, 38–50.

Chen, S., Li, L., Xu, B., & Liu, J. (2009). Insular cortex involvement in declarative memory deficits in patients with post-traumatic stress disorder. *BMC Psychiatry, 9*, 39.

Chen, S., Xia, W., Li, L., Liu, J., He, Z., Zhang, Z., et al. (2006). Gray matter density reduction in the insula in fire survivors with posttraumatic stress disorder: A voxel-based morphometric study. *Psychiatry Research, 146*(1), 65–72.

Christensen, B. K., & Bilder, R. M. (2000). Dual cytoarchitectonic trends: An evolutionary model of frontal lobe functioning and its application to psychopathology. *Canadian Journal of Psychiatry, 45*(3), 247–256.

Chung, Y. A., Kim, S. H., Chung, S. K., et al. (2006). Alterations in cerebral perfusion in posttraumatic stress disorder patients without re-exposure to accident-related stimuli. *Clinical Neurophysiology, 117*(3), 637–642.

Clark, C. R., McFarlane, A. C., Morris, P., et al. (2003). Cerebral function in posttraumatic stress disorder during verbal working memory updating: A positron emission tomography study. *Biological Psychiatry, 53*(6), 474–481.

Cohen, R. A., Grieve, S., Hoth, K. F., Paul, R. H., Sweet, L., Tate, D., et al. (2006). Early life stress and morphometry of the adult anterior cingulate cortex and caudate nuclei. *Biological Psychiatry, 59*(10), 975–982.

Corbo, V., Clement, M. H., Armony, J. L., Pruessner, J. C., & Brunet, A. (2005). Size versus shape differences: Contrasting voxel-based and volumetric analyses of the anterior cingulate cortex in individuals with acute posttraumatic stress disorder. *Biological Psychiatry, 58*(2), 119–124.

De Bellis, M. D., Hall, J., Boring, A. M., Frustaci, K., & Moritz, G. (2001). A pilot longitudinal study of hippocampal volumes in pediatric maltreatment-related posttraumatic stress disorder. *Biological Psychiatry, 50*(4), 305–309.

De Bellis, M. D., & Keshavan, M. S. (2003). Sex differences in brain maturation in maltreatment-related pediatric posttraumatic stress disorder. *Neuroscience and Biobehavioral Reviews, 27*(1–2), 103–117.

De Bellis, M. D., Keshavan, M. S., Shifflett, H., Iyengar, S., Beers, S. R., Hall, J., et al. (2002). Brain structures in pediatric maltreatment-related posttraumatic stress disorder: A sociodemographically matched study. *Biological Psychiatry, 52*(11), 1066–1078.

Deckersbach, T., Dougherty, D. D., & Rauch, S. L. (2006). Functional imaging of mood and anxiety disorders. *Journal of Neuroimaging, 16*(1), 1–10.

Delgado, M. R., Nearing, K. I., LeDoux, J. E., & Phelps, E. A. (2008). Neural circuitry underlying the regulation of conditioned fear and its relation to extinction. *Neuron, 59*(5), 829–838.

Driessen, M., Beblo, T., Mertens, M., et al. (2004). Posttraumatic stress disorder and fMRI activation patterns of traumatic memory in patients with borderline personality disorder. *Biological Psychiatry, 55*(6), 603–611.

Emdad, R., Bonekamp, D., Sondergaard, H. P., Bjorklund, T., Agartz, I., Ingvar, M., et al. (2006). Morphometric and psychometric comparisons between non-substance-abusing patients with posttraumatic stress disorder and normal controls. *Psychotherapy and Psychosomatics, 75*(2), 122–132.

Etkin, A., & Wager, T. D. (2007). Functional neuroimaging of anxiety: A meta-analysis of emotional processing in PTSD, social anxiety disorder, and specific phobia. *The American Journal of Psychiatry, 164*(10), 1476–1488.

Felmingham, K., Williams, L. M., Whitford, T. J., Falconer, E., Kemp, A. H., Peduto, A., et al. (2009). Duration of posttraumatic stress disorder predicts hippocampal grey matter loss. *Neuroreport, 20*(16), 1402–1406.

Fennema-Notestine, C., Stein, M. B., Kennedy, C. M., Archibald, S. L., & Jernigan, T. L. (2002). Brain morphometry in female victims of intimate partner violence with and without posttraumatic stress disorder. *Biological Psychiatry, 52*(11), 1089–1101.

Francati, V., Vermetten, E., & Bremner, J. D. (2007). Functional neuroimaging studies in posttraumatic stress disorder: Review of current methods and findings. *Depression and Anxiety, 24*(3), 202–218.

Geuze, E., Westenberg, H. G., Jochims, A., et al. (2007). Altered pain processing in veterans with posttraumatic stress disorder. *Archives of General Psychiatry, 64*(1), 76–85.

Giaccio, R. G. (2006). The dual origin hypothesis: An evolutionary brain-behavior framework for analyzing psychiatric disorders. *Neuroscience and Biobehavioral Reviews, 30*(4), 526–550.

Gilbertson, M. W., Shenton, M. E., Ciszewski, A., Kasai, K., Lasko, N. B., Orr, S. P., et al. (2002). Smaller hippocampal volume predicts pathologic vulnerability to psychological trauma. *Nature Neuroscience, 5*(11), 1242–1247.

Gilbertson, M. W., Williston, S. K., Paulus, L. A., Lasko, N. B., Gurvits, T. V., Shenton, M. E., et al. (2007). Configural cue performance in identical twins discordant for posttraumatic stress disorder: Theoretical implications for the role of hippocampal function. *Biological Psychiatry, 62*(5), 513–520.

Gilboa, A., Shalev, A. Y., Laor, L., Lester, H., Louzoun, Y., Chisin, R., et al. (2004). Functional connectivity of the prefrontal cortex and the amygdala in posttraumatic stress disorder. *Biological Psychiatry, 55*(3), 263–272.

Gold, J. J., & Squire, L. R. (2005). Quantifying medial temporal lobe damage in memory-impaired patients. *Hippocampus, 15*(1), 79–85.

Goldberg, G. (1985). Supplementary motor area structure and function: Review and hypotheses. *Behavioral and Brain Sciences, 8*(567–616).

Golier, J. A., Yehuda, R., De Santi, S., Segal, S., Dolan, S., & de Leon, M. J. (2005). Absence of hippocampal volume differences in survivors of the Nazi Holocaust with and without posttraumatic stress disorder. *Psychiatry Research, 139*(1), 53–64.

Grillon, C., Southwick, S. M., & Charney, D. S. (1996). The psychobiological basis of posttraumatic stress disorder. *Molecular Psychiatry, 1*(4), 278–297.

Gurvits, T. V., Shenton, M. E., Hokama, H., Ohta, H., Lasko, N. B., Gilbertson, M. W., et al. (1996). Magnetic resonance imaging study of hippocampal volume in chronic, combat-related posttraumatic stress disorder. *Biological Psychiatry, 40*(11), 1091–1099.

Hara, E., Matsuoka, Y., Hakamata, Y., Nagamine, M., Inagaki, M., Imoto, S., et al. (2008). Hippocampal and amygdalar volumes in breast cancer survivors with posttraumatic stress disorder. *The Journal of Neuropsychiatry and Clinical Neurosciences, 20*(3), 302–308.

Hassabis, D., & Maguire, E. A. (2007). Deconstructing episodic memory with construction. *Trends in Cognitive Sciences, 11*(7), 299–306.

Hedges, D. W., Allen, S., Tate, D. F., Thatcher, G. W., Miller, M. J., Rice, S. A., et al. (2003). Reduced hippocampal volume in alcohol and substance naive Vietnam combat veterans with posttraumatic stress disorder. *Cognitive and Behavioral Neurology, 16*(4), 219–224.

Hedges, D. W., & Woon, F. L. (2010). Alcohol use and hippocampal volume deficits in adults with posttraumatic stress disorder: A meta-analysis. *Biological Psychology, 84*(2), 163–168.

Hendler, T., Rotshtein, P., Yeshurun, Y., Weizmann, T., Kahn, I., Ben-Bashat, D., et al. (2003). Sensing the invisible: Differential sensitivity of visual cortex and amygdala to traumatic context. *NeuroImage, 19*(3), 587–600.

Hou, C., Liu, J., Wang, K., et al. (2007). Brain responses to symptom provocation and trauma-related short-term memory recall in coal mining accident survivors with acute severe PTSD. *Brain Research, 1144*, 165–174.

Isaac, C. L., Cushway, D., & Jones, G. V. (2006). Is posttraumatic stress disorder associated with specific deficits in episodic memory? *Clinical Psychology Review, 26*(8), 939–955.

Isaacs, E. B., Vargha-Khadem, F., Watkins, K. E., Lucas, A., Mishkin, M., & Gadian, D. G. (2003). Developmental amnesia and its relationship to degree of hippocampal atrophy. *Proceedings of the National Academy of Sciences of the United States of America, 100*(22), 13060–13063.

Jackowski, A. P., Douglas-Palumberi, H., Jackowski, M., Win, L., Schultz, R. T., Staib, L. W., et al. (2008). Corpus callosum in maltreated children with posttraumatic stress disorder: A diffusion tensor imaging study. *Psychiatry Research, 162*(3), 256–261.

Jatzko, A., Rothenhofer, S., Schmitt, A., Gaser, C., Demirakca, T., Weber-Fahr, W., et al. (2006). Hippocampal volume in chronic posttraumatic stress disorder (PTSD): MRI study using two different evaluation methods. *Journal of Affective Disorders, 94*(1–3), 121–126.

Karl, A., Schaefer, M., Malta, L. S., Dorfel, D., Rohleder, N., & Werner, A. (2006). A meta-analysis of structural brain abnormalities in PTSD. *Neuroscience and Biobehavioral Reviews, 30*(7), 1004–1031.

Kasai, K., Yamasue, H., Gilbertson, M. W., Shenton, M. E., Rauch, S. L., & Pitman, R. K. (2008). Evidence for acquired pregenual anterior cingulate gray matter loss from a twin study of combat-related posttraumatic stress disorder. *Biological Psychiatry, 63*(6), 550–556.

Kemp, A. H., Felmingham, K. L., Falconer, E., et al. (2009). Heterogeneity of non-conscious fear perception in posttraumatic stress disorder as a function of physiological arousal: An fMRI study. *Psychiatry Research, 174*(2), 158–161.

Kim, J. J., & Jung, M. W. (2006). Neural circuits and mechanisms involved in Pavlovian fear conditioning: A critical review. *Neuroscience and Biobehavioral Reviews, 30*(2), 188–202.

Kitayama, N., Brummer, M., Hertz, L., Quinn, S., Kim, Y., & Bremner, J. D. (2007). Morphologic alterations in the corpus callosum in abuse-related posttraumatic stress disorder: A preliminary study. *The Journal of Nervous and Mental Disease, 195*(12), 1027–1029.

Kitayama, N., Quinn, S., & Bremner, J. D. (2006). Smaller volume of anterior cingulate cortex in abuse-related posttraumatic stress disorder. *Journal of Affective Disorders, 90*(2–3), 171–174.

Lanius, R. A., Williamson, P. C., Densmore, M., et al. (2001). Neural correlates of traumatic memories in posttraumatic stress disorder: A functional MRI investigation. *American Journal of Psychiatry, 158*(11), 1920–1922.

Lanius, R. A., Williamson, P. C., Boksman, K., et al. (2002). Brain activation during script-driven imagery induced dissociative responses in PTSD: A functional magnetic resonance imaging investigation. *Biological Psychiatry, 52*(4), 305–311.

Lanius, R. A., Williamson, P. C., Hopper, J., et al. (2003). Recall of emotional states in posttraumatic stress disorder: An fMRI investigation. *Biological Psychiatry, 53*(3), 204–210.

Lanius, R. A., Williamson, P. C., Bluhm, R. L., et al. (2005). Functional connectivity of dissociative responses in posttraumatic stress disorder: A functional magnetic resonance imaging investigation. *Biological Psychiatry, 57*(8), 873–884.

Lanius, R. A., Bluhm, R., Lanius, U., & Pain, C. (2006). A review of neuroimaging studies in PTSD: Heterogeneity of response to symptom provocation. *Journal of Psychiatric Research, 40*(8), 709–729.

Lanius, R. A., Vermetten, E., Loewenstein, R. J., Brand, B., Schmahl, C., Bremner, J. D., et al. (2010). Emotion modulation in PTSD: Clinical and neurobiological evidence for a dissociative subtype. *The American Journal of Psychiatry, 167*(6), 640–647.

Lanius, R. A., Williamson, P. C., Densmore, M., Boksman, K., Neufeld, R. W., Gati, J. S., et al. (2004). The nature of traumatic memories: A 4-T FMRI functional connectivity analysis. *The American Journal of Psychiatry, 161*(1), 36–44.

Liberzon, I., Taylor, S. F., Amdur, R., et al. (1999). Brain activation in PTSD in response to trauma-related stimuli. *Biological Psychiatry, 45*(7), 817–826.

Liberzon, I., Britton, J. C., & Phan, K. L. (2003). Neural correlates of traumatic recall in posttraumatic stress disorder. *Stress, 6*(3), 151–156.

Lebron, K., Milad, M. R., & Quirk, G. J. (2004). Delayed recall of fear extinction in rats with lesions of ventral medial prefrontal cortex. *Learning & Memory, 11*(5), 544–548.

Liberzon, I., & Sripada, C. S. (2008). The functional neuroanatomy of PTSD: A critical review. *Progress in Brain Research, 167*, 151–169.

Lindauer, R. J., Vlieger, E. J., Jalink, M., Olff, M., Carlier, I. V., Majoie, C. B., et al. (2004). Smaller hippocampal volume in Dutch police officers with posttraumatic stress disorder. *Biological Psychiatry, 56*(5), 356–363.

Maren, S. (2001). Neurobiology of Pavlovian fear conditioning. *Annual Review of Neuroscience, 24*, 897–931.

Marx, B. P., Doron-Lamarca, S., Proctor, S. P., & Vasterling, J. J. (2009). The influence of pre-deployment neurocognitive functioning on post-deployment PTSD symptom outcomes among Iraq-deployed army soldiers. *Journal of the International Neuropsychological Society, 15*(6), 840–852.

Matsuoka, Y., Yamawaki, S., Inagaki, M., Akechi, T., & Uchitomi, Y. (2003). A volumetric study of amygdala in cancer survivors with intrusive recollections. *Biological Psychiatry, 54*(7), 736–743.

Mega, M. S., Cummings, J. L., Salloway, S., & Malloy, P. (1997). The limbic system: An anatomic, phylogenetic, and clinical perspective. *Journal of Neuropsychiatry, 9*, 315–330.

Milad, M. R., Orr, S. P., Lasko, N. B., Chang, Y., Rauch, S. L., & Pitman, R. K. (2008). Presence and acquired origin of reduced recall for fear extinction in PTSD: Results of a twin study. *Journal of Psychiatric Research, 42*(7), 515–520.

Milad, M. R., Pitman, R. K., Ellis, C. B., Gold, A. L., Shin, L. M., Lasko, N. B., et al. (2009). Neurobiological basis of failure to recall extinction memory in posttraumatic stress disorder. *Biological Psychiatry, 66*(12), 1075–1082.

Milad, M. R., & Quirk, G. J. (2002). Neurons in medial prefrontal cortex signal memory for fear extinction. *Nature, 420*(6911), 70–74.

Milad, M. R., Rauch, S. L., Pitman, R. K., & Quirk, G. J. (2006). Fear extinction in rats: Implications for human brain imaging and anxiety disorders. *Biological Psychology, 73*(1), 61–71.

Osuch, E. A., Willis, M. W., Bluhm, R., Ursano, R. J., & Drevets, W. C. (2008). Neurophysiological responses to traumatic reminders in the acute aftermath of serious motor vehicle collisions using [15O]-H2O positron emission tomography. *Biological Psychiatry, 64*(4), 327–335.

Pandya, D. N., Seltzer, B., & Barbas, H. (1988). Input–output organization of the primate cerebral cortex. In H. D. Steklis & J. Erwin (Eds.), *Comparative primate biology* (Neuroscience, Vol. 4, pp. 39–80). New York: Alan R. Liss Inc.

Pardo, J., Fahnhorst, S., Lee, J. T., et al. (2009). PET study of script-driven fear imagery: Combat veterans with active vs. remitted PTSD. *Neuroimage, 47*, S70.

Pare, D. (2002). Mechanisms of Pavlovian fear conditioning: Has the engram been located? *Trends in Neurosciences, 25*(9), 436–437. discussion 437–438.

Parslow, R. A., & Jorm, A. F. (2007). Pretrauma and posttrauma neurocognitive functioning and PTSD symptoms in a community sample of young adults. *The American Journal of Psychiatry, 164*(3), 509–515.

Petrides, M., & Pandya, D. N. (1994). Comparative architectonic analysis of the human and the macaque frontal cortex. In F. Boller & J. Grafman (Eds.), *Handbook of neuropsychology* (Vol. 9, pp. 17–58). Amsterdam: Elsevier.

Phelps, E. A., Delgado, M. R., Nearing, K. I., & LeDoux, J. E. (2004). Extinction learning in humans: Role of the amygdala and vmPFC. *Neuron, 43*(6), 897–905.

Pribram, K. H. (1991). *Brain and perception: Holonomy and structure in figural processing*. Hove: Psychology Press.

Protopopescu, X., Pan, H., Tuescher, O., et al. (2005). Differential time courses and specificity of amygdala activity in posttraumatic stress disorder subjects and normal control subjects. *Biological Psychiatry, 57*(5), 464–473.

Quirk, G. J., & Beer, J. S. (2006). Prefrontal involvement in the regulation of emotion: Convergence of rat and human studies. *Current Opinion in Neurobiology, 16*(6), 723–727.

Qingling, H., Guangming, L., & Zhiqiang, Z. (2009). Resting-state fMRI study of posttraumatic stress disorder. *Journal of Clinical Radiology*

Rauch, S. L., Whalen, P. J., Shin, L. M., et al. (2000). Exaggerated amygdala response to masked facial stimuli in posttraumatic stress disorder: A functional MRI study. *Biological Psychiatry, 47*(9), 769–776.

Rauch, S. L., Shin, L. M., Segal, E., Pitman, R. K., Carson, M. A., McMullin, K., et al. (2003). Selectively reduced regional cortical volumes in post-traumatic stress disorder. *Neuroreport, 14*(7), 913–916.

Rauch, S. L., Shin, L. M., & Phelps, E. A. (2006). Neurocircuitry models of posttraumatic stress disorder and extinction: Human neuroimaging research–past, present, and future. *Biological Psychiatry, 60*(4), 376–382.

Resick, P. A., & Miller, M. W. (2009). Posttraumatic stress disorder: Anxiety or traumatic stress disorder? *Journal of Traumatic Stress, 22*(5), 384–390.

Ressler, K. J., & Mayberg, H. S. (2007). Targeting abnormal neural circuits in mood and anxiety disorders: From the laboratory to the clinic. *Nature Neuroscience, 10*(9), 1116–1124.

Rogers, M. A., Yamasue, H., Abe, O., Yamada, H., Ohtani, T., Iwanami, A., et al. (2009). Smaller amygdala volume and reduced anterior cingulate gray matter density associated with history of post-traumatic stress disorder. *Psychiatry Research, 174*(3), 210–216.

Sachinvala, N., Kling, A., Suffin, S., et al. (2000). Increased regional cerebral perfusion by 99mTc hexamethyl propylene amine oxime single photon emission computed tomography in post-traumatic stress disorder. *Military Medicine, 165*(6), 473–479.

Semple, W. E., Goyer, P. F., McCormick, R., et al. (1996). Attention and regional cerebral blood flow in posttraumatic stress disorder patients with substance abuse histories. *Psychiatry Research, 67*(1), 17–28.

Semple, W. E., Goyer, P. F., McCormick, R., et al. (2000). Higher brain blood flow at amygdala and lower frontal cortex blood flow in PTSD patients with comorbid cocaine and alcohol abuse compared with normals. *Psychiatry, 63*(1), 65–74.

Sanides, F. (1962). Structure and function of the human frontal lobe. *Neuropsychologia, 2*(3), 209–219.

Sanides, F. (1970). Functional architecture of motor and sensory cortices in primates in the light of a new concept of neocortex evolution. In C. R. Noback & W. Montagna (Eds.), *Advances in primatology* (The primate brain, Vol. 1, pp. 137–208). New York: Appleton-Century-Crofts, Meredith Corporation.

Sapolsky, R. M., Krey, L. C., & McEwen, B. S. (1986). The neuroendocrinology of stress and aging: The glucocorticoid cascade hypothesis. *Endocrine Reviews, 7*(3), 284–301.

Schiller, D., & Delgado, M. R. (2010). Overlapping neural systems mediating extinction, reversal and regulation of fear. *Trends in Cognitive Sciences, 14*(6), 268–276.

Sehlmeyer, C., Schoning, S., Zwitserlood, P., Pfleiderer, B., Kircher, T., Arolt, V., et al. (2009). Human fear conditioning and extinction in neuroimaging: A systematic review. *PLoS ONE, 4*(6), e5865.

Shalev, A. Y., Gilboa, A., & Rasmusson, A. M. (2011). Neurobiology of PTSD. In J. Stein & C. Blanco (Eds.), *Post-traumatic stress disorder*. Chichester: John Wiley.

Shaw, M. E., Strother, S. C., McFarlane, A. C., et al. (2002). Abnormal functional connectivity in posttraumatic stress disorder. *Neuroimage, 15*(3), 661–674.

Shin, L. M., Kosslyn, S. M., McNally, R. J., et al. (1997). Visual imagery and perception in posttraumatic stress disorder. A positron emission tomographic investigation. *Archives of General Psychiatry, 54*(3), 233–241.

Shin, L. M., McNally, R. J., Kosslyn, S. M., et al. (1999). Regional cerebral blood flow during script-driven imagery in childhood sexual abuse-related PTSD: A PET investigation. *American Journal of Psychiatry, 156*(4), 575–584.

Shin, L. M., Whalen, P. J., Pitman, R. K., et al. (2001). An fMRI study of anterior cingulate function in posttraumatic stress disorder. *Biological Psychiatry, 50*(12), 932–942.

Shin, L. M., Shin, P. S., Heckers, S., et al. (2004). Hippocampal function in posttraumatic stress disorder. *Hippocampus, 14*(3), 292–300.

Shin, L. M., & Handwerger, K. (2009). Is posttraumatic stress disorder a stress-induced fear circuitry disorder? *Journal of Traumatic Stress, 22*, 409–415.

Shin, L. M., Orr, S. P., Carson, M. A., Rauch, S. L., Macklin, M. L., Lasko, N. B., et al. (2004). Regional cerebral blood flow in the amygdala and medial prefrontal cortex during traumatic imagery in male and female Vietnam veterans with PTSD. *Archives of General Psychiatry, 61*(2), 168–176.

Shin, L. M., Rauch, S. L., & Pitman, R. K. (2006). Amygdala, medial prefrontal cortex, and hippocampal function in PTSD. *Annals of the New York Academy of Sciences, 1071*, 67–79.

Shin, L. M., Shin, P. S., Heckers, S., Krangel, T. S., Macklin, M. L., Orr, S. P., et al. (2004). Hippocampal function in posttraumatic stress disorder. *Hippocampus, 14*(3), 292–300.

Shin, L. M., Wright, C. I., Cannistraro, P. A., Wedig, M. M., McMullin, K., Martis, B., et al. (2005). A functional magnetic resonance imaging study of amygdala and medial prefrontal cortex responses to overtly presented fearful faces in posttraumatic stress disorder. *Archives of General Psychiatry, 62*(3), 273–281.

Simmons, A. N., Paulus, M. P., Thorp, S. R., Matthews, S. C., Norman, S. B., & Stein, M. B. (2008). Functional activation and neural networks in women with posttraumatic stress disorder related to intimate partner violence. *Biological Psychiatry, 64*(8), 681–690.

Squire, L. R. (1992). Memory and the hippocampus: A synthesis from findings with rats, monkeys, and humans. *Psychological Review, 99*(2), 195–231.

Squire, L. R. (1998). Memory systems. *Comptes Rendus de l'Académie des Sciences. Série III, 321*(2–3), 153–156.

Stein, M. B., Koverola, C., Hanna, C., Torchia, M. G., & McClarty, B. (1997). Hippocampal volume in women victimized by childhood sexual abuse. *Psychological Medicine, 27*(4), 951–959.

Stuss, D. T., Alexander, M. P., Floden, D., Binns, M. A., Levine, B., McIntosh, A. R., et al. (2002). Fractionation and localization of distinct frontal lobe processes: evidence from focal lesions in humans. In D. T. Stuss & R. T. Knight (Eds.), *Principles of frontal lobe functions* (pp. 392–407). New York: Oxford University Press.

Thomaes, K., Dorrepaal, E., Draijer, N. P., et al. (2009). Increased activation of the left hippocampus region in complex PTSD during encoding and recognition of emotional words: A pilot study. *Psychiatry Research, 171*(1), 44–53.

Vasterling, J. J., Brailey, K., Constans, J. I., & Sutker, P. B. (1998). Attention and memory dysfunction in posttraumatic stress disorder. *Neuropsychology, 12*(1), 125–133.

Vermetten, E., Vythilingam, M., Southwick, S. M., Charney, D. S., & Bremner, J. D. (2003). Long-term treatment with paroxetine increases verbal declarative memory and hippocampal volume in posttraumatic stress disorder. *Biological Psychiatry, 54*(7), 693–702.

Vermetten, E., Schmahl, C., Southwick, S. M., et al. (2007). Positron tomographic emission study of olfactory induced emotional recall in veterans with and without combat-related posttraumatic stress disorder. *Psychopharmacology Bulletin, 40*(1), 8–30.

Vertes, R. P. (2004). Differential projections of the infralimbic and prelimbic cortex in the rat. *Synapse, 51*(1), 32–58.

Videbech, P., & Ravnkilde, B. (2004). Hippocampal volume and depression: A meta-analysis of MRI studies. *The American Journal of Psychiatry, 161*(11), 1957–1966.

Villarreal, G., Hamilton, D. A., Graham, D. P., Driscoll, I., Qualls, C., Petropoulos, H., et al. (2004). Reduced area of the corpus callosum in posttraumatic stress disorder. *Psychiatry Research, 131*(3), 227–235.

Villarreal, G., Hamilton, D. A., Petropoulos, H., Driscoll, I., Rowland, L. M., Griego, J. A., et al. (2002). Reduced hippocampal volume and total white matter volume in posttraumatic stress disorder. *Biological Psychiatry, 52*(2), 119–125.

Vythilingam, M., Luckenbaugh, D. A., Lam, T., Morgan, C. A., 3rd, Lipschitz, D., Charney, D. S., et al. (2005). Smaller head of the hippocampus in Gulf War-related posttraumatic stress disorder. *Psychiatry Research, 139*(2), 89–99.

Wang, Z., Neylan, T. C., Mueller, S. G., Lenoci, M., Truran, D., Marmar, C. R., et al. (2010). Magnetic resonance imaging of hippocampal subfields in posttraumatic stress disorder. *Archives of General Psychiatry, 67*(3), 296–303.

Werner, N. S., Meindl, T., Engel, R. R., et al. (2009). Hippocampal function during associative learning in patients with posttraumatic stress disorder. *Journal of Psychiatric Research, 43*(3), 309–318.

Whalley, M. G., Rugg, M. D., Smith, A. P., et al. (2009). Incidental retrieval of emotional contexts in post-traumatic stress disorder and depression: An fMRI study. *Brain and Cognition, 69*(1), 98–107.

Wignall, E. L., Dickson, J. M., Vaughan, P., Farrow, T. F., Wilkinson, I. D., Hunter, M. D., et al. (2004). Smaller hippocampal volume in patients with recent-onset posttraumatic stress disorder. *Biological Psychiatry, 56*(11), 832–836.

Woodward, S. H., Kaloupek, D. G., Streeter, C. C., Martinez, C., Schaer, M., & Eliez, S. (2006). Decreased anterior cingulate volume in combat-related PTSD. *Biological Psychiatry, 59*(7), 582–587.

Woon, F. L., & Hedges, D. W. (2008). Hippocampal and amygdala volumes in children and adults with childhood maltreatment-related posttraumatic stress disorder: A meta-analysis. *Hippocampus, 18*(8), 729–736.

Woon, F. L., & Hedges, D. W. (2009). Amygdala volume in adults with posttraumatic stress disorder: A meta-analysis. *The Journal of Neuropsychiatry and Clinical Neurosciences, 21*(1), 5–12.

Yamasue, H., Kasai, K., Iwanami, A., Ohtani, T., Yamada, H., Abe, O., et al. (2003). Voxel-based analysis of MRI reveals anterior cingulate gray-matter volume reduction in posttraumatic stress disorder due to terrorism. *Proceedings of the National Academy of Sciences of the United States of America, 100*(15), 9039–9043.

Zubieta, J. K., Chinitz, J. A., Lombardi, U., et al. (1999). Medial frontal cortex involvement in PTSD symptoms: A SPECT study. *Journal of Psychiatric Research, 33*(3), 259–264.

Part IV
The Development of Evidence-Based Treatment for PTSD

Chapter 11
Prolonged Exposure Treatment

Nitsa Nacasch, Lilach Rachamim, and Edna B. Foa

Introduction

A large body of evidence supports the efficacy of exposure therapy for posttraumatic stress disorder (PTSD) (Cahill, Rothbaum, Resick, & Follette, 2009). Exposure therapy has been recommended as the first-line treatment for PTSD in several treatment guidelines (e.g., American Psychiatric Association, 2006), and the Institute of Medicine concluded that "the evidence is sufficient to conclude the efficacy of exposure therapies in the treatment of PTSD" (Institute of Medicine, 2008, p. 97).

Prolonged Exposure therapy is a specific exposure therapy protocol that has been successfully used with patients suffering from PTSD from various types of trauma (e.g., sexual and nonsexual assault, combat, MVA, natural disaster, and terror). It is aimed to reduce PTSD symptoms and related problems (e.g., depression, guilt) by helping patients confront their trauma-related memories, feelings, and stimuli that evoke fear and anxiety, because they are perceived as dangerous and/or are reminders of the traumatic events.

N. Nacasch, M.D. (✉)
Brill Community Mental Health Center, Hatsvi 9, Tel Aviv, Israel
e-mail: nitsana@clalit.org.il

L. Rachamim, Ph.D.
Interdisciplinary Center, Herzliya, Israel

Schneider Children's Medical Center of Israel, Petah Tikva, Israel
e-mail: lilach.rachamim7@gmail.com

E.B. Foa, Ph.D.
Center for Treatment and Study of Anxiety, University of Pennsylvania,
3535 Market Street, Philadelphia, PA 19104, USA
e-mail: Foa@ail.med.upenn.edu

M.P. Safir et al. (eds.), *Future Directions in Post-Traumatic Stress Disorder*,
DOI 10.1007/978-1-4899-7522-5_11

Emotional Processing Theory

PE treatment is based on emotional processing theory that was developed by Foa and Kozak (1985, 1986) to explain anxiety disorders including PTSD and the treatment for such disorders. The theory rests on two basic premises. The first premise is that anxiety disorders including PTSD reflect the presence of pathological fear structures in memory. A fear structure includes representations of fear stimuli (e.g., tiger in the jungle), fear responses (e.g., heart beats, sweating), and the meanings associated with them (e.g., tiger is a dangerous animal and the physiological responses are the result of fear). A fear structure is activated when information in the environment matches some of the information represented in the structure resulting in producing cognitive, behavioral, and physiological anxiety reactions. For example, when a person is crossing the street and suddenly a car is approaching quickly, the fear structure accurately represents a dangerous situation so that the person runs fast to escape from danger. However, a fear structure becomes pathological when (1) associations among stimulus elements do not accurately represent the world, (2) physiological and escape/avoidance responses are evoked by harmless stimuli, (3) excessive responses interfere with adaptive behavior, and (4) quiet and safe stimulus and responses are erroneously associated with danger.

The second basic premise of emotional processing theory is that successful treatment modifies the pathological elements of the fear structure. Two conditions are necessary for the modification of the fear structure: (1) the activation of the fear structure; and (2) the availability of new corrective information. The new information is incorporated into the fear structure and, consequently, maladaptive beliefs are disconfirmed.

Within the framework of emotional processing theory, the development of chronic PTSD is conceptualized as a failure to adequately process the traumatic memory. In chronic PTSD the pathological fear structure includes a large number of stimuli that are associated with danger, excessive responses of fear, and maladaptive behaviors. Individuals with PTSD perceive the world as completely dangerous. They also perceive their behavior during the traumatic event and their subsequent symptoms as indicative of self-incompetence. These negative cognitions (the world is entirely dangerous, I am completely incompetent) lead to avoidance and escape behavior and thus worsen the severity of PTSD symptoms, which in turn support the erroneous cognitions (for more details, see Foa & Rothbaum, 1998).

Overview of PE Protocol

PE treatment protocol consists of 9–15 weekly sessions, lasting 90 min each. The treatment has four components: relaxation through breathing retraining, education about common reactions to trauma, in vivo exposure to trauma-related situations and objects, and imaginal exposure in which the patient recounts the traumatic memory.

In the first treatment session the therapist presents an overview of the treatment. The therapist explains that the treatment focus is on PTSD symptoms. The rationale for treatment is presented emphasizing the role of avoidance in the maintenance of PTSD: "three main factors maintain PTSD symptoms. (1) The avoidance of thoughts and memories of the traumatic event prevents emotional processing of the trauma; (2) the avoidance of trauma-related situations and stimuli prevents disconfirmation of beliefs that safe situations are dangerous; (3) the presence of dysfunctional cognitions: the world is extremely dangerous and I am extremely incompetent promotes avoidance and thereby further prevents disconfirmation of danger and of the person's ability to cope with stress". Following this explanation, the therapist discusses the two main procedures in PE therapy: in vivo exposure and imaginal exposure.

After presenting the treatment rationale, a trauma history is obtained in order to identify the traumas that require processing. Breathing retraining is then practiced to reduce severe distress that might ensue from the discussion about the traumatic events. In the second session the therapist provides psycho-education about common reactions to trauma (e.g., intrusive thoughts about the trauma and avoidance) and gathers information about the patient's symptoms. Psycho-education helps to normalize and validate PTSD symptoms. In this session the therapist discusses the rationale for in vivo exposure. This rationale includes the following points: In vivo exposure will help break your habit of reducing your distress by avoidance or escape from the distressing situation; it will disconfirm your expectations that the situation is dangerous and that it will cause you harm; it will provide you with the experience that distress does not remain forever, but rather distress and anxiety decrease while you are in the situation; and it will teach you that you can successfully cope with distress. Following the presentation of the rationale a hierarchical list of avoided trauma-related situations and objects is built. Three types of activities are commonly included in this hierarchical list: (a) situations, activities, places, and objects the patient is avoiding because he perceives them as dangerous (e.g., going to crowded places); (b) situations, activities, and places that are avoided because they trigger trauma-related distressing memories or feelings (i.e., certain odors); (c) activities that the patient tends to avoid due to lack of interest and pleasure (behavioral activation exercises such as seeing friends or listening to music). As a homework assignment the patient is requested to gradually expose himself to these situations, objects, activities, and places. Examples of in vivo homework are going to safe places after dark, or shopping in a mall during the day when it is crowded.

In session three the therapist presents the rationale for imaginal exposure. Prolonged and repeated recounting of the traumatic memory helps the following: Revisiting and recounting your most upsetting traumatic memory will help you process and organize the memory of the trauma and gain new perspective on it; It will also help you distinguish between thinking about the trauma and actually re-encountering it; it results in habituation of the distress associated with the memory so that the trauma can be remembered without intense anxiety; it helps you realize that thinking about the trauma will not cause you to "go crazy" or "fall apart"; and finally, it will help enhance your sense of self-control and personal competence.

After presenting the rationale, the patient is asked to recount the traumatic memory with eyes closed, in present tense. The patient recounts the traumatic memory for 30–40 min. The recounting of the memory is recorded and the patient is asked to listen to it as homework assignments every day in the same manner that he does during the session. Following exposure, the therapist and the patient process the traumatic memory by directing the patients to express their experience during the imaginal exposure and discuss any new insight that they gained during the imaginal exposure.

From session six the imaginal exposure is conducted focusing on "hot spots" (the most distressing parts of the traumatic memory) and repeating them again and again for about 30 min. In the last session, patient and therapist review the progress that has been made and discuss how the perception of the trauma and the world and oneself has changed. Specifically, the therapist and the patient discuss how the patient's ability to revisit the traumatic memories without "falling apart" have changed their perception of themselves as weak and unable to cope with stress to a perception that they are able to successfully deal with stress. Similarly, they discuss how in vivo exposure taught the patient that they are able to cope successfully with distress and that the situations they avoided are not dangerous, thus replacing their view that the world is entirely dangerous with the view that the world can be sometimes dangerous, but for the most part it is safe.

Effectiveness and Efficacy of PE

PE therapy for PTSD has been found effective in reducing PTSD symptoms in many RCTs in a wide range of trauma (e.g., rape, nonsexual violence, combat, terror, motor vehicle accidents, etc., see Cahill et al., 2009). PE is effective for both chronic PTSD even decades after the traumatic event (e.g., Foa et al., 1999, 2005; Nacasch et al., 2010) and acute stress disorder (Bryant, Sackville, Dang, Moulds, & Guthrie, 1999; Foa, Zoellner, & Feeny, 2006). Patients treated with PE generally maintain their gains at follow-ups of a year or more (e.g., Foa et al., 2005; Nacasch et al., 2007, 2010). PE is effective for both single and multiple traumas (e.g., combat, child sexual abuse) (Foa, 2011; Schnurr et al., 2007). PE is more effective in reducing PTSD symptoms compared to relaxation training (Marks, Lovell, Noshirvani, Livanou, & Thrasher, 1998; Taylor et al., 2003; Vaughan et al., 1994), supportive counseling (Bryant, Moulds, & Nixon, 2003; Schnurr et al., 2007), "treatment as usual" including pharmacotherapy (Asukai, Saito, Tsuruta, Kishimoto, & Nishikawa, 2010; Nacasch et al., 2010), and a non-exposure-based individual psychotherapy (Boudewyns, Hyer, Woods, Harrison, & McCranie, 1990).

The combination of PE with other techniques (stress inoculation training, cognitive restructuring) did not augment the effectiveness of PE alone (Foa et al., 1999, 2005).

Resick, Nishith, Weaver, Astin, and Feuer (2002), compared 9 sessions of PE to 12 sessions of cognitive processing therapy (CPT) and to a wait-list. Both PE and CPT were superior to wait-list, but there was no significant difference in outcome between PE and CPT.

Several randomized controlled trials (RCTs) which compared EMDR to PE found no significant difference between the two (e.g., Power et al., 2002; Rothbaum, Astin, & Marsteller, 2005) while other studies found PE superior to EMDR (Taylor et al., 2003). Others found that EMDR was only as effective as PE when in vivo exposure was added to the standard EMDR protocol (Forbes et al., 2007). Still other comparative treatment studies failed to find significant differences between PE and cognitive therapy (Bryant et al., 2003, 2008; Marks et al., 1998). In conclusion, a large number of RCTs—the largest number of any psychological treatment for PTSD, indicate that PE is effective in reducing PTSD symptoms in a wide range of populations and across various countries and cultures (Cahill et al., 2009). Moreover, its efficacy was shown in studies conducted by independent research groups from different countries and cultures (Asukai, Saito, Tsuruta, Ogami, & Kishimoto, 2008). In addition, it is effective also with patients who suffer from comorbid diagnoses such as depression, personality disorders, and alcohol dependence (Foa, Hembree, & Rothbaum, 2007). The structured and simple manual of PE treatment can be easily taught to clinicians with no CBT background following a 3–4 day workshop along with weekly supervision. Foa (2006) trained community therapists in an organization "Woman Organized Against Rape" (WOAR). These therapists were as effective in their delivery of PE as were therapists at the Center for the Treatment and Study of Anxiety (CTSA). In the past decade PE has been successfully disseminated worldwide (Asukai et al., 2010; Nacasch et al., 2010) and was chosen to be one of the two treatments disseminated in the veterans administration (VA) in the USA. This was as a result of the finding that the war in Afghanistan and Iraq has raised the need for effective and short treatment for large number of veterans who suffer from PTSD. Studies indicate successful dissemination in the VA (Schnurr et al., 2007; Tuerk et al., 2011).

Recent meta-analyses were conducted under the auspices of the Institute of Medicine (2008). The review committee considered 24 controlled studies of some form of exposure therapy: alone, or in combination with SIT or CT; 10 studies of EMDR; three studies of CT; and four studies of coping skills training, which included SIT treatment and relaxation control conditions. Consistent with the previous reviews, the IOM concluded regarding exposure therapy that "the evidence is sufficient to conclude the efficacy of exposure therapies in the treatment of PTSD" (p. 8).

References

American Psychiatric Association. (2006). *American Psychiatric Association practice guidelines for the treatment of psychiatric disorders: Compendium 2006*. Arlington, VA: Author.

Asukai, N., Saito, A., Tsuruta, N., Kishimoto, J., & Nishikawa, T. (2010). Efficacy of exposure therapy for Japanese patients with posttraumatic stress disorder due to mixed traumatic events: A randomized controlled study. *Journal of Traumatic Stress, 21*(3), 340–343.

Asukai, N., Saito, A., Tsuruta, N., Ogami, R., & Kishimoto, J. (2008). Pilot study on prolonged exposure of Japanese patients with posttraumatic stress disorder due to mixed traumatic events. *Journal of Traumatic Stress, 21*, 340–343.

Boudewyns, P. A., Hyer, L., Woods, M. G., Harrison, W. R., & McCranie, E. (1990). PTSD among Vietnam veterans: An early look at treatment outcome using direct therapeutic exposure. *Journal of Traumatic Stress, 3*, 359–368.

Bryant, R. A., Mastrodomenico, J., Felmingham, K. L., Hopwood, S., Kenny, L., Kandris, E., et al. (2008). Treatment of acute stress disorder: A randomized controlled trial. *Archives of General Psychiatry, 65*, 659–667.

Bryant, R. A., Moulds, M. L., & Nixon, R. V. D. (2003). Cognitive behaviour therapy of acute stress disorder: A four-year follow-up. *Behaviour Research and Therapy, 41*, 489–494.

Bryant, R. A., Sackville, T., Dang, S. T., Moulds, M., & Guthrie, R. (1999). Treating acute stress disorder: An evaluation of cognitive behavior therapy and supportive counseling techniques. *American Journal of Psychiatry, 156*, 1780–1786.

Cahill, S. P., Rothbaum, B. O., Resick, P. A., & Follette, V. M. (2009). Cognitive behavioral therapy for adults. In E. B. Foa, T. M. Keane, M. J. Friedman, & J. A. Cohen (Eds.), *Effective treatments for PTSD: Practice guidelines from the International Society for Traumatic Stress Studies* (pp. 139–222). New York: Guilford.

Foa, E. B. (2006). Psychosocial therapy for posttraumatic stress disorder. *Journal of Clinical Psychiatry, 67*, 40–45.

Foa, E. B. (2011, October). *Prolonged exposure for PTSD*. Workshop presented at the University of Pennsylvania, Philadelphia, PA.

Foa, E. B., Dancu, C. V., Hembree, E. A., Jaycox, L. H., Meadows, E. A., & Street, G. P. (1999). A comparison of exposure therapy, stress inoculation training, and their combination for reducing posttraumatic stress disorder in female assault victims. *Journal of Consulting and Clinical Psychology, 67*, 194–200.

Foa, E. B., Hembree, E. A., Cahill, S. P., Rauch, S. A., Riggs, D. S., Feeny, N. C., et al. (2005). Randomized trial of prolonged exposure for PTSD with and without cognitive restructuring: Outcome at academic and community clinics. *Journal of Consulting and Clinical Psychology, 73*, 953–964.

Foa, E. B., Hembree, E. A., & Rothbaum, B. O. (2007). *Prolonged exposure for PTSD: Emotional processing of traumatic experiences*. New York: Oxford University Press.

Foa, E. B., & Kozak, M. J. (1985). Treatment of anxiety disorders: Implications for psychopathology. In E. H. Tuma & J. D. Maser (Eds.), *Anxiety and the anxiety disorders* (pp. 421–452). Hillsdale, NJ: Erlbaum.

Foa, E. B., & Kozak, M. J. (1986). Emotional processing of fear: Exposure to corrective information. *Psychological Bulletin, 99*, 20–35.

Foa, E. B., & Rothbaum, B. O. (1998). *Treating the trauma of rape: Cognitive behavioral therapy for PTSD*. New York: Guilford Press.

Foa, E. B., Zoellner, L. A., & Feeny, N. C. (2006). An evaluation of three brief programs for facilitating recovery after assault. *Journal of Traumatic Stress, 19*(1), 29–43.

Forbes, D., Creamer, M., Phelps, A., Bryant, R., McFarlane, A., Devilly, G. J., et al. (2007). Australian guidelines for the treatment of adults with acute stress disorder and post-traumatic stress disorder. *Australian and New Zealand Journal of Psychiatry, 41*, 637–648.

Institute of Medicine. (2008). *Treatment of posttraumatic stress disorder: An assessment of the evidence*. Washington, DC: National Academies Press.

Marks, I., Lovell, K., Noshirvani, H., Livanou, M., & Thrasher, S. (1998). Treatment of posttraumatic stress disorder by exposure and/or cognitive restructuring: A controlled study. *Archives of General Psychiatry, 55*, 317–325.

Nacasch, N., Foa, E. B., Fostick, L., Polliack, M., Dinstein, Y., Tzur, D., et al. (2007). Prolonged exposure therapy for chronic combat-related PTSD: A case report of five veterans. *CNS Spectrums, 12*, 690–695.

Nacasch, N., Foa, E. B., Huppert, J. D., Tzur, D., Fostick, L., Dinstein, Y., et al. (2010). Prolonged exposure therapy for combat and terror-related posttraumatic stress disorder: A randomized control comparison with treatment as usual. *Journal of Clinical Psychiatry, 72*, 1174–1180.

Power, K., McGoldrick, T., Brown, K., Buchanan, R., Sharp, D., Swanson, V., et al. (2002). A controlled comparison of eye movement desensitization and reprocessing versus exposure plus cognitive restructuring versus waiting list in the treatment of post-traumatic stress disorder. *Clinical Psychology and Psychotherapy, 9*, 299–318.

Resick, P. A., Nishith, P., Weaver, T. L., Astin, M. C., & Feuer, C. A. (2002). A comparison of cognitive processing therapy with prolonged exposure and a waiting condition for the treatment of chronic posttraumatic stress disorder in female rape victims. *Journal of Consulting and Clinical Psychology, 70*, 867–879.

Rothbaum, B. O., Astin, M. C., & Marsteller, F. (2005). Prolonged exposure versus eye movement desensitization and reprocessing (EMDR) for PTSD rape victims. *Journal of Traumatic Stress, 18*, 607–616.

Schnurr, P. P., Friedman, M. J., Engel, C. C., Foa, E. B., Shea, M. T., Chow, B. K., et al. (2007). Cognitive behavioral therapy for posttraumatic stress disorder in women: A randomized controlled trial. *Journal of the American Medical Association, 297*, 820–830.

Taylor, S., Thordarson, D. S., Maxfield, L., Federoff, I. C., Lovell, K., & Ogrodniczuk, J. (2003). Efficacy, speed, and adverse effects of three PTSD treatments: Exposure therapy, relaxation training, and EMDR. *Journal of Consulting and Clinical Psychology, 71*, 330–338.

Tuerk, P. W., Yoder, M., Grubaugh, A., Myrick, H., Hamner, M., & Acierno, R. (2011). Prolonged exposure therapy for combat-related posttraumatic stress disorder: An examination of treatment effectiveness for veterans of the wars in Afghanistan and Iraq. *Journal of Anxiety Disorders, 25*, 397–403.

Vaughan, K., Armstrong, M. S., Gold, R., O'Connor, N., Jenneke, W., & Tarrier, N. (1994). A trial of eye movement desensitization compared to image habituation training and applied muscle relaxation in posttraumatic stress disorder. *Journal of Behavior Therapy and Experimental Psychiatry, 25*, 283–291.

Chapter 12
Cognitive Processing Therapy: Beyond the Basics

Kathleen M. Chard and Kristen H. Walter

Within the past 20 years substantial research has emerged suggesting that brief cognitive-behavioral (CBT) interventions for posttraumatic stress disorder (PTSD) can yield long-term gains in patients' psychosocial, psychological, and even physical functioning (Schnurr et al., 2008). In fact, recent studies have shown that 12–20 sessions of CBT appear to be effective in helping patients manage their distress not only during treatment, but also up to 5 years after completing therapy (Resick et al., 2008; Tarrier & Sommerfield, 2004). The purpose of this chapter is to review the literature regarding one form of CBT, cognitive processing therapy (CPT), including an overview of the therapy, randomized controlled trials, effectiveness data, theoretical implications, and dissemination data.

CPT was created in 1988 as a manualized cognitive-behavioral protocol to treat PTSD and related symptoms in rape survivors (Resick & Schnicke, 1992). CPT consists of 12 weekly sessions delivered in a manualized, serial format. In sessions

K.M. Chard, Ph.D. (✉)
Trauma Recovery Center, Cincinnati VA Medical Center – Ft. Thomas Division, 1000 South Fort Thomas Avenue, Ft. Thomas, KY 41075, USA

PTSD & Anxiety Disorders Clinic, Cincinnati VA Medical Center, 1000 S. Ft. Thomas Avenue, Ft. Thomas, KY 41075, USA

Department of Psychiatry and Behavioral Neuroscience, University of Cincinnati College of Medicine, 3235 Eden Avenue, CARE/Crawley Building Suite E-870, Cincinnati, OH 45267, USA

Cincinnati VA Medical Center, Cincinnati, OH, USA
e-mail: Kathleen.Chard@va.gov

K.H. Walter, Ph.D.
Veterans Medical Research Foundation, VA San Diego Healthcare System, 3350 La Jolla Village Dr. (111N-1), Building 13, San Diego, CA 92161, USA

Cincinnati VA Medical Center, Cincinnati, OH, USA
e-mail: Kristen.Walter@va.gov

M.P. Safir et al. (eds.), *Future Directions in Post-Traumatic Stress Disorder*, DOI 10.1007/978-1-4899-7522-5_12

1–4 the individual is given information regarding the theory behind CPT and is asked to write an impact statement discussing why they believe the traumatic event occurred and how the event has shaped their beliefs about self, others, and the world, particularly in the areas related to safety, trust, power/control, esteem, and intimacy. Next, the individual learns about the connection between events, thoughts, and feelings through the use of the A-B-C Sheet, and they begin to identify places where they have become "stuck" in their thinking. Clients are taught the ways in which people can become derailed in their thinking about traumatic events, and the underlying concepts of assimilation (taking in the new information without changing preexisting beliefs), over-accommodation (changing beliefs about the self and the world to extremes), and accommodation (modifying preexisting beliefs to incorporate new information) are introduced to clients in lay language. Finally, the client writes detailed accounts of the most traumatic incident including sensory details, thoughts, and feelings. [Note: in the CPT—cognitive only version no traumatic accounts are written]. The therapist employs Socratic dialogue to help the client begin to analyze their "stuck points" and to view past events with a more balanced interpretation.

In sessions 5–7, the core cognitive therapy skills are taught, including using the Challenging Questions Worksheet to examine a single belief. The Patterns of Problematic Thinking Sheet is then introduced to allow the client to become familiar with common faulty thinking patterns that can interfere with recovery from PTSD. Finally, the client is taught the Challenging Beliefs Worksheet which brings all of the prior worksheets together and allows the client to look at their original beliefs, challenge them, and provide alternative beliefs while also noting their change in emotions.

Sessions 8–12 allow the individual to focus their thought examination in each of five key areas including safety, trust, power/control, esteem, and intimacy using the Challenging Beliefs Worksheets. For session 12 the individual rewrites their impact statement and compares it to the version written for session two. This allows the client to clearly recognize the changes in their thoughts, feelings, and behaviors. Finally, the therapist and client look to the future and identify any areas that may continue to be problematic for the client and discuss ways that the client can manage these issues.

The first study of CPT was published in 1992 comparing group CPT to a naturally occurring wait-list and the first therapist manual, *Cognitive Processing Therapy for Rape Victims*, was published in 1992 (Resick & Schnicke, 1992). Since that time numerous controlled and clinic efficacy-based studies have been performed using CPT to treat PTSD related to a variety of traumatic incidents.

The Efficacy of CPT for Reducing PTSD and Trauma-Related Symptoms

Randomized clinical trials are considered the gold standard approach for investigating the efficacy of a treatment. CPT has been examined in rigorous studies and shown to be efficacious in reducing symptoms of PTSD and related symptoms, such as depression, and support the delivery of CPT in individual, group, and group and individual modalities. In the first controlled trial examining CPT in an individualized format, Resick et al. (2002) compared CPT, prolonged exposure (PE), and a minimal attention wait-list among female rape victims. The study demonstrated that among all women intended to be treated in the study, individuals receiving CPT and PE significantly decreased their symptoms of PTSD and depression over the course of treatment. However, individuals receiving CPT showed a greater decrease in PTSD symptoms, albeit a small difference. The findings were even more pronounced for individuals who received a full dose of treatment. Individuals receiving CPT and PE again evidenced significant differences in symptom reduction as compared to the minimal attention wait-list; however, there were no differences between CPT and PE. Overall, CPT and PE did not significantly differ from one another with regard to decreasing PTSD and depression symptoms. There was a trend for CPT to have greater effect sizes for good end-state functioning (at or below 20 on the PSS and at or below 10 on the BDI) at assessments until the 9-month assessment, where no difference emerged between the two active treatment conditions.

CPT has also been shown to significantly reduce PTSD symptom severity among veterans. Monson et al. (2006) compared CPT to a wait-list condition and found that CPT resulted in a significantly greater reduction in PTSD symptom severity across time. Furthermore, individuals who received CPT were significantly less likely to meet diagnostic criteria for PTSD following treatment. Further examination of the PTSD symptom clusters indicated that re-experiencing and numbing symptoms improved; however, behavioral avoidance and hyperarousal symptoms did not improve as compared to wait-list. Thus, CPT appears to be particularly effective for reducing re-experiencing and emotional numbing symptoms of PTSD.

In addition to reducing clinical symptoms of PTSD and depression, studies have demonstrated that CPT reduces trauma-related emotions and symptoms, such as guilt, affect control, social adjustment, and physical health complaints. Resick et al. (2002) in their randomized controlled trial showed that CPT and PE differed from the minimal attention wait-list on guilt subscales of global guilt, hindsight bias, lack of justification, and wrongdoing. Individuals receiving CPT reported greater decreases in hindsight bias and lack of justification than the PE or the minimal attention groups following treatment. CPT evidenced a large effect for guilt cognitions and PE revealed a medium effect size among the intent-to-treat sample. Among treatment completers, CPT demonstrated very large effects for reducing guilt cognitions and moderate to large effects for CPT as compared to PE at posttreatment and 9 months following treatment. Further analysis of this data revealed that CPT was effective in reducing guilt among participants with only a diagnosis of PTSD and those with a diagnosis of PTSD and major depressive disorder. Additionally, findings indicate that CPT was more effective than PE in reducing guilt-related distress among these clinical subgroups.

Similar results were noted among veterans, as Monson et al. (2006) found that participants who received CPT, as compared to a wait-list condition, had significant reductions in trauma-related guilt distress. This finding supports those by Resick et al. (2008), who showed that participants with high guilt cognition ratings at pretreatment had a greater rate of change in PTSD severity over the course of the study. These findings suggest that the cognitive restructuring component of CPT may specifically target guilt-related cognitions and distress by challenging over-accommodated beliefs. Of note, the Monson et al. (2006) study examined veterans, which is a population that may particularly benefit from therapy addressing guilt-related cognitions resulting from combat experience.

CPT has also yielded improvements in other important areas of psychological functioning and physical health. Monson et al. (2006) revealed that veterans receiving CPT significantly improved their affect control, alexithymia, and social adjustment as compared to the wait-list condition. Research also supports the use of CPT in reducing health complaints among treated individuals. Galovski, Monson, Bruce, and Resick (2009) compared participants who completed either CPT or PE. Both groups evidenced significant improvement on health-related complaints. However, CPT treatment completers showed significantly more physical health improvements than the PE condition, yielding a moderate effect size. The study also explored the effects of treatment on sleep quality and results showed that there were significant improvements across assessments, but no significant differences emerged between the CPT and PE conditions. Thus, results suggest that CPT is superior to PE in reduction health-related complaints but comparable to PE in improving sleep quality.

Identifying the Active Components of CPT

After the randomized clinical trial comparing CPT, PE, and a wait-list control condition, a dismantling study was conducted to determine the relative value of the active components in CPT (Resick et al., 2008). This study compared three conditions: cognitive therapy only (CPT-C), written accounts only (WA), and the full CPT protocol. Participants received 2 h of therapy per week for 6 weeks. The sample consisted of 150 women who met criteria for PTSD based on a sexual or physical assault. Exclusionary criteria included current psychosis, danger to self or others, current substance dependence, or medication changes within the 3 months prior to entering the study.

Several findings emerged from the CPT dismantling study. It is important to note that the three conditions did not differ on pretreatment symptom measures and that, overall, symptoms of PTSD and depression significantly improved across all three treatment condition. Despite global improvement, several notable differences were evident. First, no significant differences emerged between individuals who received the full CPT protocol and those who received CPT-C over the course of the study. Second, CPT differed from the WA condition on self-reported PTSD symptoms only at the posttreatment assessment, with those receiving CPT having significantly lower scores. Third, participants receiving CPT-C significantly differed from the WA conditions at most assessments during treatment on self-reported PTSD symptoms and evidenced a trend on self-reported symptoms of depression, with those in the CPT-C condition reporting lower symptom scores.

Table 12.1 Comparison of CPT versus CPT-C session flow

CPT	CPT-C
1. Introduction and education	1. Introduction and education
2. Meaning of the event	2. Meaning of the event
3. Identification of thoughts and feelings (ABC)	3. Identification of thoughts and feelings (ABC)
4. Remembering traumatic events	4. Identification of stuck points (ABC)
5. Remembering traumatic events	5. Challenging questions
6. Challenging questions	6. Patterns of problematic thinking
7. Patterns of problematic thinking	7. Challenging beliefs
8. CBW safety issues	8. Safety issues
9. Trust issues	9. Trust issues
10. Power/control issues	10. Power/control issues
11. Esteem issues	11. Esteem issues
12. Intimacy issues and meaning of the event	12. Intimacy issues and meaning of the event

Diagnostic status and treatment completion were also evaluated in this study. Among the intent-to-treatment sample, participants receiving CPT-C were slightly more likely to no longer meet criteria for PTSD at posttreatment. However, the groups did not differ with regard to PTSD diagnostic status at 6-month follow-up. Among individuals who completed treatment, there were no significant differences between the treatment groups at any assessment time point. The study also examined the magnitude of the differences between the conditions, which yielded small effect sizes for participants only receiving assessments, medium effect sizes for participants who received partial treatment, and large effect sizes for the intent-to-treat and completer samples. Overall, the study demonstrated that the combination of cognitive therapy and written account (CPT) did not incrementally improve upon the results of each component alone. Individuals in the CPT-C treatment condition reported lower symptom scores than the WA condition; this finding suggests that the cognitive component appears to be the factor contributing to the greatest symptom reduction. Furthermore, the greatest symptom reduction was associated with receiving a full dose of treatment among the three conditions. A comparison of the session flow for CPT and CPT-C is included in Table 12.1.

Consistent with the finding that the cognitive restructuring appears to be the primary active components of CPT, Sobel, Resick, and Rabalais (2009) assessed the change in cognitions among rape survivors over the course of CPT. The investigators assessed this change by comparing the content of the two impact statements. This study indicated that there was a significant increase in the number of accommodated clauses in the final impact statement; and the number and percent of accommodated clauses were significantly negatively related to a change in self-reported PTSD symptoms. In other words, the more an individual is able to change their thinking to accommodate new information, the greater their decrease of PTSD symptoms. The study also showed a significant decrease in the number of over-accommodated, assimilated, informational, and total clauses. The percent of over-accommodated clauses were significantly positively related to a change in self-reported PTSD symptoms. Thus, the better able individuals are to alter their drastic change of beliefs, the greater their decrease in PTSD symptoms. Findings from this study provide support for the theoretical rationale for CPT in that modifying existing beliefs to more accurately reflect the traumatic experience results in a decrease PTSD symptoms.

Who Does CPT Work for?

Several studies have examined predictor variables regarding treatment outcome, including treatment dropout. Rizvi, Vogt, and Resick (2009) investigated factors related to cognition (level of education, intelligence, and age) and mood states associated with PTSD (anger, guilt, and depression) on treatment outcome. These variables were examined as they were hypothesized to affect the ability to adopt new ways of thinking and that negative mood states may interfere with the processing of traumatic memories. The study demonstrated that level of education, intelligence, and age did not affect treatment efficacy for the entire sample. Furthermore, age was related to treatment outcome when analyzed by treatment condition (CPT and PE). Younger age was associated with the best outcomes in CPT, whereas older age was related to the best outcomes in PE. These findings are consistent with those of Resick et al.'s (2008), whose additional findings revealed a trend for older age to be related to poorer treatment outcome in CPT.

Results also indicated that comorbid negative mood states did not affect treatment efficacy, suggesting that these mood states do not interfere with the emotional and cognitive processing of traumatic memories. Although higher depression and guilt scores were associated with higher PTSD symptom scores, participants evidenced a proportional reduction in PTSD over time, resulting in comparable scores to those with lower levels of depression and guilt. These findings again were similar to those of Resick et al. (2008), suggesting that higher scores on negative comorbid mood states were still able to show improvement in PTSD symptom scores.

Several factors emerged in relation to treatment dropout. Younger age and lower intelligence were related to treatment dropout, which is consistent with findings by Resick et al. (2008). Participants with lower education also trended towards greater rates of treatment dropout. Higher trait anger did not impact CPT; however, participants with higher trait anger were more likely to drop out of PE.

Iverson, Resick, Suvak, Walling, and Taft (2011) examined the influence of current interpersonal violence (IPV), which was defined as experiencing an act of IPV within the past year, on treatment outcome among women. The study showed that those who experienced current IPV were less likely to begin treatment than those who did not experience current IPV. However, if women who experienced current IPV did begin treatment, IPV was not predictive of treatment completion. Results also indicated that women who experienced more frequent IPV showed greater reductions in PTSD and depression symptoms over the course of treatment. However, their symptom levels at the 6-month follow-up were comparable to those who experienced less frequent IPV. Collectively, these findings suggest that if women who experienced current IPV engage in CPT—including those who experience frequent IPV—are able to reduce their PTSD and depression symptoms over the course of the study and at follow-up.

Modifications of CPT for Specific Populations

Alterations have been made to the original CPT format to accommodate various populations. As the dismantling study (Resick et al., 2008) illustrated, CPT (cognitive therapy and the written account) did not improve upon the results of either component alone and the cognitive aspect of CPT (CPT-C) yielded significantly lower scores than the written account condition. In sum, this finding indicates that CPT-C is an effective modification of CPT for treating PTSD. CPT-C may be the preferred treatment option when individuals are noncompliant with the written account, lack a clear memory of the traumatic event, or have significant writing difficulties. Furthermore, CPT-C has been demonstrated to be effective for veterans with PTSD and a history of traumatic brain injury (TBI; Chard, Schumm, McIlvain, Bailey, & Parkinson, 2011), particularly with moderate to severe histories of TBI where lasting impairments are more commonly experienced.

CPT has also been adapted for child abuse survivors (CPT-SA; Chard, 2005). This adaptation was developed to address particular issues often presented by child abuse survivors, including attachment and developmental history. Topic areas added to the adapted protocol include sexual intimacy, assertiveness/communication, and social support. The CPT-SA protocol includes seventeen 90-min group therapy sessions and 60-min individual therapy sessions for the first 9 weeks of treatment and then again during the last week (session 17). The format is designed to allow patients to fully process their traumatic events with their individual therapist, which also decreases the risk of vicarious traumatization in group therapy sessions. Furthermore, individual therapy sessions are not scheduled from weeks 10 to 16, which encourages the patient to rely on the group and their own coping strategies—rather than the therapist. The group format also encourages appropriate social interactions and the opportunities to practice skills learned in the context of therapy.

Chard (2005) compared CPT-SA to a minimal attention wait-list control group. Results indicated that individuals who received CPT-SA showed significant improvement on clinician-assessed PTSD symptoms and self-reported PTSD, depressive, and dissociation symptoms. Furthermore, findings showed large effect sizes for change for the CPT-SA group as compared to the minimal attention group. In addition to changes from pre- to posttreatment, positive treatment outcomes regarding PTSD, depression, and dissociation remained for at least 1 year following treatment completion.

CPT has also been employed as a treatment modality for traumatized refugees in a community setting and shown to be an effective treatment (Schulz, Resick, Huber, & Griffin, 2006). This finding is particularly noteworthy as traumatized refugees often experience numerous and severe traumatic events, increasing their risk for developing psychological problems (Nicholl & Thompson, 2004). The Schulz et al. (2006) study evaluated 53 refugees who had pre- and posttreatment data. None of the participants were fluent in English and interpreters were utilized for approximately half of the participants. Several modifications were made to accommodate special considerations for this population. First, the majority of treatment sessions (83 %) occurred in the participant's homes. A second modification was that the length of treatment and duration of sessions were negotiated. The average length of sessions was 1.5–2 h and the average number of sessions was 17 (which included 3–4 assessment sessions). It should be noted that the number of sessions negotiated was comparable to the established 12 sessions in the CPT manual although the duration of sessions differed.

Results from the Schulz et al. (2006) study showed a significant decrease in PTSD symptom scores from pre- to posttreatment (effect size 2.6) for the entire sample. Additionally, participants who received CPT with the use of an interpreter were compared to those participants who did not have an interpreter involved in their treatment. These findings indicated that these groups did not differ on age, education, or the mean number of sessions. However, participants who received treatment without the use of an interpreter received more hours of therapy and also had a greater decrease in PTSD symptom scores (effect size 3.4) compared to participants whose treatment was delivered through the use of an interpreter (effect size 2.0). Overall, results indicated that CPT was highly effective for the overall sample, but that participants who received CPT without the use of an interpreter evidenced greater gains than those whose treatment involved an interpreter.

Implications for Trauma Theory

Many clinicians have hypothesized that exposure to the traumatic memory is necessary for a successful treatment outcome and that the mechanism of change was through habituation of the fear network and extinction of the traumatic response (i.e., the amygdala hijacking hypothesis; Gurvits et al. 2000). The findings regarding cognitive therapy without exposure bring this into question and suggest that there may be other mechanisms of change. An alternative route might be through cognitive therapy and a distanced perspective taking. For example, Kross and Ayduk (2008) compared a self-immersed versus self-distanced perspective on emotion (e.g., what versus why). The distanced perspective allowed "cool" reflection and less "hot" negative emotions. Those who had a distanced perspective reported lower negative affect, less rumination, and lower blood pressure. This research might explain why guilt and anger have been associated with poorer outcome with exposure therapy and a better outcome with cognitive therapy, including CPT. Several studies are under way that will examine this and other treatment issues in more detail, including CPT for PTSD and chronic pain, CPT combined with hypnosis, group versus individual CPT, variable length CPT, and CPT via telemedicine to name a few.

Dissemination of CPT

The United States Department of Veterans Affairs (VA) began an initiative disseminating CPT across the VA system in 2007 as collaboration between the VA Office of Mental Health Services (OMHS) and the National Center for PTSD (NCPTSD) (Karlin et al., 2010). The goal of these efforts is to increase access for all interested veterans seeking CPT treatment by ensuring that all veterans have access to CPT at their VA clinic.

In Phase I, a Military/Veteran version of the treatment manual was created, followed by a Trainer's Manual and a Consultant's Manual. Training videos demonstrating CPT with actual patients were created and a Train the Trainers conference led by Drs. Patricia Resick, Candice Monson, and Kathleen Chard was held with 15 trainers. In Phase II, 22 conferences were held and consultation calls were made available 25 h a week. A website was created hosting downloadable materials, a discussion board, and the consultation call schedule. Finally advanced lectures were held via teleconferencing. Program evaluation was conducted in May of 2009 showing that 2,469 individuals had been trained and 244 individuals had signed up for consultation calls. When asked how often individuals utilized the full protocol 25.6 % said Always, 47.5 % said Usually, 15.6 % said Sometimes, and 11.3 % said Never. In Phase III, the CPT Veteran/Military: Group Manual (Chard, Resick, Monson, & Kattar, 2008) and related training videos were created and another 16 workshops were conducted, including an optional third day of group training. A web-based CPT enhancement course was also developed to facilitate adoption. Finally in Phase IV in addition to 3-day workshops, the training staff offered two 4-day regional Train the Trainer workshops to 30 VA clinicians and four 2-day refresher courses for clinicians who were unable to implement CPT after their initial training.

To date there have been 2,106 official rollout participants, 233 who have attended rollout refreshers, 748 attended non-rollout VA workshops, 171 Vet Center workshops, and 416 community attendees, for a total of 3,674 total workshop participants. Furthermore, 1,543 individuals have attended consultation calls since October of 2007 and 762 participants have completed all training and consultation requirements and are considered "CPT providers." Future goals for the initiative include additional national and regional trainers and the addition of more regional trainers to make the access to training and consultation even easier for therapists throughout the United States. In addition, an online enrichment course will be launched in 2011 offering advanced education in the session by session content of CPT. Last, a similar dissemination initiative was also started in 2010 in the Canadian Veterans Affairs system. Through these efforts veterans all over North America will have access to a gold standard, evidence-based treatment that can help to improve the quality of their life in addition to improving their PTSD.

References

Chard, K. M. (2005). An evaluation of cognitive processing therapy for the treatment of posttraumatic stress disorder related to childhood sexual abuse. *Journal of Consulting and Clinical Psychology, 73*, 965–971.

Chard, K. M., Resick, P. A., Monson, C. M., & Kattar, K. (2008). *Cognitive processing therapy: Veteran/military group manual*. Washington, DC: Department of Veterans Affairs.

Chard, K. M., Schumm, J. A., McIlvain, S. M., Bailey, G. W., & Parkinson, R. B. (2011). Exploring the efficacy of a residential treatment program incorporating cognitive processing therapy-cognitive for veterans with PTSD and traumatic brain injury. *Journal of Traumatic Stress, 24*(3), 347–351.

Galovski, T. E., Monson, C. A., Bruce, S., & Resick, P. A. (2009). Does cognitive-behavioral therapy for PTSD improve perceived health? *Journal of Traumatic Stress, 22*(3), 197–204.

Gurvits, T. V., Gilbertson, M. W., Lasko, N. B., Tarhan, A. S., Simeon, D., Macklin, M. L., et al. (2000). Neurologic soft signs in chronic posttraumatic stress disorder. *Archives of General Psychiatry, 57*, 181–186.

Iverson, K. M., Resick, P. A., Suvak, M. K., Walling, S., & Taft, C. T. (2011). Intimate partner violence exposure predicts PTSD treatment engagement and outcome in cognitive processing therapy. *Behavior Therapy, 42*, 236–248.

Karlin, B. E., Ruzek, J. I., Chard, K. M., Eftekari, A., Monson, C. M., Hembree, E. A., et al. (2010). Dissemination of evidence-based psychological treatments for posttraumatic stress disorder in the Veterans Health Administration. *Journal of Traumatic Stress, 23*, 663–673.

Kross, E., & Ayduk, O. (2008). Facilitating adaptive emotional analysis: Distinguishing distanced-analysis of depressive experiences from immersed-analysis and distraction. *Personality and Social Psychology Bulletin, 34*, 924–938.

Monson, C. M., Schnurr, P. P., Resick, P. A., Friedman, M. J., Young-Xu, Y., & Stevens, S. P. (2006). Cognitive processing therapy for veterans with military-related posttraumatic stress disorder. *Journal of Consulting and Clinical Psychology, 74*, 898–907.

Nicholl, C., & Thompson, A. (2004). The psychological treatment of post traumatic stress disorder (PTSD) in adult refugees: A review of the current state of psychological therapies. *Journal of Mental Health, 13*, 351–362.

Resick, P. A., Galovski, T. E., Uhlmansiek, M. O., Scher, C. D., Clum, G. A., & Young-Xu, Y. (2008). A randomized clinical trial to dismantle components of cognitive processing therapy for posttraumatic stress disorder in female victims of interpersonal violence. *Journal of Consulting and Clinical Psychology, 76*, 243–258.

Resick, P. A., Nishith, P., Weaver, T. L., Astin, M. C., & Feuer, C. A. (2002). A comparison of cognitive processing therapy with prolonged exposure therapy and a waiting list condition for the treatment of chronic posttraumatic stress disorder in female rape victims. *Journal of Consulting and Clinical Psychology, 70*, 867–879.

Resick, P. A., & Schnicke, M. K. (1992). Cognitive processing therapy for sexual assault victims. *Journal of Consulting and Clinical Psychology, 60*, 748–756.

Resick, P. A., Williams, L. F., Suvak, M. K., Monson, C. M., & Gradus, J. L. (2012). Long-term outcomes of cognitive-behavioral treatments for posttraumatic stress disorder among female rape survivors. *Journal of Consulting and Clinical Psychology, 80*(2), 201–210.

Rizvi, S. L., Vogt, D. S., & Resick, P. A. (2009). Cognitive and affective predictors of treatment outcome in cognitive processing therapy and prolonged exposure for posttraumatic stress disorder. *Behaviour Research and Therapy, 47*(9), 737–743.

Schnurr, P. P., Green, B. L., & Kaltman, S. (2008). Trauma exposure and physical health. In M. Friedman, T. Keane, & P. Resick (Eds.), *Handbook of PTSD*. New York: Guilford.

Schulz, P. M., Resick, P. A., Huber, L. C., & Griffin, M. G. (2006). The effectiveness of cognitive processing therapy for PTSD with refugees in a community setting. *Cognitive and Behavioral Practice, 13*, 322–331.

Sobel, A., Resick, P., & Rabalais, A. (2009). The effect of cognitive processing therapy on cognitions: Impact statement coding. *Journal of Traumatic Stress, 22*(3), 205–211.

Tarrier, N., & Sommerfield, C. (2004). Treatment of chronic PTSD by cognitive therapy and exposure: 5-year follow-up. *Behavior Therapy, 35*, 231–246.

Chapter 13
Interpersonal Psychotherapy for PTSD

Alexandra Klein Rafaeli and John C. Markowitz

Introduction

Interpersonal psychotherapy (IPT) is a time-limited, evidence-based treatment that focuses on patients' social and interpersonal functioning, affect, and current life events. IPT helps patients explore affective experiences through the lens of the social and the interpersonal, and offers techniques to help the patient translate feelings into interpersonal interventions that ameliorate functioning in those domains.

The late Gerald Klerman, MD, and Myrna Weissman, PhD, developed the original IPT protocol intending to operationalize a form of psychotherapy for major depressive disorder. In developing this approach, Klerman and Weisman followed theorists such as Adolf Meyer, Harry Stack Sulllivan, and John Bowlby, who viewed social interactions with others as a profound source of understanding one's psychological distress. They were equally interested in the psychosocial data linking life circumstances and mood (Markowitz & Weissman, 2012a, 2012b; Weissman, 2006). IPT focused on helping patients name their emotions and translate them into interpersonal behaviors with other people. This approach both relieved depressive symptoms and improved social skills.

A.K. Rafaeli, Psy.D. (✉)
The Ruth and Allen Ziegler Student Services Division, Tel Aviv University, Tel Aviv, Israel

The New School of Psychotherapy, Tel Aviv, Israel
e-mail: alexandrar@post.tau.ac.il

J.C. Markowitz, M.D.
New York State Psychiatric Institute, New York, NY, USA

Columbia University College of Physicians & Surgeons,
1051 Riverside Drive, Unit #129, New York, NY 10032, USA
e-mail: jcm42@columbia.edu

M.P. Safir et al. (eds.), *Future Directions in Post-Traumatic Stress Disorder*,
DOI 10.1007/978-1-4899-7522-5_13

Since Klerman and Weissman's development of the original IPT protocol, there has been growing evidence that social support is important for both physical and psychological health, and in fact, is shown to help people reduce psychological distress (Markowitz, Milrod, Blieberg, & Randall, 2009; Taylor, 2011), yet supportive networks are not necessarily beneficial. For one to have the perception of being cared for, the urge to reciprocate support, and the desire to be included in a supportive social network, the desired social support has to match the support received (Cutrona & Russell, 1990). Thus, the aim in IPT is to guide the patient to recent interpersonal incidents and to explore them in the patient's life outside the office—both for emotional content and practical options that might produce constructive change.

IPT has been supported by numerous clinical trials over the last 40 years, and it continues to be applied and adapted across cultures, pathologies, and modalities (Markowitz & Weissman, 2012a, 2012b; Verdeli et al., 2003; Weissman et al., 2006). Specifically, IPT has demonstrated efficacy in treating a spectrum of depressive disorders, (Frank, 2005; Markowitz, 1996; Weissman & Markowitz, 1998) as well as Bulimia Nervosa (Fairburn, Jones, Peveler, Hope, & O'Connor, 1993; Weissman & Markowitz, 1998) and has been modified for use with adolescents (Mufson et al., 1993) and older adults (Hinrichsen, 1999). IPT is also currently included in both American and International guidelines as a recommended first-line treatment for major depression and bulimia nervosa (American Psychiatric Association, 2004; National Collaborating Centre for Mental Health, 2004). Among the many contemporary adaptations, is the use of IPT for PTSD, for which there is promising pilot data (Bleiberg & Markowitz, 2005; Campanini et al., 2010; Graf & Markowitz, 2012; Krupnick et al., 2008; Rafaeli & Markowitz, 2011; Ray & Webster, 2010; Robertson, Rushton, Bartrum, Moore, & Morris, 2007; Robertson, Rushton, Bartrum, & Ray, 2004).

We will trace the theories that influenced the design, research, and practice of IPT as we describe in more detail the approach and its recent application to posttraumatic stress disorder (PTSD) in this chapter.

Theoretical and Empirical Bases for IPT

Dr. Gerald Klerman was a renaissance psychiatrist: not only a psychopharmacologist and psychotherapist but also an epidemiologist and community mental health advocate. Although he considered depression fundamentally a biological illness, he observed clinically how social and interpersonal stressors could aggravate his patients' symptoms. As he said, "One of the great features of the brain is that it responds to its environment" (Weissman, 2006). Klerman was trained in psychoanalysis but also influenced by Aaron Beck's evidence-based cognitive therapy and valued supportive therapy (Weissman, 2006). He and Myrna Weissman aimed to design a brief treatment that could be defined, practical, and efficacious. Their basic assumption was that a relationship existed between the patient's psychiatric symptoms and his or her social and interpersonal relationships: symptoms arise not in a vacuum but in an interpersonal context (Weissman, Markowitz, & Klerman, 2000).

A few key theorists informed Klerman and Weismann's thinking about psychotherapy throughout their own training and practice, and helped shape the principles and techniques for IPT.

Adolf Meyer, a Swiss-born psychiatrist who became president of the American Psychiatric Association, played a leading role in developing ideas in psychiatry in the early twentieth century. Meyer believed in applying a scientific approach to understanding mental illness. He was known for collecting comprehensive case histories of his patients which integrated biological, psychological, and social factors relevant to their lives. Meyer's psychobiological model for understanding pathology stressed the importance of the patient's relationship to his or her environment (Meyer, 1957).

Echoing Meyer's social worldview, Harry Stack Sullivan believed that an individual's interpersonal world was paramount to understanding psychiatric illness (Perry, 1982; Evans, 1996). Sullivan, an American psychiatrist, also practicing during the first half of the twentieth century, aimed to broaden Freudian psychoanalysis to serve patients with severe mental disorders, particularly schizophrenia. He hypothesized that maladaptive interpersonal relationships lay at the root of severe mental illnesses, characterizing loneliness as the most painful of human experiences. Therefore, clinical treatment needed to focus on developing an understanding of the individual based on the network of relationships in which he or she is enmeshed; to focus not only on the "intrapsychic, but the interactional" (Perry, 1982). Subsequently, Sullivan, along with Karen Horney, Erich Fromm, Erik H. Erikson, and others, laid the groundwork for understanding individuals based on their networks of social relationships (Perry, 1982).

Meyer's and Sullivan's viewpoints are congruent with the extensive literature on attachment theory, which posits that interpersonal relations are the most basic of mammalian biological needs (Bowlby & King, 2004). Attachment theorists recognize that social and emotional development starts at infancy, and that secure attachments form through having at least one strong, nourishing, and consistent connection with a caregiver. This first reciprocal relationship then shapes the dynamics of future relationships. Securely attached infants, for example, tend to become more socially skilled than their insecure peers (Bowlby, 1988).

John Bowlby, a British psychiatrist and near contemporary of Meyer and Sullivan, investigated social support in adult psychopathology by studying the effects of secure and insecure childhood attachment (Bowlby, 1988). He deduced that attachment behavior was innately biological, and that parental responses lead the child to develop attachment patterns that in turn lead to "internal working models," which predict patterns in later relationships (Bowlby, 1988). Bolby's theory is extremely important to the understanding of clinical depression and anxiety: whereas secure attachment can afford the individual confidence to explore and elicit support from others, any conflicts within the early caregiving connection may lead to vulnerability, mistrust in others, and avoidance of painful or fearful reactions (Kobak & Madsen, 2008; Manassis, Bradley, Goldberg, Hood, & Swinson, 1995; Warren, Huston, Byron, & Sroufe, 1997). Concerning PTSD, secure attachment should strengthen the ability to ward off negative and long-lasting effects of trauma, presumably in part through activating his or her social support network

(Markowitz et al., 2009), whereas an insecurely attached individual attachment would be less likely to seek out social support, and ultimately overcome initial fearful reactions (Declercq & Palmans, 2006; Stovall-McClough & Cloitre, 2006). In fact, differing attachment styles is among the strongest predictors to date of whether an individual shows resilience after a traumatic experience or develops PTSD (Brewin, Andrews, & Valentine, 2000; Ozer, Best, Lipsey, & Weiss, 2003).

At least as much as theory, an empirical basis for understanding psychosocial aspects of depression guided the development and subsequent growth and adaptations of IPT. One of Klerman and Weissman's goals was to educate patients about their illness and its consequences for relationships; through this understanding, a sense of purpose and motivation can emerge, helping patients to realize their own relationship difficulties and improve interpersonal problem areas. Thus, IPT was built on the relevant research literature, with an eye towards integrating key psychosocial concepts into clinical practice.

Klerman and Weissman turned to studies associating stress and life events with the onset and clinical course of depression to determine key factors to address short term psychotherapy. For example, how intimacy and social support act as protection against depression (Brown & Harris, 1978), the impact chronic, social, and interpersonal stress have on depressive onset (Pearlin & Lieberman, 1979), and epidemiological data strongly associating marital disputes and major depression (Henderson et al., 1978; Weissman, 1987). Klerman and Weissman synthesized these findings and applied them directly to their protocol, crafting the four IPT interpersonal problem areas—grief, role dispute, role transition, and interpersonal deficit—to reflect empirical findings.

By design, IPT reflected the theoretical ideas and empirical data described in this section. From the initial phase of treatment, when the therapist conducts a detailed interpersonal inventory and presents a biopsychosocial formulation, to focus on interpersonal problem areas, to techniques and tactics designed to improve social interactions, and to mobilize the patient's social support, the treatment's constant focus is on interpersonal targets and how they change in mood and relationships.

Description of the IPT Approach

IPT's distinctive qualities include: linking the individual's psychiatric symptoms to an interpersonal crisis, understanding these symptoms as a medical illness distinct from personality or temperament, and balancing between affect-focused psychotherapy and functional application to provide opportunities for enhanced social and emotional functioning. Most psychotherapy approaches aim to help the patient reduce psychiatric symptoms, reduce social isolation, and restore a general sense of self-belief and self-reliance. However, IPT differs in its explicit attention to present functioning and interpersonal relationships. IPT does not claim to address personality functioning or character pathology, but focuses attention on alleviating symptoms through exploring, identifying, and improving problem areas within interpersonal relations (Weissman & Markowitz, 1998).

The IPT therapist frames the patient's symptoms using a medical model, which posits that a patient should not be held responsible for his/her diagnosis, is excused for functioning at a suboptimal level while ill, and needs to work to regain his or her health (Parsons, 1951). The message remains clear throughout the treatment protocol: The patient is suffering from a treatable condition. The symptoms which make up the diagnosis are the problem, not the person. The method aims to reduce any self-blame the patient may be experiencing. The therapist encourages hope towards recovery.

IPT protocols are manually *guided*, but not driven by session-to-session agendas. Instead, the approach is comprised of three phases. The initial phase requires the therapist to identify the target diagnosis and the interpersonal context in which it presents. The therapist then elicits an "interpersonal inventory," a review of the patient's patterns in relationships, capacity for intimacy, and particularly an evaluation of current relationships. From there, the four theoretical IPT interpersonal problem areas—grief, role dispute, role transition, and interpersonal deficit—are rendered to create a focus for treatment: someone important may have died (*complicated bereavement*), there may be a struggle with a significant other (*role dispute*), the patient may have undergone some other important life change (*role transition*), or the individual, absent of an actual or current life event, may have trouble connecting or relating to others (*interpersonal deficits*).

A formulation detailing this interpersonal focus then drives the remainder of the therapy. In the middle phase of treatment, the therapist uses specific strategies to deal with the problem area. This might involve appropriate mourning in complicated bereavement, resolving an interpersonal struggle in a role dispute, helping a patient to mourn the loss of an old role and assume a new one in a role transition, or develop and practice skills that will address interpersonal deficits and enhance communication with others.

In the last few sessions, termination is addressed as an essential element towards closure. Termination is a significant segment of the IPT protocol, for it underscores the necessity of viewing the patient's outside environment as more important than the therapy itself; reinforcing healthy interpersonal skills, analyzing what went wrong in a social situation, brainstorming and role playing new interpersonal options are all strategies hopefully gained from the treatment. These strategies will ultimately be applied in the patient's real life.

As illustrated in greater detail in the case presentation chapter, the symptoms of PTSD often compromise interpersonal functioning. The individual withdraws from people and places as a means of avoiding intense mood reactions, and as a result loses sight of the importance of interpersonal connections. In IPT, the therapist would first help the patient with PTSD see these symptoms as a condition rather than a characterological defect and then guide him or her to focus on identifying interpersonal problem areas, before re-mobilizing the social support that can help them get well. The focus of the therapy is less about the trauma the patients have experienced and more about the assured ways they can work towards pulling through their personal tragedy.

Underlying Principles for Applying IPT to PTSD

Initial evidence suggests that IPT may benefit patients with PTSD (Bleiberg & Markowitz, 2005; Campanini et al., 2010; Graf & Markowitz, 2012; Krupnick et al., 2008; Rafaeli & Markowitz, 2011; Ray & Webster, 2010; Robertson et al., 2004, 2007). There are at least three rationales for testing IPT for this population. First, IPT does not expose patients to trauma reminders. Although extensive evidence supports the efficacy of exposure-based therapies for PTSD APA, 2004, IPT offers an alternative for patients who refuse or do not respond to exposure techniques. Second, IPT improves patients' affect tolerance and interpersonal functioning (Markowitz, 2010; Markowitz et al., 2006, 2009), which are commonly impaired in PTSD (APA, 2000) and thus an important target for change. A recent review suggested that highly traumatized patients who dissociate may fare better receiving an affect-focused therapy than exposure-based therapy (Lanius et al., 2010). Third, social support, which IPT helps patients activate and maintain, has repeatedly been shown to be a key factor in preventing and recovering from PTSD (Brewin et al., 2000; Ozer et al., 2003).

In contrast to CBT approaches, IPT eschews focusing on reminders of traumas, concentrating on the patient's current life events, particularly on social and interpersonal aspects. The basic IPT premise for PTSD is that trauma shatters the patient's sense of interpersonal safety, leading to withdrawal from interpersonal relationships and impaired ability to use social supports to process the traumatic event (Markowitz et al., 2009). By withdrawing, individuals with PTSD cut off the vital social supports needed when they are most vulnerable. Interpersonally hypervigilant, patients with PTSD mistrust relationships (Bleiberg & Markowitz, 2005). IPT helps the patient to understand rather than avoid his or her feelings, to recognize them as social cues (anger means someone is bothering you; it's a normal emotion, not something "bad"), to use them to enhance communication and effectively manage interactions with others, and thereby to rebuild interpersonal trust. Finding ways to meaningfully reconnect to one's surrounding world may reinstate severed social networks, provide a sense of control over one's interpersonal environment, and reduce PTSD symptoms.

IPT defines an interpersonal crisis and helps the patient to resolve it. In IPT for PTSD, one of the following problem areas is used for case conceptualization: grief (mourning the death of a significant other), role dispute (a struggle with a significant other, which the patient is inevitably losing), or role transition (any major life change, including having suffered a traumatic event or events) (Markowitz et al., 2009). The fourth problem area, interpersonal deficits, which can be found in the research, has been used to denote the absence of a current life event. This problem area was not included in the IPT-PTSD protocol as it focuses on interpersonal problems which stem from "no-life" events, such as loneliness or isolation. In the case of a PTSD diagnosis however, the individual indeed has experienced "life-events", and any loneliness or isolation is symptomatic of the disorder, not the individual. Treatment helps the patient to identify one of these problem areas and develop skills, as well as new interpersonal opportunities, which can renew their much needed social support system. The goal of the time-limited (14 weekly 50-min sessions) treatment is for the patient to resolve this focal interpersonal crisis. The patient approaches this goal at his or her own pace: IPT involves no week-to-week assigned homework, thereby obviating the risk of the patient failing to do it.

Empirical Support for IPT-PTSD

Although considerable evidence supports exposure to reminders of trauma as an effective core principle for treating PTSD (Cahill & Foa, 2004; Ehlers et al., 2010), a focus on attachment styles and interpersonal relationships may be an alternative approach to ameliorating PTSD symptoms (Markowitz, 2010; Markowitz et al., 2009). Research suggests that parenting styles and primary childhood relationships increase later risk of developing anxiety disorders. In addition, differing attachment styles in adulthood influence how individuals seek and benefit from social support (Hirshfeld-Becker et al., 2004; Manassis et al., 1995).

Two initial studies applying IPT to PTSD patients show encouraging preliminary findings. Using a manualized modification of individual IPT for PTSD, focusing on interpersonal sequelae of PTSD rather than exposure to its traumatic triggers, a small open trial treated 14 patients with chronic PTSD, yielding large effect size (≥1.8) improvements across the three PTSD DSM-IV-TR symptom clusters as well as reductions in depression and anger and improved social functioning (Bleiberg & Markowitz, 2005; Krupnick et al., 2008). An NIMH-funded, randomized controlled study is currently comparing three 14-week psychotherapies that employ very different mechanisms for treating chronic PTSD: (1) prolonged exposure (Foa & Rothbaum, 1998); (2) IPT, focusing on interpersonal sequelae of PTSD rather than exposure to its traumatic triggers; and (3) relaxation, emphasizing reduction of anxiety through relief of physical tension (Jacobson, 1938). This study will evaluate not only the efficacy of IPT for PTSD but potential mediators and moderators of treatment outcome, such as interpersonal awareness measured by reflective function (Fonagy, Steele, Moran, Steele, & Higgitt, 1991; Meehan, Levy, Reynoso, Hill, & Clarkin, 2009). Mediators and moderators are key research variables because they may elucidate differential treatment selection and mechanisms of psychotherapy efficacy. One baseline finding is that study patients tend to prefer IPT to prolonged exposure, even though they are told that the latter has a stronger evidence base (Markowitz, 2010).

Conclusion

IPT has been shown to enhance interpersonal functioning through identifying problem areas in relationships, helping patients to tolerate and express their feelings in relationships, thereby improving social skills, and building a community of support and connection. Focusing on incidents from the patient's current life, IPT emphasizes the recognition and repair of interpersonal difficulties. IPT for the treatment of patients with PTSD provides opportunities to reverse interpersonal avoidance, increase social support, undergo corrective emotional experiences with others that potentially will modulate trauma-related interpersonal distortions, and improve demoralization and helplessness that inhibit motivation to overcome trauma-related fears.

A manualized treatment protocol has adapted the original IPT approach for PTSD. Unlike exposure-based therapies, which focus on relieving symptoms through direct contact or experience with the trauma, IPT's view of treatment is that trauma impairs the individual's ability to trust their social environment. Experiencing the environment and the relationships within as dangerous then triggers maladaptive social functioning, which helps to perpetuate PTSD. PTSD symptoms, in turn, reinforce social detachment and dysfunction. Treatment counters the perceived helplessness and shamefulness of PTSD with a sense of interpersonal competence, and redirects the patient's attention from inner preoccupation with past trauma to coping with the immediate interpersonal outer world.

Some patients with PTSD refuse exposure-based therapies, an unsurprising consequence of their anxious avoidance: "Some trauma survivors are reluctant to confront trauma reminders and to tolerate the high anxiety and temporarily increased symptoms that sometimes accompany exposure. Thus, not everyone may be a candidate for exposure-based treatment" (Markowitz et al., 2009). Indeed, no one treatment benefits all patients with any specific psychiatric disorder. A non-exposure-based, interpersonal model might effectively engage such patients in treatment.

References

American Psychiatric Association. (2004). Practice guideline for the treatment of patients with acute stress disorder and posttraumatic stress disorder. *American Journal of Psychiatry, 161*, 3–31.

American Psychiatric Association. (2000). Diagnostic and statistical manual of mental disorders, 4th edition, text revision. Washington, DC: American Psychiatric Association.

Bowlby, J. (1988). *A secure base: Parent-child attachment and healthy human development*. London: Routledge.

Bleiberg, K. L., & Markowitz, J. C. (2005). Interpersonal psychotherapy for posttraumatic stress disorder. *American Journal of Psychiatry, 162*, 181–183.

Bowlby, R., & King, P. (2004). *Fifty years of attachment theory: Recollections of Donald Winnicott and John Bowlby*. London: Karnac.

Brewin, C. R., Andrews, B., & Valentine, J. D. (2000). Meta-analysis of risk factors for posttraumatic stress disorder in trauma-exposed adults. *Journal of Consulting Clinical Psychology, 68*(5), 748–766.

Brom, D., Kleber, R. J., & Defares, P. B. (1989). Brief psychotherapy for posttraumatic stress disorders. *Journal of Consulting Clinical Psychology, 57*(5), 607–612.

Brown, G. W., & Harris, T. O. (1978). *Social origins of depression*. London: Tavistock.

Cahill, S. P., & Foa, E. B. (2004). A glass half empty or half full? "Where we are and directions for future research in the treatment of PTSD". In S. Taylor (Ed.), *Advances in the treatment of posttraumatic stress disorder: Cognitive-behavioral perspectives* (pp. 267–313). New York: Springer.

Campanini, R. F., Schoedl, A. F., Pupo, M. C., Costa, A. C., Krupnick, J. L., & Melo, M. F. (2010). Efficacy of interpersonal therapy-group format adapted to post-traumatic stress disorder: an open-label add-on trial. *Depression and Anxiety, 27*, 72–77.

Cutrona, C. E., & Russell, D. W. (1990). Types of social support and specific stress: Toward a theory of optimal matching. In B. R. Sarason, I. G. Sarason, & G. R. Pierce (Eds.), *Social support: An interactional view* (pp. 319–366). New York: Wiley.

Declercq, F., & Palmans, V. (2006). Two subjective factors as moderators between critical incidents and the occurrence of post traumatic stress disorders: Adult attachment and perception of social support. *Psychology and Psychotherapy: Theory, Research and Practice, 79*, 323–337.

Ehlers, A., Bisson, J., Clark, D. M., Creamer, M., Pilling, S., Richards, D., et al. (2010). Do all psychological treatments really work the same in posttraumatic stress disorder? *Clinical Psychological Review, 30*(2), 269–276.

Evans, F. B. (1996). *Harry Stack Sullivan: Interpersonal theory and psychotherapy*. London: Routledge.

Fairburn, C. G., Jones, R., Peveler, R., Hope, R., & O'Connor, M. (1993). Psychotherapy and bulimia nervosa: Longer-term effects of interpersonal psychotherapy, behavior therapy, and cognitive behavior therapy. *Archives of General Psychiatry, 50*, 419–428.

Foa, E. B., & Rothbaum, B. O. (1998). *Treating the trauma of rape: Cognitive-behavioral therapy for PTSD*. New York: Guilford Press.

Fonagy, P., Steele, H., Moran, G., Steele, M., & Higgitt, A. (1991). The capacity for understanding mental states: The reflective self in parent and child and its significance for security of attachment. *Infant Mental Health Journal, 13*, 200–217.

Frank, E. (2005). *Treating bipolar disorder: A clinician's guide to interpersonal and social rhythm therapy*. New York: Guilford.

Graf, E. P., & Markowitz, J. C. (2012). IPT for posttraumatic stress disorder. In J. C. Markowitz & M. M. Weismann (Eds.), *Casebook of interpersonal psychotherapy* (pp. 149–168). New York: Oxford University Press.

Henderson, S., Byrne, D. G., Duncan-Jones, P., Adock, S., Scott, R., & Steele, G. P. (1978). Social bonds in the epidemiology of neurosis. *British Journal of Psychiatry, 132*, 463–466.

Hinrichsen, G. A. (1999). Treating older adults with interpersonal psychotherapy for depression. *Psychotherapy in Practice, 55*(8), 949–960.

Hirshfeld-Becker, D. R., Biederman, J., Faraone, S. V., Segool, B. A., Buchwald, B. A., Jerrold, F., et al. (2004). Lack of association between behavioral inhibition and psychosocial adversity factors in children at risk for anxiety disorders. *American Journal of Psychiatry, 161*(3), 547–555.

Jacobson, E. (1938). *Progressive relaxation*. Chicago: University of Chicago Press.

Kobak, R., & Madsen, S. (2008). Disruption in attachment bonds. In J. Cassidy & P. R. Shaver (Eds.), *Handbook of attachment: Theory, research and clinical applications* (pp. 23–47). New York: Guilford Press.

Krupnick, J. L., Green, B. L., Stockton, P., Miranda, J., Krause, E., & Mete, M. (2008). Group interpersonal psychotherapy with low-income women with posttraumatic stress disorder. *Psychotherapy Research, 18*, 497–507.

Lanius, R. A., Vermetten, E., Loewenstein, R. J., Brand, B., Schmal, C., Bremner, J. D., et al. (2010). Emotion modulation in PTSD: Clinical and neurobiological evidence for a dissociative subtype. *American Journal of Psychiatry, 167*, 640–647.

Manassis, K., Bradley, S., Goldberg, S., Hood, J., & Swinson, R. P. (1995). Behavioural inhibition, attachment and anxiety in children of mothers with anxiety disorders. *Canadian Journal of Psychiatry, 40*(2), 87–92.

Markowitz, J. C. (1996). Psychotherapy for dysthymic disorder. *Psychiatric Clinics of North America, 19*, 133–149.

Markowitz, J. C., Bleiberg, K. L., Christos, P., & Levitan, E. (2006). Solving interpersonal problems correlates with symptom improvement in interpersonal psychotherapy: preliminary findings. *Journal of Nervous and Mental Disease, 194*, 15–20.

Markowitz, J. C. (2010). IPT and PTSD. *Depression and Anxiety, 27*(10), 879–881.

Markowitz, J. C., Milrod, B., Blieberg, K., & Randall, D. (2009). Interpersonal factors in understanding and treating posttraumatic stress disorder. *Journal of Psychiatric Practice, 15*, 133–140.

Markowitz, J. C., & Weissman, M. M. (2012a). IPT: Past, present, and future. *Clinical Psychology and Psychotherapy, 19*, 99–105.

Markowitz, J. C., & Weissman, M. M. (Eds.). (2012b). *Casebook of interpersonal psychotherapy*. New York: Oxford University Press.

Meehan, K. B., Levy, K. N., Reynoso, J. S., Hill, L. L., & Clarkin, J. F. (2009). Measuring reflective function with a multidimensional rating scale: Comparison with scoring reflective function on the AAI. *Journal of American Psychoanalytic Association, 57*, 208–213.

Meyer, A. (1957). *Psychobiology: A science of man*. Springfield, IL: Thomas, C.T.

Mufson, L., Moreau, D., Weissman, M. M., et al. (1993). Interpersonal Psychotherapy for Depressed Adolescents. New York: Guilford Press.

National Collaborating Centre for Mental Health. (2004). *Eating disorders: Core interventions in the treatment and management of anorexia nervosa. Bulimia nervosa, and related eating disorders developed by National Collaborating centre for Mental Health*. London: British Psychological Society and Gaskell.

Ozer, E. J., Best, S. R., Lipsey, T. L., & Weiss, D. S. (2003). Predictors of posttraumatic stress disorder and symptoms in adults: A meta-analysis. *Psychological Bulletin, 129*, 52–73.

Parsons, T. (1951). Illness and the role of the physician: A sociological perspective. *The American Journal of Orthopsychiatry, 21*, 452–460.

Pearlin, L. I., & Lieberman, M. A. (1979). Social sources of emotional distress. *Research in Community Mental Health, 1*, 217–248.

Perry, H. S. (1982). *Psychiatrist of America. The life of Harry Stack Sullivan*. Cambridge: Belknap Press.

Rafaeli, A. K., & Markowitz, J. C. (2011). Interpersonal psychotherapy (IPT) for PTSD: A case study. *American Journal of Psychotherapy, 65*, 205–223.

Ray, R. D., & Webster, R. (2010). Group interpersonal psychotherapy for veterans with posttraumatic stress disorder: A pilot study. *International Journal of Group Psychotherapy, 60*, 131–140.

Robertson, M., Rushton, P., Bartrum, D., Moore, E., & Morris, P. (2007). Open trial of interpersonal psychotherapy for posttraumatic stress disorder. *Australian Psychiatry, 15*, 375–379.

Robertson, M., Rushton, P. J., Bartrum, M. D., & Ray, R. (2004). Group-based interpersonal psychotherapy for posttraumatic stress disorder: Theoretical and clinical aspects. *International Journal of Group Psychotherapy, 54*, 145–175.

Stovall-McClough, K. C., & Cloitre, M. (2006). Unresolved attachment, PTSD, and dissociation in women with childhood abuse histories. *Journal of Consulting Clinical Psychology, 74*, 219–228.

Taylor, S. E. (2011). Social support: A review. In M. S. Friedman (Ed.), *The handbook of health psychology* (pp. 189–214). New York: Oxford University Press.

Verdeli, H., Clougherty, K. F., Bolton, P., Speelman, L., Ndogoni, L., Bass, J., et al. (2003). Adapting group interpersonal psychotherapy for a developing country: Experience in rural Uganda. *World Psychiatry, 2*(2), 114–120.

Warren, S. L., Huston, L., Byron, E., & Sroufe, L. A. (1997). Child and adolescent anxiety disorders and early attachment. *Journal of the American Academy of Child & Adolescent Psychiatry, 36*(5), 637–644.

Weissman, M. M. (1987). Advances in psychiatric epidemiology: Rates and risks for major depression. *American Journal of Public Health, 77*, 445–451.

Weissman, M. (2006). A brief history of interpersonal therapy (IPT). *Psychiatric Annals, 36*(8), 553–557.

Weissman, M. M., & Markowitz, J. C. (1998). An overview of interpersonal psychotherapy. In J. Markowitz (Ed.), *Interpersonal psychotherapy* (pp. 1–33). Washington, DC: American Psychiatric Press.

Weissman, M. M., Markowitz, J. C., & Klerman, G. L. (2000). *Comprehensive guide to interpersonal psychotherapy*. New York: Basic Books.

Weissman, M. M., Verdeli, H., Gameroff, M. J., Bledsoe, S. E., Betts, K., Mufson, L., et al. (2006). A national survey of psychotherapy training in psychiatry, psychology and social work. *Archives of General Psychiatry, 63*(8), 925–934.

Part V
Modifications of PTSD Treatment

Chapter 14
Inclusion of Virtual Reality: A Rationale for the Use of VR in the Treatment of PTSD

Azucena García-Palacios, Cristina Botella, Rosa Baños, Verónica Guillén, and Maria Vicenta Navarro

Exposure Therapy for PTSD

Posttraumatic Stress Disorder (PTSD) was introduced in the Diagnostic and Statistical Manual (DSM) of mental disorders as a diagnostic category in 1980 (APA 1980). Since then, there has been an increased emphasis on the study of its psychopathology and treatment given the significant personal distress and interpersonal/occupational impairment associated with this condition.

PTSD is concerned with a natural human condition, reaction to adversity (Herbert & Sageman, 2004). Human beings have long tried to cope with adversity using a

A. García-Palacios, Ph.D. (✉) • C. Botella, Ph.D.
Universitat Jaume I, Castellon, Spain

Ciber Fisiopatología Obesidad y Nutrición CIBERobn, CB06/03, Instituto Salud Carlos III, Madrid, Spain
e-mail: azucena@uji.es; botella@uji.es

R. Baños, Ph.D.
Ciber Fisiopatología Obesidad y Nutrición CIBERobn, CB06/03, Instituto Salud Carlos III, Madrid, Spain

Universitat de Valencia, Valencia, Spain
e-mail: banos@uv.es

V. Guillén, Ph.D.
Universitat Jaume I, Castellon, Spain

Centro Clínico PREVI, València, Spain
e-mail: vguillen@previsl.com

M.V. Navarro, Ph.D.
University of Washington, Seattle, WA, USA
e-mail: Marna82@u.washington.edu

M.P. Safir et al. (eds.), *Future Directions in Post-Traumatic Stress Disorder*,
DOI 10.1007/978-1-4899-7522-5_14

multitude of strategies that are usually effective. History is filled with examples of the resilience of humans and their capacity to overcome severe traumas such as war, terrorist attacks, and physical assault.

PTSD occurs when the strategies to overcome traumas do not work. In that case, a typical reaction is increased arousal, avoidance of reminders of the trauma in many forms (situations, emotions, activities, etc.), and reexperiencing symptoms in several forms (flashbacks, nightmares, repetitive thoughts or images, etc.). These three clusters of symptoms constitute the core of PTSD that can become a complex and chronic psychological problem.

At the current time, evidence-based approaches for the treatment of this condition are available. Cognitive behavior therapy (CBT) programs have been demonstrated to be effective in the treatment of this problem. In fact, exposure therapy is considered the first-line treatment for PTSD, given the amount of empirical evidence that has been generated in support of its clinical efficacy (i.e., Foa, Rothbaum, & Furr, 2003).

Exposure therapy is based on the notion that people are able to adjust to distressing, but not dangerous, stimuli through repeated confrontation with these situations. By repeatedly confronting the anxiety-provoking situation in a safe, therapeutic environment, unrealistic cognitions are disconfirmed and the situations cease to arouse excessive distress. Through repeated practice, exposure therapy helps the person generate new and adaptable patterns of thinking and feeling. One process involved in the efficacy of exposure is emotional processing. Foa and Kozak (1986) used this concept to explain fear reduction during exposure. Emotional processing theory proposes that anxiety disorders reflect fear structures that contain pathological and unrealistic associations among the elements that constitute the experience (physiological, cognitive, and behavioral). Foa and Kozak suggested that exposure to feared stimuli allow: (a) the activation of the fear structure and (b) the presentation of corrective information incompatible with the pathological elements of the fear structure. Foa and McNally (1996) suggested that exposure therapy helps to form a new structure that contains more realistic associations among the elements. This process is especially relevant in the case of PTSD.

Exposure may occur through imagining the anxiety-arousing stimuli or in vivo where the person confronts the real life situation, object, or person that arouses the anxiety. The therapeutic strategy involves identification of the stimulus cues that activate fears associated with the traumatic events. The individual is then exposed to those cues through prolonged and repeated imaginal and in vivo exposure. With the support of the therapist, the individual learns how to self-manage the unwanted responses in the presence of a variety of stimulus cues.

Exposure-based techniques provide participants with opportunities to learn to control their own responses when confronted with stimuli related to the traumatic experience. The treatment program for PTSD with the most empirical support is Prolonged Exposure (PE), developed by Foa and Rothbaum (1998), which involves imaginal exposure to the traumatic experience. The aim of this intervention is to evoke the stressful event and to work on processing it in an adaptive way.

Exposure may also involve real life situations, objects, or people that arouse the anxiety. The individual can also receive training in self-regulation skills like breathing, training, and reframing interpretations of events.

Limitations of Exposure Therapy for PTSD

Despite these encouraging findings, exposure appears to be under-utilized in clinical practice. Becker et al. (2004) found that only a small minority of a sample of psychologists used exposure to treat PTSD. Although around half of the sample reported being familiar with imaginal exposure (IE), only 17 % used it to treat PTSD. One of the main reasons for not using IE was lack of training and experience with PTSD. However, of those who were trained and had experience in treating PTSD, less than 50 % used it to treat at least half of their PTSD patients. When asking therapists about the barriers to using IE, they indicated contraindications not empirically based, like a worsening in symptoms or an increased desire to drop out of therapy. These views were independent of training, familiarity, or theoretical orientation. Becker et al. expressed their concern with these findings given that as they stated "many patients who could benefit from exposure are inappropriately being excluded based on clinicians' beliefs that IE is associated with an extensive list of contraindications" (p. 289). The conclusion to this study is that IE has an important problem concerning dissemination among clinicians.

Empirical evidence does not support such contraindications. Hembree et al. (2003) offered data about the dropout rate of exposure therapy for PTSD. These authors reviewed 25 controlled studies exploring the efficacy of CBT for PTSD. The results did not support the hypothesis that dropout rates for exposure therapy will be higher than from other treatments that do not include the more direct confrontation of trauma memory that is characteristic of IE (Cognitive Restructuring, Stress Inoculation Training, and Eye Movement Desensitization and Reprocessing). The dropout rate for exposure therapy was 20.5 %, similar to the dropout rates of the other forms of CBT for PTSD and similar to the dropout rates of exposure therapy for other diagnostic groups.

Another concern about exposure therapy is symptom exacerbation. Foa, Zoellner, Feeny, Hembree, and Alvarez-Conrad (2002) explored symptom exacerbation in a sample of women diagnosed with PTSD and treated with exposure therapy. They found that only a minority of patients (11 %) showed an exacerbation of PTSD symptoms that was temporary. As well, such exacerbation was not related to dropout or treatment response. Another barrier for dissemination of exposure therapy for PTSD could be patients' preferences. Becker et al. (2004) conducted a survey with an analog sample with varying degrees of trauma history (7 % met self-reported criteria of PTSD). They were asked to imagine experiencing a traumatic event, developing PTSD symptoms, and seeking treatment. They evaluated seven descriptions of different treatments (Exposure, CBT, Eye Movement Desensitization and Reprocessing, Psychodynamic, Thought-field therapy, Sertraline, My Therapy

Buddy) and rated their most and least preferred treatment. Most participants chose exposure therapy and CBTs the most preferred treatment, which contradicts the general view that exposure therapy will be rejected by PTSD patients. The preference rates were similar in participants meeting PTSD criteria, although it is important to obtain results from clinical samples to strengthen these results. These authors conclude that the problem of underutilization of exposure therapy may be due to more therapists' factors than to patients' preferences. These findings support that exposure therapy is not only an efficacious approach to treat PTSD, but also more tolerable than many clinicians think.

Alternatively, it is important to take into consideration the concerns raised by clinicians. An interesting study conducted by Zayfert et al. (2005) points out the differences in dropout rates in randomized clinical trials similar to those reviewed by Hembree et al. (2003) and in naturalistic clinical settings. In this setting they found that the completion rate of CBT (28 %) was markedly lower than rates reported in randomized trials (60 %). When studying the relationship between IE and dropout they found that most dropouts occurred before starting IE and that initiating IE was associated with greater likelihood of completion. Avoidance and depression were the unique predictors of non-completion. These findings indicate that individuals who are more avoidant and depressed are more likely to show reluctance to begin IE or show behaviors that inhibit clinicians from initiating IE. The problem is not the efficacy of IE, given that once the patient starts IE they are more prone to complete the treatment. Zayfert et al. concluded that it is important to explore the factors affecting treatment engagement and develop means to help clinicians to be able to better apply IE.

Avoidance of the feared stimuli is a central diagnostic feature of anxiety disorders and PTSD. Thus, the need to confront the trauma in therapy can present a significant challenge for these patients. Some patients are able to think about their trauma, but are emotionally detached from the experience. The lack of emotional engagement can hinder anxiety reduction, resulting in poor treatment outcomes Jaycox, Foa, and Morral (1998). Potential negative effects on treatment response can also occur as a result of the patient's inability to imagine.

Finally, we would like to mention the study by Bradley, Greene, Russ, Dutra, and Westen (2005) who conducted a meta-analysis of 26 efficacy studies of psychotherapy for PTSD and found that 56 % of those following a psychological treatment and 67 % of completers did not meet criteria for PTSD at posttreatment. Although these findings are very encouraging, pointing out that we have at our disposal good psychological treatments for PTSD (exposure therapy being the most supported by the scientific evidence), there is still room for improvement in order to reach and benefit a larger number of PTSD patients.

Emerging Treatments for PTSD

Based on the scientific literature, exposure therapy is considered to be the gold standard treatment for PTSD. However, despite the impressive efficacy data of this approach there are still limitations and not all people who need treatment could benefit.

With this in mind, several approaches have been recently designed and tested with the aim of improving psychological treatments for PTSD. Cukor, Spitalnick, Difede, Rizzo, and Rothbaum (2009) reviewed these emerging treatments for PTSD. They divided the different therapies in the following categories: (a) Social and family-based treatments (couple and family therapy and interpersonal psychotherapy); (b) behavioral treatments (behavioral activation, trauma management therapy, interoceptive exposure, mindfulness, and yoga and acupuncture); (c) imagery-based treatments (imagery rescripting and imagery rehearsal therapy); (d) therapies focusing on distress tolerance (dialectical behavior therapy, DBT, and acceptance and commitment therapy, ACT); (e) power therapy (thought field therapy, trauma incident reduction, and Visio kinesthetic disassociation); and finally (f) technological-based treatments (Internet and computer-based treatment and virtual reality).

After performing this review the authors concluded that there is a growing effort by clinicians and researchers to develop alternative treatment approaches. However, sufficient evidence to draw conclusions about their efficacy has not been generated thus far. It seems that some of these approaches can help to augment an already well-established treatment such as IE by addressing specific symptoms and problematic areas like interpersonal therapy for social impairment linked to PTSD or behavioral treatments such as behavioral activation and mindfulness to improve depression or increase distress tolerance. In other cases (i.e., power therapy), the review concludes that there is not any evidence of efficacy. Finally, of all the approaches reviewed, technology-based treatments offer the strongest preliminary evidence. In the following section we will address the use of one of these technologies, virtual reality, in the treatment of anxiety disorders and PTSD.

Virtual Reality (VR)

Virtual reality is an Information and Communication Technology (ICT) which utilizes adjustable computer-generated simulations of reality to engage the patient in trauma-relevant scenarios. The typical VR setting involves VR software, a Head Mounted Display (HMD), a tracker, and an interaction device (such as a joystick). The user is immersed in a 3-D environment where he/she can interact with the virtual objects and experience a sense of presence, as if they were "there" in the virtual world.

The capacity of simulating reality in such a unique way has appealed to health professionals since its first developments. VR has been used to address a variety of health conditions such as pain, addiction, cognitive/physical rehabilitation, and most prominently, anxiety disorders.

Given its immersive features, VR is a powerful distraction technique that has been used for acute pain control mainly with burn patients during wound care or physical therapy (Hoffman, Doctor, Patterson, Carrougher, & Furness, 2000; Hoffman, Patterson, & Carrougher, 2000, see Keefe et al., 2012 for a review).

By far the largest body of work in the clinical application of VR has been with anxiety disorders, especially phobias. Since the publication of the pioneer work by Rothbaum, Hodges, Opdyke, Willifor, and North (1995), describing a case study of the use of VR exposure for fear of heights, VR has been demonstrated to be effective in the treatment of a wide diversity of specific phobias, including fear of flying, arachnophobia, acrophobia, claustrophobia, and driving phobia. It has also been used for the delivery of exposure in other more complex anxiety disorders like panic disorder with agoraphobia, social phobia, or PTSD. Two meta-analyses (Parsons & Rizzo, 2008; Powers & Emmelkamp, 2008) explored the efficacy of VR for anxiety disorders and Parsons et al. found an average effect size of 0.96, concluding that VR exposure is an effective treatment for a variety of anxiety disorders. In a more recent meta-analysis, Opris et al. (2012) compared the efficacy of VR exposure with traditional evidence-based treatments for anxiety disorders finding a similar efficacy at short- and long-term and a similar dropout rate.

The features of VR make this technology an attractive means to deliver exposure therapy. The key element of exposure therapy is to confront the feared objects or situations, in vivo (real situations) or using imagination. VR environments could be viewed as scenarios between real and imagined situations. VR constitutes a tool that can be used as an adjunct to in vivo or imaginal exposure or as a means to increase the acceptability of the traditional ways of applying exposure therapy.

The main advantage of using VR environments for the delivery of exposure in the treatment of anxiety disorders is the high degree of control over the feared objects or situations that is not always possible with in vivo or imaginal exposure. The VR software can prevent the occurrence of unpredictable events allowing an accurate gradation of the exposure to the feared object or situation. We can add more and more difficult feared cues to the computer-generated environment in a very progressive way, respecting the rhythm of a specific individual. This can result in the patient being more willing to start and complete the exposure program. For example, an individual with agoraphobia can be exposed to a feared situation like a trip in a train while the therapist can control moderators like the number of people present in the train. The therapist can expose the individual first to an empty train, then add a few people, then gradually increase number of people, increasing the provocative elements in the hierarchy until reaching a train that is completely crowded. VR exposure also helps in terms of being able to provoke situations for exposure tasks that would be difficult to control and deliver in the real world (e.g., a break down in an elevator). Another advantage of VR is that we can repeat the same exposure task as many times as needed without having to wait for the real situation to naturally occur again. This advantage facilitates "overlearning," one of the processes that increases the efficacy of exposure (Marks, 1987). For example, we can repeat an airplane take-off over and over with an individual with fear of flying in a single exposure session. Also, compared to in vivo exposure VR offers a more confidential setting, given that there is no need to go out of the therapist's office to conduct exposure tasks. That is, patients do not need to be afraid that their problem might be known to others.

In summary, VR can be a useful way of deliver exposure that can increase the acceptability of exposure therapy. In fact, there are studies exploring the acceptability of VR therapy. Garcia-Palacios, Botella, Hoffman, and Fabregat (2007) conducted a survey among people diagnosed of specific phobia. After reading a description of VR exposure or in vivo exposure, most of them reported to be more willing to be involved in VR exposure, and when making them choosing between VR or in vivo exposure, 76 % chose VR exposure. Therapists also seem to like VR therapy. Richard and Gloster (2007) conducted a survey of professional members of the Anxiety Disorders Association of America, and found that VR exposure was viewed as more acceptable, helpful, and ethical than traditional exposure-based therapies.

In this line, VR could also be a more attractive way of offering therapy to anxiety disordered people. For example, younger generations who have grown up with technology as a natural part of everyday life may be more inclined to seek treatment in this format. Thus, a therapeutic approach supported by technology could increase the acceptability of being involved in it and serve to break down barriers to care.

In summary, VR exposure has proven to be a valid and effective means of delivering exposure therapy in the treatment of anxiety disorders. Its good efficacy data and acceptability make VR exposure an alternative for applying exposure approaches with PTSD patients. In the next section we will discuss the use of this technology in the treatment of this condition.

Rationale for the Use of Virtual Reality in the Treatment of Posttraumatic Stress Disorder

VR has developed rapidly in the past 15 years and offers a promising alternative to imaginal and in vivo exposure. It may be a valuable approach to overcoming the limitations of relying solely upon the individual's imagination and memory to recall the traumatic experience.

One of the central features of VR is the increase in focused attention. The capacity of the VR environment to draw the individual into the virtual world is described as creating "presence," a sense of being "there" in the virtual world (Hoffman, Prothero, Wells, & Groen, 1998). Virtual reality affords opportunities to enhance the sense of presence with visual, auditory, and even haptic computer-generated experiences. The experience of presence may be a critical factor in the utility of VR exposure treatment for PTSD because it has the capacity to immerse the individual in an environment that will help recreate the situation where the trauma first occurred. VR offers rich sensory simulations of the traumatic event. This augments the imaginative capacities of the individual that may prevent cognitive avoidance and therefore enhance emotional engagement, an essential issue in the efficacy of exposure. Thus, for patients who are reluctant to engage in recollections of feared memories, the sensory-rich virtual world creates an evocative therapeutic environment which may enhance the patient's emotional engagement.

Additionally, as in the case of other anxiety disorders, VR technology allows for graded exposure in increasingly feared virtual environments, objects, or events that can be carefully monitored and tailored to the individual patient. VR provides a safe and protected therapeutic context where there is a very accurate control over the computer-generated stimuli. The VR world could include several steps in order for the patient to progress from lower to higher levels of distress, being exposed to parts of the traumatic event in a very progressive way. For example, the world developed by Difede and Hoffman for September 11th victims includes different levels of the attack, starting from views of the World Trade Center and going up the hierarchy including, for example, the view of people jumping from the towers, all in a 3-D environment that gives the participant a first-person view. As a result of the possibility of customized and graduated exposure tasks, VR therapy experiences may increase a patient's feelings of self-efficacy and of being an active agent of their own experience.

VR environments can also be used to include other strategies in order to go beyond the reduction of symptoms and promote resilience in order to face the future. There is already evidence of the efficacy of VR in the treatment of PTSD. Rothbaum et al. (1999) published the first case study where VR exposure was used in the treatment of PTSD with a Vietnam veteran. This team also reported data from an open trial with 16 Vietnam-era veterans (Rothbaum, Hodges, Ready, Graap, & Alarcon, 2001), revealing a trend towards reduction in some PTSD symptoms and maintenance of the therapeutic gains at 6-month follow-up. The virtual world developed for these studies was "Virtual Vietnam" and it simulated scenarios representing situations experienced by the veterans of the Vietnam War, including a rice paddy and a helicopter ride. It is important to highlight that the patients included in these studies suffered from a chronic PTSD of more than 20 years of duration. Also, the authors pointed out that the treatment did not have adverse effects. None of the patients decompensated or had to be hospitalized during the application of the treatment or follow-up.

Difede and Hoffman (2002) presented a case study on the use of VR exposure for the treatment of PTSD in a victim of the September 11th attack with positive results. Later, this group conducted a clinical trial comparing VR exposure with a waiting list condition (Difede et al., 2007), with very good results at posttreatment (effect size of 1.54) that were maintained at 6-month follow-up. It must be underlined that these authors included in their studies patients who did not respond to the traditional imaginal exposure. Therefore, they showed that VR could be a useful alternative for those patients who have not been treated successfully with imaginal exposure.

In the area of terrorism with civilian victims, another group in Israel developed a virtual world simulating a "Bus Bombing" terrorist attack (Josman et al., 2006). They tested the preliminary efficacy of this VR environment in a case study (Freedman et al., 2010) showing significant reductions of PTSD symptoms at post-test that were maintained at 6-month follow-up.

Beck, Palyo, Winer, Schwagler, and Ang (2007) reported data of an uncontrolled trial of six patients suffering PTSD resulting from motor vehicle accidents (MVA) and treated with virtual driving scenarios. The results showed reductions in PTSD symptoms as well as higher sense of presence and satisfaction with the treatment.

A line of research that is being expanding in the last few years is the use of VR exposure for the treatment of PTSD in military personnel returning from Iraq and Afghanistan. There is preliminary evidence of the efficacy of VR in this population.

Rizzo et al. (2010) found that 16 out of 20 treatment completers participating in an open trial did not meet PTSD criteria after the treatment. Reger et al. (2011) conducted an open trial in a naturalistic setting reporting significant reductions of PTSD symptoms in 24 active duty soldiers. McLay et al. (2011) published data of a small randomized clinical trial comparing VR exposure to a treatment as usual condition (TAU), reporting also positive results.

These results are still preliminary, but very encouraging. All the virtual worlds described thus far for the treatment of PTSD have been designed and addressed to very specific populations that have experienced the same traumatic event. The virtual scenario was very similar for all patients. A possible limitation of this approach is that it could be difficult to reach all patients suffering different traumatic experiences. In a research setting or in specific clinical settings (i.e., mental health care for veterans), it is more common to have such specific populations. However, in a clinical setting providing general mental health care, it is typical to encounter different people with a wider variety of trauma experiences. In this case it would be more suitable to use a different approach with more flexible virtual worlds in order to be able to customize the virtual environments for different PTSD populations like assault victims, terrorism victims, sexual aggression victims, MVA, etc.

This approach is addressed by Botella's research team in Spain. The focus in designing such flexible and tailored VR environments is not on realism, but on using customized symbols and stimuli to evoke an emotional reaction in the participant to help achieve the needed emotional processing of the trauma. The aim of this work is to design clinically significant environments for each participant, while attending to the meaning of the trauma for the individual. At the same time, the process creates a safe and protective environment that helps the patient to recover and improve their functioning in his/her life. This line of research has been conducted within the Engaging Media for Mental Health Applications (EMMA) project, a research project funded by the European Union. In this project, a VR application using an adaptive display was designed (EMMA's world). In this world the therapist and patient work in exposure therapy going though the trauma and processing negative emotions related to it (anxiety, fear, anger, sadness). EMMA's world is a natural environment where it is possible to change the landscape and weather in order to represent the patient's emotions (a desert, a green countryside, snow, rain, storms, etc.). In Fig. 14.1 we offer some pictures of the different landscapes. There is also an architectural space where the patient and therapist can use different virtual elements: objects, pictures, videos, music, etc. in order to represent and work on processing the traumatic event. Patients are also given access to the "Book of Life," a virtual book where all the patient's virtual elements can be placed in order to help them to construct and "narrate" the trauma and its meaning in a dynamic way progressing from session to session. This VR world can be used for the treatment of PTSD and also for other stress-related disorders like adjustment disorders or pathological grief. Baños et al. (2011) published preliminary data from a controlled trial with 39 participants comparing the use of EMMA for the treatment of stress-related disorders compared to standard CBT. The results at posttreatment indicated that both

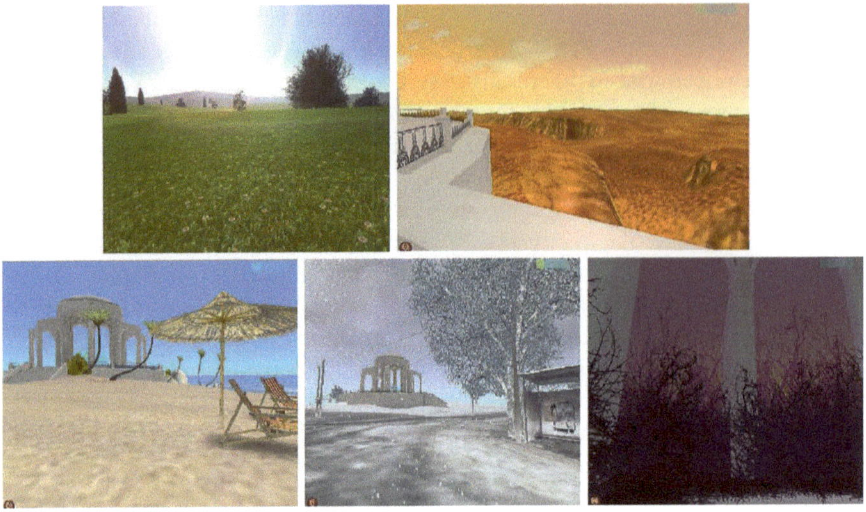

Fig. 14.1 Images of EMMA's world landscapes

treatment conditions were equally efficacious in the main outcome variables. The EMMA condition was also reported to be slightly, but significantly superior in social impairment ($p < 0.034$) and depression ($p < 0.044$).

Although the data are still preliminary, the EMMA approach could be a useful alternative to other VR systems that have a specific trauma approach in settings where the patients present different traumas and there is a need of a higher customization of the stimuli to conduct VR exposure.

Closing Remarks

There has been an impressive progress in the understanding and treatment of PTSD since its inclusion in DSM-III in 1980. And the research literature supports the view that CBT approaches including exposure therapy constitute the first-line treatment for this disorder.

Despite this existing evidence, there is still room for improvement given that exposure therapy in the field of PTSD seems to have a dissemination problem. As we have seen, therapists do not use exposure therapy as often as it should be recommended. There are misconceptions that are not empirically supported which suggest that exposure could exacerbate symptoms or increase treatment dropout. This seems to be more a problem for therapists who are unaware of the state of the literature, than for patients. One important direction for this work is to disseminate the benefits of exposure therapy in a more effective way. Rigorous research and training may not be enough. Perhaps better dissemination of the research data in a more "friendly" or personalized way, for example including the views and opinions of patients who had benefited from this form of treatment, could be a way to reach patients and therapists and support its effective implementation.

Another approach is to design new treatment programs for PTSD. There are a wide variety of emerging psychological treatments for this disorder. However, the results are still preliminary and none of them have been demonstrated to be superior to exposure-based approaches. It seems that some of these new programs could be used as an adjunct to exposure therapy in order to treat other comorbid symptoms like depression or social impairment.

It is also important to highlight that exposure therapy is supported by consistent findings from a number of randomized clinical trials and rigorous research. Thus, any emerging treatment should demonstrate to be at least equally effective as standard exposure therapy before recommending it as an alternative for the treatment of PTSD.

Finally, another approach could be to improve the way to deliver exposure therapy. This is the goal of VR exposure programs. VR can help to enhance the effectiveness and acceptability of exposure therapy. VR can simulate the stressful event with a high degree of realism and, therefore, help the patients regardless of their ability to imagine or engage with the trauma experience. It also permits precise control in the presentation of the feared stimuli or situations to the patient. This may prevent cognitive avoidance and therefore enhance emotional engagement, an essential issue in the efficacy of exposure. In the review by Cukor et al. (2009) about emerging treatments for PTSD, the authors concluded that technological-based approaches (VR) obtained the strongest efficacy support. We believe it is worth to continue exploring the efficacy and effectiveness of this way of delivering exposure in the treatment of PTSD. It is important to conduct randomized clinical trials comparing the efficacy of VR exposure with the gold standard, imaginal exposure, in order to determine if VR exposure is as efficacious as imaginal exposure. If that is the case (as it has been demonstrated with other anxiety disorders, cf. Parsons & Rizzo, 2008) another line of work should be to investigate if VR could have better acceptability than the traditional imaginal exposure. A possible benefit of using VR exposure would be seen in an increase in the number of people willing to start an exposure-based program. Finally, the work done by Difede et al. (2007) is another important line of research that has explored the use of VR for those individuals who do not respond to imaginal exposure. Difede and her collaborators have offered preliminary data supporting this fact.

In summary, information and communication technology, and specifically VR has significant potential as an innovative way of applying exposure therapy that could help to reach a larger number of individuals who suffer from a severe and chronic condition like PTSD. VR exposure for PTSD is an example of the progress of cognitive-behavioral therapy in the search of innovation and improvement of existing strategies for this disorder.

References

American Psychiatric Association (APA). (1980). *Diagnostic and statistical manual of mental disorders (DSM-III)* (3rd ed.). Washington, DC: American Psychiatric Association.

Baños, R. M., Guillén, V., Quero, S., García-Palacios, A., Alcañiz, M., & Botella, C. (2011). A virtual reality system for the treatment of stress-related disorders: A preliminary analysis of efficacy compared to a standard cognitive behavioral program. *International Journal of Human-Computer Studies, 69*, 602–613.

Beck, J. G., Palyo, S. A., Winer, E. H., Schwagler, B. E., & Ang, E. J. (2007). Virtual reality exposure therapy for PTSD symptoms after a road accident: An uncontrolled case series. *Behavior Therapy, 38*(1), 39–48.

Becker, C. B., Darius, E., & Schaumberg, K. (2007). An analog study of patient preferences for exposure versus alternative treatments for posttraumatic stress disorder. *Behaviour Research and Therapy, 45*, 2861–2873.

Becker, C. B., Zayfert, C., & Anderson, E. (2004). A survey of psychologists' attitudes towards and utilization of exposure therapy for PTSD. *Behaviour Research and Therapy, 42*, 277–292.

Bradley, R., Greene, J., Russ, E., Dutra, L., & Westen, D. (2005). A multidimensional metaanalysis of psychotherapy for PTSD. *American Journal of Psychiatry, 162*(2), 214–227.

Cukor, J., Spitalnick, J., Difede, J., Rizzo, A., & Rothbaum, B. O. (2009). Emerging treatments for PTSD. *Clinical Psychology Review, 29*(8), 715–726.

Difede, J., Cukor, J., Jayasinghe, N., Patt, I., Jedel, S., Spielman, L., et al. (2007). Virtual reality exposure therapy for the treatment of posttraumatic stress disorder following September 11, 2001. *Journal of Clinical Psychiatry, 68*(11), 1639–1647.

Difede, J., & Hoffman, H. G. (2002). Virtual reality exposure therapy for world trade center posttraumatic stress disorder: A case report. *Cyberpsychology and Behavior, 5*, 529–535.

Foa, E. B., & Kozak, M. J. (1986). Emotional processing of fear. Exposure to corrective information. *Psychological Bulletin, 99*, 20–35.

Foa, E. B., & McNally, R. (1996). Mechanisms of change in exposure therapy. In R. M. Rapee (Ed.), *Current controversies in anxiety disorders* (pp. 329–343). New York: Guilford.

Foa, E. B., & Rothbaum, B. O. (1998). *Treating the trauma of rape. Cognitive-behavioral therapy for PTSD*. New York: Guilford Press.

Foa, E. B., Rothbaum, B. O., & Furr, J. M. (2003). Augmenting exposure therapy with other CBT procedures. *Psychiatric Annals, 33*(1), 47–53.

Foa, E. B., Zoellner, L. A., Feeny, N. C., Hembree, E. A., & Alvarez-Conrad, J. (2002). Does imaginal exposure exacerbate PTSD symptoms? *Journal of Consulting and Clinical Psychology, 70*, 1022–1028.

Freedman, S. A., Hoffman, H. G., Garcia-Palacios, A., Weiss, P. L., Avitzour, S., & Josman, N. (2010). Prolonged exposure and virtual reality–enhanced imaginal exposure for PTSD following a terrorist bulldozer attack: A case study. *Cyberpsychology, Behavior and Social Networking, 13*, 95–101.

Garcia-Palacios, A., Botella, C., Hoffman, H., & Fabregat, S. (2007). Comparing acceptance and refusal rates of virtual reality exposure vs. in vivo exposure by patients with specific phobias. *Cyberpsychology and Behavior, 10*, 722–724.

Hembree, E. A., Foa, E. B., Dorfan, N. M., Street, G. P., Kowalski, J., & Tu, X. (2003). Do patients drop out prematurely from exposure therapy for PTSD? *Journal of Traumatic Stress, 16*, 555–562.

Herbert, J. D., & Sageman, M. (2004). "First do not harm:" Emerging guidelines for the treatment of posttraumatic reactions. In G. M. Rosen (Ed.), *Posttraumatic stress disorder. Issues and controversies*. New York: Wiley.

Hoffman, H. G., Doctor, J. N., Patterson, D. R., Carrougher, G. J., & Furness, T. A. (2000). Use of virtual reality for adjunctive treatment of adolescent burn pain during wound care: A case report. *Pain, 85*, 305–309.

Hoffman, H. G., Patterson, D. R., & Carrougher, G. J. (2000). Use of virtual reality for adjunctive treatment of adult burn pain during physical therapy: A controlled study. *The Clinical Journal of Pain, 16*(3), 244–250.

Hoffman, H. G., Prothero, J., Wells, M. J., & Groen, J. (1998). Virtual chess: Meaning enhances users' sense of presence in virtual environments. *International Journal of Human-Computer Interaction, 10*, 251–263.

Jaycox, L. H., Foa, E. B., & Morral, A. R. (1998). Influence of emotional engagement and habituation on exposure therapy for PTSD. *Journal of Consulting and Clinical Psychology, 66*(1), 185–192.

Josman, N., Somer, E., Reisberg, A., Weiss, P. L. T., Garcia-Palacios, A., & Hoffman, H. (2006). BusWorld: Designing a virtual environment for post-traumatic stress disorder in Israel: A protocol. *Cyberpsychology & Behavior, 9*(2), 241–244.

Keefe, F. J., Huling, D. A., Coggins, M. J., Keefe, D. F., Rosenthal, M. Z., Herr, N. R., et al. (2012). Virtual reality for persistent pain: A new direction for behavioural pain management. *Pain, 153*, 2163–2166.

Marks, I. M. (1987). *Fears, phobias and rituals*. Nueva York: Oxford University.

McLay, R. N., Wood, D. P., Webb-Murphy, J. A., Spira, J. L., Wiederhold, M. D., Pyne, J. M., et al. (2011). A randomized, controlled trial of virtual reality-graded exposure therapy for post-traumatic stress disorder in active duty service members with combat-related post-traumatic stress disorder. *Cyberpsychology, Behavior and Social Networking, 14*, 223–229.

Opris, D., Pintea, S., García-Palacios, A., Botella, C., Szamosközi, S., & David, D. (2012). Virtual reality exposure therapy in anxiety disorders: A quantitative meta-analysis. *Depression and Anxiety, 29*, 85–93.

Parsons, T. D., & Rizzo, A. A. (2008). Affective outcomes of virtual reality exposure therapy for anxiety and specific phobias: A meta-analysis. *Journal of Behavior Therapy and Experimental Psychiatry, 39*(3), 250–261.

Powers, M. B., & Emmelkamp, P. M. G. (2008). Virtual reality exposure therapy for anxiety disorders: A meta-analysis. *Journal of Anxiety Disorders, 22*(3), 561–569.

Reger, G. M., Holloway, K. M., Candy, C., Rothbaum, B. O., Difede, J., Rizzo, A. A., et al. (2011). Effectiveness of virtual reality exposure therapy for active duty soldiers in a military mental health clinic. *Journal of Traumatic Stress, 24*(1), 93–96.

Richard, D. C. S., & Gloster, A. T. (2007). Exposure therapy has a public relations problem: A dearth of litigation amid a wealth of concern. In D. C. S. Richard & D. Lauterbach (Eds.), *Handbook of exposure therapies* (pp. 409–425). New York: Academic Press/Elsevier.

Rizzo, A., Difede, J., Rothbaum, B. O., Reger, G., Spitalnick, J., Cukor, J., et al. (2010). Development and early evaluation of the virtual Iraq/Afghanistan exposure therapy system for combat-related PTSD. *Annals of the New York Academy of Sciences, 1208*, 114–125.

Rothbaum, B. O., Hodges, L., Alarcon, R. D., Ready, D., Shahar, F., Graap, K., et al. (1999). Virtual reality exposure therapy for Vietnam veterans with posttraumatic stress disorder. *Journal of Traumatic Stress, 12*, 263–271.

Rothbaum, B., Hodges, L., Opdyke, D., Willifor, M., & North, M. (1995). Effectiveness of computer-generated (virtual reality) graded exposure in the treatment of acrophobia. *American Journal of Psychiatry, 152*, 626–628.

Rothbaum, B. O., Hodges, L., Ready, D., Graap, K., & Alarcon, R. D. (2001). Virtual reality exposure therapy for Vietnam veterans with posttraumatic stress disorder. *Journal of Clinical Psychiatry, 62*, 617–622.

Zayfert, C., DeViva, J. C., Becker, C. B., Pike, J. L., Gillock, K. L., & Hayes, S. A. (2005). Exposure utilization and completion of cognitive behavioral therapy for PTSD in a "real world" clinical practice. *Journal of Traumatic Stress, 18*(6), 637–645.

Chapter 15
Initial Development and Dissemination of Virtual Reality Exposure Therapy for Combat-Related PTSD

Greg M. Reger, Albert A. Rizzo, and Gregory A. Gahm

Introduction

US military operations in Iraq and Afghanistan have resulted in the deployment of millions of military service members (American Psychiatric Association, 2007). These deployments include inherent risks of exposure to combat and other potentially traumatic events (Hoge et al., 2004). Accordingly, research has found an increased risk of mental health disorders among military personnel (Hoge et al., 2004; Hoge, Auchterlonie, & Milliken, 2006; Milliken, Auchterlonie, & Hoge, 2007; Thomas et al., 2010). Rates of posttraumatic stress disorder (PTSD) have been particularly noteworthy. Studies have found that approximately 12–20 % of Army combat soldiers and Marines screen positive for the disorder following deployment (Hoge et al., 2004; Milliken et al., 2007; Thomas et al., 2010).

Fortunately, effective treatments are available. Cognitive behavioral treatments are among the most researched interventions and have robust evidence supporting

---

DOD Disclaimer: The opinions or assertions contained herein are the private views of the authors and are not to be construed as official or as reflecting the views of the Department of the Army or the Department of Defense.

G.M. Reger, Ph.D. (✉)
National Center for Telehealth and Technology, Joint Base Lewis-McChard, Tacoma, WA 99431, USA

VA Puget Sound Health Care System, Seattle, WA 98108, USA
e-mail: Greg.Reger@va.gov

A.A. Rizzo, Ph.D.
Institute for Creative Technologies, University of Southern California, Playa Vista, CA, USA
e-mail: Rizzo@ict.usc.edu

G.A. Gahm, Ph.D.
National Center for Telehealth and Technology, Joint Base Lewis-McChord, Tacoma, WA 98431, USA
e-mail: gregory.a.gahm.civ@mail.mil

M.P. Safir et al. (eds.), *Future Directions in Post-Traumatic Stress Disorder*,
DOI 10.1007/978-1-4899-7522-5_15

their efficacy (American Psychiatric Association, 2004; Foa, Keane, Friedman, & Cohen, 2009). Among these treatments, exposure therapy in particular has received empirical support (Institute of Medicine, 2008; Powers, Halpern, Ferenschak, Gillihan, & Foa, 2010). However, based on smaller effect sizes for survivors of combat trauma (Bradley, Greene, Russ, Dutra, & Westen, 2005) and the need for treatment choices that can mitigate stigma (Reger & Gahm, 2008), innovative treatment options for military personnel have been pursued.

One promising innovative treatment is virtual reality exposure therapy (VRET). VRET is a form of exposure therapy that builds on emotional processing theory (Foa & Kozak, 1986) by seeking to leverage multisensory virtual reality stimuli that are relevant to the patient's trauma memory in order to activate the related fear structure and modulate emotional engagement. Previous research shows preliminary support in the use of VRET to treat Vietnam veterans (Rothbaum, Hodges, Ready, Graap, & Alarcon, 2001), survivors of 9/11 (Difede et al., 2007), motor vehicle accidents (Beck, Palyo, Winer, Schwagler, & Ang, 2007), and active duty soldiers (Reger et al., 2011). However, at the time of this writing, there are no head-to-head randomized controlled trials comparing VRET to an evidence-based treatment for PTSD. Particular interest has been paid in recent years to the development of VRET systems that could be effectively used to treat service members with PTSD following deployments to Iraq and Afghanistan.

There are specific challenges related to the development and dissemination of any computer-based psychological intervention. First, the development of a useful and effective solution requires focused consideration of the end user, in this case the soldier, sailor, airman, or marine. Doing so requires the implementation of a user-centered approach to the design of the tool. Second, the technical and clinical skill set related to the use of the tool must be disseminated to those practitioners who need it. The most effective treatment in the world is of little value if it is not used by those conducting research on the treatment of patients with the disorder. This chapter reviews work done to incorporate the feedback of military personnel into the early development of a Virtual Iraq/Afghanistan system and also reviews efforts to disseminate this promising treatment to DoD and VA researchers and behavioral health providers.

Soldiers Reactions and Feedback

The fact that software developers believe a technology solution is useful has little relevance to the prediction of what end users will think (Barnum, 2002). User-centered design places the expected user of a technology, in this case the U.S. service member, at the heart of the design process (Rubin & Chisnell, 2008). Keeping the end user in mind during development helps to ensure that the solution being considered is wanted by users, is useful, efficient, effective, and is satisfactory (Barnum, 2002). Indeed, the gathering of user feedback should be repeated in an iterative fashion; doing so helps to ensure that the limited resources available will be applied in a fashion that will meet the defined needs. The current economic landscape demands efficient use of resources and a user-centered approach is essential to cost-effective execution (Nielsen, 1994). When usability is not taken into account, technology solutions frustrate, developed health interventions are not used, resources are wasted, and ultimately, military personnel do not receive the help they need.

User feedback may be particularly important for a trauma-focused psychological intervention. Exposure-based treatments aim to activate a theoretically optimal level of emotional engagement (Foa, Huppert, & Cahill, 2006). This is accomplished by asking the patient to confront difficult memories and feared situations/circumstances in their day-to-day lives (Foa, Hembree, & Rothbaum, 2007). Accordingly, exposure is inherently difficult for the patient. A minority of patients actually experience a temporary symptom exacerbation prior to improvement (Foa, Zoellner, Feeny, Hembree, & Alvarez-Conrad, 2002). Incorporating a poorly designed virtual reality tool that augments exposure with multisensory cues could increase emotional engagement and discomfort to the point that new learning is not taking place. Alternatively, the video game like appearance of a virtual environment may not represent the highly emotional combat trauma with enough fidelity to activate the fear structure. If unrealistic, VRET could distract the patient from their memory, decrease emotional engagement, and possibly reduce clinical outcomes. Similarly, although VRET is presumed to offer an appealing form of treatment for a young, technologically savvy population of military personnel (Reger, Gahm, Rizzo, Swanson, & Duma, 2009), without user feedback the developed environments may be judged negatively by patients, potentially impacting decisions to access care, rates of treatment compliance, or treatment satisfaction.

Feedback from Deployed Soldiers

In March 2005, the first author was assigned to a combat stress control detachment that deployed in support of Operation Iraqi Freedom. Shortly after the initiation of this deployment, a portable prototype Virtual Iraq system was acquired and shipped into theater. The system included two XPS Dell notebook computers, a head-mounted display (HMD) with head orientation tracking, a USB gaming joystick, and a crossover cable to connect the two computers. One of these computers delivered the virtual environment to the HMD that the patient interacted with and the other computer enabled a clinician's interface that allowed real time customization of the virtual environment in order to match a trauma memory. The Virtual Iraq software was at an early stage of development and the purpose of sending the system to Iraq was to obtain feedback from service members actually located in the country represented by the virtual environment. In addition, the delivery of timely, exposure-based treatments to personnel who are still deployed is of growing interest (Cigrang, Peterson, & Schobitz, 2005; McLay, McBrien, Wiederhold, & Wiederhold, 2010). Although no VRET was delivered in theater, we were interested in the durability of the computer hardware and VR peripherals in an austere environment as well as the relevance of graphic imagery delivered by the system (See Fig. 15.1).

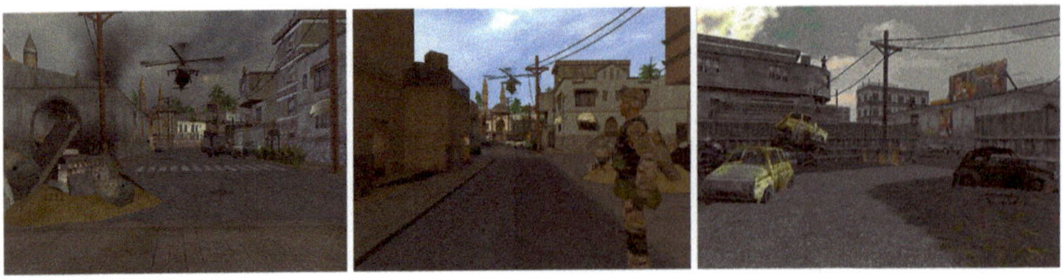

Fig. 15.1 Virtual Iraq prototype system, circa 2004–2005

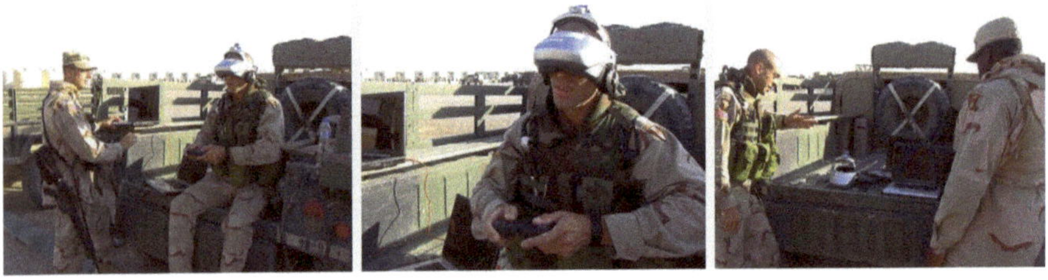

Fig. 15.2 SM User in Iraq experiencing virtual Iraq and providing feedback

Dozens of deployed soldiers used the environment (see Fig. 15.2) and were asked to provide feedback and recommendations for improvement. Initial feedback suggested general satisfaction with the realism of the auditory stimuli based on their deployment experiences. However, soldiers recommended three-dimensional sounds that would adjust according to head movements or location (e.g., when located in a virtual building interior). Soldiers also recommended that auditory stimuli representing small arms fire include a representation of impact with a vehicle or building.

Problematic features of the Virtual Iraq were also identified. For example, unrealistic visual intrusions distracted users from a sense of realistic participation. An Iraqi voice saying the unrealistic phrase "Go home cowboy!," unrealistic Saddam statue, geographically dispersed building structures instead of clusters of structures with miles of vacant desert, too many destroyed vehicles, and too many clouds in the sky were all potential distractions. On the other hand, certain expected stimuli were noted to be absent. For example, soldiers reported that the Virtual Iraq would better represent their experience if it included significant civilian traffic and more pedestrians, clusters of garbage on sides of the road, and children begging. The addition of animals (dead and alive), improvised explosive devices, crowds of teenage rock throwers, and the ability to drive on the opposite side of the road were also recommended.

Similarly, deployed soldiers did not like the navigation available at that time. Soldiers found foot patrol movement in the city environment somewhat awkward as it required the user to look in the direction he or she wanted to move. This resulted in unusual and strained head positions to navigate to the desired destination. Soldiers were also frustrated by the inability to steer the vehicle in the convoy or adjust speed

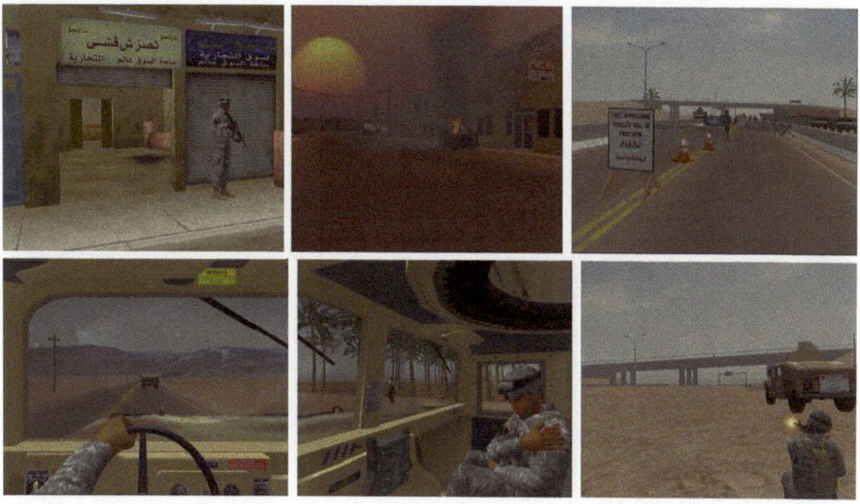

Fig. 15.3 Virtual Iraq/Afghanistan system, circa 2007, Middle Eastern City and driving scenarios

of movement in both scenarios. Although some of these recommendations were not surprising given the early stage of development, the soldiers' feedback was helpful for the development team to prioritize their efforts and avoid wasting limited resources on features irrelevant to intended users.

Feedback from Previously Deployed Soldiers

Based on the need for continued, iterative soldier feedback and a desire to formalize a data collection methodology, the authors launched a study of previously deployed soldiers' feedback (Reger et al., 2009) of the evolving Virtual Iraq/Afghanistan VRET system, the design of which was informed by the initial feedback from soldiers in Iraq. Soldiers who had been home from Iraq or Afghanistan for less than a year were recruited to use and evaluate the current system.

The Virtual Iraq/Afghanistan application developed at the time (2006–2007) comprised of a series of virtual scenarios including a Middle-East themed city and roadway environments (See Fig. 15.3). The scenarios were designed to resemble the general contexts that most SMs would have experienced during a deployment to Iraq or Afghanistan. The 18-square block City setting had a variety of elements including a marketplace, desolate streets, old buildings, ramshackle apartments, warehouses, mosques, shops, and dirt lots strewn with junk. Access to building interiors and rooftops was available and the backdrop surrounding the navigable exposure zone created the illusion of being embedded within a section of a sprawling densely populated desert city. Vehicles were active in streets and animated virtual pedestrians (civilian and military) could be added or eliminated from the scenes.

Users could be teleported to specific locations within the city, based on a determination as to which environments most closely matched their experiences.

The Iraq Desert road scenario consisted of a roadway through an expansive desert area with sand dunes, occasional areas of vegetation, intact and broken down structures, bridges, battle wreckage, a checkpoint, debris, and virtual human figures. The system also had an Afghanistan-themed road scenario that contained similar elements but within a more mountainous terrain context that included Afghan style architectural and cultural elements. In both the Iraq and Afghanistan roadways, the user could be positioned inside of a HUMVEE that supported the perception of travel within a convoy or as a lone vehicle with selectable positions as a driver, passenger, or from the more exposed turret position above the roof of the vehicle. Both the city and HUMVEE scenarios were adjustable for time of day or night, weather conditions, night vision, illumination, and ambient sound (wind, motors, city noise, prayer call, etc.). Users could navigate in both scenarios via the use of a standard gamepad controller.

In addition to the visual stimuli presented in the VR Head-Mounted Display (HMD), directional 3D audio, vibrotactile and olfactory stimuli could be delivered into the VR scenarios in real time by the clinician. The presentation of additive, combat-relevant stimuli in the VR scenarios could be controlled via a "Wizard of Oz" control panel, while the clinician was in full audio contact with the patient. This clinical "interface" provided the clinician with the capacity to customize the therapy experience to the individual needs of the patient. The patient could be placed by the clinician in VR scenario locations that resembled a setting relevant to their trauma experience and modify ambient light and sound conditions to match the patient's description of their experience. The interface also allowed the clinician to gradually introduce and control trigger stimuli in real time to foster the anxiety modulation needed for therapeutic habituation and emotional processing in a customized fashion according to the patient's past experience and treatment progress. Such options for real time stimulus delivery flexibility and user experience customization were considered to be key elements for this application. Trigger stimuli included a variety of auditory stimuli (e.g., incoming mortars, weapons fire, voices, wind), dynamic audiovisual events including helicopter flyovers, bridge attacks, exploding vehicles and IEDs, and olfactory stimuli (e.g., burning rubber, gunpowder, garbage, diesel fuel). In contrast to the VR system taken to Iraq, this study added a platform with bass shaker speakers. These speakers enabled low frequency sounds (e.g., virtual explosions or the idle of the vehicle) to also be experienced as vibrations by participants.

Soldiers responded to a series of likert scale items ranging from 1 (*poor*) to 10 (*excellent*), with the midpoint of 5 representing an *adequate* rating. Ninety-three soldiers provided feedback. Although the average evaluation was between adequate and excellent for all rated aspects (see Table 15.1), additional needed improvements were identified. For example, soldiers felt it was unrealistic to stand on a platform and navigate in a foot patrol scenario holding a gaming joystick. A number of participants reported that realism would be enhanced if they were holding their weapon. Both environments were judged too clean. Soldiers recommended more

Table 15.1 Means and standard deviations for soldier evaluations of the virtual reality Iraq

	City environment		Convoy environment	
	Mean	SD	Mean	SD
Overall realism	6.02	1.81	6.42	1.95
Sense of being in Iraq	6.09	2.40	6.48	2.25
Quality of visual scenery	6.75	1.88	7.08	1.84
Realism of visual scenery	6.55	2.08	6.61	2.08
Quality of sounds	7.72	1.79	7.99	1.70
Realism of sounds	7.66	1.70	7.81	1.81
Ability to move	5.45	2.37	6.30	2.44
Comfort of the head-mounted display	8.18	1.71	8.19	1.72
Quality of computer graphics update	8.43	1.53	8.52	1.58

Note Reprinted with permission from Reger et al. (2009)
Evaluations were made on a scale ranging from 0 to 10 with anchors of 0 (poor), 5 (adequate), and 10 (excellent)

debris, dirt, and garbage. Soldiers also found it unrealistic to be seated in a virtual vehicle or walking through an Iraqi city alone. They requested the presence of additional soldiers. Additional Iraqi civilian pedestrians were requested and the possibility of more congested traffic was recommended. Soldiers also suggested the development of a library of tactical vehicles and weapons that could be selected based on the personal experience of the soldier.

The Resulting Virtual Iraq/Afghanistan System

These two efforts resulted in a number of key improvements to the Virtual Iraq/Afghanistan system. Changes included the adaptation of a mock M4 rifle with a mounted mini joystick, allowing soldiers to navigate through the virtual city in a naturalistic fashion, while holding the physical prop of a realistic weapon. Truck commanders, turret gunners, and passengers were added and both environments were improved with additional pedestrian and vehicle traffic. Among other improvements, recommendations regarding the inclusion of animal carcasses, dirt, and garbage were implemented.

Feedback received from the intended end users was essential to the development of a useful Virtual Iraq/Afghanistan system. More importantly, the development of an improved system enabled successful treatment protocol development and clinical application. The VR Iraq/Afghanistan system has been used for the effective exposure therapy treatment of members of the National Guard (Gerardi, Rothbaum, Ressler, Heekin, & Rizzo, 2008) as well as active component soldiers (Reger et al., 2011; Reger & Gahm, 2008; Rizzo et al., 2011). Well-designed randomized controlled trials are currently underway to determine the efficacy of VRET relative to existing standards of care. Based on the initial success of the use of this approach for the delivery of exposure therapy using VR, the U.S. Department of Defense has funded the development of an updated and expanded version of the Virtual Iraq/Afghanistan system built from currently available software. This work will be detailed in the chapter by Rizzo et al. (2014) in this volume.

Dissemination of Virtual Reality Exposure in the Treatment of PTSD

Change is difficult. This appears to be as true of mental health practitioners as anyone. Research has demonstrated that adoption of evidence-based psychotherapies by clinicians is slow, despite significant research supporting efficacy (Frueh, Grubaugh, Cusack, & Elhai, 2009). A survey of 207 licensed psychologists found that only 9 % reported using imaginal exposure with 50 % or more of their PTSD patients (Becker, Zayfert, & Anderson, 2004). The primary factor limiting use of imaginal exposure was limited training (Becker et al., 2004). Similarly, when 296 trauma experts were asked to what extent they agreed with the statement that they had received good training in imaginal exposure, their average response was lukewarm. On a scale from 1 to 10, with 10 representing strong agreement, the average response was 3.76 ($SD = 3.03$, van Minnen, Hendriks, & Olff, 2010). It is not surprising that only a minority of these therapists used exposure to treat their PTSD patients.

Development of a new, promising innovative treatment does not guarantee adoption and implementation, even by interested early adopters and researchers. Adequate training is required. Furthermore, researchers or clinicians seeking to study or implement VRET need training to build on existing best practices. In October 2008, we had received enough requests for VRET training that we began hosting clinical training workshops to assist Veterans Administration (VA) and Department of Defense (DoD) researchers and providers who were seeking to learn current best practices for this promising emerging treatment.

The training approach was carefully considered with an eye towards the likely audience, necessary prerequisite knowledge, and common factors affecting implementation (Ruzek & Rosen, 2009). According to Fixsen and colleagues, as cited in Ruzek and Rosen (2009), the impact of training workshops increases when skill demonstration and rehearsal are included. We also wanted to build in opportunities for post-training consultation and supervision to support an ethical model of new skill acquisition (American Psychological Association, 2002) and to assist with post-training consolidation of learned skills (Ruzek & Rosen, 2009).

The resulting VRET training program included the prerequisite that attendees have prior formal training in prolonged exposure. This requirement was established because the skills necessary for the VRET treatment protocol (Rothbaum, Difede, & Rizzo, 2008) resemble many of those required by other exposure therapy protocols (Foa et al., 2007). Foundational exposure therapy skills were judged essential as a prerequisite for training competent VRET therapists. The workshops were also planned to dedicate significant time to demonstrations of VRET skills

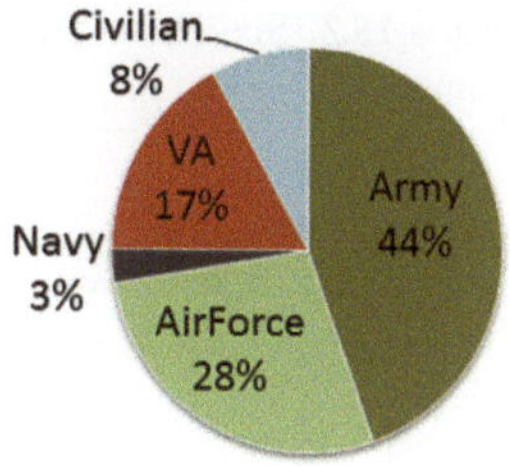

Fig. 15.4 Organizational and service representation of VRET trainees (*N*=148)

Table 15.2 Student evaluations of virtual reality exposure therapy training (*N*=120)

Item	Percent of trainees who "Strongly Agree"[a] (%)
Teaching strategies and methods used in the program were appropriate and effective	94
The overall training was worthwhile	94
The training objectives were relevant to your professional needs and interests	84
I would recommend this program to a friend or coworker	96

[a]On a 5-point likert scale, Strongly Agree=5

and hands-on rehearsal. Over the course of a 2-day workshop, as much as half of the training time is dedicated to hands-on experience with the Virtual Iraq/Afghanistan software, virtual reality hardware, trouble shooting, and role plays with faculty and other students. Trainees are divided into breakout groups of approximately five trainees and one faculty member to rehearse the instructed skills. Finally, from the outset we included the opportunity for 6 months of weekly telephone consultation with faculty.

At the time of writing, we have hosted seven training workshops, which have disseminated VRET to 148 individuals from 35 locations. Providers from all three military services and the VA have been trained (Fig. 15.4). Trainees have included primarily psychologists, although social workers and psychiatrists have also attended. All workshops included student evaluations as part of the continuing education program evaluation. Over this period of time, the institutional survey items have unfortunately changed but 6 of the 7 workshops had key items that remained constant.

As is evident in Table 15.2, the trainings have been very well regarded by the trained clinicians. The vast majority of workshop attendees found the training relevant, worthwhile, and well instructed. The fact that 96 % of attendees "strongly agreed" (5/5 on a 5-point likert item) that they would recommend the training to their peers speaks volumes about the perceived value by those in attendance.

To support the program evaluation of the longer term impact of the workshops, attendees were provided a brief survey 6 months following each training. Specifically, we were interested in whether trained clinicians were using or planning to use VRET in research or clinical practice. To date, we have followed up with 107 of the

Table 15.3 Six-month program evaluation survey of virtual reality exposure therapy workshop trainees ($N=67$)

Item	Percent of previous trainees responding "yes" (%)
Do you have equipment for VRET with PTSD patients?	61
Have you used VR in research with PTSD patients?	7
Have you used VR in clinical practice with PTSD patients?	18
Are you planning VR research with PTSD patients?	36
Are you planning to use VRET in clinical practice with PTSD patients?	57

148 trained clinicians. Of these, we received responses from 67 (63 % response rate). The results were somewhat disheartening (see Table 15.3). Although slightly more than half of the previous participants who responded had the computer hardware and peripherals to use VRET, only a small percentage of prior trainees had used VRET in research or clinical practice 6-month post-training. Relative to their reported current use, prior trainees reported moderately higher rates of planned VRET use. It is not known what proportion of these plans were carried out.

Our program evaluation did not ask providers to identify barriers to implementation. However, our experience across these training efforts suggests a number of likely factors that could be considered. First, VRET requires acquisition of computer hardware and related VR equipment. The cost of this equipment has decreased significantly in recent years (Rizzo et al., 2011). Regardless, in a challenging economic landscape, implementation of VRET in a VA or DoD organization requires purchasing equipment within a context of already strained budgets. Indeed, our program evaluation found that 39 % of previous trainees did not have the equipment necessary for VRET 6-month post-training. It is possible that current requests for budget increases are not likely to be supported and some managers may have been unwilling to invest in VRET.

Second, the current absence of randomized controlled trials of VRET relative to other PTSD treatment options impedes evaluations of the return on investment for this treatment choice. Although research has demonstrated the effectiveness of VRET (Difede et al., 2007; Reger et al., 2011; Reger & Gahm, 2008; Rizzo, Difede, Rothbaum, & Reger, 2010; Rothbaum et al., 2001) and VRET appears to be a more appealing treatment than traditional approaches for some soldiers (Wilson, Onorati, Mishkind, Reger, & Gahm, 2008), responsible cost-benefit analysis cannot currently be conducted based on the existing literature. Quality head-to-head clinical trials are needed.

Third, based on the requests for VRET training we received, we expected research to make up a significant proportion of post-training VRET use. The fact that this was not the case within 6-months is perhaps not surprising. The writing, review, and approval of research grants and protocols by funding agencies and Institutional Review Boards can be a lengthy process. We understand that this is particularly true for some VA and DoD researchers. Several former trainees who reported planned research noted that the process had been started but was early in development or still under review. Such administration processes can be a particularly time consuming process for providers who are not allocated any dedicated research hours.

Fourth, implementation of new PTSD training is often impacted by system factors (Ruzek & Rosen, 2009). Previous researchers identified barriers to the implementation of PTSD treatments in public sector settings (Frueh et al., 2009), which may be relevant to the current discussion. For example, high patient case loads, too few clinicians, and inadequate knowledge of PTSD and its treatment among supervisors and administrators can all affect implementation (Frueh et al., 2009). Although we do not have an assessment of trainee's system support for VRET, it is noteworthy that the opportunity for weekly consultation with the faculty was only rarely accessed. It was not unusual to have only one or two trainees take advantage of this consultation, even though the vast majority of trainees rated the teaching of the faculty as excellent (see Table 15.2). It may be that the priority for rapid access to care for service members and veterans and a shortage of behavioral health providers in these organizations resulted in clinician schedules dedicated to patient care as opposed to consolidation of new skills.

Finally, although it may be surprising to some readers, a number of trained clinicians reported limited opportunities to treat PTSD. Service-related differences in mission may affect the population risk of exposure to deployment-related trauma. Several Air Force clinicians stated that they had not encountered many cases of PTSD in their clinic and had not been able to use VRET despite their intentions.

Conclusions

Virtual reality opens up revolutionary potential to transform psychological education, training, assessment, and treatment. Military personnel are active consumers of personal technologies (Bush, Fullerton, Crumpton, Metzger-Abamukong, & Fantelli, 2012) and service members present a patient population that is well suited to the adoption of innovative technology treatments. VRET in particular offers the promising capability to deliver customized virtual environments to support the exposure therapy of service members with PTSD. This innovative tool is consistent with current theories of PTSD acquisition and treatment (Foa & Kozak, 1986) and is showing promise in the research literature. However, as a relatively new technology tool, it faces a mix of new and old challenges.

Psychologists are not software developers or engineers and the discussion of user feedback above highlights the inherently multidisciplinary nature of work in VRET. As innovative psychologists continue to seek creative solutions that leverage virtual reality, they must reach out to partner with others that have a range of skill sets, including expertise in interface design, user experience, software development, usability, and ergonomics to name a few. Overlooking this need could be costly. Failure to incorporate end user considerations into the design from the outset will result in frustrations, delays, and failures. Engaging this challenge, however, can create new, better ideas and improved tools and solutions. This engagement will push creative behavioral health providers and researchers out of their clinics and labs and into the realms of other disciplines. This requires a teachable spirit and humility. The expert behavioral health provider is a neophyte in these new disciplines. However, the synergy potentially created by these multidisciplinary collaborations sets the stage for a new era in the psychological support of service members.

Unfortunately, the longstanding challenge of dissemination and implementation of any PTSD treatment also persists. To date, dissemination of VRET has been primarily to support early adopters of an emerging treatment and to support researchers seeking to study this promising, innovative approach. If current randomized controlled trials find VRET to be as effective as existing standards of care (or more effective), dissemination could become a more urgent issue. If this comes to pass, the dissemination efforts discussed above suggest the need for careful attention to prior lessons learned in PTSD treatment dissemination (Frueh et al., 2009; Karlin et al., 2010; Ruzek & Rosen, 2009).

References

American Psychiatric Association. (2002). *Ethical principles of psychologists and code of conduct.* Retrieved September 28, 2011, from http://www.apa.org/ethics/code/index.aspx

American Psychiatric Association. (2004). *Practice guideline for the treatment of patients with acute stress disorder and posttraumatic stress disorder.* Washington, D.C.: American Psychiatric Association.

American Psychiatric Association. (2007). *The psychological needs of U.S. military service members and their families: A preliminary report.* Retrieved September 30, 2011, from http://www.ptsd.ne.gov/publications/military-deployment-task-force-report.pdf

Barnum, C. M. (2002). *Usability testing and research.* New York: Longman.

Beck, J. G., Palyo, S. A., Winer, E. H., Schwagler, B. E., & Ang, E. J. (2007). Virtual reality exposure therapy for PTSD symptoms after a road accident: An uncontrolled case series. *Behavior Therapy, 38*(1), 39–48.

Becker, C. B., Zayfert, C., & Anderson, E. (2004). A survey of psychologists' attitudes towards and utilization of exposure therapy for PTSD. *Behaviour Research and Therapy, 42*(3), 277–292.

Bradley, R., Greene, J., Russ, E., Dutra, L., & Westen, D. (2005). A multidimensional meta-analysis of psychotherapy for PTSD. *The American Journal of Psychiatry, 162*(2), 214–227.

Bush, N., Fullerton, N., Crumpton, R., Metzger-Abamukong, M., & Fantelli, E. (2012). Soldiers' personal technologies on deployment and at home. *Telemedicine and e-Health, 18*, 253–263.

Cigrang, J. A., Peterson, A. L., & Schobitz, R. P. (2005). Three American troops in Iraq: Evaluation of a brief exposure therapy treatment for the secondary prevention of combat-related PTSD. *Pragmatic Case Studies in Psychotherapy, 1*(2), 1–25.

Difede, J., Cukor, J., Jayasinghe, N., Patt, I., Jedel, S., Spielman, L., et al. (2007). Virtual reality exposure therapy for the treatment of posttraumatic stress disorder following September 11, 2001. *Journal of Clinical Psychiatry, 68*(11), 1639–1647.

Foa, E. B., Huppert, J. D., & Cahill, S. P. (2006). Emotional processing theory: An update, In B.O. Rothbaum (Ed.), Pathological Anxiety (3–24). New York: Guilford.

Foa, E. B., Hembree, E. A., & Rothbaum, B. O. (2007). *Prolonged exposure therapy for PTSD: Emotional processing of traumatic experiences: Therapist guide.* New York, NY: Oxford University Press.

Foa, E. B., Keane, T. M., Friedman, M. J., & Cohen, J. A. (Eds.). (2009). *Effective treatments for PTSD: Practice guidelines from the international society for traumatic stress studies*. New York: Guilford Press.

Foa, E. B., & Kozak, M. J. (1986). Emotional processing of fear: Exposure to corrective information. *Psychological Bulletin, 99*(1), 20–35.

Foa, E. B., Zoellner, L. A., Feeny, N. C., Hembree, E. A., & Alvarez-Conrad, J. (2002). Does imaginal exposure exacerbate PTSD symptoms? *Journal of Consulting and Clinical Psychology, 70*(4), 1022–1028.

Frueh, B. C., Grubaugh, A. L., Cusack, K. J., & Elhai, J. D. (2009). Disseminating evidence-based practices for adults with PTSD and severe mental illness in public-sector mental health agencies. *Behavior Modification, 33*(1), 66–81.

Gerardi, M., Rothbaum, B. O., Ressler, K., Heekin, M., & Rizzo, A. (2008). Virtual reality exposure therapy using a virtual Iraq: Case report. *Journal of Traumatic Stress, 21*(2), 209–213.

Hoge, C. W., Auchterlonie, J. L., & Milliken, C. S. (2006). Mental health problems, use of mental health services, and attrition from military service after returning from deployment to Iraq or Afghanistan. *Journal of the American Medical Association, 295*(9), 1023–1032.

Hoge, C. W., Castro, C. A., Messer, S. C., McGurk, D., Cotting, D. I., & Koffman, R. L. (2004). Combat duty in Iraq and Afghanistan, mental health problems, and barriers to care. *The New England Journal of Medicine, 351*(1), 13–22.

Institute of Medicine. (2008). *Treatment of posttraumatic stress disorder: An assessment of the evidence*. Washington, DC: National Academies Press.

Karlin, B. E., Ruzek, J. I., Chard, K. M., Eftekhari, A., Monson, C. M., Hembree, E. A., et al. (2010). Dissemination of evidence-based psychological treatments for posttraumatic stress disorder in the Veterans Health Administration. *Journal of Traumatic Stress, 23*(6), 663–673.

McLay, R. N., McBrien, C., Wiederhold, M. D., & Wiederhold, B. K. (2010). Exposure therapy with and without virtual reality to treat PTSD while in the combat theater: A parallel case series. *Cyberpsychology, Behavior and Social Networking, 13*(1), 37–42.

Milliken, C. S., Auchterlonie, J. L., & Hoge, C. W. (2007). Longitudinal assessment of mental health problems among active and reserve component soldiers returning from the Iraq war. *Journal of the American Medical Association, 298*(18), 2141–2148.

Nielsen, J. (1994). *Guerrilla HCI: Using discount usability engineering to penetrate the intimidation barrier*. Retrieved September 15, 2011, from http://www.useit.com/papers/guerrilla_hci.html

Powers, M. B., Halpern, J. M., Ferenschak, M. P., Gillihan, S. J., & Foa, E. B. (2010). A meta-analytic review of prolonged exposure for posttraumatic stress disorder. *Clinical Psychology Review, 30*(6), 635–641.

Reger, G. M., & Gahm, G. A. (2008). Virtual reality exposure therapy for active duty soldiers. *Journal of Clinical Psychology, 64*(8), 940–946.

Reger, G. M., Gahm, G. A., Rizzo, A. A., Swanson, R., & Duma, S. (2009). Soldier evaluation of the virtual reality Iraq. *Telemedicine Journal and E-Health: The Official Journal of the American Telemedicine Association, 15*(1), 101–104.

Reger, G. M., Holloway, K. M., Candy, C., Rothbaum, B. O., Difede, J., Rizzo, A. A., et al. (2011). Effectiveness of virtual reality exposure therapy for active duty soldiers in a military mental health clinic. *Journal of Traumatic Stress, 24*(1), 93–96.

Rizzo, A., Difede, J., Rothbaum, B. O., & Reger, G. (2010). Virtual Iraq/Afghanistan: Development and early evaluation of a virtual reality exposure therapy system for combat-related PTSD. *Annals of the New York Academy of Sciences, 1208*, 114–125.

Rizzo, A., Parsons, T. D., Lange, B., Kenny, P., Buckwalter, J. G., Rothbaum, B., et al. (2011). Virtual reality goes to war: A brief review of the future of military behavioral healthcare. *Journal of Clinical Psychology in Medical Settings, 18*(2), 176–187.

Rothbaum, B. O., Difede, J., & Rizzo, A. A. (2008). *Therapist treatment manual for virtual reality expsoure therapy: Posttraumatic stress disroder in Iraq combat vetnerans*. Atlanta: Virtually Better.

Rothbaum, B. O., Hodges, L. F., Ready, D., Graap, K., & Alarcon, R. D. (2001). Virtual reality exposure therapy for Vietnam veterans with posttraumatic stress disorder. *Journal of Clinical Psychiatry, 62*(8), 617–622.

Rubin, J., & Chisnell, D. (2008). *Handbook of usability testing*. Indianapolis: Wiley.

Ruzek, J. I., & Rosen, R. C. (2009). Disseminating evidence-based treatments for PTSD in organizational settings: A high priority focus area. *Behaviour Research and Therapy, 47*(11), 980–989.

Thomas, J. L., Wilk, J. E., Riviere, L. A., McGurk, D., Castro, C. A., & Hoge, C. W. (2010). Prevalence of mental health problems and functional impairment among Active Component and National Guard soldiers 3 and 12 months following combat in Iraq. *Archives of General Psychiatry, 67*(6), 614–623.

van Minnen, A., Hendriks, L., & Olff, M. (2010). When do trauma experts choose exposure therapy for PTSD patients? A controlled study of therapist and patient factors. *Behaviour Research and Therapy, 48*(4), 312–320.

Wilson, J. A. B., Onorati, K., Mishkind, M., Reger, M. A., & Gahm, G. A. (2008). Soldier attitudes about technology-based approaches to mental health care. *CyberPsychology and Behavior, 11*(6), 767–769.

Chapter 16
Update and Expansion of the Virtual Iraq/Afghanistan PTSD Exposure Therapy System

Albert Rizzo, JoAnn Difede, Barbara Olasov Rothbaum, J. Galen Buckwalter, J. Martin Daughtry, and Greg M. Reger

Introduction

War is perhaps one of the most challenging situations that a human being can experience. The physical, emotional, cognitive, and psychological demands of a combat environment place enormous stress on even the best-prepared military personnel. Thus, it is no surprise that the stressful experiences that have been characteristic of the Operation Enduring Freedom/Operation Iraqi Freedom (OEF/OIF) combat theaters have produced significant numbers of returning service members (SMs) at risk for developing posttraumatic stress disorder (PTSD) and other psychosocial/behavioral health conditions. For example, as of December 2012, the

A. Rizzo (✉) • J.G. Buckwalter
Institute for Creative Technologies, University of Southern California, Los Angeles, CA, USA
e-mail: rizzo@ict.usc.edu; jgbuckwalter@gmail.com

J. Difede
Department of Psychiatry, Weill Cornell Medical College, New York, NY, USA
e-mail: jdifede@med.cornell.edu

B.O. Rothbaum
Emory University School of Medicine, Emory University, Atlanta, GA, USA
e-mail: brothba@emory.edu

J.M. Daughtry
Department of Music, New York University, New York, NY, USA
e-mail: martin.daughtry@gmail.com

G.M. Reger
National Center for Telehealth and Technology, Joint Base Lewis-McChord, Tacoma, WA, USA

VA Puget Sound Health Care System, Seattle, WA, USA
e-mail: Greg.Reger@va.gov

M.P. Safir et al. (eds.), *Future Directions in Post-Traumatic Stress Disorder*,
DOI 10.1007/978-1-4899-7522-5_16

Defense Medical Surveillance System reported that 131,341 active duty SMs have been diagnosed with PTSD (Fischer, 2013). As well, Hoge (2013) reported that 13.2 % of OEF/OIF operational infantry units met criteria for PTSD in a meta-analysis across studies since 2001 (Kok, Herrell, Thomas, & Hoge, 2012) with the PTSD incidence rising dramatically, ranging from 25 to 30 %, in infantry units with the highest levels of direct combat (Kok et al., 2012; Thomas et al., 2010). During this same time period, the prevalence of PTSD among discharged Veterans receiving treatment at Veteran Health Affairs clinics has been reported to be 29 % (Fischer, 2013). These findings make a compelling case for a continued focus on developing and enhancing the availability of diverse evidence-based treatment options to address this military behavioral healthcare challenge.

This chapter will describe a set of projects that are developing content for inclusion in a newly updated "Virtual Iraq/Afghanistan" virtual reality (VR) system for the delivery of VR exposure therapy (VRET). The chapter presupposes that the reader has read and understands the history and rationale for VRET use with Anxiety Disorders and PTSD as presented by Garcia-Palacios, Botella, Baños, Guillén, and Navarro (2014) and the early development and dissemination of the initial treatment version of the Virtual Iraq/Afghanistan system presented in Reger et al. (2014), earlier in this volume. The present chapter will start with a brief detailing of the factors that led to the initial development of Virtual Iraq/Afghanistan VRET system and the clinical outcomes that have been reported with its use. We will then discuss the current efforts to update the VRET system with more advanced software to expand the VR content and features based on input from clinical users of the previous 2007 version of the system. Following a description of this new Virtual Iraq/Afghanistan application (now referred to as "BRAVEMIND"), we will then focus on a general overview of two new projects that aim to provide relevant and customizable options for conducting VRET with users having a wider range of military trauma experiences, combat medics/corpsmen, and victims of military sexual assault. The chapter will conclude with a description of the further expansion of the system to create a VR tool for use to prevent the incidence of combat-related PTSD via pre-deployment resilience training.

Context and Rationale for Military Adoption of VRET for Combat-Related PTSD

It was during the "computer revolution" in the 1990s that promising technologically driven innovations in behavioral healthcare had begun to be considered and prototyped. Primordial efforts from this period can be seen in research and development (R&D) that aimed to use computers to enhance productivity in patient documentation and record-keeping, to deliver "drill and practice" cognitive rehabilitation, to improve access to care via internet-based teletherapy, and in the use of virtual reality simulations to deliver exposure therapy for specific phobias. These and other computer and internet driven behavioral health applications gradually evolved as the technology got faster, better, and cheaper moving into the twenty-first century. However, it was the onset of OEF/OIF and the subsequent need to provide optimal care for the significant numbers of U.S. SMs returning from the battlefront with traumatic injuries that really drove an intensive focus (and significant funding) on how technology could be marshaled to enhance, expand, and extend the reach of behavioral healthcare. Thus, the urgency of war essentially led to increased U.S. government funding levels that has substantially driven innovative R&D in behavioral healthcare technology. Primarily supported through the U.S. Department of Defense (DoD) and the Department of Veteran Affairs (VA), this increased focus and support has been most dramatically seen in research efforts to enhance the treatment of PTSD and comorbid health conditions. It is within this historical context that the DoD/VA have driven advances in behavioral healthcare technology by supporting R&D to (1) advance the development and delivery of evidence-based treatments for behavioral health conditions and (2) reduce "barriers to care" by investigating ways to improve the awareness, availability, access, appeal, acceptance, and adherence of/to evidence-based treatments and services (IOM, 2012).

This R&D funding supported a range of technology-based efforts at advancing behavioral healthcare including: teletherapy, online informational and self-help Web sites, mobile smartphone apps, virtual reality and online virtual worlds, intelligent healthcare agents, and interactive clinical training systems. However, one would be mistaken to assume that this level of DoD/VA support emerged from a naïve view or belief that technology, in and of itself, could actually "fix" anyone. In spite of the pressure at the time to address a growing behavioral healthcare challenge, funding agencies in the USA took a measured approach to funding some of the many novel systems that were being proposed at the time. Consequently, one can observe that the most promising first efforts at applying technology to address the psychological "wounds of war" were typically seen to meet two criteria: (1). They did not require the imposition of a new theoretical model of clinical care—technology-based approaches were best seen as tools to support and advance the delivery of already known and evidence-based clinical methods (e.g., Virtual Reality delivery of Prolonged Exposure), and (2). each technologic approach needed to clearly specify its rationale for targeting some recognized barrier to care. For example, most technology-based systems that were initially supported during this time also made the case that some element of the care *process* would also be enhanced to: Promote *Awareness* of care options (e.g., online resources/Web sites, Social Media), improve *Access* to care (e.g., teletherapy), support treatment *Appeal* and *Acceptability* to reduce stigma (e.g., VRET and other approaches that leverage compelling game technologies), increase the *Availability* of well-trained providers (e.g., Online training, virtual patient training), and to support *Adherence* to treatment (e.g., mobile phone apps, teletherapy). By making this secondary case, the complexity and cost of new technology-based systems could be more easily justified for support by these agencies.

The use of VR to deliver exposure-based interventions for PTSD clearly met these criteria, and consequently within this wartime zeitgeist, the DoD/VA significantly supported R&D to develop and evaluate VRET applications. The rationale for this was clear and compelling. Prolonged exposure (PE) (Foa, Hembree, &

Rothbaum, 2007) had been documented to be an effective "evidence-based" treatment for PTSD across a spectrum of trauma experiences due to combat, terrorist attacks, sexual assault, and motor vehicle accidents (IOM, 2007, 2012). However, while the efficacy of imaginal PE was established in multiple studies with diverse trauma populations, many patients were observed to be unable or unwilling to effectively visualize traumatic events and memories. In fact, avoidance of trauma reminders is inherent in PTSD and is one of the cardinal symptoms of the condition. To address this challenge, the VR delivery of an evidence-based PE protocol was seen as a way to immerse users in simulations of trauma-relevant environments in which the emotional intensity of the scenes could be precisely controlled by the clinician to personalize the exposure for the individual patient. In this fashion, VRET offered a way to circumvent the natural avoidance tendency by directly delivering multisensory and context-relevant cues that aided in the confrontation and processing of traumatic memories. Previous success in similarly using VR to deliver exposure therapy for persons with anxiety disorders such as specific phobias had been documented in at least three independent meta-analyses of the literature (Powers and Emmelkamp, 2008; Parsons & Rizzo, 2008; Opris et al., 2012) and this literature is extensively detailed in Garcia-Palacios et al. (2014). As well, three publications reported positive outcomes with non-OEF/OIF PTSD using VRET with patients who were unresponsive to a previous course of *imaginal-only* PE treatment (Difede et al., 2007; Difede & Hoffman, 2002; Rothbaum, Hodges, Ready, Graap, & Alarcon, 2001).

Moreover, the use of VR as a PE delivery system may also have potential advantages for breaking down barriers to care by improving treatment appeal, acceptability, and adherence by SMs and Veterans in need of care. The current generation of young military SMs, many having grown up with digital gaming technology, may actually be more attracted to and comfortable with participation in a VR therapy application approach and this could lead to increased access of care by those in need (Reger, Gahm, Rizzo, Swanson, and Duma, 2009; Wilson, Onorati, Mishkind, Reger, & Gahm, 2008). Additionally, in spite of DoD and VA efforts to foster adoption of PE as a first-line treatment, challenges have been noted in the dissemination of PE in part due to clinician hesitancy to adopt and use it (Becker, Zayfert, & Anderson, 2004; IOM, 2012). This challenge might be reduced with a VR system that allows a care provider to more easily create customized simulated scenarios to support patient trauma narratives with a computer control interface and thus support PE adoption by empowering clinicians with a VR tool that is readily learnable. VR also provides an objective and consistent format for documenting the sensory stimuli that the patient is exposed to that is not possible when operating exclusively within the unseen world of the patient's imagination. However, these speculations on VRET attraction and adoption still require controlled research to determine how and to what extent a VR approach may break down barriers to care and enhance dissemination.

Development and Research Outcomes from the Initial Virtual Iraq/Afghanistan VRET System

In view of the military behavioral health needs at the time and supported by a clear theoretical rationale and the extant literature, the USC Institute for Creative Technologies developed an initial prototype Virtual Iraq system in 2004 to run user tests to determine feasibility (*Video 1–2004 Virtual Iraq Prototype:* http://www.youtube.com/watch?v=zTtaK6mK3_c). A full Virtual Iraq/Afghanistan VRET simulation for PTSD treatment was developed and evaluated during 2005–2007, funded by the U.S. Office of Naval Research (cf. Fig. 15.3 in Reger et al., 2014). The 2007 system consisted of four customizable scenarios designed to represent relevant contexts for VRET: three Humvee driving scenarios within Iraq, Afghanistan, and USA-themed settings (*Video 2–2007 Virtual Iraq Humvee Driving with Attack Stimuli*: http://youtu.be/cdtqHxdjPnM) and a 24-block middle-eastern city (*Video 3–2007 Virtual Middle Eastern City Zones:* http://youtu.be/oT1iyT63au0) that was navigable in a dismounted patrol format (*Video 4–2007 Virtual Middle Eastern City Dismounted Patrol*: http://www.youtube.com/watch?v=s9MXM9RllWo). The creation of these VRET scenarios was the product of both theory-driven design and iterative user-centered feedback cycles with OEF/OIF service members to maximize the content-relevance for these clinical users (cf. Reger et al., 2014). Since that time, the system was disseminated to over 50 "early-adopter" clinical sites for use as a tool to deliver PE and to collect outcome data on its effectiveness. A detailed description of this Virtual Iraq/Afghanistan system and the methodology for a standard VRET clinical protocol can be found elsewhere (Rothbaum, Difede, & Rizzo, 2008).

Initial clinical tests of the system produced encouraging results. Three case study reports initially documented its feasibility and safety, and produced positive clinical outcomes with use of the system (Gerardi, Rothbaum, Ressler, Heekin, & Rizzo, 2008; Reger & Gahm, 2008; Rizzo et al., 2007). These were followed by an open clinical trial with 20 active duty treatment completers (19 male, 1 female, Mean Age = 28, Age Range: 21–51) which also reported positive clinical outcomes (Rizzo, Difede, Rothbaum, & Reger, 2010). Results reported from this open trial indicated that mean pre/post PCL-M (Blanchard, Jones-Alexander, Buckley, & Forneris, 1996) scores decreased in a statistical and clinically meaningful fashion from 54.4 (SD = 9.7) to 35.6 (SD = 17.4). Paired pre/post t-test analysis showed these differences to be significant ($t = 5.99$, $df = 19$, $p < 0.001$) with 16 of the 20 completers no longer meeting PCL-M criteria for PTSD at posttreatment (see Fig. 16.1) and an average 50 % decrease in symptoms. Five participants in this group with PTSD diagnoses had pretreatment baseline scores below the conservative cutoff value of 50 (prescores = 49, 46, 42, 36, 38) and reported decreased values at posttreatment (post-scores = 23, 19, 22, 22, 24, respectively) suggesting improvements for subthreshold PTSD users as well. Beck Anxiety Inventory (BAI) (Beck, Epstein, Brown, & Steer, 1988) scores significantly decreased 33 % from 18.6 ($SD = 9.5$) to 11.9 ($SD = 13.6$), ($t = 3.37$, $df = 19$, $p < 0.003$) and mean PHQ-9 (Kroenke & Spitzer, 2002) depression scores decreased 49 % from 13.3 ($SD = 5.4$) to 7.1 ($SD = 6.7$),

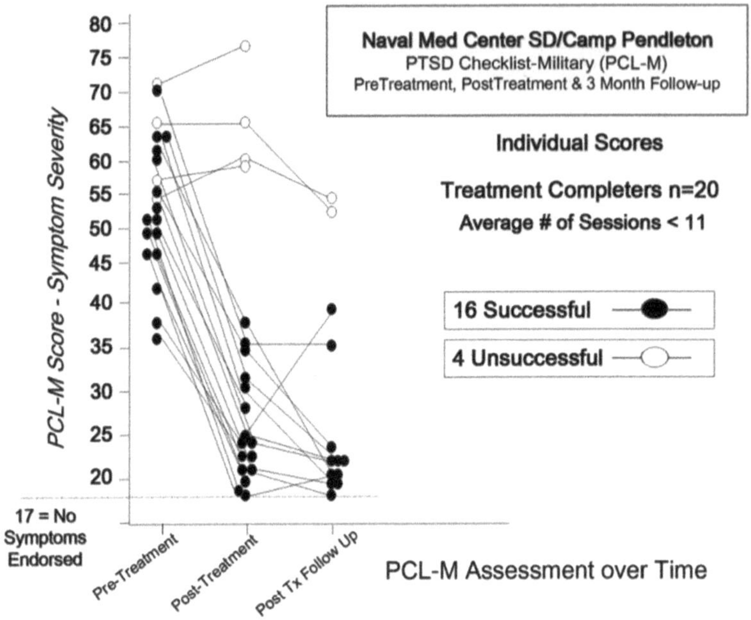

Fig. 16.1 PCL-M scores across treatment

($t=3.68$, $df=19$, $p<0.002$) (see Fig. 16.2). Treatment gains were maintained at 3-month posttreatment follow-up and anecdotal patient reports suggested that they saw improvements in everyday life functioning. The average number of sessions for this study was just under 11.

Another open clinical trial with active duty soldiers ($n=24$) produced significant pre-/post-reductions in PCL-M scores and a large treatment effect size (Cohen's $d=1.17$) (Reger et al., 2011a). After an average of 7 sessions, 45 % of those treated no longer screened positive for PTSD and 62 % had reliably improved. In a small preliminary quasi-randomized controlled trial (McLay et al., 2011), 7 of 10 participants with PTSD showed a 30 % or greater improvement with VR, while only 1 of 9 participants in a "treatment as usual" group showed similar improvement. While the results of this study are limited by its small sample size, lack of blinding, a single therapist, and treatment comparison with a relatively uncontrolled care as usual condition, these results do add to the incremental evidence suggesting VR to be a safe and effective approach for delivering PE for combat-related PTSD. Finally, at the 2012 American Psychiatric Association Convention, McLay (2012) presented data from an ongoing comparison of VRET with the traditional, evidence-based PE approach in active duty SMs. The results showed significantly better maintenance of positive treatment outcomes at 3-month follow-up for VRET compared to traditional PE (McLay 2012). The overall trend of these positive findings (in the absence of any reports of negative findings) is encouraging for the view that VRET is safe

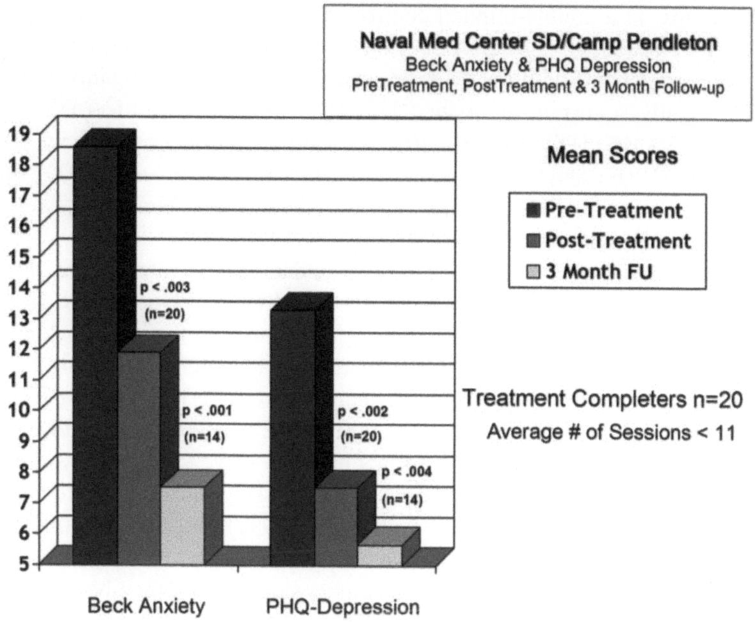

Fig. 16.2 BAI and PHQ-9 depression scores

and may be an effective approach for delivering an evidence-based treatment (PE) for PTSD.

Currently, five randomized controlled trials (RCTs) are ongoing using the Virtual Iraq/Afghanistan system with active duty SM and Veteran populations. Two RCTs are focusing on comparisons of treatment efficacy between VRET and prolonged imaginal exposure (PE) (Reger & Gahm, 2010, 2011b) and another is testing VRET compared with VRET + a supplemental care approach (Beidel, Frueh, & Uhde, 2010). Two more RCTs (Difede, Rothbaum, & Rizzo, 2010; Rothbaum et al., 2008) are investigating the additive value of supplementing VRET and imaginal PE with a cognitive enhancer called D-Cycloserine (DCS). DCS, an N-methyl-d-aspartate partial agonist, has been shown to facilitate extinction learning in laboratory animals when infused bilaterally within the amygdala prior to extinction training (Walker, Ressler, Lu, & Davis, 2002). The first clinical test in humans combined orally administered DCS with VRET (Ressler et al., 2004) with participants diagnosed with acrophobia ($n = 28$). Participants who received DCS + VRET experienced significant decreases in fear within the virtual environment 1 week and 3 months posttreatment, and reported significantly more improvement than the placebo group in their overall acrophobic symptoms at 3-month follow-up. The DCS group achieved lower scores on a psychophysiological measure of anxiety than the placebo group. Further evidence of both VRET and DCS effectiveness has recently been reported by Difede et al. (2013) in a clinical trial with World Trade Center

PTSD patients. In a double-blinded controlled comparison between VRET + DCS and VRET + Placebo, both groups had clinically meaningful and statistically significant positive outcomes with the DCS group achieving equivalent gains with fewer sessions. Finally, a current multisite PTSD RCT (NICoE, Weill-Cornell, and the Long Beach VAMC) (Difede et al., 2010) is testing the effect of DCS vs. placebo when added to VRET and PE with active duty and veteran samples ($n = 300$). Further details on DCS and PTSD can be found in the Burton, Youngner, McCarthy, Rothbaum, and Rothbaum (2014).

Significant funding support for these RCTs underscore the interest that the DOD/VA has in exploring this innovative approach for delivering PE using VR. However, while RCTs are the gold standard for gaining acceptance by the scientific and clinical communities for the use of emerging treatment approaches, it should be noted that at its core, the therapeutic model/principle that underlies VRET (CBT with exposure) is in fact evidence-based (IOM, 2007, 2012). VRET is simply the delivery of this evidence-based treatment in a format that may serve to engage a wider range of patients in the necessary confrontation and processing of traumatic memories or "fear-structures" (cf. Foa, Davidson, & Frances, 1999) needed for positive clinical outcomes. Thus, even equivalent "non-inferior" positive results with PE in these RCTs would validate the use of VRET as another safe and evidence-based treatment option. Moreover, the VRET approach could serve to draw SMs and Veterans into treatment, many of whom have grown up "digital" and may be more likely to seek care in this format compared to what they perceive as traditional talk therapy.

Project BRAVEMIND: Updating and Expanding the Virtual Iraq/Afghanistan VRET System

Based on the initial encouraging outcomes to date using VRET to treat combat-related PTSD and the urgency of the need for diverse evidence-based treatment options for the growing numbers of those reporting PTSD symptoms, the U.S. Army has funded the development of an updated and expanded version of Virtual Iraq/Afghanistan system, now referred to as BRAVEMIND. One of the primary goals for this project was to update and expand the diversity of the VR scenario content and functionality to improve the customizability of stimulus delivery to meet the needs of users having had a diverse range of trauma experiences. These aims were supported by drawing on patient and clinician feedback that has now come from a large number of SM and Veterans who were treated with the previous version of the VRET system. The system has been updated using the Unity Game Engine, an advanced state-of-the art VR development software platform that supports full 3D graphic rendering, physics, and a wide variety of interaction device options.

The current BRAVEMIND system now consists of 14 diverse scenarios. The original system contained four: a foot patrol navigable 18-block middle eastern city and 3 Humvee driving scenarios within Iraq, Afghanistan, and USA-themed settings (cf. Reger et al., 2014). The four original 2007 environments have been completely rebuilt

(*Video 5–2013 Bravemind Humvee Turret Attack Mix Scenes*: https://www.youtube.com/watch?v=8ZQjrfTqvDs&feature=youtu.be) and 10 additional scenarios have been added for a total of 14 (*Videos 6 and 7–2013 Bravemind Collected Scenes*: https://www.youtube.com/watch?v=iMeEuSdJ7EU&list=UUQrbzaW3x9wWoZPl4-l4GSA&index=1 and https://www.youtube.com/watch?v=_XO4nq4XUcA), including: separate Iraq and Afghanistan cities, a rural Afghan village, an industrial zone, a roadway checkpoint, slum and high-end residential areas, a mountainous forward operating base, and a Bagram Air Force Base setting (see Fig. 16.1). New features include selectable Humvee/MRAP/Helicopter vehicles, vehicle-to-foot patrol transitioning, expanded weather and time of day controls, customizable sound trigger profiles, and an updated clinical interface designed with clinician feedback to enhance usability. The Unity Game Engine and higher fidelity graphic art/animation have been used to enhance the realism and credibility of the stimulus content while presenting an experience that is uniquely designed to differentiate it from a commercial video game. The system was also designed to use off the shelf components (e.g., standard laptop, head mounted display, tracking/interface technology, etc.) that require only one computer with the aim to reduce equipment costs to well under $5,000. The BRAVEMIND VRET system is currently undergoing beta testing and has been designed to provide a flexible software architecture that will support the efficient addition of new content for the expansion and diversification of the system as new clinical needs are specified. More information on the BRAVEMIND system components is available in a detailed equipment/software manual available from the first author and an 18-min media story with new BRAVEMIND content and a former patient can be seen here (*Video 8*): https://www.youtube.com/watch?v=glIxXwT0cK4&list=UUQrbzaW3x9wWoZPl4-l4GSA. More videos of various PTSD system content, media pieces, and patient interviews can be accessed here: https://www.youtube.com/playlist?feature=edit_ok&list=PLMuMO5eoYy_BDmAfZrFSLBLlniAtvAdad.

The rebuilding of this VRET system has now provided the architecture to support the flexible and efficient expansion of the system's content and functionality to support new customizable and relevant options for conducting VRET with a wider range of relevant trauma experiences. The BRAVEMIND VRET system is now being further evolved to address the unique therapeutic needs of combat medics/corpsmen and in persons who have experienced military sexual trauma (MST) with PTSD. As well, the software has now been reconfigured to provide a VR tool that is being tested for its use for providing psychological resilience training prior to a combat deployment (Buckwalter & Rizzo, 2011; Rizzo et al., 2013) (Figs. 16.3, 16.4, 16.5, 16.6, 16.7, and 16.8).

Combat Medics/Corpsman VRET Project

Observations from our existing clinical work and from reports by medics (Cannady, 2012) indicate that there is a growing need to address PTSD in combat medics & corpsman. This will require specialized VR content that is more relevant to their

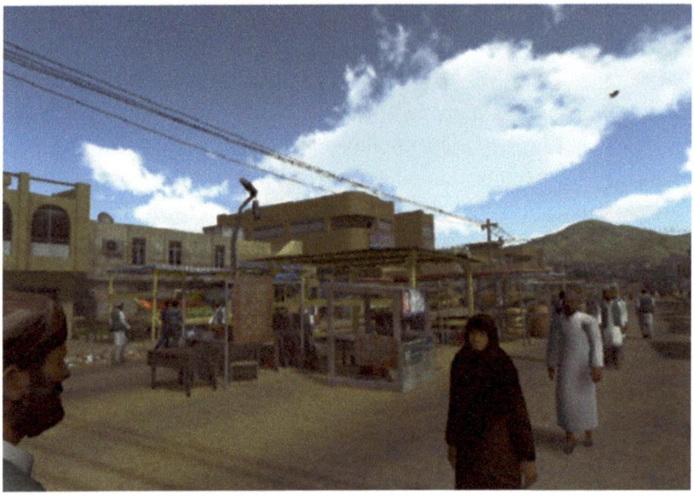

Fig. 16.3 Afghanistan city market

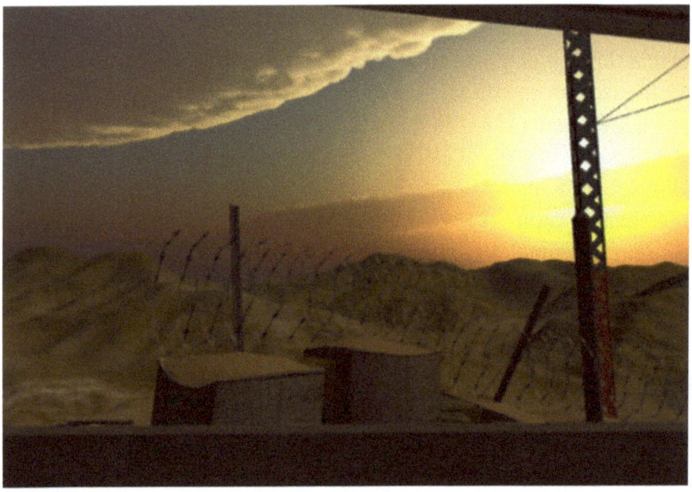

Fig. 16.4 Afghanistan FOB

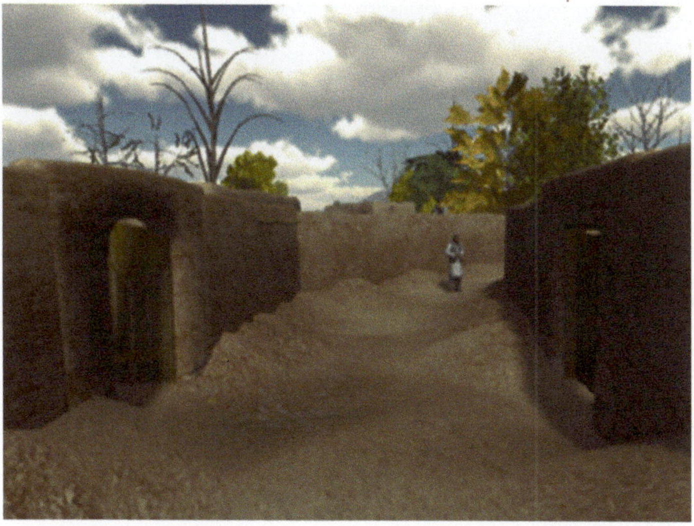

Fig. 16.5 Afghanistan rural village

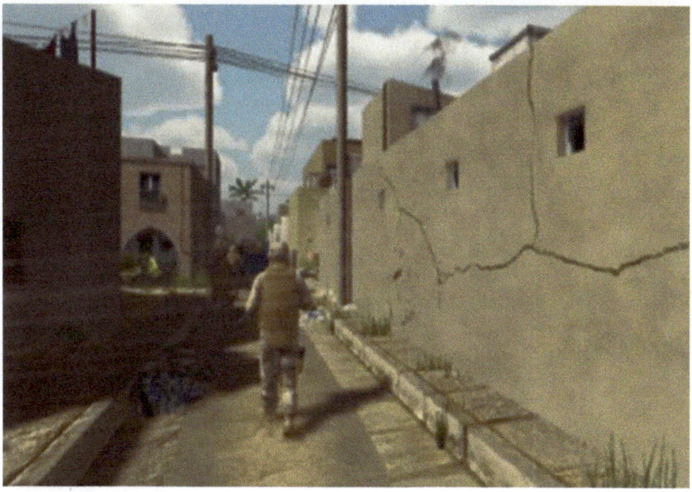

Fig. 16.6 Iraq Alley patrol

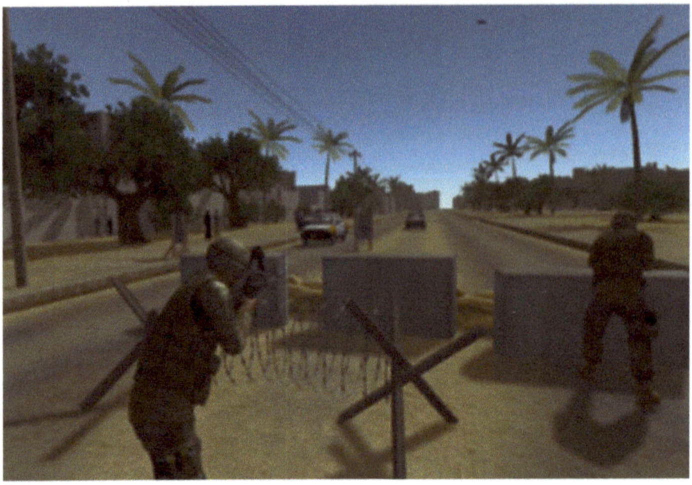

Fig. 16.7 Checkpoint zone

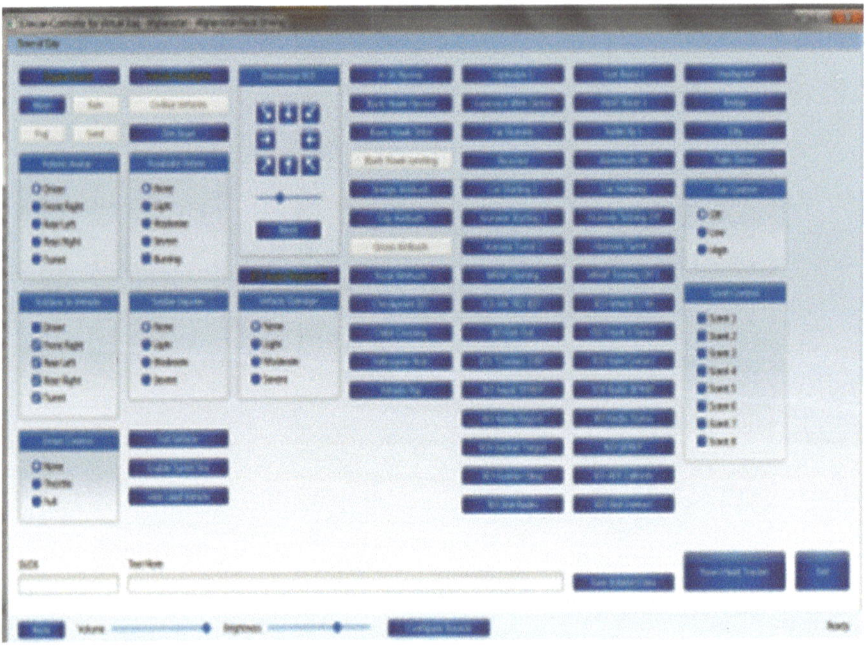

Fig. 16.8 Clinician control panel

experiences with emotionally challenging situations that are fundamentally different from what has been effective with other SMs. The primary role of the combat medic (Army and Air Force) and corpsmen (Navy and Marines) is to provide medical treatment to the wounded in a combat environment. Often they are assigned one to platoon or equivalent unit and this is mandatory due to their importance to the success of the unit's mission (Cabrera, Figley, & Yarvis, 2012). Combat medics/corpsmen are a unique population within the ranks of deployed SMs. They serve double duty, both professionally and psychologically. In addition to bearing all the responsibilities of soldiering, medics must calmly treat the devastating wounds of modern warfare: legs and arms mangled by roadside bombs, bodies peppered with shrapnel, arteries severed by high-velocity bullets. They are more exposed than other soldiers to seriously wounded or dead fellow SMs. Unlike hospital doctors or nurses, who rarely know their patients, medics have the added pressure of being close to the soldiers they are trying to keep alive. And when one dies, medics often face self-doubt—an emotion they must hide or risk losing the platoon's confidence.

While very preliminary findings have suggested that medics might be more resilient and less likely than other soldiers to have symptoms of PTSD, a small survey study looked at medics only 3 and 12 months after their deployments and reported PTSD symptoms that were seen to develop over time (Chapman, 2011). Cabrera et al. (2012) are currently studying this issue longitudinally in more detail. However, regardless of the limitations of the extant data on relative comparative rates of PTSD, there is no doubt that there is a clinical need for optimal treatment for this group and it has been the aim of this project to create the content required to meet that need.

This effort has required the tailoring of the existing scenarios to include more wounded virtual humans that can display a range of wounds/burns and manifest realistic injury behaviors. Helicopter insertion and extraction scenarios and a Bagram Air Force Base hospital setting for medic "first receivers" have been developed (see Figs. 16.9, 16.10, and 16.11). This effort has required the creation of significant new graphic art, motion capture animation, airborne vehicle integration, and a library of virtual human content that emulates the wounds and injuries common to the combat environment in order to offer relevant VRET for combat medics/corpsmen with PTSD. This system is currently nearing completion and will be available for use in early 2014.

Military Sexual Trauma

PTSD can result from exposure to actual or threatened death, serious injury, or sexual violation (APA, 2013). New to the APA DSM-5 is the explicit reference to a sexual violation as a possible source of trauma. This is of particular relevance for SMs who may face trauma from both the threat that is naturally inherent in the combat theater, as well as from the possible additive occurrence of sexual violations from within the ranks. Thus, military sexual trauma (MST) that is experienced as a result of an occurrence (or threat of an occurrence) of a sexual violation or assault within a military context can produce additional risk for the development of PTSD in a population that is already at high risk due to the existing occupational hazards present in the combat environment.

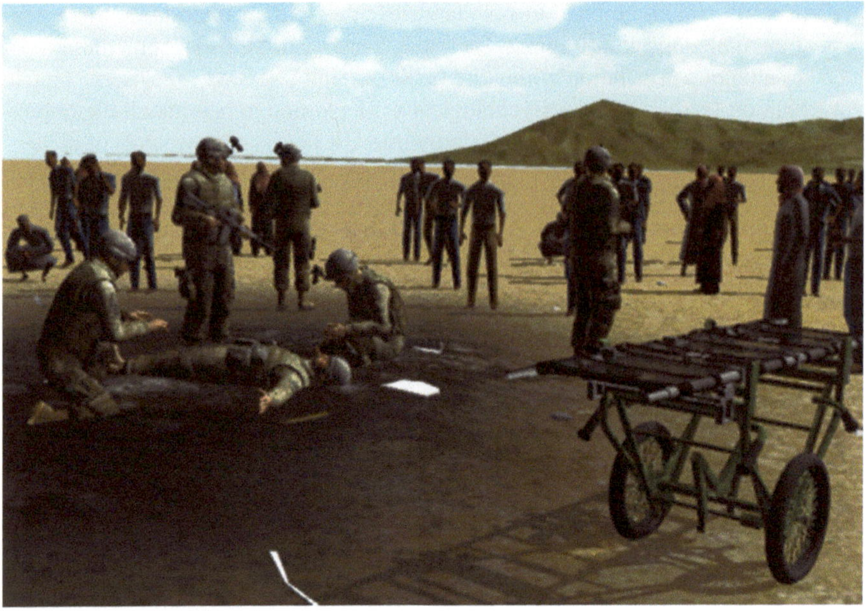

Fig. 16.9 Combat injury site

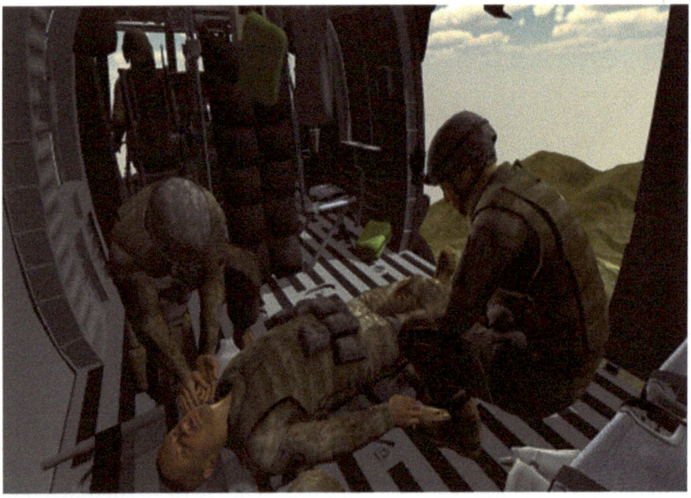

Fig. 16.10 Helicopter evacuation

In a recent report issued by the Joint Chiefs and Commandant of the Coast Guard, together with the DoD Sexual Assault Prevention and Response Program (SAPR) (DoD, 2012a), sexual assault has been defined "as intentional sexual contact, characterized by the use of force, threats, intimidation, abuse of authority, or

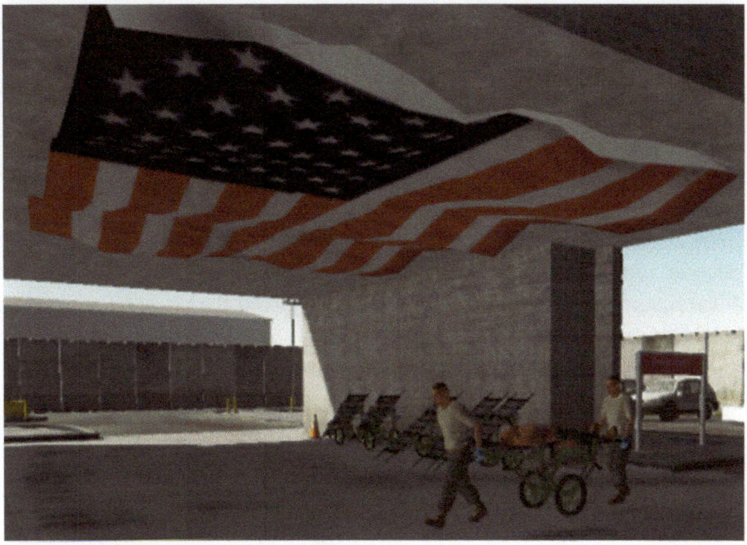

Fig. 16.11 Bagram first receiver area

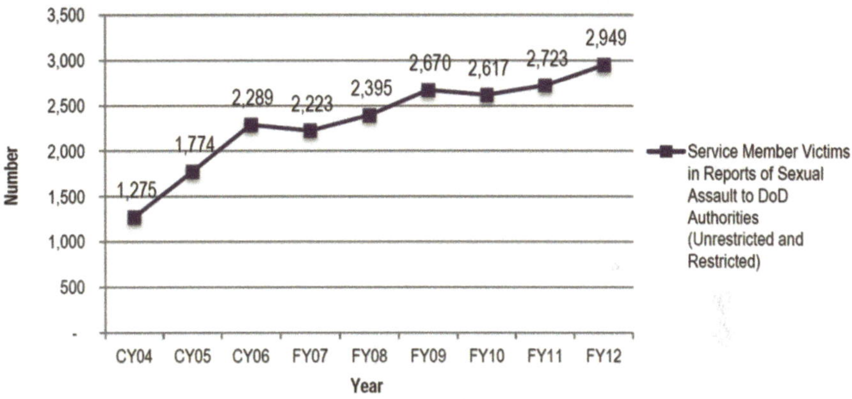

Fig. 16.12 Service member victims in DoD sexual assault reports, CY04–FY12 (from DoD2012c)

when the victim does not or cannot consent. Sexual assault includes rape, forcible sodomy, and other unwanted sexual contact that is aggravated, abusive, or wrongful (to include unwanted and inappropriate sexual contact), or attempts to commit these acts." (p. 5). The report further specifies the need for improvements in, "...advocacy coordination, medical services, legal support and [**behavioral health**] **counseling for the victim**" (p. 13). This has become an issue of grave concern within the military, as reports of sexual violations and assaults have not only been on the rise over the last 10 years (see Fig. 16.12), but have also garnered significant popular media attention (Kime, 2013; Valencia, 2013). Overall, 6.1 % of women and 1.2 % of men (active duty SMs) indicated they experienced unwanted sexual contact in 2012. For women, this rate is statistically significantly higher in 2012 than in 2010 (6.1 vs. 4.4 %) (DoD, 2012b).

A bleaker picture of the problem emerges when reports from post-discharge Veteran surveys are considered. Underreporting of MST by SMs while on active duty may occur due to fear of reprisal, concern for military careers, shame, or because they didn't want anyone to know while in the service and this additional threat may be lessened once the person transitions to Veteran status. For example, retrospective reports of sexual assault and harassment during active duty—by female Veterans following discharge—have suggested higher MST incidence than what has been reported in active duty samples. In a nationwide randomly selected sample of women seeking care through VA medical centers, approximately 1 out of 4 reported experiencing a sexual trauma while on active duty (Skinner et al., 2000). The reported prevalence rates of MST in women were 20–25 % for sexual assault and 24–60 % for sexual harassment and more recent indicators suggest that this problem is expected to grow exponentially in the future (Department of Veterans Affairs, 2007). The implication that MST can be a primary factor for the development of PTSD has also been supported by multiple studies that indicate that many women who report experiencing a MST also experience mental health problems, with the most frequently reported being PTSD (Kimerling et al., 2010; Street, Gradus, Stafford, & Kelly, 2007; Street, Stafford, Mahan, & Hendricks, 2008). For example, within a sample of women seeking PTSD-related services within the VA system, 71 % reported MST experiences (Murdoch, Polusny, Hodges, & O'Brien, 2004). Moreover, as with PTSD, MST is associated with a variety of comorbid mental and physical health disorders (Brewin, Andrews, & Valentine, 2000; Sadler, Booth, Nielson, & Doebbeling, 2000; Zinzow, Grubaugh, Monnier, Suffoletta-Maierle, & Frueh, 2007) as well as impairments in both social functioning and quality of life (Rheingold, Acierno, & Resnick, 2004; Surıs, Lind, Kaashner, & Borman, 2007). Thus, while the DoD is mobilizing to reduce the incidence of MST with novel education and prevention programs (DoD 2012a, 2012b, 2012c), a significant effort is also required to develop and disseminate effective treatment approaches to address the existing problem of PTSD due to MST.

The current project is developing content for inclusion in BRAVEMIND that will provide new customizable options for conducting VRET with persons who have experienced MST. The novel component of the current project involves the creation of new content that will be embedded within the existing BRAVEMIND scenarios such as barracks, tents, other living and work quarters, latrines, and other contexts that have been reported by MST victims as locations where their sexual assault occurred. This system will ***not*** attempt to recreate the sexual assault, but rather set up the contexts surrounding the assault, in which users can be supported in the therapeutic confrontation and processing of MST memories in accordance with the protocol that has been used previously that implements PE within the simulations (Rothbaum et al., 2008). When the new content is complete (summer 2014) a pilot waitlist RCT will commence with 34 male and female participants. This has not been attempted previously with immersive VRET and the unique challenges for creating such unique and sensitive content are significant. While both men and women can experience MST, the urgent need for this work is underscored by the growing role of women transitioning into full combat roles in the combat theater, an area that up to now has been primarily the domain of men.

Virtual Reality Resilience Training

Resilience is the dynamic process by which individuals exhibit positive adaptation when they encounter significant adversity, trauma, tragedy, threats, or other sources of stress (McEwen & Stellar, 1993). The core aim of resilience training is to promote psychological fitness through self-awareness, self-esteem, emotional regulation, and social support. This multidimensional approach to resilience training is designed to better prepare SMs for the psychological stressors that they may experience during a combat deployment and to provide them with the tools needed to resolve the inevitable reactivity they experience after trauma/stress. There is a powerful rationale for developing methods that promote SM resilience and psychological fitness prior to a combat deployment. The current urgency in efforts to address the psychological wounds of war in SMs and Veterans has also driven an emerging focus within the military on emphasizing a proactive approach for better preparing SMs for the emotional challenges they may face during a combat deployment to reduce the potential for later adverse psychological reactions such as PTSD, suicidality, and depression. This focus on resilience training prior to deployment represents no less than a quantum shift in military culture and can now be seen emanating from the highest levels of command in the military. For example, in an American Psychologist article, Army General George Casey (2011) stated that "...soldiers can "be" better before deploying to combat so they will not have to "get" better after they return." (p. 1), and he then calls for a shift in the military "...to a culture in which psychological fitness is recognized as every bit as important as physical fitness." (p. 2).

This level of endorsement can be seen in practice by way of the significant funding and resources applied to a variety of resilience training programs across all branches of the U.S. Military (Cornum, Matthews, & Seligman, 2011; Hovar, 2010; Luthar, Cicchetti, & Becker, 2000). Perhaps the program that is attempting to influence the largest number of SMs is the Comprehensive Soldier Fitness (CSF) program (Cornum et al., 2011). This project has created and disseminated training that aims to improve emotional coping skills and ultimate resilience across all Army SMs. One element of this program draws input from principles of cognitive-behavioral science, which generally advances the view that it is not the *event* that causes an emotion, but rather how a person *appraises* the event (based on how they think about the event) that leads to the emotion (Ortony, Clore, & Collins, 1988). From this theoretical base, it then follows that internal thinking or appraisals about combat events can be "taught" in a way that leads to more healthy and resilient reactions to stress. This approach does not imply that people with effective coping skills do not feel some level of "rational" emotional pain when confronted with a challenging event that would normally be stressful to any individual. Instead, the aim is to teach skills that may assist soldiers in an effort to cope with traumatic stressors more successfully.

The core motive with such efforts is to provide resilience training that would serve to promote psychological fitness and reduce the later incidence of PTSD and other psychological health conditions upon redeployment home (e.g., depression, suicide, substance abuse). A recent study on the Comprehensive Soldier Fitness program reported results from a longitudinal study over 18 months with 22,000 soldiers indicating positive outcomes (Lester, Harms, Herian, Krasikova, & Beal, 2011), but this report has been criticized for its exclusive reliance on self-report data and on other methodological grounds (PBS, 2012). Regardless of those academic "battles," the post-deployment psychological health statistics are alarming and provide a compelling justification for continued efforts to better prepare SMs for the onslaught of emotional challenges that they may face during a combat deployment.

Recently, the USC Institute for Creative Technologies has begun development of the STress Resilience In Virtual Environments (STRIVE) project which expands on the Virtual Iraq/Afghanistan simulations developed for VRET. The STRIVE project aims to foster psychological resilience by creating a set of combat simulations that can be used as contexts for SMs to experientially learn stress reduction tactics and cognitive-behavioral emotional coping strategies prior to deployment. This approach involves immersing and engaging SMs within a variety of virtual "mission" episodes where they are confronted with emotionally challenging situations that are inherent to the OEF/OIF combat environment. Interaction by SMs within such emotionally challenging scenarios aims to provide a more meaningful context in which to engage with psychoeducational information and to learn and practice stress reduction tactics and cognitive coping strategies that are believed to better prepare a SM for the psychological challenges that may occur during a combat deployment.

To accomplish this, STRIVE is being designed as a 30-episode interactive narrative in VR, akin to being immersed within a "Band of Brothers" type storyline that spans a typical deployment cycle. Within these episodes, SMs will get to know the distinct personalities of the virtual human characters in their squad and interact within an immersive digital narrative that employs cinematic strategies for enhancing engagement with the evolving storyline (e.g., strategic use of narration, montage shots, and dynamic camera direction). At the end of each of the graded 10-min episodes, an emotionally challenging event occurs, designed in part from feedback provided by SMs undergoing PTSD treatment (e.g., seeing/handling human remains, death/injury of a squad member, killing someone, the death/injury of a civilian child). At that point in the episode, the virtual world "freezes in place" and a virtual human "mentor" character emerges from the midst of the chaotic VR scenario to guide the user through stress-reduction tactics. These include psychoeducational animations, affect awareness and regulation strategies, moral appraisal discussions, "positive psychology"-based self-management tactics, as well as rational restructuring exercises for appraising and processing the virtual experience. The resilience training component is drawing on evidence-based content that has been endorsed as part of standard classroom-delivered DoD stress resilience training programs, as well as content that has been successfully applied in nonmilitary contexts (e.g., humanitarian aid worker training, sports psychology).

In this fashion, STRIVE provides a digital "emotional obstacle course" that can be used as a tool for providing context-relevant learning of emotional coping strategies under very tightly controlled and scripted simulated conditions. Training in this format is hypothesized to improve generalization to real world situations via a state dependent learning component (Godden & Baddeley, 1980) and further support resilience by leveraging the learning theory process of latent inhibition. Latent inhibition refers to the delayed learning that occurs as a result of pre-exposure to a stimulus without a consequence (Feldner, Monson, & Friedman, 2007; Lubow & Moore, 1959). Thus, the exposure to a simulated combat context is believed to decrease the likelihood of fear conditioning during the real event (Sones, Thorp, & Raskind, 2011).

Six episodes have been created thus far that expose SMs to the following stressors/trauma: the moral quandaries implicit in being a warrior in a less developed society, threat to self via an IED, the need to respect vastly different, even immoral, cultural actions through an episode where the patrolling squad comes upon a civilian woman is being beaten by men enforcing a local code of punishment, the death of an innocent child in which some unintentional, indirect responsibility can be in inferred to one of the members of your squad, the death of an inspirational Unit Leader, and an episode that reveals the varied stages in the grieving responses of individual squad members in the aftermath of the death of the leader. Several of these issues were selected given the frequency with which they are reported to be pivotal events in the development of PTSD (and on common themes that appeared in the narratives of patients previously treated with our VRET system). For example, the death of a local civilian child that a squad member had a relationship with is an event that resonates time and again as the service member tries to reengage in civilian life. Moral relativistic challenges are also presented in the episodes. This occurs specifically in a horrific event (the beating of a civilian woman by locals) where the culturally based systems of morality that one must accept to live resiliently as a warrior are presented in a way designed to challenge the psychological underpinnings of even the most resolute person. These moral issues are not part of the usual training that SMs receive and these episodes are designed to prepare SMs to consider such "what if" questions in advance of their possible occurrence during actual missions. Similarly, the act of killing is one that many soldiers never truly contemplate until it has occurred. And while we do not yet fully know how we can best train SMs to be psychologically resilient warriors on the battlefield and concerned civilians off, we do know from the increasing numbers of SMs returning from combat with "moral injuries," or psychological distress experienced from transgressing some moral value, that we need to acknowledge the need to study and improve the process of resilience training for the entire range of psychological challenges we find associated with the hellish demands of modern warfare.

The STRIVE project also incorporates a novel basic science protocol. While other stress resilience research efforts typically incorporate one or two biomarkers of stress and or resilience, the STRIVE projects will measure what we refer to as the "physiological fingerprint of stress," commonly called Allostatic Load (AL). The theoretical construct of AL, initially developed by one of the STRIVE collaborators, Bruce McEwen, is a measure of cumulative wear and tear on physiological symptoms due to chronic stress (McEwen & Stellar, 1993). As a theoretical construct, it is a preliminary attempt to formulate the relationship between environmental stressors and disease, by hypothesizing mechanisms whereby multiple kinds of stressors confer risk simultaneously in multiple physiological systems.

The construct of AL is based on the widely accepted response called allostasis. Sterling and Eyer (1988) defined allostasis as the body's set points for various physiological mechanisms, such as blood pressure or heart rate, which vary to meet specific external demands, e.g., emotional stress. McEwen and Stellar (1993) furthered our understanding of allostasis by broadening its scope. Rather than discuss allostasis in terms of a single set point that changed in response to a stressor, they described allostasis as the combination of all physiological coping mechanisms that are required to maintain equilibrium of the entire system. Thus, allostasis is the reaction and adaptation to stressors by multiple physiological systems that brings the system back to equilibrium. The related concept of homeostasis refers specifically to system parameters essential for survival (McEwen, 2002). To place AL into the context of allostasis, requires the view that allostasis does not always proceed in a normal manner. Any of the major physiological systems (e.g., inflammatory, metabolic, immune, neuroendocrine, cardiovascular, respiratory) in the process of responding to stress can exact a cost, or an allostatic load that can result in some form of physiological or psychological disturbance. McEwen (2000) identified four types of AL. The first is frequent activation of allostatic systems; second is a prolonged failure to shut off allostatic activity after stress; third is a lack of adaptation to stress, and fourth is an inadequate response of allostatic systems leading to elevated activity of other, normally counter-regulated allostatic systems after stress (e.g., inadequate secretion of glucocorticoid resulting in increased cytokines normally countered by glucocorticoids). Any of these types of AL intervene with the normal stress response of allostasis thus increasing the negative health impact from stress. This will increase one's risk for disease in the long term and may preclude the short-term development of physical hardiness and psychological resilience.

The STRIVE system will be empirically tested to determine if AL can predict acute response to stress (e.g., EEG, GSR, ECG, pupil dilation, etc.), when participants are exposed to the stressful simulated VR missions. Further analyses will determine if AL can predict participants' responses to virtual mentor instructions on how the participants can cope with stress through resilience training. Pilot research on this project will commence in January 2014 with a National Guard Special Operations Unit that will be deployed to Afghanistan in March 2014. We have the rare opportunity with this unit to have them participate in a 6-episode STRIVE experience and to follow their mental health status immediately upon the return home and at 6-month follow-up. If we find that AL is capable of predicting either short-term response to stress or the ability to learn stress resilience, there would be numerous implications for the future use of AL, including identification of leadership profiles and for informing the development of appropriate training systems for all SMs. This project is noteworthy in that it represents the direct application of a novel VR development effort (psychological resilience training) with a system that also serves as an "ultimate Skinner-Box" for the scientific study of stress reactions using objective physiological assessment measures.

Conclusions

This chapter has detailed the history and rationale for the updating of the Virtual Iraq/Afghanistan VRET system with the aim to expand the system's content and functionality to more widely address the range of possible trauma experiences that may occur during a military deployment. Previous research with this VRET system to address combat-related PTSD has produced positive results, yet the absence of relevant content that uniquely addresses the needs of combat medics/corpsmen and those who have experienced MST was seen as a gap in the provision of evidence-based PTSD care. Upon completion of this content, the system will immediately undergo tests within an existing clinical trial with medics/corpsmen and a new trial with male and female SMs and Veterans who have experienced MST. If these new applications produce positive clinical outcomes similar to what has emerged thus far with the existing Virtual Iraq/Afghanistan system, then support for a broader general use of VRET could also potentially drive increased adoption of this method of PE delivery within the civilian sector.

The BRAVEMIND VRET project has been updated with the use of an advanced VR software development platform (the Unity Game Engine). The capabilities of this state-of-the-art software have also driven the reconfiguration of VRET assets to create a tool designed to prevent the incidence of combat-related PTSD via pre-deployment psychological resilience/coping training. The STRIVE program is designed to both create a VR application for enhancing SM resilience and to provide a highly controllable laboratory test bed for investigating stress responding in provocative simulated contexts. Success in this area could have significant impact on the nature of military training as well as for the prevention of combat stress-related disorders.

Another option for use of the STRIVE system could involve its application as a tool for emotional assessment at the time of recruitment into the military. The larger question regarding such an application involves whether it would be possible (and ethical) to assess prospective SMs in a series of challenging combat-relevant emotional environments delivered in the STRIVE system to predict their potential risk for developing PTSD or other mental health difficulties based on their verbal, behavioral, and physiological/hormonal reactions recorded during these virtual engagements. To use such information for recruitment decisions would require a change from current military thinking, where doctrine dictates that anyone can be made into an infantryman. However, practical implementation of such an approach could advise that those who display reactions that were found to predict higher risk for a negative stress reaction post-combat, could either be assigned non-combat duties, not accepted into the services, or more preferably, presented with the opportunity to participate in a personally tailored psychological resilience training program that could minimize their identified risk to post-trauma dysfunction. This is not a new concept. Since the early days of the Army Alpha/Beta, assessments have been routinely conducted that are designed to predict what role is best suited to the unique characteristics and talent of a given recruit. Moreover, potential recruits are not accepted into the military for many reasons that are more easily measurable (e.g., having a criminal record, poor physical fitness, significant health conditions).

If one reviews the history of the impact of war on advances in clinical care, it could be suggested that Clinical VR may be an idea whose time has come. For example, during WW I, the Army Alpha/Beta Classification Test emerged from the need for better cognitive ability assessment; that development later set the stage for the civilian psychometric testing movement during the mid-twentieth century. As well, the birth of clinical psychology as a treatment-oriented profession was borne from the need to provide care to the many Veterans returning from WW II with "shell shock" or "battle fatigue." The Vietnam War then drove the recognition of PTSD as a definable and treatable clinical disorder. In similar fashion, one of the clinical "game changing" outcomes of the OIF/OEF conflicts could derive from the military's support for research and development that has advanced clinical systems that leverage new interactive and immersive technologies such as VR. If the positive findings seen in the early research is borne out in larger controlled trials, those results could potentially drive increased recognition and adoption within the civilian sector. As we have seen throughout history, innovations that emerge in military health care, driven by the urgency of war, typically have a lasting influence on civilian health care long after the last shot is fired.

References

APA. (2013). *Diagnostic and statistical manual of mental disorders*. Washington, DC: American Psychiatric Association (DSM-5).

Beck, A. T., Epstein, N., Brown, G., & Steer, R. A. (1988). An inventory for measuring clinical anxiety: Psychometric properties. *Journal of Consulting and Clinical Psychology, 56*, 893–897.

Becker, C. B., Zayfert, C., & Anderson, E. (2004). A survey of psychologists' attitudes towards and utilization of exposure therapy for PTSD. *Behaviour Research and Therapy, 42*, 277–292.

Beidel, D. C., Frueh, B. C., & Uhde, T. W. (2010). *Trauma management therapy for OIF/OEF veterans*. Department of Defense United States Army Military Operational Medical Research Program: http://www.psych.ucf.edu/faculty_beidel.php

Blanchard, E. B., Jones-Alexander, J., Buckley, T. C., & Forneris, C. A. (1996). Psychometric properties of the PTSD checklist (PCL). *Behaviour Research and Therapy, 34*(8), 669–673.

Brewin, C. R., Andrews, B., & Valentine, J. D. (2000). Meta-analysis of risk factors for posttraumatic stress disorder in trauma-exposed adults. *Journal of Consulting and Clinical Psychology, 68*, 748–766.

Buckwalter, J. G., & Rizzo, A. A. (2011). Stress resilience, virtual environments and allostatic load. *Proceedings of the Interservice/Industry Training, Simulation and Education Conference.*

Burton, M. S., Youngner, C. G., McCarthy, A. J., Rothbaum, A. O., & Rothbaum, B. O. (2014). Enhancing exposure therapy for PTSD using D-cycloserine. In M. Safir, H. Wallach, & A. A. Rizzo (Eds.), *Future directions in posttraumatic stress disorder: Prevention, diagnosis and treatment*. New York, NY: Springer.

Cabrera, D., Figley, C. R., & Yarvis, J. S. (2012). Helping the combat medic and corpsman: Adapting to both primary and secondary traumatic stress down range and beyond. In J. Beder (Ed.), *Advances in social work practice with the military* (pp. 112–118). New York, NY: Routledge.

Cannady, V. (2012, June 1). *Combat medics suffer from a high rate of PTSD*. Retrieved from: http://voices.yahoo.com/combat-medics-suffer-high-rate-ptsd-11398322.html?cat=31

Casey, G. W. (2011). Comprehensive soldier fitness: A vision for psychological resilience in the U.S. army. *American Psychologist, 66*(1), 1–3.

Chapman, P. (2011, September 16). *Study looks at psychological effects suffered by combat medics*. Retrieved from: http://www.stripes.com/news/study-looks-at-psychological-effects-suffered-by-combat-medics-1.155272)

Cornum, R., Matthews, M. D., & Seligman, M. E. P. (2011). Comprehensive soldier fitness: Building resilience in a challenging institutional context. *American Psychologist, 66*(1), 4–9.

Department of Veterans Affairs. (2007). *Women veterans: Past, present and future: Office of policy and planning*. Washington, DC: Government Printing Office.

Difede, J., Cukor, J., Jayasinghe, N., Patt, I., Jedel, S., Spielman, L., et al. (2007). Virtual reality exposure therapy for the treatment of posttraumatic stress disorder following September 11, 2001. *Journal of Clinical Psychiatry, 68*, 1639–1647.

Difede, J., Cukor, J., Wyka, K., Olden, M., Hoffman, H., Lee, F. S. & Altemus, M. (2013 November, 12). D-cycloserine augmentation of exposure therapy for posttraumatic stress disorder: A pilot randomized clinical trial. *Neuropsychopharmacology*. doi: 10.1038/npp.2013.317

Difede, J., & Hoffman, H. G. (2002). Virtual reality exposure therapy for world trade center post-traumatic stress disorder: A case report. *Cyberpsychology and Behavior, 5*, 529–535.

Difede, J., Rothbaum, B. O. & Rizzo, A. (2010–2013). Enhancing exposure therapy for PTSD: Virtual reality and imaginal exposure with a cognitive enhancer. *Randomized Controlled Trial*. http://clinicaltrials.gov/ct2/show/NCT01352637

DoD. (2012a). *Strategic direction to the joint force on sexual assault prevention and response*. Downloaded from: http://www.jcs.mil/content/files/2012-05/050812085404_Joint_Strategic_Direction_on_Sexual_Assault_(7_May_12).pdf

DoD. (2012b). *DoD FY12 annual report on sexual assault in the military, Vol. 2*. Downloaded from: http://www.sapr.mil/public/docs/reports/FY12_DoD_SAPRO_Annual_Report_on_Sexual_Assault-VOLUME_TWO.pdf

DoD. (2012c). *DoD FY12 annual report on sexual assault in the military, Vol. 1*. Downloaded from: http://www.sapr.mil/public/docs/reports/FY12_DoD_SAPRO_Annual_Report_on_Sexual_Assault-VOLUME_ONE.pdf

Feldner, M. T., Monson, C. M., & Friedman, M. J. (2007). A critical analysis of approaches to targeted PTSD prevention: Current status and theoretically derived future directions. *Behavior Modification, 31*, 80–116.

Fischer, H. (2013, February 5). United States military casualty statistics: Operation New Dawn, operation Iraqi freedom, and operation enduring freedom. *Congressional Research Service 7–5700*, RS22452. Retrieved from: http://www.fas.org/sgp/crs/natsec/RS22452.pdf

Foa, E. B., Davidson, R. T., & Frances, A. (1999). Expert consensus guideline series: Treatment of posttraumatic stress disorder. *American Journal of Clinical Psychiatry, 60*, 5–76.

Foa, E. B., Hembree, E., & Rothbaum, B. O. (2007). *Prolonged exposure therapy for PTSD: Emotional processing of traumatic experiences, therapist guide*. New York: Oxford University Press.

Garcia-Palacios, A., Botella, C., Baños, R., Guillén, V., & Navarro, M. V. (2014). Modifications of PTSD treatment. Inclusion of virtual reality A rationale for the use of VR in the treatment of PTSD. In M. Safir, H. Wallach, & A. A. Rizzo (Eds.), *Future directions in posttraumatic stress disorder: Prevention, diagnosis and treatment*. New York, NY: Springer.

Gerardi, M., Rothbaum, B. O., Ressler, K., Heekin, M., & Rizzo, A. A. (2008). Virtual reality exposure therapy using a virtual Iraq: Case report. *Journal of Traumatic Stress, 21*(2), 209–213.

Godden, D. R., & Baddeley, A. D. (1980). When does context influence recognition memory? *British Journal of Psychology, 71*, 99–104.

Hoge, C. W. (2013). Risks associated with untreated PTSD in veterans: Implications for improving mental health care engagement and treatment. *Federal Practitioner* (June), 5S–9S.

Hovar, C. (2010, December 10). *The military operational medicine research program for the US army*. Retrieved from: http://www.donhcs.com/hsr/21_march/doc/presentations/Carl%20Hover%20MRMC%20MOMRP%208%20slides.pdf

Institute of Medicine (IOM). (2007). *Treatment of posttraumatic stress disorder: An assessment of the evidence*. Washington, DC: The National Academies Press, 200 p. ISBN: 0-309-10925-6. Downloaded from: http://www.nap.edu/catalog/11955.html

Institute of Medicine (IOM). (2012). *Treatment for posttraumatic stress disorder in military and veteran populations: Initial assessment.* Washington, DC: The National Academies Press, 396 p. ISBN: 978-0-309-25421-2. Downloaded from: http://www.nap.edu/catalog.php?record_id=13364

Kime, P. (2013). *DoD, VA failing to treat military sexual trauma, veterans testify*. Army Times. Accessed on July 20, 2013 at: http://www.armytimes.com/article/20130719/NEWS05/307190039/DoD-VA-failing-treat-military-sexual-trauma-veterans-testify

Kimerling, R., Street, A., Pavao, J., Smith, M. W., Cronkite, R. C., Holmes, T. H., et al. (2010). Military-related sexual trauma among Veterans health administration patients returning from Afghanistan and Iraq. *American Journal of Public Health, 100*, 1409–1412.

Kok, B. C., Herrell, R. K., Thomas, J. L., & Hoge, C. W. (2012). Posttraumatic stress disorder associated with combat service in Iraq or Afghanistan: Reconciling prevalence difference between studies. *The Journal of Nervous and Mental Disease, 200*(5), 444–450.

Kroenke, K., & Spitzer, R. L. (2002). The PHQ-9: A new depression and diagnostic severity measure. *Psychiatric Annals, 32*, 509–521.

Lester, P. B., Harms, P. D., Herian, M. N., Krasikova, D. V. & Beal, S. J. (2011). *The comprehensive soldier fitness program evaluation.* Report #3: Longitudinal Analysis of the Impact of Master Resilience Training on Self-Reported Resilience and Psychological Health Data. Retrieved August 14, 2012, from: http://dma.wi.gov/dma/news/2012news/csf-tech-report.pdf

Lubow, R. E., & Moore, A. U. (1959). Latent inhibition: The effect of non-reinforced exposure to the conditioned stimulus. *Journal of Comparative and Physiological Psychology, 52*, 415–419.

Luthar, S. S., Cicchetti, D., & Becker, B. (2000). The construct of resilience: A critical evaluation and guidelines for future work. *Child Development, 71*, 543–562.

McEwen, B. S. (2000). Allostasis and allostatic load: Implications for neuropsychopharmacology. *Neuropsychopharmacology, 22*, 108–124. doi:10.1016/S0893-133X(99)00129-3.

McEwen, B. S. (2002). Sex, stress and the hippocampus: Allostasis, allostatic load and the aging process. *Neurology of Aging, 23*, 921–939.

McEwen, B. S., & Stellar, E. (1993). Stress and the individual: Mechanism leading to disease. *Archives of Internal Medicine, 153*, 2093–2101.

McLay , R. N. (2012). *New technology to treat post traumatic stress disorder*. Paper presented at the American Psychiatric Association Convention. May 8, 2012. Philadelphia, PA.

McLay, R. N., Wood, D. P., Webb-Murphy, J. A., Spira, J. L., Weiderhold, M. D., Pyne, J. M., & Weiderhold, B. K. (2011). A randomized, controlled trial of virtual reality exposure therapy for post-traumatic stress disorder in active duty service members with combat-related post-traumatic stress disorder. *Cyberpsychology, Behavior and Social Networking, 14*, 223–229.

Murdoch, M., Polusny, M. A., Hodges, J., & O'Brien, N. (2004). Prevalence of in-service and postservice sexual assault among combat and noncombat veterans applying for Department of Veterans Affairs posttraumatic stress disorder disability benefits. *Military Medicine, 169*, 392–395.

Opris, D., et al. (2012). Virtual reality exposure therapy in anxiety disorders: A quantitative meta-analysis. *Depression and Anxiety, 29*(2), 85–93.

Ortony, A., Clore, G., & Collins, A. (1988). *The cognitive structure of emotions*. Cambridge: Cambridge University Press.

Parsons, T., & Rizzo, A. A. (2008). Affective outcomes of virtual reality exposure therapy for anxiety and specific phobias: A meta-analysis. *Journal of Behavior Therapy and Experimental Psychiatry, 39*, 250–261.

Powers, M & Emmelkamp, P. M. G. (2008). Virtual reality exposure therapy for anxiety disorders: A meta-analysis. *Journal of Anxiety Disorders, 22*, 561–569.

Public Broadcasting System (PBS). (2012). *Health experts question army report on psychological training*. Retrieved August 14, 2012, from: http://www.pbs.org/newshour/updates/military/jan-june12/csf_training_01-02.html

Reger, G., & Gahm, G. (2008). Virtual reality exposure therapy for active duty soldiers. *Journal of Clinical Psychology, 64*, 940–946.

Reger, G. & Gahm, G. (2010). Comparing virtual reality exposure therapy to prolonged exposure (VRPE extension).*Randomized Controlled Trial*: http://clinicaltrials.gov/ct2/show/NCT01193725?term=Reger&rank=2

Reger, G. & Gahm, G. (2011b). Comparing virtual reality exposure therapy to prolonged exposure (VRPE extension). *Randomized Controlled Trial*: http://clinicaltrials.gov/ct2/show/NCT01352637

Reger, G. M., Gahm, G. A., Rizzo, A. A., Swanson, R.A., & Duma, S. (2009). Soldier evaluation of the virtual reality Iraq. *Telemedicine and e-Health Journal, 15*, 100–103.

Reger, G. M., Holloway, K. M., Rothbaum, B. O., Difede, J., Rizzo, A. A., & Gahm, G. A. (2011). Effectiveness of virtual reality exposure therapy for active duty soldiers in a military mental health clinic. *Journal of Traumatic Stress, 24*(1), 93–96.

Reger, G. M., Rizzo, A. A., & Gahm, G. A. (2014). Development and dissemination of virtual reality exposure therapy for combat related PTSD. In M. Safir, H. Wallach, & A. A. Rizzo (Eds.), *Future directions in posttraumatic stress disorder: Prevention, diagnosis and treatment*. New York, NY: Springer.

Ressler, K. J., Rothbaum, B. O., Tannenbaum, L., Anderson, P., Zimand, E., Hodges, L., et al. (2004). Facilitation of psychotherapy with D-cycloserine, a putative cognitive enhancer. *Archives of General Psychiatry, 61*, 1136–1144.

Rheingold, A. A., Acierno, R., & Resnick, H. (2004). Trauma, post-traumatic stress disorder, and health risk behaviors. In P. P. Schnurr & B. L. Green (Eds.), *Trauma and health: Physical health consequences of exposure to extreme stress* (pp. 217–243). Washington, DC: American Psychological Association.

Rizzo, A. A., Buckwalter, J. G., Forbell, E., Difede, J., Rothbaum, B. O., Lange, B., et al. (2013). Virtual reality applications to address the wounds of war. *Psychiatric Annals, 43*(3), 123–138.

Rizzo, A., Difede, J., Rothbaum, B. O., & Reger, G. (2010). Virtual Iraq/Afghanistan: Development and early evaluation of a virtual reality exposure therapy system for combat-related PTSD. *Annals of the New York Academy of Sciences, 1208*, 114–125.

Rizzo, A. A., Graap, K., Mclay, R. N., Perlman, K., Rothbaum, B., Reger, G., et al. (2007). Initial case reports from a VR exposure therapy application for combat-related post traumatic stress disorder. *IEEE XPlore Virtual Rehabilitation International Conference*, 2007, pp. 124–130.

Rothbaum, B., Difede, J., & Rizzo, A. (2008). *Therapist treatment manual for virtual reality exposure therapy: Posttraumatic stress disorder in Iraq combat veterans*. Atlanta: Virtually Better.

Rothbaum, B. O., Hodges, L., Ready, D., Graap, K., & Alarcon, R. (2001). Virtual reality exposure therapy for Vietnam veterans with posttraumatic stress disorder. *Journal of Clinical Psychiatry, 62*, 617–622.

Rothbaum, B.O., & Ressler, K.J. (2008). *D-cycloserine and virtual reality exposure to treat Iraq war veterans with TSD*: http://clinicaltrials.gov/ct2/show/NCT00356278?term=Barbara+Rothbaum&rank=4

Sadler, A. G., Booth, B. M., Nielson, D., & Doebbeling, B. N. (2000). Health-related consequences of physical and sexual violence: Women in the military. *Obstetrics & Gynecology, 96*, 473–480.

Skinner, K. M., Kressin, N., Frayne, S., Tripp, T. J., Hankin, C. S., Miller, D. R., et al. (2000). The prevalence of military sexual assault among female Veterans' Administration outpatients. *Journal of Interpersonal Violence, 15*, 291–310.

Sones, H. M., Thorp, S. R., & Raskind, M. (2011). Prevention of posttraumatic stress disorder. *Psychiatric Clinics of North America, 34*, 79–94.

Sterling, P., & Eyer, J. (1988). Allostasis: A new paradigm to explain arousal pathology. In S. Fisher & J. Reason (Eds.), *Handbook of life stress, cognition and health* (pp. 629–639). New York, NY: Wiley.

Street, A. E., Gradus, J. L., Stafford, J., & Kelly, K. (2007). Gender differences in experiences of sexual harassment: Data from a male-dominated environment. *Journal of Consulting and Clinical Psychology, 75*, 464–474.

Street, A. E., Stafford, J., Mahan, C. M., & Hendricks, A. (2008). Sexual harassment and assault experienced by reservists during military service: Prevalence and health correlates. *Journal of Rehabilitation Research and Development, 45*, 409–419.

Surıs, A., Lind, L., Kaashner, T. M., & Borman, P. D. (2007). Mental health, quality of life, and health functioning in women veterans: Differential outcomes associated with military and civilian sexual assault. *Journal of Interpersonal Violence, 22*, 179–197.

Thomas, J. L., Wilk, J. E., Riviere, L. A., McGurk, D., Castro, C. A., & Hoge, C. W. (2010). Prevalence of mental health problems and functional impairment among active component and National Guard soldiers 3 and 12 months following combat in Iraq. *Archives of General Psychiatry, 67*(6), 614–623.

Valencia, O. (2013). Veterans seek resources to treat military sexual trauma. *Talk Radio News Service*. Accessed on July 20, 2013 at: http://www.talkradionews.com/pentagon/2013/07/19/veterans-seek-resources-to-treat-military-sexual-trauma.html#.UerSFfPn9ow

Walker, D. L., Ressler, K. J., Lu, K. T., & Davis, M. (2002). Facilitation of conditioned fear extinction by systemic administration or intra-amygdala infusions of D-cycloserine as assessed with fear-potentiated startle in rats. *Journal of Neuroscience, 22*, 2343–2351.

Wilson, J., Onorati, K., Mishkind, M., Reger, M., & Gahm, G. A. (2008). Soldier attitudes about technology-based approaches to mental healthcare. *Cyberpsychology and Behavior, 11*, 767–769.

Zinzow, H. M., Grubaugh, A. L., Monnier, J., Suffoletta-Maierle, S., & Frueh, B. C. (2007). Trauma among female veterans: A critical review. *Trauma, Violence & Abuse, 8*, 384–400.

Chapter 17
Mental Health Problems and Treatment Utilization of Iraq and Afghanistan Veterans Enrolled in Department of Veterans Affairs Health Care

Karen H. Seal, Shira Maguen, and Beth E. Cohen

Mental Health Problems in Iraq and Afghanistan Veterans

It has been over a decade since the current conflicts began and roughly 2.5 million service members have served in Operation Enduring Freedom (OEF, principally Afghanistan), Operation Iraqi Freedom (OIF, principally Iraq), and Operation New Dawn (OND). Of these, 1.5 million have separated from active duty service and have become eligible for Department of Veterans Affairs (VA) healthcare services. Many soldiers have endured multiple tours of duty and most have experienced "front-line" combat. Making the transition from warzone to home has been challenging, especially for veterans who have sustained physical injuries, as well as for those who have developed mental health problems.

The VA is the single largest provider of health care for returning Iraq and Afghanistan veterans. The mental health prevalence estimates our research group provides are based on data acquired from VA national administrative databases which contain mental health diagnostic codes associated with VA clinical visits. The use of diagnostic codes has been shown to be a valid proxy for estimating disease prevalence, but is subject to reporting biases and some misclassification errors. Our findings are based on the entire population of OEF/OIF/OND veterans who

K.H. Seal, M.D., M.P.H. (✉) • S. Maguen, Ph.D. • B.E. Cohen, M.D., M.A.S.
Department of Medicine, University of California, San Francisco, CA, USA

Department Psychiatry, University of California, San Francisco, CA, USA

General Internal Medicine, San Francisco VA Medical Center,
111A-1, 4150 Clement St., San Francisco, CA 94121, USA
e-mail: karen.seal@ucsf.edu; karen.seal@va.gov;
shira.maguen@ucsf.edu; beth.cohen@ucsf.edu

M.P. Safir et al. (eds.), *Future Directions in Post-Traumatic Stress Disorder*,
DOI 10.1007/978-1-4899-7522-5_17

sought VA health care nationwide and thus, are not based on a nationally representative sample of OEF/OIF/OND veterans. Nevertheless, our findings have been consistent with other published studies of nationally representative samples of OEF/OIF veterans (Milliken, Auchterlonie, & Hoge, 2007; Tanielian & Jaycox, 2008).

These VA administrative data confirm that the burden of mental health diagnoses has continued to increase since the conflicts began in 2001. In one of our earlier studies (Seal et al., 2009), of 289,328 Iraq and Afghanistan veterans who were first-time users of VA health care after separation from OEF and/or OIF military service, new mental health diagnoses increased sixfold from 6 % in April 2002 to 37 % by March 31, 2008, with rates of PTSD increasing most rapidly (Fig. 17.1a, b). Thus, by 2008 over one of every three veterans enrolled in VA health care had received one or more mental health diagnoses. Moreover, with each additional year that a Veteran was followed in care, we observed the accrual of additional mental health diagnoses in individual veterans (Fig. 17.2). The most recent data released from the VA Environmental Epidemiology Service (March 31, 2012) indicate that 424,803 (53 %) of 804,704 VA-enrolled veterans have received mental health diagnoses and 228, 361 (28 %) have received posttraumatic stress (PTSD) diagnoses. Similarly, Milliken and colleagues demonstrated increases in mental health problems among OEF/OIF/OND soldiers who were screened again several months after returning home compared to rates immediately after returning (Milliken et al., 2007).

There are several factors that contribute to delayed onset of mental health diagnoses. There may be stigma leading to reluctance to disclose mental health problems until those problems interfere with functioning (Hoge et al., 2004). Some military service-related mental health problems only appear months to years after combat (Solomon & Mikulincer, 2006) and somatization or comorbidity often confound accurate mental health diagnosis (Kessler, Sonnega, Bromet, Hughes, & Nelson, 1995). The VA policy change that extended free VA military service-related health care to 5 years from 2 years post-discharge has likely increased VA's ability to detect mental illness in OEF/OIF veterans. Now the challenge for VA is to engage Veterans with mental health problems in care (Fig. 17.3).

Several key findings regarding the prevalence of mental health disorders have emerged from our recently published studies (Maguen, Ren, Bosch, Marmar, & Seal, 2010; Seal et al., 2009; Seal et al., 2011):

- Among OEF/OIF/OND veterans with mental health diagnoses, two-thirds had two or more co-occurring mental health diagnoses, increasing diagnostic complexity and complicating treatment.
- PTSD and depression have proved highly comorbid with as many as 70 % of veterans suffering from both conditions.
- Overall, from 2002 to 2011, the rate of PTSD increased by a factor of over 100 times, with the most rapid increase in PTSD following the invasion of Iraq in 2003.
- Overall, over 11 % of OEF/OIF Veterans received substance use disorder diagnoses. Male veterans had over twice the risk for substance use disorders as female veterans. Among veterans with substance use disorders, 55–75 % had comorbid PTSD or depression diagnoses.

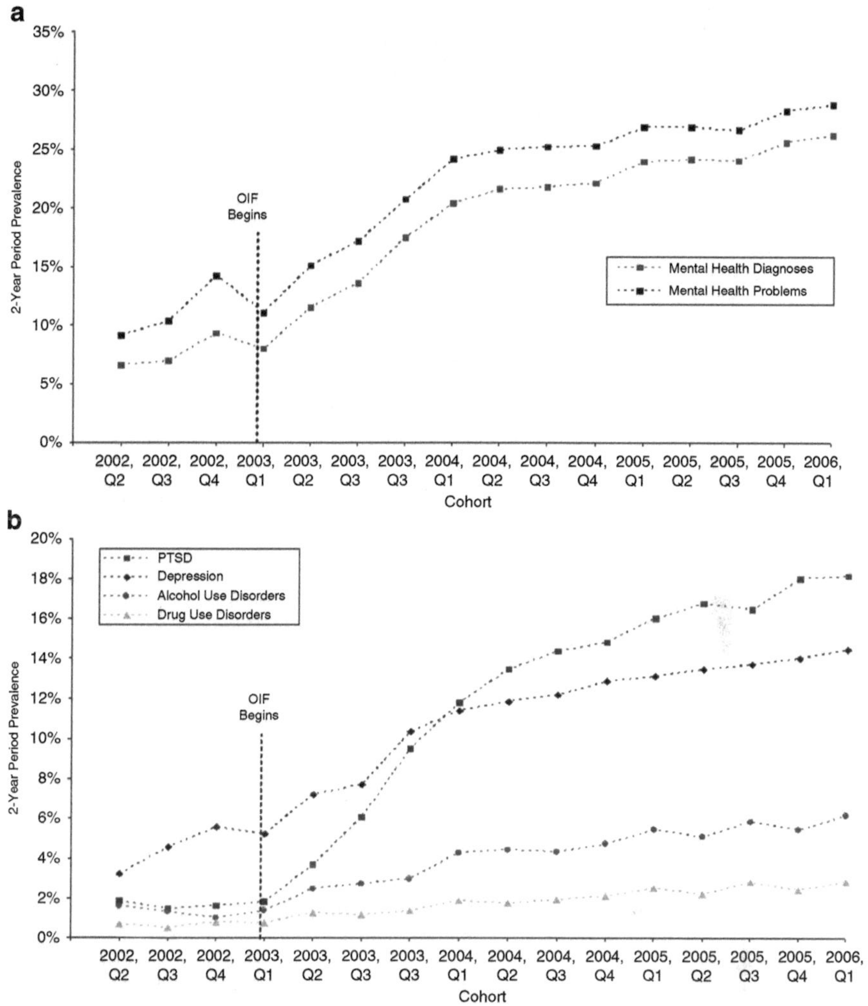

Fig. 17.1 (**a** and **b**) Two-year period prevalence of mental health diagnoses (based on *International Classification of Diseases, Ninth Revision, Clinical Modification* codes ICD-9 codes 290.0-319.0 that correspond to *Diagnostic and Statistical Manual of Mental Disorders, Fourth Edition, Revised (DSM-IV-R)* diagnostic codes for mental illness) and problems (includes V-Codes (see "Methods" section) indicating psychosocial or behavioral problem: V15.40–V15.49; V60.0–V60.2; V60.4; V61.0–V61.22; V61.80–V61.83; V61.90; V62.0; V62.2; V62.5; V62.80–V62.89; V63.0; V63.9; V65.2; V65.5; V69.2–V69.8; V70.1–V70.2; V71.0–V71.01; V71.5; V71.81; V79.0–V79.1 in addition to ICD-9-CM mental health diagnoses 290.0-319.0) (2a) and specific mental health diagnoses (the ICD-9 CM code for "PTSD" is 309.81, for "depressive disorders" are 296.20–296.25, and 296.30–296.35, 300.4, and 311 (excludes depression in remission and depression in conjunction with bipolar disorders), for "alcohol use disorders" are 305.00-305.03 (alcohol abuse) and 303 (alcohol dependence), and for "drug use disorders" are 305.20–305.93 (drug abuse), 304 (drug dependence), excluding code for nicotine dependence, 305.1) (2b) in Distinct Cohorts of OEF/OIF/OND Veterans Entering VA in successive calendar quarters and followed for 2 years, April 1, 2002–March 31, 2006

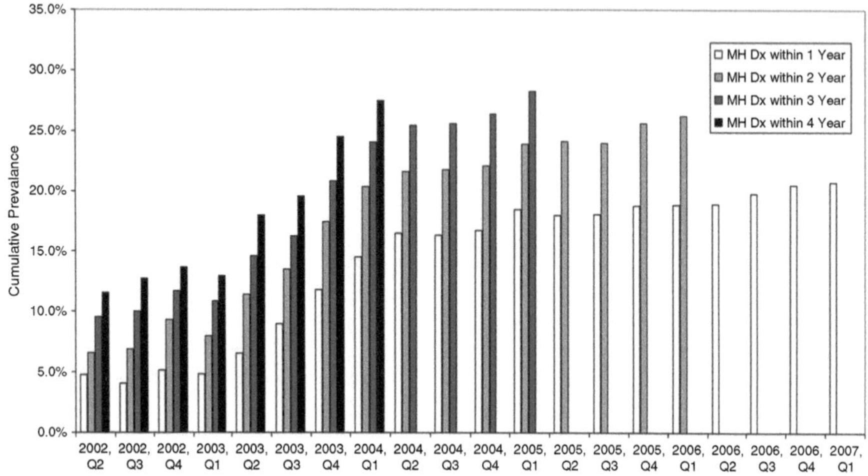

Fig. 17.2 Cumulative prevalence of new mental health diagnoses (MH Dx) in successive cohorts of OEF/OIF/OND Veterans Entering VA Healthcare and followed for increasing lengths of time from 1 to 4 years. Permission from Am J Public to reproduce these figures

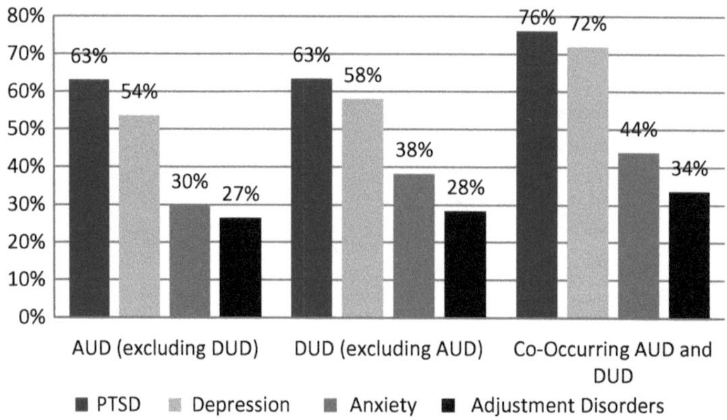

Fig. 17.3 Unadjusted prevalence of comorbid military service-related mental health diagnoses (PTSD, depression, anxiety, and adjustment disorders) associated with alcohol use disorders (AUD), drug use disorders (DUD), and both among active duty and National Guard and Reserve veterans of Iraq and Afghanistan

- Age and component type mattered: ***Active duty*** veterans **<u>less than age 25</u>** years had 2–5 times higher rates of PTSD and alcohol and drug use disorder diagnoses compared to active duty veterans **<u>over age 40</u>**. In contrast, among ***National Guard/Reserve*** veterans, risk for PTSD and depression was significantly higher in veterans **<u>over age 40</u>** compared to their younger counterparts **<u>less than age 25</u>**.
- Women OEF/OIF veterans were at significantly higher risk for depression than men; women veterans were also at significantly higher risk for anxiety disorders and eating disorders than their male counterparts.

- 31 % of women with PTSD compared 1 % of men with PTSD screened positive for a history of military sexual trauma (MST). Women veterans with MST were over four times more likely to develop PTSD than OEF/OIF female veterans without MST.

In summary, PTSD rates in treatment-seeking veterans in VA health care have increased steadily since the conflicts began, closely followed by increasing rates of depression diagnoses. Particular subgroups of Iraq and Afghanistan veterans appear at higher risk for mental health diagnoses. Younger, active duty veterans appear to be at particularly high risk for PTSD likely due to higher combat exposure. In contrast, older National Guard and Reserve veterans were at higher risk for PTSD and depression than younger National Guard/Reserve veterans. Further investigation of the causes of mental health diagnoses in older Guard/Reserve veterans is warranted because measures of greater combat exposure were not consistently associated with mental health diagnoses. One explanation is that when called to arms, older Guard/Reserve members are more established in civilian life and may be less well prepared for combat, making their transition to warzone and home again more challenging. Regarding the relatively low prevalence rates of drug use disorders in combat veterans in our sample, stigma, fear of negative repercussions, and lack of universal screening for illicit substances in VA may have reduced the number of drug use disorders reported and detected. Finally, there are pronounced gender differences in military service-related mental health disorders: Rates of depression, anxiety, and eating disorders were elevated in women compared to men; female veterans who experienced MST were at extremely high risk for developing PTSD. Appreciating subgroup differences in the prevalences and types of mental health disorders can help guide more targeted interventions and treatments, as well as future research efforts.

Mental Health Services Utilization in OEF/OIF Veterans

Overview

Over 50 % of all returned combat Veterans have enrolled in VA health care. This is historically high for VA; only 10 % of Vietnam veterans enrolled in VA health care (Kulka et al., 1990). Since 2001, the VA had provided OEF/OIF Veterans 2 years of free military service-related health care from the time of service separation, a benefit which was extended to 5 years in 2008 ("National Defense Authorization Act of 2008"). Most of the over 150 VA medical centers in the United States offer a complete spectrum of mental health services, including over 140 PTSD specialty clinics. For rural veterans living far from a VA medical center, over 900 VA community-based outpatient clinics offer basic health care and some offer basic mental health services. After the 5-year period of combat-related health coverage, OEF/OIF/OND veterans are eligible to continue to use VA healthcare services without charge (if they have a service-connected disability) or they are assessed a nominal co-pay scaled to income. Of note, Iraq and Afghanistan veterans who have health insurance through employment, school, or otherwise, may seek non-VA reimbursed healthcare services in their communities, and VA data systems do not capture this non-VA healthcare utilization.

Early, adequate evidence-based mental health treatment has been shown to prevent mental health disorders, such as PTSD, from becoming chronic (Bryant, Moulds, Guthrie, & Nixon, 2003). Multiple studies of veterans and civilians reveal however that a substantial proportion of those suffering from mental health problems either do not access, delay, or fail to complete an adequate course of specialty mental health treatment (Hoge et al., 2004; Tanielian & Jaycox, 2008; Wang et al., 2005). Studies have shown that mental health disorders other than PTSD, such as depression and substance use disorders, may be managed in primary care as opposed to specialty mental health clinics (Batten & Pollack, 2008). Some specific symptoms of PTSD, such as insomnia, may be managed by primary care clinicians in primary care. However, consistent with the Institute of Medicine's finding that only two trauma-focused therapies have demonstrated efficacy for PTSD, Cognitive Processing Therapy and Prolonged Exposure Therapy, the VA mandates that veterans with a PTSD diagnosis have access to treatment by mental health providers trained in these evidence-based therapies, which typically occurs in specialty mental health clinics (Department of Veterans Affairs Uniformed Mental Health Services Handbook, 2008).

Mental Health Services Utilization in OEF/OIF Veterans Using VA Health Care (2002–2008) (Seal et al., 2010)

Evidence-based PTSD treatments require a minimum of nine or more sessions, ideally spaced at weekly intervals (Foa, Hembree, & Rothbaum, 2007; Monson et al., 2006). We found that of nearly 50,000 Iraq and Afghanistan veterans with newly diagnosed PTSD, 80 % compared to 49 % of those receiving mental health diagnoses other than PTSD had at least one VA mental health visit in the first year of diagnosis (Seal et al., 2010). Nevertheless, only 9.5 % with new PTSD diagnoses attended nine or more follow-up sessions in 15 weeks or less after receiving their diagnosis. When the follow-up period was extended to 1 year, a larger proportion, 27 % attended nine or more mental health sessions. Among OEF/OIF/OND veterans receiving mental health diagnoses other than PTSD (e.g., depression), only 4 % attended nine or more follow-up sessions in 15 weeks or less and slightly more, and 9 % attended nine or more sessions when the follow-up period was extended to 1 year (Fig. 17.4a, b). Our study was limited in that we lacked information about non-VA mental health treatment utilization and the specific type of mental health treatment received. Thus, we can draw no firm conclusions about the adequacy and intensity of mental health care for OEF/OIF/OND veterans since we lack data on care received outside the VA system. Nevertheless, VA is currently the single largest

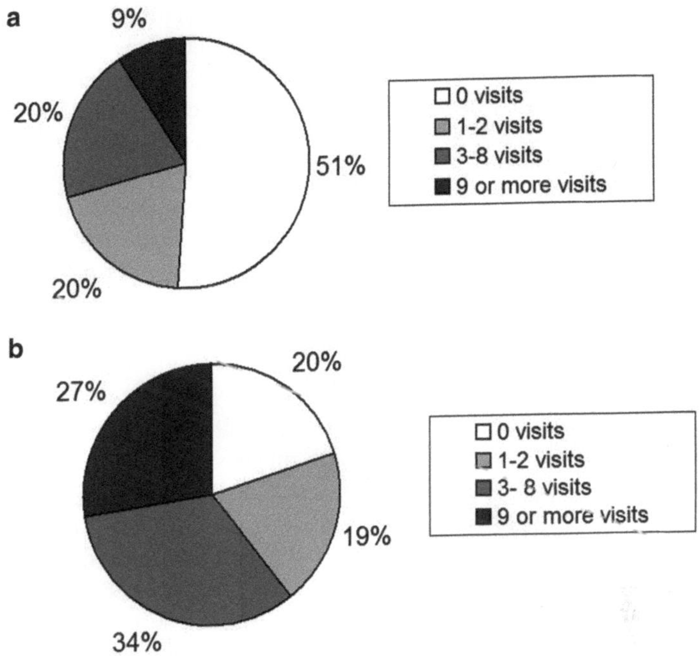

Fig. 17.4 (**a**) Number of follow-up VA mental health (MH) visits among OEF/OIF veterans in the first year of non-PTSD MH diagnoses. (**b**) Number of follow-up VA mental health (MH) visits among OEF/OIF veterans within the first year of receiving new PTSD diagnoses

provider of health care for OEF/OIF veterans and, of those with new PTSD diagnoses, in the first year of diagnosis, at the time the study that was conducted under 10 % appear to have received what would approximate evidence-based mental health treatment for PTSD at a VA facility, and those with other mental health diagnoses received an even lower intensity of VA care.

Our study revealed that factors such as being young (under age 25) and male, factors linked to a greater likelihood of receiving a PTSD diagnosis, were also associated with a failure to receive minimally adequate PTSD treatment (Seal et al., 2010). These findings may reflect the symptoms of PTSD itself, including avoidance, denial, and comorbid disorders such as depression and substance abuse. In young male veterans, stigma surrounding health care likely also plays a major role (Hoge et al., 2004). In addition, we found that having received a mental health diagnosis from a nonmental health clinic (i.e., primary care) and living far from a VA facility (>25 miles) were associated with failing to receive adequate PTSD treatment. Veterans who receive PTSD diagnoses from VA primary care may be less symptomatic than those receiving diagnoses from mental health clinics and less in need of specialty mental health treatment or prefer primary care-based treatments. Indeed, many mental health problems of combat veterans other than

PTSD, such as depression, may be effectively managed in primary care. In fact, we found that among veterans receiving mental health diagnoses other than PTSD, more than 85 % had attended at least one primary care visit in the year following diagnosis, the majority of which were coded to indicate that a mental health concern had been discussed. It is also possible that veterans who receive PTSD diagnoses from nonmental health clinics or who live far from VA services fall through the cracks in the referral for specialty mental health care. Indeed, rural veterans experience significantly greater mental health morbidity than their urban counterparts. (Wallace, Weeks, Wang, Lee, & Kazis, 2006) In sum, our research findings support ongoing implementation efforts by VA leadership to promote expanded access and adherence to specialty mental health care, especially for rural veterans (Zeiss & Karlin, 2008).

Our results suggest that OEF/OIF/OND veterans may, in fact, be more likely than Vietnam-era veterans to have had ***at least one*** initial VA mental health follow-up visit after receiving a new mental health diagnosis. In the National Vietnam Veterans Readjustment Study (NVVRS), a nationally representative sample of Vietnam-era veterans, a much lower proportion of Vietnam Veterans (30 %) reported having sought any mental health treatment and only 7.5 % used VA mental health services (Kulka et al., 1990). A more recent study demonstrated that after adjustments for potential confounding, variables such as age and the complexity of mental health disorders were more important predictors of whether veterans received mental health treatment as opposed to the era during which they served (Harpaz-Rotem & Rosenheck, 2011).

It stands to reason that Iraq and Afghanistan veterans would be more likely than prior-era veterans to have had at least an ***initial*** mental health visit. In comparison to Vietnam-era veterans, a higher proportion of OEF/OIF/OND veterans have experienced "front-line" combat exposure and have survived their injuries (Gawande, 2004). These factors have been associated with the development of mental health disorders and increased need for mental health services (Hoge, Terhakopian, Castro, Messer, & Engel, 2007). Unlike in prior eras, Congress extended health coverage for OEF/OIF/OND veterans to 5 years after service separation. Thus, many newly returned veterans facing economic hardship have taken advantage of blanket VA healthcare coverage and have used VA services. Also, different from prior eras, the Department of Defense, in an effort to reduce stigma, now openly discusses combat-related stress with active duty service members. Similarly, widespread media attention focused on mental health disorders in Iraq and Afghanistan veterans has likely lowered the threshold for recently returned veterans to seek care. Finally, both the VA and the military have implemented population-based post-deployment mental health screening programs and routinely refer veterans who screen positive for further mental health assessment and/or treatment (Hoge, Auchterlonie, & Milliken, 2006; Seal et al., 2008), all factors which support ***initial*** VA mental health services utilization.

Nevertheless, despite ***initial*** use of VA mental health services among returned combat veterans, ***retention*** in VA mental health services appears less robust. The strongest predictor of retention in VA mental health treatment services in our study, as in others, was "need" for mental health treatment (Spoont, Murdoch, Hodges, & Nugent, 2010). Veterans receiving PTSD diagnoses (as opposed to other mental health diagnoses) and those receiving additional comorbid mental health diagnoses in conjunction with PTSD were more likely to remain in care and receive minimally adequate PTSD treatment. Unfortunately, compared to studies of civilians however, retention in VA mental health treatment appears inferior. For instance, the National Comorbidity Survey Replication Study, a population-based survey of 9,282 US civilian adults, found that 48 % of patients with any mental disorder (including PTSD) reported having received at least "minimally adequate therapy," defined by evidence-based national mental health treatment guidelines, within the first year of diagnosis (Wang et al., 2005). In contrast, similar to our findings, a RAND Corporation study reported that a much lower proportion, 25 % of a nationally representative sample of Iraq and Afghanistan veterans with PTSD and depression, received "minimally adequate therapy" within the first year of diagnosis (Tanielian & Jaycox, 2008).

In summary, we found that the majority of Iraq and Afghanistan veterans that were enrolled in VA care and received new mental health diagnoses, including PTSD, attended at least one mental health follow-up visit in the year after mental health diagnosis. However, the vast majority of OEF/OIF/OND veterans with new PTSD diagnoses failed to attend a minimum number of mental health sessions within a recommended time frame required for evidence-based PTSD treatment. Because early, evidence-based PTSD treatment may prevent chronic PTSD, it will be important that the VA, in its mission to provide the best care for returning combat veterans, continue to develop and implement interventions to improve retention in mental health treatment, with particular attention to the needs of more vulnerable combat veterans.

Barriers to VA Mental Health Care

Patient Barriers

There have been numerous reports of barriers to mental health care for Iraq and Afghanistan veterans. Our data and the work of others indicate that while there are indeed barriers to access and initiation of mental health treatment, longer-term retention in mental health treatment is far more problematic (Harpaz-Rotem & Rosenheck, 2011; Seal et al., 2010; Seal et al., 2011). Barriers to engagement in mental health treatment have generally been categorized into patient-related barriers and system barriers. Patient barriers have been well described and include: (1) Stigma regarding mental illness concerns about being perceived as weak by family, friends, colleagues, or within one's culture for coming forward with mental health problems, (2) "Battlemind"—not perceiving that behaviors such as hypervigilance and sleeping minimally, behaviors that were adaptive in the warzone, are "mental health symptoms" and therefore not seeking or accepting mental health treatment,

(3) Beliefs and attitudes that mental health treatment, including psychoactive medication, is not effective or even dangerous, (4) Logistical barriers such as job, school, family obligations, and geographical distance (rurality), (5) Symptoms of mental health disorders themselves, such as avoidance in PTSD, apathy in depression, and denial in drug and alcohol abuse, and (6) Self-medication with illicit drugs, alcohol, and prescription medication (polypharmacy) that may temporarily mask symptoms (Hoge, 2011).

VA System Goals and Residual System Barriers

The Institute of Medicine (IOM) identified six goals to improve the quality of mental health care. These included safety, effectiveness, patient-centeredness, timeliness, efficiency, and equity. Consistent with these goals, the VA has made numerous strides toward improving the delivery of mental health treatment for Iraq and Afghanistan veterans by greatly increasing mental health capacity and services. For instance, in order to improve identification and treatment of veterans with mental health disorders, since 2004, the VA has conducted universal post-deployment mental health screening of OEF/OIF/OND veterans, although it should be noted that mental health screening has not been shown to improve mental health outcomes (Seal et al., 2008). In addition, in 2007, the VA initiated an expansion of mental health services capacity, which included an increase in the number of mental health staff assigned to more rural VA clinics, an increase in the use of video-teleconferencing services ("telemental health") to increase access to specialty mental health care for rural Veterans, and the implementation of the Primary Care Mental Health Integration initiative to colocate mental health providers in primary care settings (Zeiss & Karlin, 2008). Indeed, most recently, the VA has rolled out the Patient Aligned Care Team (PACT) model which organizes primary care providers into coordinated teams supported by a nurse care manager at the center. In addition, PACT more closely affiliates mental health clinicians with primary care providers and patients to provide more timely and coordinated mental health care services for veterans.

Nevertheless, with ever-increasing numbers of Iraq and Afghanistan veterans presenting with mental health problems, VA has not always been able to keep pace with the demand for services, particularly in more rural VA facilities. There are several VA system barriers which are remediable and require our attention:

- There are shortages of mental health staff (psychologists and social workers) who are trained in evidence-based therapies for PTSD, particularly in more rural VA community-based outpatient clinics.
- There is a lack of training in military cultural competency to help VA clinicians (primarily civilians) foster solid therapeutic alliances and continued engagement with former warriors who may not perceive themselves as having mental health problems.

- There is a lack of universal access to telemental health services (video teleconferencing) to provide access to specialty mental health clinicians based at VA medical centers for veterans who receive their care at rural VA community-based outpatient clinics.
- Information technology (IT) security is important, yet overconcern about IT security may hinder the development and use of more novel web- and telephone-based mental health treatment options that may especially appeal to younger veterans.
- Veterans continue to complain about difficulties navigating the VA system to schedule appointments, long wait times for appointments, and shortages of drop-in appointments, which limit access to care.
- Most mental health treatment programs at VA do not include family or significant others, who could otherwise be mobilized to support the veteran's adherence to mental health treatment. A related problem is that there are very limited mental health treatment resources for families and children of veterans at VA.
- In the VA and Department of Defense's effort to share medical information, some veterans are concerned that their confidential VA electronic medical records will be viewed by the Department of Defense, which cause reluctance to disclose sensitive, but medically important information, such as substance abuse concerns and interpersonal violence, which limits their ability to receive treatment for these problems.

Utilization of VA Primary Care in OEF/OIF Veterans with Mental Health Problems

Despite underutilization of ***mental health services***, Iraq and Afghanistan veterans with mental health disorders disproportionately use VA ***primary care medical services*** compared to those without mental health problems. Frayne et al. (2011) examined nonmental health medical care among 90,558 veterans from 2005 through 2006 and found that those with a diagnosis of PTSD had a greater number of medical diagnoses and greater primary care service utilization than those without a mental health diagnosis. Another article published by Cohen et al. (2010) found an increased prevalence of cardiovascular risk factors (i.e., hypertension, high cholesterol, smoking, and obesity) in OEF/OIF veterans with PTSD compared to those with mental health conditions other than PTSD, or no mental health conditions (Fig. 17.5). In a related study, Cohen et al. (2010) reported that Iraq and Afghanistan veterans with PTSD consumed almost twice as much primary medical care as those without a mental health diagnosis (Fig. 17.6).

There are several possible explanations for this disproportionate use of primary care medical services in veterans with PTSD. The traumatic events that caused PTSD might have also caused physical injury requiring medical attention; somatic symptoms coupled with stigma associated with PTSD symptoms may have led some veterans to preferentially seek VA primary care (instead of mental health

	No MH Dx N=182,151	MH Dx (not PTSD) N=48,502	PTSD (±other MH Dx) N=72,873
Tobacco Use	1.0	3.0 (3.0-3.1)	3.6 (3.6-3.7)
Hypertension	1.0	2.4 (2.3-2.5)	2.9 (2.8-3.0)
High cholesterol	1.0	2.3 (2.2-2.4)	2.7 (2.6-2.8)
Obesity	1.0	2.1 (2.1-2.2)	2.4 (2.4-2.5)
Diabetes	1.0	2.5 (2.4-2.8)	2.6 (2.4-2.8)

*** Adjusted for age, sex, race, active duty status, branch, multiple deployments**

Fig. 17.5 Association of mental health (MH) status and cardiovascular disease risk factors (adjusted for age, sex, race, active duty status, branch, multiple deployments)

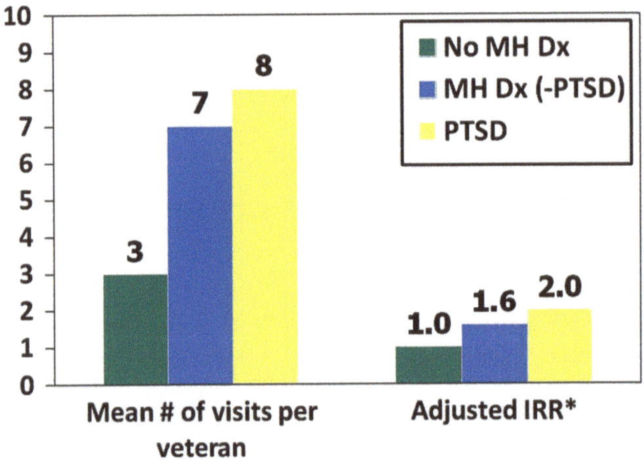

Fig. 17.6 Total outpatient medical service utilization in the first year of VA entry by mental health (MH) category (incidence rate ratio (IRR) adjusted for age, sex, race, marital status, active duty status, rank, branch, multiple deployments, distance to VA)

care), and increased contact with the medical system through PTSD treatment may have led to increased detection of other physical problems and thus more primary care utilization. In addition, in a recent editorial, Hoge posits that veterans with PTSD, given their recent combat and warzone exposure (in addition to the effects of PTSD), may have added dysregulation of the autonomic nervous system and the hypothalamic–pituitary–adrenal axis resulting in disturbed sleep patterns, chronic pain syndromes, post-concussive symptoms, neurocognitive impairments, and self-medication with alcohol and other substances (Hoge, 2011). To the extent that VA and other healthcare systems fail to engage and retain veterans in specialty mental health treatment however, veterans may continue to seek care for these chronic psychosomatic symptoms in primary care clinics. Because most individuals with PTSD, including OEF/OIF/OND veterans, pursue medical treatment in primary care, new care models that integrate primary care and mental health treatment may improve both engagement and retention of patients in mental health care, while simultaneously addressing co-occurring physical complaints.

Enhancing Access to and Retention in Mental Health Treatment for Iraq and Afghanistan Veterans

Capitalizing on the propensity for OEF/OIF/OND Veterans to receive care in VA primary care settings, one strategy to further enhance engagement in mental health services is to further colocate and integrate specialty mental health services, such as evidence-based PTSD treatment, within primary care. Despite the VA Primary Care Mental Health Integration initiative, even in model programs, these embedded mental health providers (many of whom are social workers) typically provide further assessment of positive mental health screens, make specialty mental health referrals, and provide medication management and brief supportive therapies, but rarely provide evidence-based mental health treatments (Possemato et al., 2011). Use of specialty mental health services has been associated with greater retention in mental health treatment, and in turn, improved clinical outcomes (Wang et al., 2005). There are several possible ways to provide greater access to specialty mental health treatment through primary care:

- Restructure health services such that specialty mental health providers trained in evidence-based mental health treatments are colocated and fully integrated within primary care. This requires a new holistic paradigm for primary care that views mental health care as part of primary care. This may even involve infrastructure changes to existing medical clinics to accommodate the co-location of more mental health clinicians in primary care to provide continuity of care primarily consisting of brief interventions. These structural change could "break down walls" that exist between medical and mental health services, overcome stigma, and narrow the gap between primary care and mental health. For instance, prescheduling specialty mental health visits to occur at the same time and place as primary care visits, as was done in our colocated, integrated primary care mental health clinic, made it significantly more likely that veterans attended an initial specialty mental health evaluation (Seal et al., 2011)
- Leverage new clinical resources available in primary care. The Medical Home Model is gaining traction in several health systems across the country, including VA.

Nurse care managers in primary care Medical Home teams are often trained to conduct motivational interventions to encourage positive health behavior changes, such as smoking cessation. Primary care nurse care managers could conceivably conduct brief telephone motivational coaching sessions to remind and motivate Veterans to attend their mental health appointments. As an alternative to the telephone, nurses could use new secure messaging systems, available in many healthcare systems, to e-mail patients about upcoming mental health visits, a communication modality that particularly appeals to younger veterans. In addition, consistent with the evidence-based collaborative care model for depression treatment, nurses could feedback relevant clinical information from patients to mental health and primary care providers to promote more efficient, coordinated, and effective care.

- Exploit new technologies to deliver mental health treatment in rural settings where there are limited or no specialty mental health services. Nurse care managers could coordinate "telemental" health visits between patients at rural health centers and specialty mental health providers based at medical centers using video teleconferencing technology available at many rural community-based outpatient clinics. For patients who need care, but are unable to travel to any clinic, there should be serious consideration given to newer technologies that bring mental health care into patients' homes. Examples include the delivery of evidence-based mental health treatments over the telephone or through computer-assisted teleconferencing "Skype," the use of mobile phone applications such as "PTSD Coach" as an adjunct to mental health treatment, and the use of the internet to deliver mental health treatments through state-of-the-art Web sites such as www.afterdeployment.org, which provides on-line evidence-based mental health treatment. These internet-based treatments could be facilitated by mental health clinicians through regular telephone or secure e-mail check-ins with patients.
- Support further research to develop and test the implementation of modified evidence-based treatments for PTSD and other mental health problems in primary care. There is a need to develop and test PTSD treatments that are briefer and better suited for primary care. PTSD is highly comorbid with other mental and physical health problems; thus integrated treatments for PTSD that simultaneously address substance abuse or other behavioral (e.g., smoking) and physical health problems (e.g., chronic pain) in the context of PTSD treatment may be more effective for multiple comorbid disorders. To date, there have been several trials of integrated PTSD treatments that have demonstrated efficacy (Brady, Dansky, Back, Foa, & Carroll, 2001; McFall et al., 2010; Najavits, Weiss, Shaw, & Muenz, 1998; Otis, Keane, & Kerns, 2003). Similarly, the incorporation of complementary and alternative modalities, such as aerobic exercise, yoga, and acupuncture in the treatment of PTSD, could be used to motivate engagement in mental health treatment and may improve overall physical and emotional well-being of veterans suffering with combat-related disorders. Finally, advanced technologies such as Virtual Reality (discussed in detail in other chapters) could be used to render evidence-based PTSD treatments, such as Exposure Therapy, more appealing and engaging to a generation of veterans raised in the digital age (Rizzo et al., 2013).

Conclusion

In summary, Iraq and Afghanistan veterans have extremely high rates of military service-related mental health problems. Despite this large burden of mental illness, because of patient and system barriers to VA mental health care, many OEF/OIF veterans do not access or receive an adequate course of mental health treatment. In contrast, despite underutilization of mental health services, combat veterans with mental health disorders disproportionately use primary care medical services. Recognizing the advances that VA has made in VA Primary Care-Mental Health Integration, and more recently, the Medical Home model, VA is poised to address many of the remaining system barriers to mental health care for OEF/OIF/OND veterans by incorporating more specialty mental health care within primary care. VA has been a pioneer in the US national healthcare system, learning and growing through its vast clinical and health services research enterprise. The current epidemic of mental health problems in Iraq and Afghanistan veterans, coupled with budgetary constraints, will undoubtedly continue to stimulate VA and other national health systems to develop and implement new systems of care, new technologies, and new services to meet the needs of this current generation of men and women who have served their country.

References

Batten, S., & Pollack, S. (2008). Integrative outpatient treatment for returning service members. *Journal of Clinical Psychology, 64*, 928–939.

Brady, K. T., Dansky, B. S., Back, S. E., Foa, E. B., & Carroll, K. M. (2001). Exposure therapy in the treatment of PTSD among cocaine-dependent individuals: Preliminary findings. *Journal of Substance Abuse Treatment, 21*, 47–54.

Bryant, R., Moulds, M., Guthrie, R., & Nixon, R. (2003). Treating acute stress disorder following mild traumatic brain injury. *American Journal of Psychiatry, 160*, 585–587.

Cohen, B. E., Gima, K., Bertenthal, D., Kim, S., Marmar, C. R., & Seal, K. H. (2010). Mental health diagnoses and utilization of VA non-mental health medical services among returning Iraq and Afghanistan veterans. *Journal of General Internal Medicine, 25*(1), 18–24.

Department of Veterans Affairs. (2008, September 11). *VHA handbook 1160.01: Uniformed mental health services in VA medical centers and clinics*. Accessed June 5, 2011, from http://www1.va.gov/vhapublications/ViewPublication.asp?pub_ID=1762

Foa, E., Hembree, E., & Rothbaum, B. (2007). *Prolonged exposure therapy for PTSD: Emotional processing of traumatic experiences: Therapist guide*. Oxford: Oxford University Press.

Frayne, S. M., Chiu, V. Y., Iqbal, S., Berg, E. A., Laungani, K. J., Cronkite, R. C., et al. (2011). Medical care needs of returning veterans with PTSD: Their other burden. *Journal of General Internal Medicine, 26*(1), 33–39.

Gawande, A. (2004). Casualties of war – Military care for the wounded from Iraq and Afghanistan. *The New England Journal of Medicine, 351*, 2471–2475.

Harpaz-Rotem, I., & Rosenheck, R. A. (2011). Serving those who served: Retention of newly returning veterans from Iraq and Afghanistan in mental health treatment. *Psychiatric Services, 62*(1), 22–27.

Hoge, C. W. (2011). Interventions for war-related posttraumatic stress disorder: Meeting veterans where they are. *JAMA, 306*(5), 549–551.

Hoge, C. W., Auchterlonie, J. L., & Milliken, C. S. (2006). Mental health problems, use of mental health services, and attrition from military service after returning from deployment to Iraq or Afghanistan. *JAMA, 295*(9), 1023–1032.

Hoge, C. W., Castro, C. A., Messer, S. C., McGurk, D., Cotting, D. I., & Koffman, R. L. (2004). Combat duty in Iraq and Afghanistan, mental health problems, and barriers to care. *The New England Journal of Medicine, 351*(1), 13–22.

Hoge, C., Terhakopian, A., Castro, C., Messer, S., & Engel, C. C. (2007). Association of posttraumatic stress disorder with somatic symptoms, health care visits, and absenteeism among Iraq war veterans. *American Journal of Psychiatry, 164*(1), 150–153.

Kessler, R. C., Sonnega, A., Bromet, E., Hughes, M., & Nelson, C. B. (1995). Posttraumatic stress disorder in the National Comorbidity Survey. *Archives of General Psychiatry, 52*(12), 1048–1060.

Kulka, R. A., Schlenger, W. E., Fiarbank, J. A., Hough, R. L., Jordan, B. K., Marmar, C. R., et al. (1990). Trauma and the Vietnam War generation: Findings from the National Vietnam Veterans Readjustment Study. New York.

Maguen, S., Ren, L., Bosch, J. O., Marmar, C. R., & Seal, K. H. (2010). Gender differences in mental health diagnoses among Iraq and Afghanistan veterans enrolled in veterans affairs health care. *American Journal of Public Health, 100*(12), 2450–2456.

McFall, M., Saxon, A. J., Malte, C. A., Chow, B., Bailey, S., Baker, D. G., et al. (2010). Integrating tobacco cessation into mental health care for posttraumatic stress disorder: A randomized controlled trial. *JAMA, 304*(22), 2485–2493.

Milliken, C. S., Auchterlonie, J. L., & Hoge, C. W. (2007). Longitudinal assessment of mental health problems among active and reserve component soldiers returning from the Iraq war. *JAMA, 298*(18), 2141–2148.

Monson, C., Schnurr, P., Resick, P., Friedman, M., Young-Xu, Y., & Stevens, S. (2006). Cognitive processing therapy for veterans with military-related posttraumatic stress disorder. *Journal of Consulting and Clinical Psychology, 74*, 898–907.

Najavits, L. M., Weiss, R. D., Shaw, S. R., & Muenz, L. R. (1998). "Seeking safety": Outcome of a new cognitive-behavioral psychotherapy for women with posttraumatic stress disorder and substance dependence. *Journal of Traumatic Stress, 11*, 437–456.

Otis, J. D., Keane, T. M., & Kerns, R. D. (2003). An examination of the relationship between chronic pain and post-traumatic stress disorder. *Journal of Rehabilitation Research and Development, 40*(5), 397–405.

Possemato, K., Ouimette, P., Lantinga, L. J., Wade, M., Coolhart, D., Schohn, M., et al. (2011). Treatment of Department of Veterans Affairs primary care patients with posttraumatic stress disorder. *Psychological Services, 8*(2), 82–93.

Rizzo, A. A., Buckwalter, J. G., Forbell, E., Difede, J., Rothbaum, B. O., Lange, B., et al. (2013). Virtual reality applications to address the wounds of war. *Psychiatric Annals, 43*(3), 123–138.

Seal, K. H., Bertenthal, D., Maguen, S., Gima, K., Chu, A., & Marmar, C. R. (2008). Getting beyond "Don't ask; don't tell": An evaluation of US Veterans Administration postdeployment mental health screening of veterans returning from Iraq and Afghanistan. *American Journal of Public Health, 98*(4), 714–720.

Seal, K. H., Cohen, G., Bertenthal, D., Cohen, B. E., Maguen, S., & Daley, A. (2011). Reducing barriers to mental health and social services for Iraq and Afghanistan veterans: Outcomes of an integrated primary care clinic. *Journal of General Internal Medicine, 26*(10), 1160–1167.

Seal, K. H., Cohen, G., Waldrop, A., Cohen, B., Maguen, S., & Ren, L. (2011). Substance use disorders in Iraq and Afghanistan Veterans in VA healthcare, 2001-2010: Implications for screening, diagnosis, and treatment. *Drug and Alcohol Dependence, 116*(1–3), 93–101.

Seal, K. H., Maguen, S., Cohen, B., Gima, K., Metzler, T. J., Ren, L., et al. (2010). VA mental health services utilization in Iraq and Afghanistan veterans in the first year of receiving new mental health diagnoses. *Journal of Traumatic Stress, 23*(1), 5–16. PMID: 20146392.

Seal, K. H., Metzler, T. J., Gima, K. S., Bertenthal, D., Maguen, S., & Marmar, C. R. (2009). Trends and risk factors for mental health diagnoses among Iraq and Afghanistan veterans using

Department of Veterans Affairs health care, 2002-2008. *American Journal of Public Health, 99*(9), 1651–1658.

Solomon, Z., & Mikulincer, M. (2006). Trajectories of PTSD: A 20-year longitudinal study. *The American Journal of Psychiatry, 163*(4), 659–666.

Spoont, M. R., Murdoch, M., Hodges, J., & Nugent, S. (2010). Treatment receipt by veterans after a PTSD diagnosis in PTSD, mental health, or general medical clinics. *Psychiatric Services, 61*(1), 58–63.

Tanielian, T. L., & Jaycox, L. H. (Eds.). (2008). *Invisible wounds of war: Psychological and cognitive injuries, their consequences, and services to assist recovery*. Santa Monica, CA: RAND.

Wallace, A. E., Weeks, W. B., Wang, S., Lee, A. F., & Kazis, L. E. (2006). Rural and urban disparities in health-related quality of life among veterans with psychiatric disorders. *Psychiatric Services, 57*(6), 851–856.

Wang, P., Berglund, P., Olfson, M., Pincus, H., Wells, K., & Kessler, R. (2005). Failure and delay in initial treatment contact after first onset of mental disorders in the National Comorbidity Survey Replication. *Archives of General Psychiatry, 62*, 603–613.

Zeiss, A., & Karlin, B. (2008). Integration of mental health and primary care services in the Department of Veterans Affairs Health Care System. *Journal of Clinical Psychology in Medical Settings, 15*, 73–78.

Chapter 18
Enhancing Exposure Therapy for PTSD Using D-Cycloserine

Mark S. Burton, Cole G. Youngner, Alexander J. McCarthy, Alex O. Rothbaum, and Barbara Olasov Rothbaum

Enhancing Treatment for PTSD

Prospective studies indicate that PTSD symptoms are almost universal in the immediate aftermath of trauma. The majority of individuals will have symptoms of reexperiencing, avoidance, and hyperarousal initially following the trauma that will extinguish over time (Rothbaum, Foa, Riggs, Murdock, & Walsh, 1992). While PTSD symptoms generally decrease over the first month following trauma, for some, after this point, they remain fairly steady across time. They don't worsen, but they don't improve. It is thought that for these individuals, PTSD develops as a result of a failure of recovery caused in part by a failure of fear extinction following the trauma. Although initially a normal response to a life-threatening situation, PTSD symptoms become problematic when the fearful response to stimuli reminiscent of the trauma remains despite the lack of an imminent threat to one's life.

Several approaches for treating PTSD, including pharmacological, psychological, and augmentation strategies, have been implemented with varying results. By exploring the results of these studies and their underlying theoretical approaches to treating PTSD and other anxiety disorders, we will uncover the need for a therapy for those who might not respond to first-line recommendations. Ultimately, in combination with the investigation of these various other strategies, our discussion of D-Cycloserine (DCS) and its application in treating anxiety disorders shows its promising potential for enhancing the efficacy of exposure therapy (ET) for PTSD.

M.S. Burton • C.G. Youngner • A.J. McCarthy • B.O. Rothbaum, Ph.D., ABPP (✉)
Emory University School of Medicine, 1256 Briarcliff Road, Atlanta, GA 30306, USA
e-mail: mark.burton@case.edu; cyoungner@emory.edu; aj.mccarthy17@gmail.com; brothba@emory.edu

A.O. Rothbaum
Virtually Better, Inc., Decatur, GA, USA
e-mail: arothba@emory.edu

M.P. Safir et al. (eds.), *Future Directions in Post-Traumatic Stress Disorder*,
DOI 10.1007/978-1-4899-7522-5_18

Pharmacotherapy

Pharmacological approaches to treating PTSD aim to correct the neurochemical imbalances in emotional processing mechanisms, such as arousal, thought to be linked to the disorder. Early studies provided mixed evidence for the use of monoamine oxidase inhibitors (MAOIs) and tricyclic antidepressants (TCAs) over placebo for the treatment of PTSD (Davidson, 1992; Kosten, Frank, Dan, McDougle, & Giller, 1991; Shestatzky, Greenberg, & Lerer, 1988), although they have fallen out of favor in lieu of selective serotonin reuptake inhibitors (SSRIs) which are thought to be better tolerated and safer (Cooper, Carty, & Creamer, 2005). Currently, the only medications to receive a Food and Drug Administration (FDA) indication for PTSD, sertraline and paroxetine, are both SSRIs (Brady et al., 2000; Davidson, Rothbaum, van der Kolk, Sikes, & Farfel, 2001; Marshall, Beebe, Oldham, & Zaninelli, 2001; Tucker et al., 2000). In support of the use of medication to treat PTSD, a meta-analysis of pharmacological treatment showed pharmacotherapy to be a more effective method than placebo, with SSRIs contributing most to the overall effect of medication on treatment response compared with other classes of antidepressants. However, this class of drug was not shown to significantly contribute to variation in symptom severity outcomes between trials, suggesting that while SSRIs have the most support in the overall literature, they are not necessarily superior to MAOIs and TCAs for the treatment of PTSD (Stein, Ipser, & Seedat, 2006). In addition to antidepressants, benzodiazepines have also been used in the treatment of PTSD, but they have not proven useful as early interventions (Gelpin, Bonne, Peri, & Brandes, 1996).

Regarding early pharmacological interventions, based on evidence that propranolol (a β-adrenergic blocker) abolishes the epinephrine enhancement of conditioning (Cahill, Prins, Weber, & McGaugh, 1994), a number of pilot studies and randomized controlled trials (RCTs) of propranolol as a preventative treatment for PTSD have been conducted which mostly show a lack of support for the intervention. Pitman et al. (2002) indicated that propranolol did not result in reduced PTSD relative to a placebo, but patients receiving propranolol displayed less psychophysiological reactivity to trauma reminders. In a non-randomized pilot study, patients who received propranolol after a trauma showed significantly less PTSD symptoms than patients who refused propranolol (Vaiva et al., 2003). A recent RCT optimized dosages of propranolol (up to 240 mg/day for 19 days) and conducted psychophysiological and clinical assessments 4 and 12 weeks post-trauma in 41 emergency department (ED) patients. Physiological reactivity during script-driven traumatic imagery, severity of PTSD symptoms, and the rate of the PTSD diagnostic outcome for the treatment group were not significantly different from placebo control (Hoge et al., 2011). One pilot study (Brunet et al., 2008) examined the effect of propranolol on psychophysiological symptoms of PTSD after mental retrieval of a past trauma event. This study indicated that for individuals already diagnosed with PTSD, propranolol given after trauma memory retrieval reduced psychophysiological symptoms 1 week later.

Ultimately, the research for treating PTSD with psychiatric medications provides mixed results at best, indicating that other therapies must be considered. A recent IOM report (2008) did not find sufficient evidence to support pharmacotherapy for PTSD. These findings indicate that much work is needed to establish effective interventions immediately following traumatic events (see Kearns et al., this volume, Chap. 6, for a more extensive review of early interventions to try to prevent the development of PTSD). Indeed, as Davidson (1992) notes, pharmacotherapy is likely to be most effective when augmented with some form of behavioral exposure therapy.

Exposure Therapy for PTSD

Cognitive behavioral therapy (CBT), specifically exposure therapy (ET), is the only treatment with sufficient empirical evidence to be recommended by the Institute of Medicine for the treatment of PTSD (IOM, 2008). Well-controlled studies in the literature examining the efficacy of exposure therapy have found that 60 % to 95 % of individuals who received exposure therapy no longer met criteria for PTSD following treatment (Foa, Rothbaum, & Furr, 2003). Other psychological interventions such as cognitive processing therapy (CPT; Resick, Nishith, Weaver, & Astin, 2002) and eye movement desensitization and reprocessing (EMDR; Shapiro, 1995) have also been shown to be beneficial for treating PTSD (Monson et al., 2006; Van Etten & Taylor, 1998). Studies suggest CPT and EMDR are likely as effective as ET (Resick et al., 2002; Rothbaum, Astin & Marsteller, 2005). The reader is referred to the most recent ISTSS treatment guidelines for a complete review of all interventions for PTSD (Foa, Keane, Friedman, & Cohen, 2009).

Exposure therapy (ET) is based on animal models of conditioning and learning which seek to reduce fear through repeated presentations of the feared stimuli without the presence of adverse consequences. This process is thought to lead to habituation and eventual extinction of fear. It is the ultimate goal of ET for the learned reduction in fear to be generalizable between sessions as well as to other contexts. During ET, feared stimuli can be presented in a number of ways including the patient's imagination (imaginal), in real life (in vivo), or in virtual reality. Each of these approaches can incorporate education, breathing relaxation, and cognitive therapy techniques with exposure (Rothbaum & Davis, 2003).

The theoretical account behind exposure therapy for PTSD is that fear and anxiety lead to avoidance which prohibits emotional processing after a trauma (Foa, Steketee, & Rothbaum, 1989). Exposure helps to process emotions by activating the avoided fear memory in order to correct false information and reduce fear and anxiety associated with that memory. In order for exposure to be therapeutic for the treatment of PTSD, anxiety associated with a fear memory must be activated using proper memory cues and then reduced with repeated exposures. During exposure therapy, we want the patient to learn that their fear is unwarranted, and their distress will decrease with continued exposure. ET has gained more empirical support than any other intervention for PTSD (Foa, Hembree, & Rothbaum, 2007; IOM, 2008).

While ET has been shown to be an effective treatment for PTSD, the nature of the disorder, specifically the avoidance of trauma memories and reminders, can make it a difficult disorder to treat. Most individuals with PTSD never seek treatment (Kessler, 2000). For those who do seek treatment, exposure may still be difficult. For example, during imaginal exposure a patient who has been avoiding his or her trauma memory may find it very difficult to actively narrate the incident. For some individuals, even though they can talk about what happened, it remains difficult to access their emotions. This emotional disengagement is particularly problematic in Veterans and active duty Service Member populations. This can lead to treatment failures and drop outs for individuals with PTSD (Cukor, Spitalnick, Difede, Rizzo, & Rothbaum, 2009).

Attempting to overcome these issues, virtual reality exposure (VRE) has been developed to assist imaginal exposure by introducing sensory cues as augmentation to the patient's imagination. Incorporating auditory, visual, and olfactory cues increases the patient's ability to more fully access the memory of the trauma and thereby engage with it. With a systematic approach that can titrate the most distressing stimuli and move at the patient's own pace, the VR environment and its multiplicity of sensory cues can act to engage the patient's emotions and the memory of the trauma in order to process those emotions in a therapeutic exposure.

One example of VRE for the treatment of combat-related PTSD comes from a recently completed trial conducted by Barbara Rothbaum and colleagues at Emory University (Rothbaum et al., 2014). The virtual environments (VE) for this study were developed with input from Veterans returning from Iraq and Afghanistan, and included not only a series of diverse *scenario settings* (i.e., humvee or city) but also options for different first person *user perspectives* (e.g., as a driver, passenger, or gunner). These options, when combined with real time clinician input via the clinical *interface*, allowed for the creation of an end-user experience that was specifically customized to the varied needs of patients who participated in treatment. This was an essential component that gave the therapist the capacity to modulate client anxiety and aided in the sense of presence experienced within the VE. Such customization and real time stimulus delivery flexibility are key elements for these types of VR exposure applications. The software has been designed such that patients can be exposed to specific scenario settings based on a determination as to which environments most closely match the patient's needs, relevant to their individual combat-related experiences.

During the virtual exposure sessions, the patient described their most traumatic event from Iraq or Afghanistan in the present tense, just as in prolonged imaginal exposure (PE: Foa et al., 2007). However, rather than having their eyes closed, as in PE, their eyes were open and they were wearing a head mounted display consisting of a helmet, visor, and headphones, which immersed them in the virtual Iraq or Afghanistan environment. The user's view in the VR changed in real time due to a position tracker in the helmet. While they were describing the event, the therapist would recreate what they described in the virtual environment. For example, if they described a humvee driving down a desert highway and an IED hitting the right front filling everything with smoke, the therapist could recreate that scenario in the virtual environment. They would see it, hear it, feel it through a bass shaker attached to the raised platform below their chair, and smell scents the therapist delivered via the computer system. This created a potent stimulus designed to hopefully break through even the strong emotional disengagement often seen in Veterans.

There are several studies that demonstrate the exciting potential of using VRE to treat PTSD. Two open label studies have utilized VRE to help combat-related PTSD and showed promising results. Rothbaum, Hodges, Ready, Graap, and Alarcon (2001) examined the benefits of VRE with Vietnam Veterans suffering from PTSD (see Fig. 18.1). Rizzo, Reger, Gahm, Difede, and Rothbaum (2009) and Rizzo, Difede, Rothbaum, and Reger (2010) used VRE to treat Veterans of Operations Iraqi and Enduring Freedom with PTSD (see Fig. 18.2), successfully decreasing PTSD symptoms in 16 of the 20 patients who completed treatment such that they were classified as treatment responders. One recently completed trial showed that 6 sessions of VRE successfully reduced symptoms of PTSD, including objective biological measures, for Veterans of the Iraq and Afghanistan wars (Rothbaum et al., 2014). Based on this promising evidence, there is an ongoing multi-cite clinical trial examining the efficacy of VRE for the treatment of PTSD in both Veteran and active duty populations. VR has also been developed to treat civilian PTSD. Specifically, VR scenarios of the World Trade Center attacks on 9/11 and an Israeli bus bombing have been implemented for the treatment of civilian PTSD for survivors from those events (Difede et al., 2007; Difede, Cukor, Patt, Giosan, & Hoffman, 2006; Josman et al., 2006). Still, VRE remains to be a relatively new form of treatment and is in need of further investigation and modification to maximize its potential.

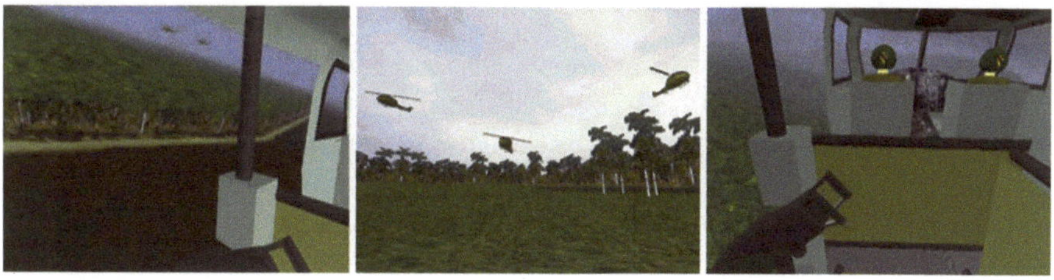

Fig. 18.1 Virtual Vietnam scenarios. Adapted from *Virtually Better* (n.d.). Retrieved January 31, 2010, from www.virtuallybetter.com

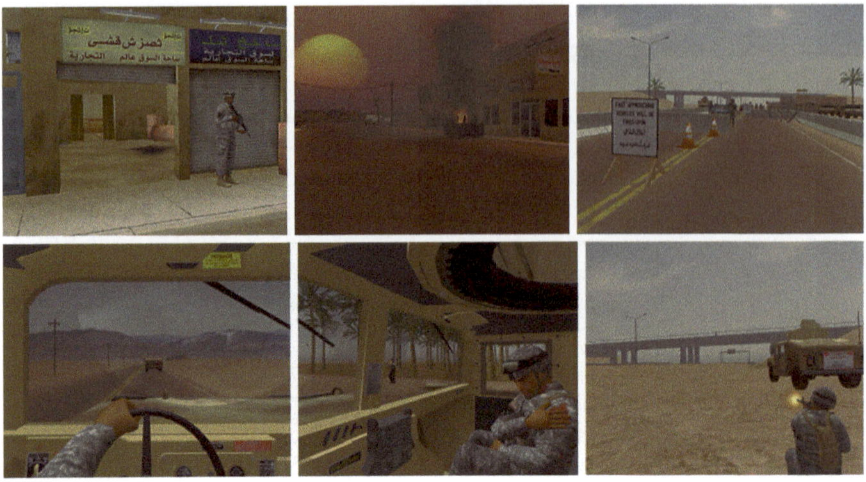

Fig. 18.2 Virtual Iraq/Afghanistan City and Desert Humvee scenarios. Adapted from *Virtually Better* and The USC Institute for Creative Technologies (n.d.). Retrieved January 31, 2010, from www.virtuallybetter.com

Augmentation Strategies

Recent literature suggests even successful psychological and pharmacological approaches are not 100 % effective (Davidson, 1992; Foa et al., 2003). So augmentation strategies may be necessary. We will discuss three augmentation strategies that have emerged for the treatment of PTSD: augmenting ongoing SSRI therapy with an antipsychotic medication, augmenting Cognitive Behavioral Therapy (CBT) with an SSRI, and augmenting prolonged exposure therapy with the medication D-Cycloserine (DCS).

Augmentation Strategy 1: Augmenting SSRI Therapy with an Antipsychotic Medication

There is growing interest in the use of atypical antipsychotics for the treatment of chronic PTSD. Due to relatively high rates of psychotic features found in more severe PTSD, such as auditory and visual hallucinations and paranoid delusions, this may be a beneficial approach. Several open label trials and RCTs have shown atypical antipsychotic mono-therapy to be a beneficial treatment for PTSD; however, some RCTs have shown no increased benefit compared to placebo (for a detailed review of the literature see Hamner & Robert, 2005). One additional study, not referenced in the Hamner and Robert review (2005), showed 6 weeks of open label treatment with risperidone significantly reduced psychotic symptoms as well as PTSD symptoms for Croatian war Veterans with psychotic PTSD (Kozarić-Kovačić, Pivac, Mück-Šeler, & Rothbaum, 2005).

In addition to positive results as a mono-therapy, there is some research to suggest that atypical antipsychotics work well as adjunctive therapy. For example, Quetiapine has been shown to reduce PTSD and psychotic symptoms when added to a concurrent medication regimen, which included Trazodone, hypnotics, anticonvulsants, and antidepressants, with most patients taking an SSRI (84.2 %) (Hamner, Deitsch et al. 2003). Similar results have been found with risperidone (Hamner, Deitsch et al. 2003; Hamner, Faldowski et al. 2003; Monnelly, Ciraulo, Knapp, & Keane, 2003).

Due to the positive results of general adjunctive therapy with antipsychotics, researchers have examined the effect of augmenting SSRIs specifically with an antipsychotic for the treatment of PTSD. Although SSRIs are the only drugs to be approved by the FDA for the treatment of PTSD, studies indicate a low remission rate for SSRIs as a mono-therapy (e.g., Davidson et al., 2001). There are only a few studies which have examined the addition of an antipsychotic for SSRI non-responders specifically. One study showed two antipsychotics to be beneficial for the treatment of PTSD for individuals who previously failed an SSRI treatment (Pivac & Kozaric-Kovacic, 2004).

There have been two placebo controlled trials examining the augmentation of concurrent SSRI therapy with an antipsychotic for the treatment of PTSD. Stein, Kline, and Matloff (2002) added Olanzepine to ongoing SSRI treatment for combat-related PTSD. Results indicated significantly greater reductions in combat PTSD symptoms, sleep disturbance, and depressive symptoms for the treatment arm as compared to placebo. Rothbaum et al. (2008) examined risperidone augmentation of SSRI therapy for civilian PTSD. In phase I of the trial, individuals were treated for 8 weeks with open label sertraline (Zoloft), an SSRI approved for the treatment of PTSD. Those who did not remit were continued on the sertraline and randomized to 8 weeks of either risperidone or placebo augmentation. Results indicated that all participants, regardless of treatment condition, saw improvement in their PTSD symptoms. More specifically, participants responded well to sertraline in phase 1 and showed a strong placebo response in phase II. Risperidone augmentation did evince beneficial effects in the areas of global improvement and positive affect and sleep. These mixed findings suggest that while atypical antipsychotics are promising as both mono-therapy and adjunctive therapy, more methodologically rigorous studies are required.

Augmentation Strategy 2: Augmenting Chronic SSRI Therapy with Psychotherapy

A second strategy for treating PTSD looks to correct the shortfalls of medication alone by combining this treatment with the most empirically supported psychotherapy, prolonged exposure (PE) (Foa et al., 2007, 2009). Rothbaum et al. (2006) examined the effect of adding PE for SSRI nonresponders. For this study, individuals diagnosed with PTSD were provided with 10 weeks of open label sertraline therapy and those who did not remit were then randomized to either receive

5 additional weeks of sertraline alone or 5 weeks of sertraline augmented with ten sessions of twice weekly PE. Results showed that the addition of 10 sessions of PE led to increased treatment gains, but only for patients who showed a partial response to phase I sertraline treatment. PE augmentation was associated with lower PTSD severity scores, more remitters at 6 month follow-up, and maintenance of treatment gains.

Simon et al. (2008) examined the mirror design of the Rothbaum et al. (2006) study described above. In phase I of this study, all participants received eight sessions of PE over 4–6 weeks. Those who were still symptomatic at the end of phase I were randomized to receive either continuing PE with an SSRI, paroxetine (Paxil) CR, or placebo. Results showed that paroxetine CR augmentation did not significantly differ from placebo for reduction in PTSD symptoms or severity of illness. It appears from these two studies that exposure therapy can augment SSRI effects, especially for the weaker medication responders (Rothbaum et al., 2006), but that SSRIs do not help boost the response to exposure therapy (Simon et al., 2008). However, a recent double-blind study by Schneier et al. (2012) reports on the combined treatment for 10 weeks using paroxetine and PE simultaneously for 27 adult survivors of the World Trade Center attacks of September 11, 2001 with PTSD. The authors concluded that treatment with combined paroxetine plus PE was more efficacious than PE plus placebo for PTSD both on response and remission rates. After 10 weeks, all patients discontinued PE and were offered 12 more weeks of continued double-blind treatment with paroxetine. The benefit of combined treatment seems to have disappeared by follow-up, with no differences between those on placebo or active treatment at follow-up.

Augmentation Strategy 3: Acute Medication Augmentation of Psychotherapy

The third augmentation strategy is one in which a medication called D-Cycloserine (DCS) is added to CBT acutely during individual exposure therapy sessions. DCS is an antibiotic which was first developed to treat tuberculosis and has been shown to be a partial agonist of the *N*-methyl D-aspartate (NMDA) receptor and a potential cognitive enhancer. In order to understand how this augmentation strategy works, it is necessary to briefly discuss the cognitive processes involved in extinction.

Unlike forgetting, extinction requires active learning, which is an NMDA-dependent process. The NMDA receptor mediates intracellular learning processes that lead to cellular changes such as enhanced synaptic activation. Pharmacological agents such as DCS are thought to augment learning processes by improving glutamate neurotransmitter activity at the NMDA receptor. Rodent studies were the first to reveal the effects of DCS on the learning process of fear extinction. Using a classical conditioning paradigm, Walker, Ressler, Lu, and Davis (2002) successfully augmented extinction trials in rodents using DCS. In this paradigm, rodents were first conditioned to fear a light source (conditioned stimulus, or CS) by pairing it with a foot shock (unconditioned stimulus, or UCS), in the fear acquisition phase. Following fear acquisition the rodents underwent extinction training in which the light was presented without the shock 30, 60, or 90 times. Results demonstrated that DCS injections into the amygdala enhanced extinction before 30 non-reinforced light exposures, reaching the level normally achieved after 60 extinction trials. Furthermore, DCS injections did not lead to a reduction in fear for rodents who did not receive extinction training, suggesting that DCS enhances the extinction training but does not independently cause extinction (or sedation). A second rodent study replicated these findings by showing that DCS significantly enhanced the extinction of conditioned fear when administered before extinction training. Furthermore, this study indicated that DCS when administered immediately after extinction training not only influences the acquisition of extinction but also memory consolidation (Ledgerwood, Richardson, & Cranney, 2003). Rodent studies have also revealed a number of additional molecular processes, such as intra-amygdala protein synthesis, which mediate the effect of DCS on extinction (Yang & Lu, 2005) and found that the effect of DCS may be related to the activation of the hippocampal glycinergic system (Yamamoto et al., 2008, 2010). In addition, While DCS seems to increase the efficacy of extinction, it does not have an impact on the renewal effect, or return of fear, when rodents are returned to the context in which fear was acquired (Woods & Bouton, 2006). This finding suggests that while DCS does facilitate extinction learning, the new learning is still dependent on context and the potential for relapse is not necessarily reduced. These rodent studies showed that DCS facilitated amygdala-dependent emotional learning, such as extinction. It is interesting to note that human studies reveal DCS also affects procedural learning. Researchers investigating the effects of DCS during a memory task found that DCS by itself as well as in conjunction with another facilitator of emotional learning, Valproic Acid (VPA), facilitated procedural memory, which was measured by a participant's ability to rapidly reproduce a series of numbers using a computer keypad. Interestingly, neither cognitive facilitator affected declarative memory, measured by a word pair learning task. The authors determined that this implicates DCS as a hippocampus-independent learning enhancer (Kuriyama, Honma, Koyama, & Kim, 2011).

For clinicians, DCS augmentation of extinction is exciting for a number of reasons. First, it is rational pharmacotherapy, based on what we know about the brain and the extinction of fear. Second, it is a novel paradigm for psychiatric medications. Rather than taken daily or in response to symptoms, DCS is taken only immediately preceding a session of exposure therapy. In the first application to humans described below (Ressler et al., 2004), patients only took two pills in total. The pill does nothing in and of itself (Heresco-Levy et al., 2002), it is only in combination with exposure therapy that it demonstrates its effects. Many patients who enter therapy do not complete a full course of treatment, so anything that makes the therapy that they do receive work faster to achieve more benefits is a huge boost to mental health care.

Initial research studying the effect of DCS augmentation of exposure therapy shows strong support for a number of psychiatric disorders. Specifically, DCS has demonstrated success in treating a variety of anxiety disorders when augmented with exposure therapy (Rothbaum, 2008). Studies included in this review employ a rigorous methodological approach of double-blind, placebo controlled treatment.

Ressler et al. (2004) first studied the effect of DCS augmentation with exposure therapy in humans with the fear of heights. Participants received two sessions of virtual reality exposure therapy (VRE) in conjunction with DCS or placebo. Medication was only taken before each VRE session, for a total of two pills. Results showed significantly greater reductions in acrophobia fears for the DCS group compared to the placebo group in the virtual environment as well as reported real life exposure to heights. The DCS group showed a decrease in spontaneous galvanic skin response (GSR) fluctuation during virtual reality exposure which was related to significantly increased real life exposure to heights after treatment and at 3-month follow-up. These preliminary data demonstrate that acute dosing of DCS can lead to increased benefit from exposure therapy for phobias. Following this study, several investigators around the world have applied the paradigm to other anxiety disorders.

Subsequent research has demonstrated that DCS can lead to increased treatment gains for individuals suffering from social anxiety disorder (SAD). In one study, individuals with a diagnosis of SAD received five exposure therapy sessions, four of which were preceded by a 50 mg dose of DCS or placebo. Results showed that individuals who received DCS compared to placebo before their exposure sessions reported significantly less anxiety symptoms as measured by the Social Phobia and Anxiety Inventory (SPAI—Turner, Beidel, Dancu, & Stanley, 1989) and the Liebowitz Social Anxiety Scale (LSAS- Liebowitz, 1987) at posttreatment and 1 month follow-up (Hofmann et al., 2006). These findings were replicated in Guastella et al. (2008). This study also found significant improvement on measures of dysfunctional cognitions and life impairment associated with SAD for the DCS group in comparison with placebo. Similar results have been found for treatment of panic disorder with 50 mg of DCS administered one hour before three of five sessions (Otto et al., 2010). This study showed DCS augmentation to reduce panic symptoms and produce higher rates of clinically significant change. However, a more recent study found that DCS augmentation did not lead to increased treatment gains for a similar population when given at the same dose and time (Siegmund et al., 2011). The evidence suggests that DCS augmentation with ET may be effective at not only combating the disorder but also at reducing highly impairing symptoms such as negative thoughts or interference with aspects of one's life such as work, family, and free time.

There have been three double-blind placebo controlled trials of DCS augmentation of ET for obsessive compulsive disorder which have demonstrated mixed results. One study measured OCD symptoms as well as depression symptoms over the course of 10 behavioral therapy sessions (exposure and response prevention). One hour before therapy, patients received either 100 mg of DCS or placebo. Results showed that OCD symptoms were significantly reduced for the DCS group at midtreatment, but not at posttreatment or 1 month follow-up. Additionally, depression symptoms were reduced at posttreatment but not at midtreatment or follow-up (Wilhelm et al., 2008). A reanalysis of the data from Wilhelm et al. (2008) determined that patients in the DCS group experienced earlier benefits to exposure therapy compared to placebo (Chasson et al., 2010). Another group reported that individuals who received 125 mg of DCS compared to placebo were less likely to drop out and showed significantly greater reductions in symptoms after four sessions of ET. Still, after ten sessions the difference between groups was not significant (Kushner et al., 2007). Coupled with the findings of Wilhelm et al. (2008) and Chasson et al. (2010), this study adds to the theory that DCS may increase the efficacy of ET leading to fewer sessions required to reach the full therapeutic effect. However, Storch et al. (2007) found that there were no significant treatment gains from DCS when individuals with OCD were given a dose of 250 mg of DCS four hours before ET. This study has been criticized for using too large a dose of DCS, too long before the session, and assessing participants only after a full course of ET. Taken together, these studies indicate that the efficacy of DCS augmentation for OCD may be greatest after brief ET (fewer than five sessions) and that dosing should be kept low as well as provided close to treatment (30–60 min prior). In general with DCS in combination with exposure therapy, less is more: lower doses of DCS, given shortly before therapy, and fewer sessions of exposure therapy.

DCS and PTSD

Due to its efficacy in augmenting exposure therapy for a number of different anxiety disorders as well as reducing fear potentiated startle in rodent populations, it stands to reason that DCS could speed the response to exposure therapy for PTSD. Recently, Dr. Barbara Rothbaum has completed a clinical trial at Emory University, in Atlanta, GA, examining the efficacy of DCS augmentation of VRE for PTSD (Rothbaum et al., 2014). Specifically, this treatment provided five sessions of manualized VRE therapy (six sessions total) for Veterans of Iraq and Afghanistan. Thirty minutes prior to each exposure session, participants received either 50 mg of DCS, .25 mg of Alprazolam (Xanax), or placebo. Alprazolam was chosen as an active comparator because it is one of the most common benzodiazepines used in clinical practice for treatment of many anxiety disorders. By providing an "active agent" control in addition to the placebo, this study aimed to directly test the clinical lore that anxiolytic medication interferes with exposure therapy, a finding that may be consistent with preclinical work showing that benzodiazepines actually interfere with extinction of fear in rodents (Bouton, Kenney, & Rosengard, 1990). The results from this type of research design are thus more externally valid since DCS as a new treatment is being tested against existing medication used in the field as opposed to the placebo's primary use in the laboratory setting.

Results from this study showed that the shortened protocol of VRE successfully reduced symptoms of PTSD in Veterans of the Iraq and Afghanistan wars. However, there was no difference between the DCS group and the placebo group in symptoms of PTSD at any time point. There was a difference between the alprazolam and placebo group in that those receiving alprazolam exhibited greater posttreatment PTSD scores and greater rates of PTSD diagnosis at 3-month follow-up compared to those receiving placebo. While an overall effect of DCS on PTSD symptoms was not found, secondary analyses showed extinction learning between sessions was associated with reduced posttreatment PTSD scores only for those receiving DCS augmentation.

Furthermore, DCS was shown to be uniquely related to reduced posttreatment startle response and cortisol reactivity. These findings suggest that alprazolam may inhibit PTSD treatment response and that DCS may be uniquely related to theorized mechanisms of change in PTSD treatment such as, between session extinction learning, cortisol reactivity and startle response.

Five additional trials have reported results of the combination of DCS and CBT for the treatment of PTSD, two with positive findings, two with null findings, and one with negative findings. Henn-Haase et al. (2010) conducted a RCT of exposure-based CBT with DCS or with placebo to investigate DCS' ability to enhance the effects of exposure therapy in treating PTSD. Both civilian and Veteran patients ($n=28$) with full or sub-syndromal PTSD (two of three symptom clusters) on DCS plus exposure therapy reported faster treatment response and greater overall improvements in PTSD symptoms at mid-treatment and posttreatment than those on placebo plus exposure therapy. Similarly, for depression and anxiety symptoms, DCS patients displayed a higher response rate at mid-treatment and posttreatment. Moreover, during the course of treatment sessions, the DCS group reported lower SUDS scores and displayed a greater rate of decrease in SUDS scores. Despite these initial, encouraging findings, the DCS group's PTSD checklist scores rebounded at 3-month follow-up, suggesting that the effectiveness of DCS is observed primarily during exposure sessions. However, when controlling for pretreatment PTSD symptoms, only the DCS group showed significant improvement in PTSD checklist scores.

In a Canadian trial, 48 civilian patients with PTSD were randomly assigned to CBT + DCS or CBT + placebo (Guay, Marchand, & Landry, 2010). Patients received 12–16 sessions of CBT that included psychoeducation, breathing retraining, imaginal exposure, in vivo exposure, and relapse prevention. From session 4, they received 50 mg of DCS or placebo one hour before each session of imaginal or in vivo exposure. Results indicated that CBT + DCS was not more efficacious than CBT + placebo in decreasing PTSD symptoms on the Clinician Administered PTSD Scale (CAPS; Blake et al., 1995) at posttreatment or 6 months following treatment. No mid-treatment or session measures were gathered, so it is not possible to ascertain if there were differences in the speed of response between the groups.

One recent study examined the effect of DCS augmentation on PE for the treatment of noncombat PTSD (de Kleine, Hendriks, Kusters, Broekman, & van Mennen, 2012). In this RCT, patients were administered DCS or placebo 1 h prior to their therapy session. Results indicated that the majority of participants showed significantly reduced CAPS and PTSD Symptom Scale, Self-Report (PSS-SR; Foa, Riggs, Dancu & Rothbaum, 1993) scores at posttreatment and DCS did not significantly impact this reduction. While this study did not find a main effect for DCS on symptom reduction, there was a significantly greater number of responders in the DCS group compared to placebo control. In addition, a session by session analysis revealed that DCS led to greater treatment gains for patients who had higher pretreatment PTSD symptoms and required longer treatment. This was not found for those who completed treatment early. The authors suggested that DCS may be most helpful for those with more severe PTSD and who do not respond as quickly to exposure therapy.

A recently completed RCT (Litz et al., 2012) showed that DCS augmentation of PE led to significantly poorer treatment outcomes on measures of PTSD and depression for combat-related PTSD. This was the first DCS augmentation trial for combat-related PTSD and the first trial to show a negative effect for DCS on treatment outcome. The authors speculated that this unexpected finding may have been the result of the effect DCS has on memory reconsolidation, which is the process by which memories become temporarily labile after being retrieved from long term memory. Furthermore, the sample size of 13 per group was fairly small, thereby limiting power and the ability to find a significant effect. In order to better understand the impact of DCS on combat-related PTSD, additional studies are needed which utilize larger military or veteran samples.

Finally, in a pilot study, Difede et al. (2013) used DCS to augment VRE for PTSD related to the World Trade Center attacks. These results showed that while those receiving DCS did not show significantly reduced symptoms of PTSD compared to placebo immediately posttreatment, they did show reduced symptoms at 6-month follow-up. Furthermore, it was shown that PTSD symptoms began to decline more rapidly for the DCS group compared to the placebo group at session six. PTSD remission rates were greater for those in the DCS group at both posttreatment and 6-month follow-up. Secondary analyses showed the same pattern of response for the DCS groups on measures of depression and anger. Several studies are ongoing comparing DCS to placebo with exposure therapy including one by Drs. Charlie Marmar and Thomas Neylan with Veterans in San Francisco, CA. A 2 × 2 three-site study is just commencing that will compare PE to VRE augmented by DCS or pill placebo using genetic markers as predictors for response to treatment that is being conducted by Drs. Rothbaum, Difede, and Rizzo in the Washington, DC area, New York, and Los Angeles. Finally, a study comparing VRE to PE for active duty Service Members is being conducted by Drs. Greg Gahm and Greg Reger at Joint Fort Lewis McChord in Tacoma, WA. We anxiously anticipate the results of all of these studies to inform us of the utility of these innovations in treatment approaches.

Conclusions

CBT, and specifically exposure therapy, is an effective treatment for anxiety disorders including PTSD. However, there is room for improvement and considering the shortfalls of medication by itself for PTSD, it is necessary to explore innovative augmentation strategies. There appears to be no advantage in combining traditional psychiatric medications with CBT for any anxiety disorder (Foa, Franklin, & Moser, 2002; Gerardi, Ressler, & Rothbaum, 2010), although there is some promise of combination strategies for more novel medications (e.g., Ressler et al., 2004). Adding a traditional medication such as an antipsychotic or SSRI to CBT to treat PTSD specifically has shown no advantage over CBT alone. This has led researchers to focus on acute DCS augmentation to increase the efficacy of exposure therapy.

Augmentation of DCS is a direct attempt to stimulate the NMDA glutamate synapses in order to enhance learning during exposure therapy. Specifically, these synapses are considered critical in supporting short term learning and memory at the same moment that CBT is being used to help the patient learn new behaviors. DCS is a unique partial agonist for this purpose because it is thought to work cooperatively with the glutamate that is presumably being released through synaptic activity associated with the patient's participation in CBT. Unlike traditional medications which aim to abate symptoms that may hamper the productivity of psychotherapy sessions, DCS directly enhances cognitive abilities in order to heighten the effectiveness of CBT and ET.

DCS has been shown to be effective in increasing the benefits of ET for anxiety disorders including panic disorder (Otto et al., 2010), social phobia (Guastella et al., 2008; Hofmann et al., 2006), and acrophobia (Ressler et al., 2004). The mixed results of DCS augmentation for treatment of obsessive compulsive disorder (Kushner et al., 2007; Storch et al., 2007; Wilhelm et al., 2008) indicate the need to further define the dosing and timing of DCS augmentation. Specifically, too early dosing may lead to the peak drug effect not being coincident with the emotional learning processes that take place during and immediately after psychotherapy sessions, while too high of a dose may activate the antagonist properties of this NMDA partial agonist. Also, future studies may need to control for a floor effect of all subjects improving from a full course of therapy which can lead to a lack of a drug by therapy effect (Rothbaum, 2008).

While CBT and ET, with their wide array of empirical and experimental support, may be the gold standard for PTSD and anxiety disorder treatment, many individuals who receive psychotherapy still suffer from PTSD. Virtual reality exposure therapy, augmented with DCS, represents a groundbreaking opportunity to improve an already potent form of therapy. Prior research suggests patients who experience difficulty in accessing emotions to immerse oneself in treatment have worse outcomes than those who have stronger emotional engagement (Jaycox, Foa, & Morral, 1998). By adding sensory cues to aid in the accessing of emotions tied to the memory of a trauma, VR may help overcome the challenge of emotional engagement. Stronger emotional engagement, along with the flexible yet systematic approach that tailors the exposure session to the individual patient's traumatic experience and idiosyncratic fear levels, may allow VRE to create a more potent exposure (Hodges, Anderson, Burdea, Hoffman, & Rothbaum, 2001). Rather than succumbing to the crippling avoidance of PTSD, patients receiving VRE augmented with DCS can encounter the fearful stimuli associated with the avoided memory in a manageable fashion that fits their needs. Thus, the burden of seeking treatment and recovering from PTSD becomes a less daunting process. Even if much progress remains to be achieved in promoting services for PTSD and raising public recognition of PTSD and its severity, for those individuals who do seek treatment, augmenting ET with DCS (and VR in particular) continues to be one of the most promising forms of therapy.

Disclosure Statement Dr. Rothbaum and Emory University own equity in *Virtually Better, Inc.*, which is developing products related to the virtual reality research described in this chapter, and Dr. Rothbaum is a consultant for *Virtually Better, Inc*. The terms of this arrangement have been reviewed and approved by Emory University in accordance with its conflict of interest policies.

References

Blake, D. D., Weathers, F. W., Nagy, L. M., Kaloupek, D. G., Gusman, F. D., Charney, D. S., et al. (1995). The development of a clinician-administered PTSD scale. *Journal of Traumatic Stress, 8*(1), 75–90.

Bouton, M. E., Kenney, F. A., & Rosengard, C. (1990). State-dependent fear extinction with two benzodiazepine tranquilizers. *Behavioral Neuroscience, 104*(1), 44–55.

Brady, K., Pearlstein, T., Asnis, G. M., Baker, D., Rothbaum, B., Sikes, C. R., et al. (2000). Efficacy and safety of sertraline treatment of posttraumatic stress disorder: A randomized controlled trial. *JAMA, 283*(14), 1837–1844.

Brunet, A., Orr, S. P., Tremblay, J., Robertson, K., Nader, K., & Pitman, R. K. (2008). Effect of post-retrieval propranolol on psychophysiologic responding during subsequent script-driven traumatic imagery in post-traumatic stress disorder. *Journal of Psychiatric Research, 42*, 503–506.

Cahill, L., Prins, B., Weber, M., & McGaugh, J. L. (1994). β-Adrenergic activation and memory for emotional events. *Nature, 371*(6499), 702–704.

Chasson, G. S., Buhlmann, U., Tolin, D. F., Rao, S. R., Reese, H. E., Rowley, T., et al. (2010). Need for speed: Evaluating slopes of OCD recovery in behavior therapy enhanced with D-cycloserine. *Behaviour Research and Therapy, 48*(7).

Cooper, J., Carty, J., & Creamer, M. (2005). Pharmacotherapy for posttraumatic stress disorder: Empirical review and clinical recommendations. *Australian and New Zealand Journal of Psychiatry, 39*(8), 674–682.

Cukor, J., Spitalnick, J., Difede, J., Rizzo, A., & Rothbaum, B. O. (2009). Emerging treatments for PTSD. *Clinical Psychology Review, 29*(8), 715–726.

Davidson, J. (1992). Drug therapy of post-traumatic stress disorder. *British Journal of Psychiatry, 160*, 309–314.

Davidson, J. T., Rothbaum, B. O., van der Kolk, B. A., Sikes, C. R., & Farfel, G. M. (2001). Multicenter, double-blind comparison of sertraline and placebo in the treatment of posttraumatic stress disorder. *Archives of General Psychiatry, 58*(5), 485–492.

de Kleine, R. A., Hendriks, G., Kusters, W. C., Broekman, T. G., & van Mennen, A. (2012). A randomized placebo-controlled trial of D-cycloserine to enhance exposure therapy for posttraumatic stress disorder. *Biological Psychiatry, 71*(11), 962–968.

Difede, J., Cukor, J., Jayasinghe, N., Patt, I., Jedel, S., Spielman, L., et al. (2007). Virtual reality exposure therapy for the treatment of posttraumatic stress disorder following September 11, 2001. *Journal of Clinical Psychiatry, 68*(11), 1639–1647.

Difede, J., Cukor, J., Patt, I., Giosan, C., & Hoffman, H. (2006). The application of virtual reality to the treatment of PTSD following the WTC attack. In R. Yehuda & R. Yehuda (Eds.), *Psychobiology of posttraumatic stress disorders: A decade of progress* (Vol. 1071, pp. 500–501). Malden: Blackwell.

Difede, J., Cukor, J., Wyka, K., Olden, M., Hoffman, H., Lee, F. S., et al. (2013). D-cycloserine augmentation of exposure therapy for post-traumatic stress disorder: A pilot randomized clinical trial. *Neuropsychopharmacology, 39*(5), 1052–1058.

Foa, E. B., Franklin, M. E., & Moser, J. (2002). Context in the clinic: How well do cognitive-behavioral therapies and medications work in combination? *Biological Psychiatry, 52*(10), 989–997.

Foa, E. B., Hembree, E. A., & Rothbaum, B. (2007). *Prolonged exposure therapy for PTSD: Emotional processing of traumatic experiences: Therapist guide*. New York, NY: Oxford University Press.

Foa, E., Keane, T., Friedman, M., & Cohen, J. (2009). *Effective treatments forPTSD: Practice guidelines from the International Society for Traumatic Stress Studies* (2nd ed.). New York, NY: Guilford Press.

Foa, E. B., Riggs, D. S., Dancu, C. V., & Rothbaum, B. O. (1993). Reliability and validity of a brief instrument for assessing post-traumatic stress disorder. *Journal of Traumatic Stress, 6*, 459–473.

Foa, E. B., Rothbaum, B. O., & Furr, J. M. (2003). Is the efficacy of exposure therapy for post-traumatic stress disorder augmented with the addition of other cognitive behavior therapy procedures? *Psychiatric Annals, 33*(1), 47–53.

Foa, E. B., Steketee, G., & Rothbaum, B. O. (1989). Behavioral/cognitive conceptualizations of post-traumatic stress disorder. *Behavior Therapy, 20*(2), 155–176.

Gelpin, E., Bonne, O., Peri, T., & Brandes, D. (1996). Treatment of recent trauma survivors with benzodiazepines: A prospective study. *Journal of Clinical Psychiatry, 57*(9), 390–394.

Gerardi, M., Ressler, K., & Rothbaum, B. (2010). Combined treatment of anxiety disorders. In D. J. Stein, E. Hollander, B. O. Rothbaum, D. J. Stein, E. Hollander, & B. O. Rothbaum (Eds.), *Textbook of anxiety disorders* (2nd ed., pp. 147–156). Arlington, VA: American Psychiatric Publishing.

Guastella, A. J., Richardson, R., Lovibond, P. F., Rapee, R. M., Gaston, J. E., Mitchell, P., et al. (2008). A randomized controlled trial of D-cycloserine enhancement of exposure therapy for social anxiety disorder. *Biological Psychiatry, 63*(6), 544–549.

Guay, S., Marchand, A., & Landry, P. (2010). Results from a 6-month follow-up of a randomized controlled trial assessing the efficacy of cognitive-behavior therapy combined with D-Cycloserine for treating PTSD. Presented at the international society for traumatic stress studies 26th annual meeting, Montreal, Canada, November 4–6, 2010.

Hamner, M. B., Deitsch, S. E., Brodrick, P. S., Ulmer, H. G., & Lorberbaum, J. P. (2003). Quetiapine treatment in patients with posttraumatic stress disorder: An open trial of adjunctive therapy. *Journal of Clinical Psychopharmacology, 23*(1), 15–20.

Hamner, M. B., Faldowski, R. A., Ulmer, H. G., Frueh, B. C., Huber, M. G., & Arana, G. W. (2003). Adjunctive risperidone treatment in post-traumatic stress disorder: A preliminary controlled trial of effects on comorbid psychotic symptoms. *International Clinical Psychopharmacology, 18*(1), 1–8.

Hamner, M. B., & Robert, S. (2005). Emerging roles for atypical antipsychotics in chronic post-traumatic stress disorder. *Neurotherapeutics, 5*(2), 267–275.

Henn-Haase, C., Best, S., Metzler, T. J., Gardner, J., Herbst, E., McCaslin, S., et al. (2010). Exposure based CBT therapy and D-cycloserine treatment for PTSD in veterans and civilians. Presented at the international society for traumatic stress studies 26th annual meeting, Montreal, Canada, November 4–6, 2010.

Heresco-Levy, U., Kremer, I., Javitt, D. C., Goichman, R., Reshef, A., Blanaru, M., et al. (2002). Pilot-controlled trial of D-cycloserine for the treatment of post-traumatic stress disorder. *International Journal of Neuropsychopharmacology, 5*, 301–307.

Hodges, L. F., Anderson, P., Burdea, G. C., Hoffman, H. G., & Rothbaum, B. O. (2001). Treating psychological and physical disorders with VR. *IEEE Computer Graphics and Applications, 21*(6), 25–33.

Hofmann, S. G., Meuret, A. E., Smits, J. J., Simon, N. M., Pollack, M. H., Eisenmenger, K., et al. (2006). Augmentation of exposure therapy with D-cycloserine for social anxiety disorder. *Archives of General Psychiatry, 63*(3), 298–304.

Hoge, E. A., Worthington, J. J., Nagurney, J. T., Chang, Y., Kay, E. B., Feterowski, C. M., et al. (2011). Effect of acute posttrauma propranolol on PTSD outcome and physiological responses during script driven imagery. *CNS Neuroscience and Therapeutics, 17*(3), 1755–5949.

Institute of Medicine. (2008). *Treatment of posttraumatic stress disorder: An assessment of the evidence*. Washington, DC: The National Academies Press.

Jaycox, L. H., Foa, E. B., & Morral, A. R. (1998). Influence of emotional engagement and habituation on exposure therapy for PTSD. *Journal of Consulting and Clinical Psychology, 66*(1), 185–192.

Josman, N., Somer, E., Reisberg, A., Weiss, P., Garcia-Palacios, A., & Hoffman, H. (2006). BusWorld: Designing a virtual environment for post-traumatic stress disorder in Israel: A protocol. *Cyberpsychology & Behavior, 9*(2), 241–244.

Kessler, R. C. (2000). Posttraumatic stress disorder: The burden to the individual and to society. *Journal of Clinical Psychiatry, 61*(Suppl 5), 4–12. discussion 13–14.

Kosten, T. R., Frank, J. B., Dan, E., McDougle, C. J., & Giller, E. L. (1991). Pharmacotherapy for posttraumatic stress disorder using phenelzine or imipramine. *Journal of Nervous and Mental Disease, 179*(6), 366–370.

Kozarić-Kovačić, D., Pivac, N., Mück-Šeler, D., & Rothbaum, B. (2005). Risperidone in psychotic combat-related posttraumatic stress disorder: An open trial. *Journal of Clinical Psychiatry, 66*(7), 922–927.

Kuriyama, K., Honma, M., Koyama, S., & Kim, Y. (2011). D-cycloserine facilitates procedural learning but not declarative learning in healthy humans: A randomized controlled trial of the effect of D-cycloserine and valproic acid on overnight properties in the performance of non-emotional memory tasks. *Neurobiology of Learning and Memory, 95*, 505–509.

Kushner, M. G., Kim, S., Donahue, C., Thuras, P., Adson, D., Kotlyar, M., et al. (2007). D-cycloserine augmented exposure therapy for obsessive-compulsive disorder. *Biological Psychiatry, 62*(8), 835–838.

Ledgerwood, L., Richardson, R., & Cranney, J. (2003). Effects of D-cycloserine on extinction of conditioned freezing. *Behavioral Neuroscience, 117*(2), 341–349.

Liebowitz, M. R. (1987). Social phobia. *Modern Problems in Pharmacopsychiatry, 22*, 141–173.

Litz, B. T., Salters-Pedneault, K., Steenkamp, M. M., Hermos, J. A., Bryant, R. A., Otto, M. W., et al. (2012). A randomized placebo-controlled trial of D-cycloserine on exposure therapy for posttraumatic stress disorder. *Journal of Psychiatric Research, 46*(9), 1184–1190.

Marshall, R. D., Beebe, K. L., Oldham, M., & Zaninelli, R. (2001). Efficacy and safety of paroxetine treatment for chronic PTSD: A fixed-dose, placebo-controlled study. *The American Journal of Psychiatry, 158*(12), 1982–1988.

Monnelly, E. P., Ciraulo, D. A., Knapp, C., & Keane, T. (2003). Low-dose risperidone as adjunctive therapy for irritable aggression in posttraumatic stress disorder. *Journal of Clinical Psychopharmacology, 23*(2), 193–196.

Monson, C. M., Schnurr, P. P., Resick, P. A., Friedman, M. J., Young-Xu, Y., & Stevens, S. P. (2006). Cognitive processing therapy for veterans with military-related posttraumatic stress disorder. *Journal of Consulting and Clinical Psychology, 74*(5), 898–907.

Otto, M. W., Tolin, D. F., Simon, N. M., Pearlson, G. D., Basden, S., Meunier, S. A., et al. (2010). Efficacy of D-cycloserine for enhancing response to cognitive-behavior therapy for panic disorder. *Biological Psychiatry, 67*(4), 365–370.

Pitman, R. K., Sanders, K. M., Zusman, R. M., Healy, A. R., Cheema, F., Lasko, N. B., et al. (2002). Pilot study of secondary prevention of posttraumatic stress disorder with propranolol. *Biological Psychiatry, 51*(2), 189–192.

Pivac, N., Kozaric-Kovacic, D., & Muck-Seler, D. (2004). Olanzapine versus fluphenazine in an open trial in patients with psychotic combat-related post-traumatic stress disorder. *Psychopharmacology, 175*(4), 451–456.

Resick, P. A., Nishith, P., Weaver, T. L., & Astin, M. C. (2002). A comparison of cognitive processing therapy, prolonged exposure, and a waiting condition for the treatment of posttraumatic stress disorder in female rape victims. *Journal of Consulting and Clinical Psychology, 70*, 867–879.

Ressler, K. J., Rothbaum, B. O., Tannenbaum, L., Anderson, P., Graap, K., Zimand, E., et al. (2004). Cognitive enhancers as adjuncts to psychotherapy: Use of D-cycloserine in phobic individuals to facilitate extinction of fear. *Archives of General Psychiatry, 61*(11), 1136–1144.

Rizzo, A., Difede, J., Rothbaum, B. O., & Reger, G. (2010). Virtual Iraq/Afghanistan: Development and early evaluation of a virtual reality exposure therapy system for combat-related PTSD. *Annals of the New York Academy of Sciences (NYAS)., 1208*, 114–125.

Rizzo, A., Reger, G., Gahm, G., Difede, J., & Rothbaum, B. O. (2009). Virtual reality exposure therapy for combat-related PTSD. In P. J. Shiromani, T. M. Keane, J. E. LeDoux, P. J. Shiromani, T. M. Keane, & J. E. LeDoux (Eds.), *Post-traumatic stress disorder: Basic science and clinical practice* (pp. 375–399). Totowa, NJ: Humana Press.

Rothbaum, B. O. (2008). Critical parameters for D-cycloserine enhancement of cognitive behavioral therapy for obsessive compulsive disorder. *American Journal of Psychiatry, 165*, 293–296.

Rothbaum, B. O., Astin, M. C., & Marsteller, F. (2005). Prolonged exposure versus eye movement desensitization and reprocessing (EMDR) for PTSD rape victims. *Journal of Traumatic Stress, 18*(6), 607–616.

Rothbaum, B. O., Cahill, S. P., Foa, E. B., Davidson, J. R. T., Compton, J., Connor, K. M., et al. (2006). Augmentation of sertraline with prolonged exposure in the treatment of posttraumatic stress disorder. *Journal of Traumatic Stress, 19*(8), 625–638.

Rothbaum, B., & Davis, M. (2003). Applying learning principles to the treatment of post-trauma reactions. In J. A. King, C. F. Ferris, I. I. Lederhendler, J. A. King, C. F. Ferris, & I. I. Lederhendler (Eds.), *Roots of mental illness in children* (pp. 112–121). New York, NY: New York Academy of Sciences.

Rothbaum, B. O., Foa, E. B., Riggs, D., Murdock, T., & Walsh, W. (1992). A prospective examination of post-traumatic stress disorder in rape victims. *Journal of Traumatic Stress, 5*, 455–475.

Rothbaum, B. O., Hodges, L. F., Ready, D., Graap, K., & Alarcon, R. D. (2001). Virtual reality exposure therapy for Vietnam veterans with posttraumatic stress disorder. *Journal of Clinical Psychiatry, 62*(8), 617–622.

Rothbaum, B. O., Killeen, T. K., Davidson, J. T., Brady, K. T., Connor, K. M., & Heekin, M. H. (2008). Placebo-controlled trial of risperidone augmentation for selective serotonin reuptake inhibitor-resistant civilian posttraumatic stress disorder. *Journal of Clinical Psychiatry, 69*(4), 520–525.

Rothbaum, B. O., Price, M., Jovanovic, T., Norrholm, S. D., Gerardi, M., Dunlop, B., et al. (2014). A randomized, double-blind evaluation of D-cycloserine or alprazolam combined with virtual reality exposure therapy for posttraumatic stress disorder in iraq and afghanistan war veterans. *American Journal of Psychiatry, 171*(6), 640–648.

Schneier, F. R., Neria, Y., Pavlicova, M., Hembree, E., Jung Suh, E., Amsel, L., et al. (2012). Combined prolonged exposure therapy and paroxetine for posttraumatic stress disorder related to the world trade center attacks: A randomized controlled trial. Presented at the international society for traumatic stress studies 26th annual meeting, Montreal, Canada, November 4–6, 2010.

Shapiro, F. (1995). *Eye movement desentization and reprocessing: Basic principles, protocols, and procedures*. New York, NY: Guilford Press.

Shestatzky, M., Greenberg, D., & Lerer, B. (1988). A controlled trial of phenelzine in posttraumatic stress disorder. *Psychiatry Research, 24*(2), 149–155.

Siegmund, A., Golfels, F., Finck, C., Halisch, A., Räth, D., Plag, J., et al. (2011). D-cycloserine does not improve but might slightly speed up the outcome of in-vivo exposure therapy in patients with severe agoraphobia and panic disorder in a randomized double blind clinical trial. *Journal of Psychiatric Research*. doi:10.1016/j.jpsychires. 2011.01.020.

Simon, N. M., Connor, K. M., Lang, A. J., Rauch, S., Krulewicz, S., LeBeau, R. T., et al. (2008). Paroxetine CR augmentation for posttraumatic stress disorder refractory to prolonged exposure therapy. *Journal of Clinical Psychiatry, 69*(3), 400–405.

Stein, D. J., Ipser, J., & Seedat, S. (2006). Pharmacotherapy for post traumatic stress disorder (PTSD). *Cochrane Database of Systematic Reviews, 25*, CD002795.

Stein, M. B., Kline, N. A., & Matloff, J. L. (2002). Adjunctive olanzapine for SSRI-resistant combat-related PTSD: A double-blind, placebo-controlled study. *The American Journal of Psychiatry, 159*(10), 1777–1779.

Storch, E. A., Merlo, L. J., Bengtson, M., Murphy, T. K., Lewis, M. H., Yang, M. C., et al. (2007). D-cycloserine does not enhance exposure-response prevention therapy in obsessive-compulsive disorder. *International Clinical Psychopharmacology, 22*(4), 230–237.

Tucker, P., Smith, K. L., Marx, B., Jones, D., Miranda, R., & Lensgraf, J. (2000). Fluvoxamine reduces physiologic reactivity to trauma scripts in posttraumatic stress disorder. *Journal of Clinical Psychopharmacology, 20*(3), 367–372.
Turner, S. M., Beidel, D. C., Dancu, C. V., & Stanley, M. A. (1989). An empirically derived inventory to measure social fears and anxiety: The Social Phobia and Anxiety Inventory. *Psychological Assessment: A Journal of Consulting and Clinical Psychology, 1*(1), 35–40.
Vaiva, G., Ducrocq, F., Jezequel, K., Averland, B., Lestavel, P., Brunet, A., et al. (2003). Immediate treatment with propranolol decreases posttraumatic stress disorder two months after trauma. *Biological Psychiatry, 54*, 947–949.
Van Etten, M., & Taylor, S. (1998). Comparative efficacy of treatments for post-traumatic stress disorder: A meta-analysis. *Clinical Psychology and Psychotherapy, 5*, 126–144.
Walker, D. L., Ressler, K. J., Lu, K., & Davis, M. (2002). Facilitation of conditioned fear extinction by systemic administration or intra-amygdala infusions of D-cycloserine as assessed with fear-potentiated startle in rats. *The Journal of Neuroscience, 22*(6), 2343–2351.
Wilhelm, S., Buhlmann, U., Tolin, D. F., Meunier, S. A., Pearlson, G. D., Reese, H. E., et al. (2008). Augmentation of behavior therapy with D-cycloserine for obsessive-compulsive disorder. *The American Journal of Psychiatry, 165*(3), 335–341.
Woods, A. M., & Bouton, M. E. (2006). D-cycloserine facilitates extinction but does not eliminate renewal of the conditioned emotional response. *Behavioral Neuroscience, 120*(5), 1159–1162.
Yamamoto, S., Morinobu, S., Fuchikami, M., Kurata, A., Kozuru, T., & Yamawaki, S. (2008). Effects of single prolonged stress and D-cycloserine on contextual fear extinction and hippocampal NMDA receptor expression in a rat model of PTSD. *Neuropsychopharmacology, 33*, 2108–2116.
Yamamoto, S., Morinobu, S., Iwamoto, Y., Ueda, Y., Takei, S., Fujita, Y., et al. (2010). Alterations in the hippocampal glycinergic system in an animal model of posttraumatic stress disorder. *Journal of Psychiatry and Research, 44*, 1069–1074.
Yang, Y. L., & Lu, K. T. (2005). Facilitation of conditioned fear extinction by D-cycloserine is mediated by mitogen-activated protein kinase and phosphatidylinositol 3-kinase cascades and requires de novo protein synthesis in basolateral nucleus of amygdala. *Neuroscience, 134*(1), 247–260.

Chapter 19
Implementation of Evidence-Based Assessment, Treatment, and Research Programs Following the World Trade Center Disaster on September 11, 2001

Megan Olden, Brittany Mello, Judith Cukor, Katarzyna Wyka, Nimali Jayasinghe, and JoAnn Difede

Overview

This chapter details the development of an evidence-based clinical assessment and treatment program following the September 11, 2001 attacks on the World Trade Center (WTC) in New York City. This unprecedented disaster resulted in a large population of disaster workers in need of psychological assessment and sometimes treatment following their deployment to Ground Zero.

Topics include an overview of what has now become the Weill Cornell Medical College Program for Anxiety and Traumatic Stress Studies and the clinical and logistical challenges involved in establishing a large-scale psychological screening and treatment program for disaster workers following the September 11th attacks. We will describe the rapid development and implementation of a well-validated, standardized psychological screening protocol of clinical interviews and self-report measures and the provision of best practices-based prolonged exposure and cognitive-behavioral treatment (CBT) for disaster workers and civilians with post-traumatic stress disorder (PTSD). In addition, we will discuss our development of a novel line of research investigating the use of virtual reality technology in the treatment of WTC-related PTSD. The rationale in embarking on this area of inquiry, the

M. Olden, Ph.D. • J. Cukor, Ph.D. • N. Jayasinghe, Ph.D. • J. Difede, Ph.D. (✉)
Psychiatry Department, Weill Correll Medical College, New York, NY, USA
e-mail: meo9011@med.cornell.edu; juc2010@med.cornell.edu;
nij2001@med.cornell.edu; jdifede@med.cornell.edu

B. Mello, B.A.
Sol Price School of Public Policy, University of Southern California, Los Angeles, CA, USA
e-mail: Brittanykmello@gmail.com

K. Wyka, Ph.D.
Public Health Department, Hunter College, City University of New York,
New York, USA
e-mail: juc2010@med.cornell.edu

M.P. Safir et al. (eds.), *Future Directions in Post-Traumatic Stress Disorder*,
DOI 10.1007/978-1-4899-7522-5_19

details of developing this program, and the clinical research outcomes of our work will be described. Finally, an overview of the potential range of mental health problems in non-rescue disaster workers consequent to the WTC attacks, as well as the larger public health implications of our findings, will be discussed.

Introduction

Disasters cause significant physical destruction and negative psychological impact. Both natural and human-made disasters have been associated with adverse consequences for affected individuals and communities: psychological problems, physical health sequelae, reduced social connectedness, and increased interpersonal, occupational, and financial stress (Norris et al., 2002). Among the psychological consequences frequently noted, multiple studies of disasters report that survivors have high rates of PTSD, major depressive disorder (MDD), and substance misuse, with the most common psychological disorder being PTSD (Galea, Nandi, & Vlahov, 2005; Neria, Nandi, & Galea, 2008; Norris et al., 2002). In an exhaustive review of the literature, Norris et al. (2002) found that PTSD was reported in 109 of 160 studies published on disaster survivors between 1981 and 2001.

Individuals suffering from PTSD are at high risk of developing additional psychological problems, such as mood, anxiety, and substance abuse disorders (Kessler, 2000). The cost to society is also large, with higher absenteeism (Alonso et al., 2010), and an estimated productivity loss in the United States of US$ 3 billion per year for the nation's economy (Kessler, 2000). Once well established, PTSD symptoms are often persistent and do not remit without treatment (Kessler, Sonnega, Bromet, Hughes, & Nelson, 1995).

Unfortunately, disasters are not rare phenomena. In 2011, there were 332 natural disasters worldwide that resulted in nearly 245 million victims, including more than 30,000 deaths, and an estimated US$ 366 billion in economic damages (Guha-Sapir, Vos, Below, & Ponserre, 2012). Although human-made disasters such as industrial accidents, shooting sprees, and terrorist attacks are less common, they take a heavy toll, resulting in approximately 6,000 deaths in 2011 (Bevere, Enz, Mehlhorn, & Tamura, 2012). Importantly, human-made disasters have been demonstrated to cause higher rates of PTSD than natural disasters (Norris et al., 2002).

Direct survivors of human-made disasters show the highest rates of PTSD, with a prevalence of 25 % to 75 %, with individuals involved in rescue and recovery work following human-made disasters exhibiting rates of PTSD symptoms ranging from 5 % to 40 % (Galea et al., 2005). Two factors that may account for these rates may be the intensity and duration of trauma exposure, two variables that have been demonstrated to significantly impact symptom development (Norris et al., 2002).

The effects of mass violence can be particularly devastating. A meta-analysis of psychological consequences following terrorism found that the prevalence of PTSD among those directly affected varied between 12 % and 16 % in the year following a terrorist incident (DiMaggio & Galea, 2006). A study of the March 11,

2004 terrorist attacks on commuter trains in downtown Madrid that claimed 192 lives and left more than 1,400 injured assessed 127 persons injured in the attack, 485 area residents, and 153 police officers who were involved in rescue efforts. These authors found that approximately 58 % of injured individuals, 26 % of area residents, and 4 % of police officers involved in rescue attempts reported symptoms consistent with a psychiatric disorder approximately 2 months following the attack (Gabriel et al., 2007). Following the 1995 Oklahoma City bombing that killed 167 people and injured 684, 45 % of the 182 direct survivors studied were found to have a psychiatric disorder approximately 6 months after the attack, and approximately 34 % met criteria for bombing-related PTSD (North et al., 1999). Additionally, 13 % of 181 male firefighters who responded to the bombing in Oklahoma City met criteria for PTSD (North et al., 2002).

The terrorist attacks of September 11, 2001 were unprecedented, killing 2,753 people in New York City, 184 individuals at the Pentagon, and 40 more aboard a hijacked plane in Shanksville, PA. The New York City Police Department (NYPD) and Fire Department (FDNY) responded with dedication and bravery on September 11th, with 23 police officers and 343 firefighters and emergency services personnel losing their lives.

In New York City, more than 10,000 people were present in the World Trade Center towers and survived. Individuals at high risk for PTSD include those who escaped from the towers, eyewitnesses to the attacks and towers' collapse, area residents displaced from their homes, and disaster workers involved in rescue and recovery efforts. An in-person screening of local residents conducted a month after the attacks found that nearly 40 % of individuals endorsed symptoms consistent with a diagnosis of PTSD (Rosenczweig, Kravitz, & Devlin, 2002). Researchers estimated that 7.5 % of all Manhattan residents, some 67,000 individuals, reported symptoms consistent with PTSD in the 2 months following the attacks on the basis of a telephone survey (Galea et al., 2002).

Symptoms of PTSD and distress appear to have persisted within diverse subpopulations. Multiple studies have documented high rates of PTSD consequent to the WTC attacks in first responders, including police officers (Bowler et al., 2012; Luft et al., 2012; Pietrzak et al., 2012), firefighters (Berninger et al., 2010; Chiu et al., 2011), and civilians (DiGrande, Neria, Brackbill, Pulliam, & Galea, 2011). In our study of 2,960 non-rescue disaster workers deployed to the WTC site following the September 11th attacks, 4.8 % of individuals met criteria for PTSD 4 years after the attacks, and 2.4 % of them continued to meet criteria 6 years after the attacks, with some individuals developing delayed-onset PTSD years later (Cukor, Wyka, Mello et al., 2011). Significant predictors of WTC-related PTSD include female gender, minority ethnicity, working for an employer that sustained fatalities, and five characteristics of direct exposure, including being on a high floor in the Twin Towers, initiating evacuation late, being caught in the dust cloud during the collapse, witnessing horror, and being physically injured (DiGrande et al., 2011). An association between PTSD and respiratory symptoms has also been reported (Luft et al., 2012; Nair et al., 2012; Webber et al., 2011).

The enormous scope of the WTC attacks and the large number of civilians, first responders, and disaster workers impacted illustrates the challenge and necessity that trauma researchers and clinicians faced in providing effective screening and treatment following the attacks. In the aftermath of a disaster, particularly one on the scale of the September 11, 2001 attacks, there is often an urgent desire among clinicians to intervene and assist those who have been affected. It is imperative, however, that these good intentions be informed by best clinical practices, namely evidence-based interventions. Although the emphasis on empirically based treatments had not yet been widely adopted in psychiatry at the time of the September 11, 2001 attacks (Torrey et al., 2001), our team was at the vanguard of recognizing the necessity of providing treatments with the strongest evidence of efficacy. Creating rigorously designed and implemented interventions while confronting vast clinical need and chaos following a large-scale disaster places unique demands on clinician-researchers aiming to provide evidence-based care in this context.

The Program for Anxiety and Traumatic Stress Studies

The Program for Anxiety and Traumatic Stress Studies (PATSS) is a specialized program within Weill Cornell Medical College's Department of Psychiatry that is comprised of licensed psychologists, psychiatrists, and postdoctoral fellows. The mission of this program is to provide state-of-the-art treatment for trauma-related psychological distress and to conduct novel research to improve treatment outcomes and contribute to the evidence base. Our group has a long-standing relationship with the FDNY and New York City's gas and electric utility company secondary to our work with burn patients at the William Randolph Hearst Burn Center at New York-Presbyterian Hospital dating back to 1997. Because of this relationship and because all burn patients were brought to New York-Presbyterian Hospital's Burn Center following the WTC attacks, we were uniquely positioned to provide critical research and clinical services to affected firefighters, police officers, utility workers, and civilians.

At the time of the September 11th attacks, we were partway through data collection for a National Institutes of Health (NIH)-funded treatment development study aimed at preventing PTSD in burn patients using prolonged imaginal exposure therapy. When the WTC attacks occurred a few months after beginning the study, this protocol provided an opportunity to treat emergency services personnel deployed to Ground Zero. Additionally, we received a National Institutes of Mental Health Rapid Assessment Postimpact of Disaster (RAPID) grant in the months after the attacks to deliver a cognitive-behavioral therapy intervention to disaster workers. The RAPID funding mechanism is designed to provide funds in the aftermath of disasters to yield results relatively quickly and aid in the design of larger scale studies on the prevention and treatment of psychological consequences of exposure to mass violence (e.g., http://grants.nih.gov/grants/guide/pa-files/PAR-12-181.html). Thus, we had multiple strains of research in place that included treating emergency services personnel and disaster workers.

Establishing a Clinical Screening and Treatment Program in the Aftermath of 9/11

Assessment Program

Immediately following the WTC attacks, the New York City utility company was asked to disable all gas and electricity to the WTC site to prevent further fires and explosions at Ground Zero and to subsequently run emergency generators and rewire the entire area. This task required thousands of utility workers to spend prolonged periods of time working at Ground Zero and its perimeter, including on the pile of rubble itself and in the empty and unstable buildings surrounding it. Many of the utility workers deployed to the WTC site arrived prior to or just as the Twin Towers were collapsing. Along with firefighters, police officers, and emergency medical workers—but without their formal training in disaster response—these utility workers were thrust into a chaotic scene filled with bodies, body parts, and fears of secondary collapses or attacks, often working 12 to 16 h days for up to a month in this dangerous environment.

Given this widespread traumatic exposure, we discussed with utility company leadership the need to create a voluntary psychological screening program for all individuals deployed to Ground Zero following the attacks. In all, approximately 3,800 utility workers were employed at some time at the WTC site and required initial and ongoing screening to assess for psychological consequences postexposure and receive clinical referrals as needed. Our mandate was to develop and implement this program in approximately 6 weeks.

Developing the Screening Program

In developing the screening program, we assigned a trauma-trained psychologist to meet individually with each utility worker to ensure maximum confidentiality and a nonthreatening environment in which to disclose all issues of concern to participants, in particular maladaptive coping.

To reduce participant burden, we combined our psychological assessments with an already scheduled annual WTC-related physical health screening through the utility company. The WTC medical screening included assessments of breathing and other physical issues and took place at the medical clinic in the company's main building. Our screenings also took place at the main medical building, and later, as the number of participants grew, in trailers at satellite sites in other New York City boroughs to accommodate the burgeoning need. In all cases, these voluntary psychological screenings were conducted in private rooms to protect confidentiality.

After speaking with other trauma experts around the country and drawing on previously formulated guidelines for establishing a screening program developed by the National Center for PTSD (National Center for Posttraumatic Stress Disorder, 2001), we selected multiple assessment measures, choosing clinical outcome research measures rather than epidemiological instruments so that the data could also be combined with ongoing treatment studies with the WTC population. With the goal of acquiring maximal information while minimizing participant burden and the practical limitation of an ongoing shortage of trauma specialists, we opted to create a battery of clinician-administered and self-report measures assessing the most relevant symptoms. Psychological interviews typically took 45–60 min and included structured interview measures including the Clinician-Administered PTSD Scale (CAPS; Blake et al., 1995), the gold standard for assessing the frequency and intensity of PTSD symptoms; the Structured Clinical Interview for DSM-IV (SCID; First, Spitzer, Williams, & Gibbon, 1997) modules for depression, panic disorder, generalized anxiety disorder, and acute stress disorder (to assess for peri-traumatic dissociation); a measure of trauma history (Green, 1993); demographic information; and a questionnaire about the extent of individuals' exposure to the WTC attacks that we developed after interviewing the first 45 individuals from the utility company. Items on the trauma exposure questionnaire included when participants first arrived at the WTC site, proximity to the pile of rubble, and whether individuals witnessed disturbing images and smells, knew someone who was killed or injured, or were present at the site of a subsequent plane crash (Flight 587) that occurred November 12, 2001, which was strongly linked in many individuals' minds to the WTC attacks.

The interview was supplemented with a battery of self-report measures completed by each participant including measures for PTSD (PTSD Checklist, PCL; Weathers, Litz, Herman, Huska, & Keane, 1993), depression (Beck Depression Inventory-II, BDI-II; Beck, Steer, & Brown, 1996), anger (State-Trait Anger Expression Inventory-2, STAXI-2; Spielberger, 1999), functioning (Sheehan Disability Scale, SDS; Sheehan, 1983), and an overview of psychological and physical symptoms (Brief Symptom Inventory, BSI; Derogatis & Spencer, 1982) (see Table 19.1).

Challenges in Implementing a Large-Scale Screening Program

One major challenge of a workplace interview format was the possibility that individuals might be motivated to minimize or deny symptoms. This factor weighed into our implementation strategy in multiple ways. For example, although we strongly considered including a formal substance use assessment in our initial interviews or self-report materials, we decided at the outset of our screening process to ask these questions indirectly as we were concerned that including these questions could cause participants to become guarded due to fear of negative work-related consequences and potentially threaten the validity of the remainder of the assessment because of social desirability bias as substance abuse was cause for termination (e.g., Klassen, Hornstra, & Anderson, 1975; Paulhus, 1991; Phillips & Clancy, 1970, 1972) or response set bias. In the third year of the screening program, once rapport had been strongly established and our presence at the workplace clinic had become routine for the employees, we added a structured assessment of alcohol intake to our clinical interviews, using the Alcohol Use Disorders Identification Test (Babor et al., 2001).

Table 19.1 Measures in WTC Screening and Treatment Program

Clinician-administered measures	*Domain*
Clinician-administered PTSD scale (CAPS; Blake et al., 1995)	PTSD
Standard clinical interview for DSM-IV (SCID; First et al., 1997)	Depression Panic disorder Generalized anxiety disorder Acute stress disorder (peri-traumatic dissociation)
WTC exposure questionnaire (developed by Weill Cornell trauma experts)	Individual's exposure to the WTC attacks
Trauma history questionnaire (Green, 1993)	Lifetime trauma history
Alcohol use disorders identification test (AUDIT; Babor, Higgins-Biddle, Saunders, & Monteiro, 2001)	Alcohol use
Self-report measures	*Domain*
PTSD checklist (PCL; Weathers et al., 1993)	PTSD
Beck depression inventory-II (BDI-II; Beck et al., 1996)	Depression
State-trait anger expression inventory-2 (STAXI-2; Spielberger, 1999)	Anger
Brief symptom inventory (BSI; Derogatis & Spencer, 1982)	Psychological and physical symptoms
Sheehan disability scale (SDS; Sheehan, 1983)	Social, occupational, and family functioning

The issue of confidentiality in a workplace interview also had to be carefully considered to allow participants adequate protection to discuss their symptoms with our clinicians. To ensure this, we arranged to provide only aggregate data to the utility company in the form of percentage of PTSD and depression in participants overall; no individual clinical information was released and all interview and self-report data was stored in our office. In the rare case when an individual reported intent to harm self or others, the incident was managed as a clinical issue between patient and therapist, following customary practices for emergencies.

The work conditions required a high degree of flexibility. Because the company was unable to give an estimate of daily expected participants (varying from 2 to 12) ahead of time, our staffing evolved from one clinician on site to two, and later to a primary clinician with a second clinician available if needed.

Our project staffing included psychologists as well as administrative staff to schedule participants, create and maintain the database, input and check the data, and photocopy the screening materials. Additional postdoctoral fellows and junior faculty members were hired and intensively trained in the CAPS, SCID, and other screening instruments. After first observing senior faculty conducting several assessments, these junior colleagues were then observed interviewing a participant and received feedback and supervision from senior faculty. Interrater reliability was continuously monitored with senior faculty observing junior faculty interviews on a random basis.

In the third year of the program, we scaled back the assessments to screen the entire group via self-report, and only interviewed a selected high-risk group and random comparison group (for a detailed description of this methodology, see Cukor, Wyka, Mello et al., 2011). This decision was made as a strategy to continue to assess those experiencing symptoms while reducing the burden on non-symptomatic participants of an additional hour-long interview for the third consecutive year. We defined high-risk individuals as those who were present at the WTC during the attacks, had a previous psychiatric history, or met criteria for PTSD or subthreshold PTSD at either of the previous assessments. Those who were not designated as high risk completed the self-report measures and then met briefly with a psychologist. If these individuals endorsed distress on self-report measures, the full assessment interview was conducted; otherwise the assessment was stopped. See Table 19.2 describing the evolution of our assessment process.

Table 19.2 WTC screening program interview format

Program year	Interview structure	PTSD prevalence and comorbid psychopathology
Year 1–2	• In-person full structured interview[a] with all participants (45–60 min, conducted by doctoral level psychologists) • Self-report measures[b] administered to all participants	Time frame: July 2002–April 2004 PTSD prevalence (CAPS-based): – Full PTSD—8 % – Subthreshold PTSD –9.3 % PTSD prevalence (PCL-based[c]): – Full PTSD—9.5 % – Subthreshold PTSD –9.3 % Comorbid psychopathology – MDD—6 % – GAD—3.5 % – Panic disorder –2.5 %
Year 3–4	• In-person full structured interview[a] with high-risk group and random comparison group (45–60 min, conducted by doctoral level psychologists), including questions on alcohol use[d] • Self-report measures[b] administered to all participants and brief meeting with a psychologist – Follow-up full interview if distress reported on self-report measures	Time frame: May 2004–Dec 2005 PTSD prevalence (CAPS-based, high-risk, and control comparison subsample): – Full PTSD—8.4 % – Subthreshold PTSD –8.9 % PTSD Prevalence (PCL-based): – Full PTSD—4.8 % – Subthreshold PTSD –3.6 % Comorbid Psychopathology – MDD—3.2 % – GAD—1.8 % – Panic disorder –2.9 %
Year 5–6	Same as above	Time frame: Jan 2007–Dec 2008 PTSD prevalence (CAPS-based, high-risk, and control comparison subsample): – Full PTSD—5.8 % – Subthreshold PTSD –7.7 % PTSD Prevalence (PCL-based): – Full PTSD—2.4 % – Subthreshold PTSD –1.8 %

[a]Clinician-administered measures: CAPS, SCID, Trauma History Questionnaire, WTC Exposure Questionnaire
[b]Self-report measures: PCL, BDI, BSI, STAXI-2, Sheehan
[c]PCL cluster scoring method
[d]AUDIT

This method provided the opportunity to meet our clinical and public health goals. At the utility company's request, we conducted screenings in this manner for 3 additional years, for a total of 7 years of assessment. Our access to this population of non-rescue disaster workers across nearly a decade has provided unique insights into the longitudinal mental health sequelae of the most significant terror attacks in the United States.

Research Findings on WTC Disaster Workers

The program we developed to assess WTC-related PTSD and other psychiatric symptomatology provided a wealth of data demonstrating the short- and long-term mental health consequences of terrorism.

Our screening program found that a substantial number of participants met criteria for comorbid psychopathology between one and 2 years following the trauma (Cukor, Wyka, Jayasinghe, et al. 2011). Within a sample of 2,960 individuals, 8 % met criteria for PTSD, 9.3 % for subthreshold PTSD,[1] 6 % reported symptoms consistent with MDD, 3.5 % met criteria for generalized anxiety disorder (GAD), and 2.5 % reported symptoms consistent with panic disorder. Thirty-nine percent of those with full PTSD reported comorbid current MDD, 14 % comorbid current GAD, and 10.5 % comorbid current panic disorder.

Several variables significantly predicted probable PTSD, including prior life trauma, prior psychopathology, and level of trauma exposure. Notably, those who perceived their lives to be in danger on the day of the attacks were twice as likely to endorse symptoms of full PTSD as the overall sample, making this the single best predictor of probable PTSD. Extent of exposure predicted 69 % of PTSD cases in the most vulnerable group (i.e., those with a psychiatric and trauma history) as well as 89 % of PTSD cases in the low-risk group (i.e., those with no such history).

Four years following the WTC attacks, probable PTSD was 4.8 % and subthreshold PTSD was 3.6 % using a PCL-based estimate for those individuals with complete data ($n=2{,}626$) (Cukor, Wyka, Mello et al., 2011). Probable PTSD was 2.4 % and subthreshold PTSD was 1.8 % 6 years post-9/11 ($n=1{,}983$). Several variables emerged as significant predictors of PTSD diagnosis at the final assessment. The presence of MDD at the initial assessment (OR=2.80, 95 % CI [1.17, 6.71]), a prior history of trauma (OR=2.27, 95 % CI [1.06, 4.85]), and extent of occupational exposure (OR=1.31, 95 % CI [1.13, 1.51]) were the strongest risk factors.

---

[1] Subthreshold PTSD in this study was defined using conservative criteria from Blanchard et al. (1996) that requires at least 2 symptom clusters to be met, while remaining distinct from full PTSD by more than one symptom. Thus, an individual must meet criteria for cluster B (reexperiencing symptoms) and for either cluster C (avoidance/ numbing symptoms) or cluster D (hyperarousal symptoms), as well as meeting duration of one month and having reported functional impairment.

This large sample allowed us to determine whether individuals with subthreshold PTSD represented a distinct group that should be the subject of research and treatment (Cukor, Wyka, Jayasinghe, & Difede, 2010). The subthreshold PTSD group displayed a moderate level of impairment between the non-PTSD group and the full PTSD group. While the largest percentage of individuals (58.8 %) had subthreshold PTSD at their first assessment and then no longer met criteria for subthreshold or full PTSD at subsequent yearly assessments, 19 % of participants had symptoms that progressed to a diagnosis of full PTSD over the next 2 years. This long-standing and considerable impairment makes a strong case for the clinical significance of subthreshold PTSD. Furthermore, 26 % of those with subthreshold PTSD had comorbid MDD, 11.4 % had GAD, and 7 % had comorbid panic disorder.

Despite these concerning findings, the majority of individuals demonstrated great resilience. Approximately 70 % of the overall sample never met criteria for full or subthreshold PTSD according to the PCL. We found a substantial reduction in PTSD symptomatology, so that improvement over time was the common course in our sample. Presumed rates of PTSD based on self-reports (using the PCL) at 6 years post-9/11 were nearly a quarter of the rates at the initial assessment, and rates had decreased by more than 50 % by 6 years for the subsample when examined using the CAPS. However, 10.6 % and 13.9 % of the subsample continued to meet criteria for full PTSD or subthreshold PTSD, respectively, on the CAPS at the final assessment 6 years post-9/11.

Treatment Program

It was evident at the inception of our assessment program that some individuals would report significant symptomatology and need treatment. Our overarching goal was to provide treatments with the strongest research demonstrating their efficacy. At the time of the September 11th terrorist attacks, there was limited agreement on the best forms of treatment for PTSD and little emphasis in the field of psychiatry on the need for evidence-based treatment in general (U.S. Department of Health and Human Services, 1999). The first expert consensus guidelines for PTSD treatment had only recently been published (Foa, Davidson, & Frances, 1999), recommending CBT with exposure therapy as the first line of treatment. Additionally, sertraline was the only medication with FDA approval to treat PTSD. As research scientists and clinicians, therefore, when asked to develop a free, formal treatment program, we sought to develop a model offering treatment with the most evidence of its effectiveness.

To increase confidentiality and the likelihood of treatment acceptance, utility company employees were offered weekly sessions in our private offices at New York-Presbyterian Hospital and were allowed to come to the appointment on work time. In an additional effort to increase confidentiality, our staff communicated all names and appointment times to a single company liaison who emailed the supervisor of each employee stating only that they had an unspecified "mandatory medical appointment" at our hospital at the designated time, a standard practice in the company for all medical appointments. Supervisors at the utility company were advised by their leadership to respect these medical appointments as well as the confidentiality of employees.

While these steps likely minimized dropout, it was initially noted that approximately half of participants did not attend their first appointment even after agreeing to come in for treatment. Speculating that a psychotherapy appointment with an unknown mental health provider might be anxiety-provoking, we altered our approach so that the psychologist performing the assessment on location could become that individual's treatment provider. In this way, the rapport that developed during the screening could be carried into future treatment, thereby increasing chances of first session attendance.

Treatment consisted of evidence-based practices, using exposure therapy as the first-line psychological treatment and sertraline as the first-line pharmacologic agent. All psychologists were trained to employ evidence-based practices to ensure patients would benefit from techniques that had been shown to work in research trials.

Given the large volume of traumatized patients seen, we developed and implemented a secondary stress prevention program to address the potential for vicarious traumatization among our program staff and the larger hospital staff treating WTC survivors. This secondary stress prevention program contained three components: (1) individual supervision, (2) group supervision, and (3) an additional wellness component in the form of yoga classes for our staff and the wider hospital community. Individual supervision was conducted strategically, with our entire group organized into teams for weekly supervision, with a senior faculty member supervising a junior faculty member who in turn supervised a postdoctoral fellow. All senior faculty were directly supervised weekly by the program director. In addition, we offered all clinicians weekly group process supervision, facilitated by the program director. Outside trauma specialists presented at a biweekly seminar series on their respective research areas to provide further discussion and support to our providers. A weekly yoga program was also developed and made available free of charge for faculty and staff across departments at Weill Cornell Medical College and New York-Presbyterian Hospital working with patients affected by the WTC attacks. The program was partially funded by a grant from the Greater New York Hospital Foundation and directed by JoAnn Difede, Ph.D., and yoga expert Beryl Bender Birch.

Pioneering a Clinical Research Program with Virtual Reality Treatment

Knowing that substantial numbers of those expected to be diagnosed with PTSD might not improve using the emerging evidence-based treatments, we sought to develop an effective alternative. While empirical evidence at the time was limited, preliminary evidence suggested that even after imaginal exposure therapy, approximately one-third of patients failed to achieve remission from PTSD (Foa et al., 1999). Effective imaginal exposure requires patients to be willing and able to describe their traumatic experience to their therapist repeatedly, in the present tense, and to actively engage their traumatic memories. Avoidance is a hallmark symptom of PTSD, leaving some patients refusing to discuss their trauma entirely and others exhibiting psychic numbing, unable to engage emotionally with their memories, which predicts poor treatment response (Jaycox, Foa, & Morral, 1998).

It is widely theorized that emotional engagement or fear activation plays a critical role in exposure therapy. Foa and Kozak (1986) proposed that in order for a reduction in fear to occur, fear relevant information associated with the patient's memory for the traumatic event (i.e., the fear structure) must be accessed and activated through emotional engagement. After the fear structure is aroused through emotional engagement, new or corrective information is incorporated into the patient's memory. These authors suggest that repeated engagement with the feared stimulus in a safe environment is necessary for the fear structures to change, thereby allowing long-term habituation to take place.

The few studies that had addressed the question of treatment failures had concluded that failure to engage emotionally predicts a poor treatment outcome. One of the few studies to examine treatment variables that mediate outcome investigated the impact of the variables emotional engagement and habituation on successful outcome of exposure therapy for chronic PTSD in female assault victims (Jaycox et al., 1998). Results showed that although all participants made treatment gains, those with high emotional engagement in the treatment and habituation to emotion-eliciting stimuli were eight times more likely to meet stringent criteria for good end-state functioning (e.g., a 50 % reduction in PTSD symptom scores and normal scores on measures of depression and anxiety).

We reasoned that virtual reality technology might provide a tool to facilitate high emotional engagement. At the time of the WTC attack, multiple studies had documented that virtual reality exposure therapy was an effective treatment for anxiety disorders other than PTSD (Carlin, Hoffman, & Weghorst, 1997; Emmelkamp, Bruynzeel, Drost, & van der Mast, 2001; Rothbaum et al., 1995, 1999; Rothbaum & Hodges, 1999; Rothbaum, Hodges, Ready, Graap, & Alarcon, 2001; Rothbaum, Hodges, Watson, Kessler, & Opdyke, 1996). Similarly to PTSD, patients with specific phobias avoid the feared stimulus but must confront it to get well. Virtual reality environments afford opportunities not only to capitalize on the patient's imaginative and memory capacities but also to augment them with visual, auditory, and even haptic computer-generated experiences. Because patients' fear-relevant cues for a specific trauma include not just thoughts and feelings but also sensory stimuli, such as the sights, sounds, and tactile sensations associated with the traumatic memory, we hypothesized that the virtual environment's ability to evoke these sensory stimuli would facilitate emotional engagement.

Development of the Virtual World Trade Center Simulation

The attack on the World Trade Center was particularly well suited to the development of a virtual scenario because those who witnessed it experienced numerous shared sensory elements (for example, survivors typically saw either or both planes hit the Twin Towers, were enveloped in the dust cloud after the collapses, and heard screams and cries from others). Virtual reality offered the opportunity to approach feared memories in a multisensory environment, rather than solely verbally, and to create a systematic, graded exposure to increasingly distressing aspects of the traumatic experience. Thus, those reluctant or unable to engage in their traumatic memories could be presented with an external, evocative environment that would allow them to process their trauma therapeutically at their own pace.

To develop the WTC virtual reality scenario, we collaborated with colleagues at the University of Washington Human Interface Technology Laboratory. As part of the software development process, 45 disaster workers who had experienced significant trauma exposure during the WTC attacks were interviewed to incorporate their diverse experiences into the creation of the virtual environment.

The initial WTC virtual world shows the Twin Towers from a distance with a clear, sunny sky as it appeared on September 11, 2001 prior to the attacks. Graded exposure to the WTC virtual scenario involves systematically progressing through multiple stages: (1) the patient sees a jet fly past the Twin Towers without crashing and hears normal New York City street noise; (2) a jet crashes into the first tower, but there is no explosion or sound effects; (3) visuals of the explosion are added; and (4) the explosion sound effects are added. Next, (5) the patient sees the first tower with fire and smoke escaping from the location where the jet hit the building but does not hear screaming sound effects; (6) screaming is added; and (7) people begin jumping from the first tower. In the final stages, (8) the second jet crashes into the second tower with the explosion and screaming sound effects; (9) the second tower collapses and creates a dust cloud; and (10) the first tower collapses and produces a dust cloud. The concluding step is when the patient views the full sequence of events in succession (11) (Fig. 19.1).

The virtual reality setup we used consisted of a Dell 530 workstation with dual 2-gigabytes CPUs, 2 gigabytes of RAM, a Wildcat 5110 video card, Windows 2000 operating system, and MultiGen-Paradigm®, Inc., VEGA VR software. A virtual reality helmet positioned two small 1,024 × 768 resolution screens with 40 degrees horizontal field of view close to the patient's eyes. Polhemus™ Fastrak position tracking devices on the helmet were used to integrate the patient's movements with the computer software in real time. Thus, the scenery changed with respect to the patient's head movements (e.g., virtual objects would get closer as the patient leaned forward), giving the sensation of immersion in the virtual environment.

The WTC virtual world itself was developed at relatively low expense. The virtual reality helmets available at that time, however, were quite costly, priced at approximately US$ 25,000 per unit; the equipment was purchased with

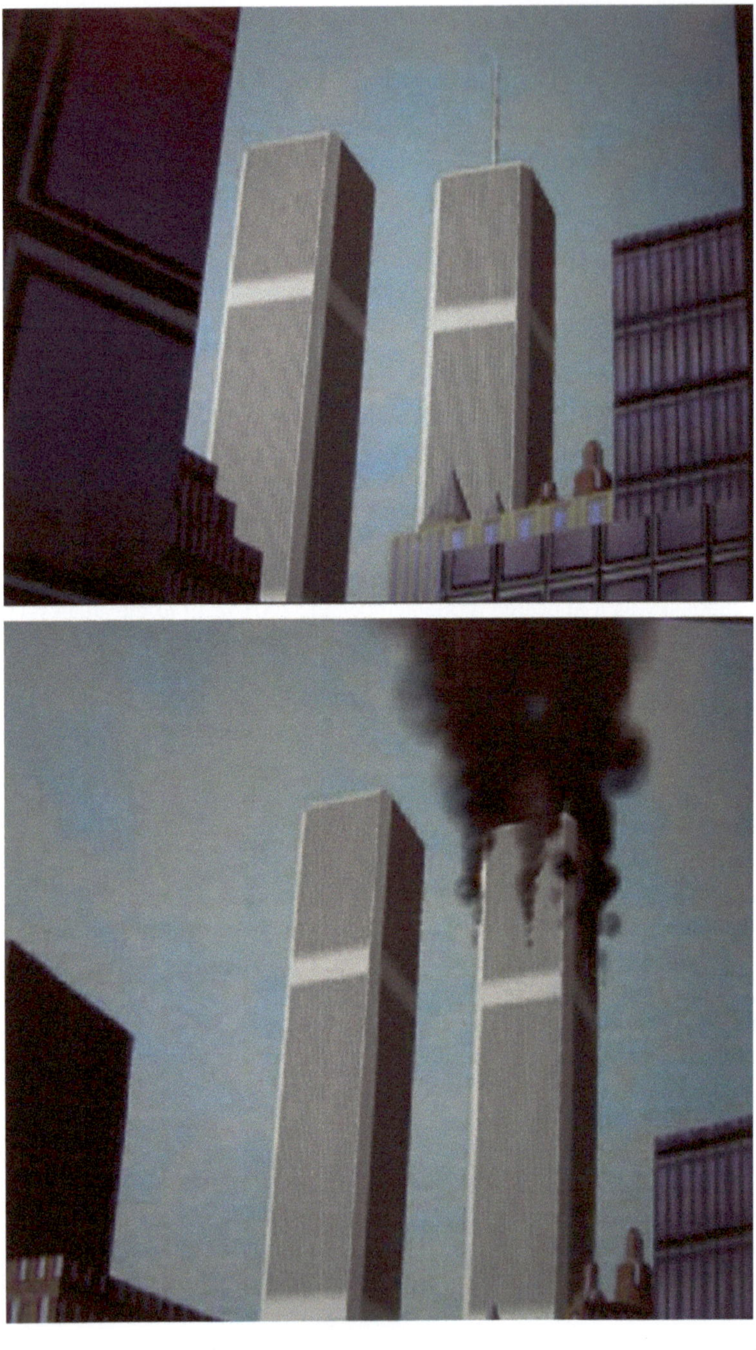

Fig. 19.1 Scenes from the WTC virtual world when the scenario begins (*top*) and after a jet has struck the first tower (*bottom*)

a community engagement grant from Pfizer Pharmaceuticals. Dell Computers, who utilized the fastest video processor available at the time, donated the high-speed processing computers necessary for our project. This high-speed processor allowed the virtual reality stimuli to be integrated in real time, thus allowing the patient to immerse in the scenario, a condition hypothesized as necessary to emotional engagement.

With great effort, the virtual environment was designed in only 3 months and ready for use in February 2002.

Creating a Virtual Reality Treatment Protocol for WTC Survivors

Our final virtual reality exposure protocol consisted of 6 to 14 weekly 75-min sessions, depending on patient need. We integrated virtual reality-based exposure with other common therapeutic techniques used in CBT, including psychoeducation, relaxation training, and cognitive restructuring. We asked an independent psychologist to conduct all clinical assessments to ensure impartiality.

The virtual reality element of the treatment followed the principles of graded behavioral exposure. During sessions in which the virtual reality apparatus was used, patients repeatedly rated their level of distress, using the Subjective Units of Distress Scale (SUDS; Wolpe, 1973), which was also used as an indicator of the patient's emotional engagement in the virtual world. All psychologists received training in using the virtual reality equipment and ongoing supervision in conducting the treatment.

Research Findings on Treatment for WTC-Related PTSD

At the time of the virtual reality WTC treatment study, the use of virtual reality technology to treat PTSD was experimental; there had only been one case study (Rothbaum et al., 1999) and one small pilot study of Vietnam Veterans that was published a month prior to the WTC attacks and showed a partial response (Rothbaum et al., 2001). The relevance of that population to acute PTSD following terrorism was not evident at the time we undertook this study. Evidence from our studies and subsequent work by others (Josman et al., 2006; Parsons & Rizzo, 2008; Rizzo et al., 2008; Walshe, Lewis, & Kim, 2003) marked a growing interest in using virtual reality to treat PTSD, and since that time there has been a proliferation of studies documenting its efficacy in the treatment of PTSD (Gerardi, Cukor, Difede, Rizzo, & Rothbaum, 2010).

The successful implementation of our WTC virtual reality treatment and resulting significant improvements in symptomatology were demonstrated first in a case study (Difede & Hoffman, 2002), and later in a controlled trial of virtual reality therapy for the treatment of WTC-related PTSD (Difede et al., 2007a). This study compared 13 participants in the virtual reality treatment group to 8 participants in a matched waitlist control group. Participants were firefighters, non-rescue disaster relief workers, and civilians with direct exposure to the WTC attacks. Of the 13 patients in the virtual reality group, there were two non-completers and one dropout, leaving 10 patients who completed the treatment protocol. The virtual reality treatment group showed statistically and clinically significant improvement on the CAPS compared to the waitlist group, and treatment gains were maintained for all nine patients who were available at the 6-month follow-up. There was a significant time by group interaction on CAPS scores, with a between-groups posttreatment effect size of 1.54 (Cohen's d). This large effect size is notable, considering the small sample size, but also because five of the 10 virtual reality exposure treatment participants had previously undergone therapy for PTSD (four of whom had failed to improve after receiving imaginal exposure therapy).

Additionally, we made several observations that supported the use of virtual reality treatment for PTSD. The treatment was well tolerated, with no one reporting becoming overwhelmed by the intensity of the sights and sounds of the virtual reality simulation. Only one participant who began the virtual reality exposure dropped out, which is promisingly low, especially for a PTSD exposure therapy study where dropout rates typically range from 20 % to 30 % (Bradley, Greene, Russ, Dutra, & Westen, 2005). The findings demonstrated that a standardized virtual reality WTC environment could be used in the treatment of WTC-related PTSD in individuals with varying types of exposure to the September 11, 2001 attacks, from first responders to civilians. Despite the many differences between individuals' traumatic experiences, the virtual simulation resonated with patients, civilians, and emergency services personnel alike. Additionally, by using virtual reality, we as clinicians were able to standardize exposure to sensory stimuli across patients. Altogether, the data yielded preliminary evidence that virtual reality simulations could be an effective tool in the treatment of PTSD, particularly for those who did not improve during imaginal exposure therapy.

In addition to our research examining the use of virtual reality to treat WTC trauma survivors, we also conducted a pilot study of CBT to address the paucity of randomized controlled clinical trials of PTSD for disaster workers in the extant literature (Difede et al., 2007b). Thirty-one disaster workers diagnosed with full or subthreshold PTSD were randomly assigned to receive either CBT with prolonged imaginal exposure or treatment as usual (TAU) through their original referral source (e.g., employee assistance program or occupational health) to determine whether CBT with exposure would be an effective treatment for this population.

Those in the CBT imaginal exposure group had a significantly greater posttreatment decline in self-report and clinician-rated PTSD symptoms, as measured by the PCL and CAPS, respectively, than in the TAU group. These preliminary data suggested that CBT may be effective for disaster workers with subthreshold or full PTSD and demonstrated the feasibility of recruiting for and conducting a brief intervention focused on common psychological outcomes post-disaster. Our dropout rate of 40 % was higher than the typical range of 20 % to 30 % for PTSD exposure therapy studies (Bradley et al., 2005), but consistent with more recent studies of combat-related PTSD (Hoge, 2011). Those who dropped out were significantly less well educated and had a lower income level than treatment completers. Dropouts were also associated with higher levels of alcohol consumption. When considered in the context of implementing interventions following large-scale disasters, special emphasis should be placed on addressing barriers to treatment retention associated with income and education.

Conclusion

Our prior relationship with New York City's utility company gave us the opportunity to assist a population with exposure to widespread devastation following the largest terrorist attack in the United States. As clinicians, we had an ethical responsibility to each of these individuals, and the potential opportunity to prevent the development of chronic PTSD in the subset of those at risk. Simultaneously, as researchers, we had a broader responsibility to collect valid, reliable, and relevant information in order to ensure that the experience of each affected individual could inform the overall PTSD knowledge base. This dual role was a constant consideration as we sought to balance our responsibilities to individuals and the public health of our community.

Faced with an urgent time frame following the WTC disaster, we worked rapidly to create a well-designed program to screen and offer treatment to thousands of non-rescue disaster recovery workers. In developing this program, we were attuned to the potential stigma attached to disclosing symptoms in the workplace and endeavored to create a sensitive and thorough evaluation process to best serve this unique population.

We found that the greatest predictors of PTSD in non-rescue disaster workers were extent of trauma exposure, prior psychopathology, and perception of life threat during the attacks, which is consistent with other research in this area. Our research also showed that a significant subset of individuals (8 %) developed full PTSD in the wake of the 9/11 attacks, while 9.3 % developed subthreshold PTSD. Many of these individuals remitted over time. In addition 70 % of individuals never developed PTSD and a very few individuals developed PTSD with a significantly delayed onset years later.

In addition, we worked quickly to create a cutting-edge treatment to best address the needs of individuals who directly witnessed the WTC attacks. Knowing that the emerging evidence-based treatments sometimes failed to successfully ameliorate PTSD symptoms (Foa, Davidson & Frances, 1999), we sought to build on the evidence base with the development of a novel virtual reality exposure treatment with the hypothesis that sensory components would more fully immerse and emotionally engage patients, thereby improving clinical outcomes. In this way, even those patients who might be unwilling or unable to confront their trauma using imaginal prolonged exposure could benefit from treatment. Our pilot and follow-up data demonstrated that this therapy was well tolerated among patients and yielded significant reductions in PTSD symptomatology.

Our work following the WTC attacks demonstrates a blend of flexibility and adherence to rigorous measurement, as well as a consideration of individual needs and the contribution to a larger public health knowledge base. We offered emerging evidence-based treatments prior to the current vanguard for empirically supported interventions, and we were additionally able to advance the knowledge base with the development of an innovative treatment study and collection of 7 years of longitudinal data on the course of PTSD in disaster workers. It was a privilege to work with thousands of non-rescue disaster workers who were witness to enormous devastation and provide information and interventions that could offer relief. From a public health perspective, it is imperative that researchers and clinicians work in concert to create and carry out well-designed psychological screening programs in the wake of future tragedies. In addition, disaster workers in need of treatment must have access to evidence-based interventions as a first-line option to reduce psychological suffering. It is in these ways that we can best honor those whose professions place their lives at risk in the service of helping others.

References

Alonso, J., Petukhova, M., Vilagut, G., Chatterji, S., Heeringa, S., Ustun, T. B., et al. (2010). Days out of role due to common physical and mental conditions: Results from the WHO World Mental Health surveys. *Molecular Psychiatry, 16*, 1–10.

Babor, T. F., Higgins-Biddle, J. C., Saunders, J. B., & Monteiro, M. G. (2001). *AUDIT: The alcohol use disorders identification test: Guidelines for use in primary care* (2nd ed.). Geneva, Switzerland: World Health Organization, Department of Mental Health and Substance Dependence.

Beck, A. T., Steer, R. A., & Brown, G. K. (1996). *Manual for the beck depression inventory-II*. San Antonio, TX: Psychological Corporation.

Berninger, A., Webber, M. P., Cohen, H. W., Gustave, J., Lee, R., Niles, J. K., et al. (2010). Trends of elevated PTSD risk in firefighters exposed to the World Trade Center disaster: 2001-2005. *Public Health Reports, 125*(4), 556–566.

Bevere, L., Enz, R., Mehlhorn, J., & Tamura, T. (2012). In J. Villat Cordova & K. Karl (Eds.), Natural catastrophes and man-made disasters in 2011: Historic losses surface from record earthquakes and floods (Vol. 2). Zurich, Switzerland: Sigma.

Blake, D. D., Weathers, F. W., Nagy, L. M., Kalopek, D. G., Charney, D. S., & Keane, T. M. (1995). *Clinician-Administered PTSD Scale for DSM-IV (CAPS-DX)*. Boston, MA: Medical Center, National Center for Posttraumatic Stress Disorder, Behavioral Science Division.

Blanchard, E. B., Hickling, E. J., Barton, K. A., Taylor, A. E., Loos, W. R., & Jones-Alexander, J. (1996). One-year prospective follow-up of motor vehicle accident victims. *Behaviour Research and Therapy, 34*(10), 775–786.

Bowler, R. M., Harris, M., Li, J., Gocheva, V., Stellman, S. D., Wilson, K., et al. (2012). Longitudinal mental health impact among police responders to the 9/11 terrorist attack. *American Journal of Industrial Medicine, 55*, 297–312.

Bradley, R., Greene, J., Russ, E., Dutra, L., & Westen, D. (2005). A multidimensional meta-analysis of psychotherapy for PTSD [erratum appears in Am J Psychiatry 2005, 162(4):832]. *American Journal of Psychiatry, 162*(2), 214–227.
Carlin, A. S., Hoffman, H. G., & Weghorst, S. (1997). Virtual reality and tactile augmentation in the treatment of spider phobia: a case report. *Behaviour Research and Therapy, 35*(2), 153–158.
Chiu, S., Webber, M. P., Zeig-Owens, R., Gustave, J., Lee, R., Kelly, K., et al. (2011). Performance characteristics of the PTSD Checklist in retired firefighters exposed to the World Trade Center disaster. *Annals of Clinical Psychiatry, 23*(2), 95–104.
Cukor, J., Wyka, K., Jayasinghe, N., Weathers, F., Giosan, C., Leck, P., et al. (2011). Prevalence and predictors of posttraumatic stress symptoms in utility workers deployed to the World Trade Center following the attacks of September 11, 2001. *Depression and Anxiety, 28*(3), 210–217. doi:10.1002/da.20776.
Cukor, J., Wyka, K., Jayasinghe, N., & Difede, J. (2010). The nature and course of subthreshold PTSD. *Journal of Anxiety Disorders, 24*(8), 918–923.
Cukor, J., Wyka, K., Mello, B., Olden, M., Jayasinghe, N., Roberts, J., Giosan, C., Crane, M., & Difede, J. (2011). The longitudinal course of PTSD among disaster workers deployed to the World Trade Center following the attacks of September 11th. *Special Issue: The September 11th 2001 Terrorist Attacks: Ten Years After. J Trauma Stress, 24*(5), 506–514.
Derogatis, L. R., & Spencer, M. S. (1982). *The Brief Symptom Inventory (BSI): Administration, scoring, and procedures manual-I.* Baltimore, MD: Johns Hopkins University School of Medicine, Clinical and Psychometrics Research Unit.
Difede, J., & Hoffman, H. G. (2002). Virtual reality exposure therapy for World Trade Center post-traumatic stress disorder: A case report. *CyberPsychology and Behavior, 5*(6), 529–535.
Difede, J., Cukor, J., Jayasinghe, N., Patt, I., Jedel, S., Spielman, L., et al. (2007a). Virtual reality exposure therapy for the treatment of posttraumatic stress disorder following September 11, 2001. *Journal of Clinical Psychiatry, 68*(11), 1639–1647.
Difede, J., Malta, L. S., Best, S., Henn-Haase, C., Metzler, T., Bryant, R., et al. (2007b). A randomized controlled clinical treatment trial for World Trade Center attack-related PTSD in disaster workers. *Journal of Nervous and Mental Disease, 195*(10), 861–865.
DiGrande, L., Neria, Y., Brackbill, R. M., Pulliam, P., & Galea, S. (2011). Long-term posttraumatic stress symptoms among 3,271 civilian survivors of the September 11, 2001, terrorist attacks on the World Trade Center. *American Journal of Epidemiology, 173*(3), 271–281.
DiMaggio, C., & Galea, S. (2006). The behavioral consequences of terrorism: A meta-analysis. *Academic Emergency Medicine, 13*, 559–566.
Emmelkamp, P. M., Bruynzeel, M., Drost, L., & van der Mast, C. A. P. G. (2001). Virtual reality treatment in acrophobia: A comparison with exposure in vivo. *CyberPsychology and Behavior, 4*(3), 335–339.
First, M. B., Spitzer, R. L., Williams, J. B. W., & Gibbon, M. (1997). *Structured clinical interview for DSM-IV SCID*. Washington, DC: American Psychiatric Association.
Foa, E. B., Dancu, C. V., Hembree, E. A., Jaycox, L. H., Meadows, E. A., & Street, G. P. (1999). A comparison of exposure therapy, stress inoculation training, and their combination for reducing posttraumatic stress disorder in female assault victims. *Journal of Consulting and Clinical Psychology, 67*(2), 194–200.
Foa, E. B., Davidson, R. T., & Frances, A. (1999). Expert consensus guideline series: Treatment of posttraumatic stress disorder. *American Journal of Clinical Psychiatry, 60*, 5–76.
Foa, E. B., & Kozak, M. J. (1986). Emotional processing of fear: Exposure to corrective information. *Psychological Bulletin, 99*(1), 20–35.
Gabriel, R., Ferrando, L., Sainz Corton, E., Mingote, C., Garcia-Camba, E., Fernandez Liria, A., et al. (2007). Psychopathological consequences after a terrorist attack: An epidemiological study among victims, the general population, and police officers. *European Psychiatry, 22*, 339–346.
Galea, S., Ahern, J., Resnick, H., Kilpatrick, D., Bucuvalas, M., Gold, J., et al. (2002). Psychological sequelae of the September 11 terrorist attacks in New York City. *The New England Journal of Medicine, 346*(13), 982–987.

Galea, S., Nandi, A., & Vlahov, D. (2005). The epidemiology of post-traumatic stress disorder after disasters. *Epidemiologic Reviews, 27*, 78–91. doi:10.1093/epirev/mxi003.

Gerardi, M., Cukor, J., Difede, J., Rizzo, A., & Rothbaum, B. (2010). Virtual reality exposure therapy for posttraumatic stress disorder and other anxiety disorders. *Current Psychiatry Reports, 12*(4), 298–305.

Green, B. L. (1993). Trauma history questionnaire. In B. H. Stamm & E. M. Varra (Eds.), *Instrumentation in stress, trauma, and adaptation* (pp. 366–369). Northbrook, IL: Research and Methodology Interest Group of the ISTSS.

Guha-Sapir, D., Vos, F., Below, R., & Ponserre, S. (2012). Annual disaster statistical review 2011: The numbers and trends. Brussels, Belgium: Centre for Research on the Epidemiology of Disasters (CRED).

Hoge, C. W. (2011). Interventions for war-related posttraumatic stress disorder: Meeting veterans where they are. *Journal of the American Medical Association, 306*(5), 549–551.

Jaycox, L. H., Foa, E. B., & Morral, A. R. (1998). Influence of emotional engagement and habituation on exposure therapy for PTSD. *Journal of Consulting and Clinical Psychology, 66*(1), 185–192.

Josman, N., Somer, E., Reisberg, A., Weiss, P. L. T., Garcia-Palacios, A., & Hoffman, H. (2006). BusWorld: Designing a virtual environment for post-traumatic stress disorder in Israel: A protocol. *Cyber Psychology and Behavior, 9*(2), 241–244.

Kessler, R. C. (2000). Posttraumatic stress disorder: the burden to the individual and to society. *Journal of Clinical Psychiatry, 61*(Suppl 5), 4–12. discussion 13–14.

Kessler, R. C., Sonnega, A., Bromet, E., Hughes, M., & Nelson, C. B. (1995). Posttraumatic stress disorder in the National Comorbidity Survey. *Archives of General Psychiatry, 52*(12), 1048–1060.

Klassen, D., Hornstra, R. K., & Anderson, P. B. (1975). Influence of social desirability on symptom and mood reporting in a community survey. *Journal of Consulting and Clinical Psychology, 43*(4), 448–452.

Luft, B. J., Schechter, C., Kotov, R., Broihier, J., Reissman, D., Guerrara, K., et al. (2012). Exposure, probable PTSD and lower respiratory illness among World Trade Center rescue, recovery and clean-up workers. *Psychological Medicine, 42*, 1069–1079.

Nair, H. P., Ekenga, C. C., Cone, J. E., Brackbill, R. M., Farfel, M. R., & Stellman, S. D. (2012). Co-occurring lower respiratory symptoms and posttraumatic stress disorder 5 to 6 years after the World Trade Center terrorist attack. *American Journal of Public Health, 102*(10), 1964–1973.

National Center for Posttraumatic Stress Disorder. (2001). Disaster rescue and response workers. 9/14/01. Retrieved Dec 08, 2003, from http://www.ncptsd.org/facts/disasters

Neria, Y., Nandi, A., & Galea, S. (2008). Post-traumatic stress disorder following disasters: A systematic review. *Psychological Medicine, 38*, 467–480. doi:10.1017/S0033291707001353.

Norris, F. H., Friedman, M. J., Watson, P. J., Byrne, C. M., Diaz, E., & Kaniasty, K. (2002). 60,000 disaster victims speak: Part I. An empirical review of the empirical literature, 1981-2001. *Psychiatry, 65*(3), 207–239.

North, C. S., Nixon, S. J., Shariat, S., Mallonee, S., McMillen, J. C., Spitznagel, E. L., et al. (1999). Psychiatric disorders among survivors of the Oklahoma City bombing. *Journal of the American Medical Association, 282*(8), 755–762.

North, C. S., Tivis, L., McMillen, J. C., Pfefferbaum, B., Spitznagel, E. L., Cox, J., et al. (2002). Psychiatric disorders in rescue workers after the Oklahoma City bombing. *American Journal of Psychiatry, 159*(5), 857–859.

Parsons, T. D., & Rizzo, A. A. (2008). Affective outcomes of virtual reality exposure therapy for anxiety and specific phobias: A meta analysis. *Journal of Behavior Therapy and Experimental Psychiatry, 39*(3), 250–261.

Paulhus, D. L. (1991). Measurement and control of response bias. In J. P. Robinson, P. R. Shaver, & L. S. Wrightsman (Eds.), *Measures of personality and social psychological attitudes* (pp. 17–59). San Diego, CA: Academic Press.

Phillips, D. L., & Clancy, K. J. (1970). Response biases in field studies of mental illness. *American Sociological Review, 35*(3), 503–515.
Phillips, D. L., & Clancy, K. J. (1972). Some effects of "social desirability" in survey studies. *American Journal of Sociology, 77*(5), 921–940.
Pietrzak, R. H., Schechter, C. B., Bromet, E. J., Katz, C. L., Reissman, D. B., Ozbay, F., et al. (2012). The burden of full and subsyndromal posttraumatic stress disorder among police involved in the World Trade Center rescue and recovery effort. *Journal of Psychiatric Research, 46*, 835–842.
Rizzo, A. A., Graap, K., Perlman, K., McLay, R. N., Rothbaum, B. O., Reger, G., et al. (2008). Virtual Iraq: initial results from a VR exposure therapy application for combat-related PTSD. *Studies in Health Technology and Informatics, 132*, 420–425.
Rosenczweig, C. C., Kravitz, J., & Devlin, E. (2002). The psychological impact of helping in a disaster—the New York City experience, September 11th, 2001. *Academic Emergency Medicine, 9*(5), 502.
Rothbaum, B. O., & Hodges, L. F. (1999). The use of virtual reality exposure in the treatment of anxiety disorders. *Behavior Modification, 23*(4), 507–525.
Rothbaum, B. O., Hodges, L., Alarcon, R., Ready, D., Shahar, F., Graap, K., et al. (1999). Virtual reality exposure therapy for PTSD Vietnam Veterans: A case study. *Journal of Traumatic Stress, 12*(2), 263–271.
Rothbaum, B. O., Hodges, L. F., Kooper, R., Obdyke, D., Williford, J. S., & North, M. (1995). Virtual reality graded exposure in the treatment of acrophobia: A case report. *Behavior Therapy, 26*(3), 547–554.
Rothbaum, B. O., Hodges, L. F., Ready, D., Graap, K., & Alarcon, R. D. (2001). Virtual reality exposure therapy for Vietnam veterans with posttraumatic stress disorder. *Journal of Clinical Psychiatry, 62*(8), 617–622.
Rothbaum, B. O., Hodges, L., Watson, B. A., Kessler, C. D., & Opdyke, D. (1996). Virtual reality exposure therapy in the treatment of fear of flying: A case report. *Behaviour Research and Therapy, 34*(5–6), 477–481.
Sheehan, D. V. (1983). *The anxiety disease*. New York, NY: Scribner's.
Spielberger, C. (1999). *STAXI-2 state-trait anger expression inventory-2: Professional manual.* Odessa, FL: Psychological Assessment Resources.
Torrey, W. C., Drake, R. E., Dixon, L., Burns, B. J., Flynn, L., Rush, A. J., et al. (2001). Implementing evidence-based practices for persons with severe mental illnesses. *Psychiatric Services, 52*(1), 45–50.
U.S. Department of Health and Human Services. (1999). *Mental Health: A report of the surgeon general.* Rockville, MD: U.S. Department of Health and Human Services, Substance Abuse and Mental Health Services Administration, Center for Mental Health Services, National Institutes of Health, National Institute of Mental Health.
Walshe, D. G., Lewis, E. J., & Kim, S. I. (2003). Exploring the use of computer games and virtual reality in exposure therapy for fear of driving following a motor vehicle accident. *Cyber Psychology and Behavior, 6*, 329–334.
Weathers, F. W., Litz, B. T., Herman, D. S., Huska, J. A., & Keane, T. M. (1993). *The PTSD Checklist (PCL). Reliability, validity, and diagnostic utility.* Paper presented at the Annual Meeting of the International Society for Traumatic Stress Studies, San Antonio, TX.
Webber, M. P., Glaser, M. S., Weakley, J., Soo, J., Ye, F., Zeig-Owens, R., et al. (2011). Physician-Diagnosed Respiratory Conditions and Mental Health Symptoms 7–9 Years Following the World Trade Center Disaster. *American Journal of Industrial Medicine, 54*, 661–671.
Wolpe, J. (1973). *The practice of behavior therapy*. New York, NY: Pergamon Press.

Part VI
Case Discussion

Chapter 20
Case Presentation of a Chronic Combat PTSD Veteran

Nitsa Nacasch, Lilach Rachamim, and Edna B. Foa

David, a 54-year-old married white man with three children, is a veteran of the 1973 Yom Kippur War in Israel. David was born in Israel, the third and the youngest child. His father was born in Poland and was a Holocaust survivor. After the war, he came to Israel and worked as a bus driver. David described his father as a very reserved person who spent hours at work. David's mother was born in Israel. David described his mother as: "a shy and quiet person, who was a housekeeper that took care of his and his brother's needs". David grew up in a city in the center of Israel. He described his childhood as happy and joyful. He was friendly and a good student at school. When he was 12 years old, he transferred to a religious boarding school together with a friend from preschool. He remembered those years as: "the best years of my life".

David and his friends loved spending time together. Mostly, they loved to hike in nature. His best friend, Ruben, grew up in the same neighborhood and was his roommate in boarding school. David graduated from high school with good grades

---

With Commentaries by: Prolonged exposure (PE): Nitsa Nacasch, Lilach Rachamim, and Edna B. Foa; Cognitive Processing Therapy (CPT): Kathleen Chard; Virtual reality (VR): Exposure therapy with D-Cycloserine (DCS): Barbara Rothbaum; Interpersonal Psychotherapy (IPT): Alexandra Klein-Rafaeli and John C. Markowitz

N. Nacasch, M.D. (✉)
Brill Community Mental Health Center, Hatsvi 9, Tel Aviv, Israel
e-mail: nitsana@clalit.org.il

L. Rachamim, Ph.D.
Interdisciplinary Center, Herzliya, Israel

Schneider Children's Medical Center of Israel, Petah Tikva, Israel
e-mail: lilach.rachamim7@gmail.com

E.B. Foa, Ph.D.
Center for Treatment and Study of Anxiety, University of Pennsylvania,
3535 Market Street, Philadelphia, PA 19104, USA
e-mail: Foa@ail.med.upenn.edu

M.P. Safir et al. (eds.), *Future Directions in Post-Traumatic Stress Disorder*,
DOI 10.1007/978-1-4899-7522-5_20

and joined the army along with Ruben. During his military service he participated in several military operations but did not exhibit any posttraumatic symptomatology. At the end of his military service he married a neighbor, and began studying accounting at the university. A half a year after getting married, his wife got pregnant and at the same time, the Yom Kippur started and he was drafted.

During the war, David served as a reserve soldier and was in severe combat many times. He was under heavy artillery over a period of 12 days, and witnessed horrific battle scenes, from seeing severely disfigured soldiers who had been wounded, or died on the battlefield, to severed body parts scattered across the fields.

On the 12th day of the war, David's tank came under fire. He was able to escape from the tank initially, but then returned when he realized his comrades had not been able to get away. None of his tank crew had survived, including his best friend, Ruben. At that moment, artillery from within the tank exploded and went up in flames. David was severely burned, but was able to escape again, only to view a vehicle with enemy soldiers advancing towards him. David was sure that he was going to be killed at that moment, but the enemy vehicle was bombarded by heavy artillery in time to prevent this from happening.

After receiving emergency care in a field hospital, David was moved to a general medical hospital where he remained for several months and where he underwent several operations and treatments for burns. While hospitalized, he began suffering from nightmares, flashbacks, and severe anxiety symptoms, but did not receive any psychological treatment.

Following the war, David continued to experience severe chronic PTSD symptoms, including frequent flashbacks and intrusive thoughts about his combat experiences—specifically the last combat event described above. He also experienced strong guilt feelings about the death of his friends and nightmares from which he would wake up with panic attacks. Subsequently, he avoided many situations and places such as malls, crowded places, and barbecues (because of the smell of the smoke and the sight of the burning meat). He tended to avoid closed places such as elevators, airplanes, and even rooms where the door was closed. Additionally, he had frequent outbursts of anger, and difficulty concentrating, hypervigilance, and exaggerated startle responses.

In addition to severe PTSD, David also suffered from complicated grief. His survival guilt had resulted in a profound depression ("I cannot enjoy life without him"). He felt his life was meaningless without Ruben, and was unable to accept his death. He was angry with himself for not taking better care of his best friend during the battle, and was generally preoccupied with his other fellow soldiers who were also killed in the war. He described a "yearning and longing" to be with them all again. He avoided numerous reminders of his loss including looking at pictures of the deceased, visiting places they used to frequent, and visiting to the deceased's parents and the cemetery.

David tried to complete his university degree after the war, but was unable to concentrate and left after several months. After several failed attempts to remain employed, he primarily stayed at home, suffering from severe depression and PTSD. David refused treatment until 2002 because he felt shame. He avoided talking about the traumatic events and did not process his trauma and grief. He felt he could not share his experiences and emotions with his parents and his wife because he did not want to cause them sorrow. “After what my father went through during the Holocaust, I did not feel I have the right to complain”. He felt ashamed because of his PTSD symptoms and felt weak that he was unemployed in comparison to his father, who managed to deal with his traumatic experiences more successfully, at least in the sense that he was able to work and support a family.

During the Intifada of 2002, David’s condition worsened, and he finally decided to seek help. He received psychodynamic therapy and medication (SSRIs) with no improvement. In 2005, he was referred to a trauma unit that specialized in cognitive-behavioral treatment (CBT). Following psychiatric assessment, he was diagnosed as suffering from severe PTSD, Major Depression Disorder (MDD), and complicated grief. His PTSD Symptom Scale Interview (PSS-I) score was 37 and Beck Depression Inventory (BDI) score was 28.

Prolonged Exposure Therapy for a Chronic Combat PTSD Veteran

Case Discussion: PE Treatment for David

Nitsa Nacaschnitsana@clalit.org.ilLilach Rachamimlilach.rachamim7@gmail.comEdna B. FoaFoa@ail.med.upenn.eduBrill Community Mental Health CenterHatsvi 9Tel AvivIsraelInterdisciplinary Center Herzliya Israel Schneider Children’s Medical Center of Israel Petah Tikva Israel Center for Treatment and Study of Anxiety University of Pennsylvania 3535 Market Street Philadelphia PA 19104 USA David, a veteran, was diagnosed as suffering from severe PTSD, MDD, and complicated grief. Forty years before, during Yom-Kipur War he served as a reserved soldier and experienced numerous severe combat events. David was severely injured and lost his best friend.

In our opinion, PE treatment is the treatment choice for this patient. We base this view on the large body of research demonstrating the high efficacy of PE. Below is a description of the treatment rationale and treatment outline for David.

Summary of the Literature

PE therapy for PTSD was found effective in reducing PTSD symptoms in randomized controlled trials (RCTs) and open trials in combat PTSD (Nacash et al., 2010; Rauch et al., 2006; Schnurr et al., 2007; Tuerk et al., 2011). PE has been found to be effective for chronic PTSD even decades following the traumatic event (e.g., Nacasch et al., 2007, 2010). Indeed PE, along with cognitive processing therapy, has been selected for wide dissemination throughout the Vetran’s Authority (VA) in the USA, and is the only Evidence-based treatment (EBT) which was studied with Israeli veterans. In addition to PTSD, David suffered from depression and survivor guilt. PE is extremely successful in ameliorating guilt, anger feelings, and depression. A variant of PE was found helpful with complicated grief, where individuals recount the story of the death using imaginal exposure, and conduct grief-related in vivo exposures in a fashion similar to PE. This treatment was found to be more effective than IPT in reduction of grief-related symptoms.

Treatment Outline

David's PE therapy would probably consist of 12–15 sessions, as the PE therapist will have to address both PTSD and complicated grief symptoms. In the first treatment session, the therapist will present an overview of PE treatment. S/he will explain the rationale for treatment, emphasizing the role of avoidance in the maintenance of PTSD and complicated grief symptoms. Since David avoided thinking and talking about the trauma, he could not emotionally process all the events of the war, nor consolidate the loss of his friends. For many years he avoided trauma-related situations and stimuli such as crowded places, elevators, and barbeques. Therefore, he could not experience disconfirmation of his dysfunctional beliefs: "the world is extremely dangerous and I am extremely incompetent." After presenting the treatment rationale, the therapist and David will establish an index trauma (the event that hurts him the most). Most probably this would be the events from the 12th day of the war when he was badly injured and lost his friends. During the second session, the therapist will discuss common reactions to trauma. This will help David to normalize and validate his symptoms, such as emotional numbness. The in vivo procedure will help him to gradually confront situations, places, people, and stimuli that were avoided because they evoke anxiety. The items in the in vivo exposure will include behavioral activation, as well as grief-related items such as looking at pictures of his deceased friend and visiting places that they used to hang out together.

An Example of Items on David's Hierarchical List

Sitting in a small restaurant
Shopping in the supermarket
Visiting a crowded moll
Smelling barbecued meat
Visiting the north of Israel
Using an elevator
Playing with his grandchildren
Inviting friends for dinner
Watching a film at the cinema theater
Taking a walk in the park
Listening to classical music
Looking at his friend's pictures

In imaginal exposure, recounting the traumatic memories will help David to process the trauma by organizing the narrative and thus to realize he could not have helped his friends. It will help him to be emotionally engaged, expressing his deep longing and extreme guilt feelings for being the survivor. Having David listening to his audiotapes as homework will provide him with the opportunity to process and to habituate to the traumatic memory.

Gradually, David might remember more and more details that will help him resolve his guilt feelings, such as the fact that he did return to the tank risking his life, in order to rescue his friend and eventually was wounded. The Therapist will encourage him to look at pictures of his dead friend, bring up pleasant memories from the past, and to say goodbye.

PE treatment will help David to change his dysfunctional beliefs about the world as a dangerous place, and himself as incompetent. It will probably decrease intrusive and hyperarousal symptoms. It will provide him with the opportunity to process the experiences he went through during the war and the loss of his friend and realize that he was not to blame.

Cognitive Processing Therapy for a Chronic Combat PTSD Veteran

Case Discussion: CPT Case Conceptualization

In the case description, "David" presents as many military combat veterans do, with survivor guilt, isolation, anger, and an inability to concentrate or focus. He also reports significant cognitive disruptions including thoughts of "not being able to enjoy life" without his best friend, believing his life was "meaningless," and believing he does not "have the right to complain" after what his father went through in the holocaust. In addition, his assessments confirm that he is suffering from PTSD related to his military experiences along with comorbid depression.

Based on this initial presentation, David appears to be an excellent candidate for Cognitive Processing Therapy (CPT, Resick, Monson, & Chard, 2010). Several randomized controlled trials and clinical effectiveness studies have shown CPT to be very effective for individuals with a variety of trauma histories, especially when the PTSD is associated with depression and guilt (Chard, 2005; Chard, Schumm, Owens, & Cottingham, 2010; Monson et al., 2006; Resick et al., 2008). In addition David has a clear memory of the trauma and there is a direct link between his disruptive thoughts and his combat experience. As David has quickly identified distressing thoughts and feelings and he is already speaking in stuck points, David will likely find the concepts of CPT easy to understand and relevant to his experiences. The therapy will allow him a safe, nonjudgmental place to share his negative thoughts about himself and also allow him to explore his natural feelings of grief and loss. CPT will also allow him to look at the evidence regarding assumptions he has made about the traumatic event and overgeneralizations he has made regarding self, others, and the world, especially in the five core areas of safety, trust, power/

control, esteem, and intimacy. Thus it is recommended that he begin the standard 12-session CPT protocol in the next week.

In the first phase of therapy David would be educated about PTSD and the theoretical model underlying CPT. He would then be asked to write about how the trauma has impacted him and he would begin looking for places where he has become "stuck" in his thinking, in both looking back at the event and looking forward to his future. He might initially identify "stuck points" such as "If I talk about my trauma, I am weak," and "Other people should not feel sorry for me." He would likely indicate that these thoughts lead to feelings of shame and loneliness. Stuck points would be recorded in each session on a log for future examination later in the therapy. Next in Phase 1 he would learn about the connection between thoughts and feelings with the therapist using the A-B-C sheets to help him see the link and generating some possible alternative thoughts.

In the middle phase of therapy David would be asked to write about the most traumatic event which will allow David to feel the natural emotions of sadness and fear that he was not able to experience and/or process after the tank incident. Second the therapist would help David identify additional stuck points related to the traumatic event such as beliefs related to hindsight bias, undoing, or self-blame. These beliefs may include "I should not have survived, when they all died" or "If only I had done X, the explosion would not have occurred" or "I could have saved them if I have done something different." The therapist would again use the A-B-C sheets and gentle Socratic Dialogue to help David being to challenge these thoughts. Finally, David would be asked to rewrite the account and write a second traumatic account on any events that he was having difficulty processing. He would also be asked to continue to feel his natural emotions and to identify additional stuck points that emerge from the trauma account.

In the third phase the therapist would help David focus more heavily on challenging his stuck points using a progression of worksheets from the Challenging Questions to the Patterns of Problematic Thinking to the Challenging Beliefs Worksheet (CBW). The (CBW) is the final worksheet and it brings all of the worksheets together in one comprehensive sheet. Using these sheets in session and at home as practice assignments will allow David to look at both his beliefs related to the event but also his beliefs related to self, others, and the world going forward. For example David would probably want to challenge his beliefs about not being able to share his trauma story with any family members, his belief that he should be able to get over the experience because his father did, and any beliefs that are preventing him from going out into public places. In addition the therapist and David will focus during part of each of the last five sessions on five core areas that commonly show disruptions in PTSD patients, namely safety, trust, power/control, esteem, and intimacy. Each week David would be asked to read a brief 2-page module related to one of these 5 themes that includes ways in which an individual might become stuck in that area, e.g., for safety they may begin to believe they can never be safe anywhere. Weeks after reading the module David would proceed to challenge any stuck points he has in each of these 5 areas, in addition to any residual stuck points from the trauma or any new stuck points he uncovers. Based on his case description some stuck points that David might identify and challenge are “Crowds are not safe”, “I am weak compared to my father,” and “ I can’t enjoy life without him.” For sessions 10 and 11 David would also be asked to add some behavioral activation activities including giving and receiving compliments and doing nice things for himself. Finally for session 12, in addition to completing the intimacy module, David would be asked to rewrite his Impact statement. In session 12 David would read his new statement and the therapist would read his old statement. This comparison will allow David to see how much change he made over the course of therapy and it will provide him with information on what he should continue to work on as part of his recovery from PTSD. Typically in an individual presenting such as David, we see significant decreases in symptoms both on clinician administered and paper-pencil measures of PTSD, depression, and related symptoms. If David attends sessions regularly and completes his homework there is every reason to believe he will leave without a diagnosis of PTSD and this improvement should be a lasting gain.

Interpersonal Therapy for a Chronic Combat PTSD Veteran

Case Discussion: Using IPT

Introduction to IPT

The Interpersonal Psychotherapy (IPT) approach to PTSD differs from other trauma-focused psychotherapies. Whereas exposure to and re-processing of reminders of the traumatic event are paramount to evidence-based cognitive and behavioral treatments, IPT focuses instead on the effect trauma has had on interpersonal functioning. IPT helps patients who have lost faith in relationships and who find interpersonal encounters dangerous to develop more adaptive methods for navigating their social-emotional world. In simplest terms, IPT operates on the premise that relationships matter: close contacts, positive interactions, and effective communication create a scaffold for the profound changes that such patients can make in their lives.

Distinct from the fear extinction model of exposure-based treatments, IPT focuses on the crucial role of social support as a protective and healing factor in PTSD (Brewin, Andrews, & Valentine, 2000; Markowitz, Milrod, Bleiberg, & Marshall, 2009; Ozer, Best, Lipsey, & Weiss, 2003). David’s case illustrates the social withdrawal that accompanies PTSD as well as major depression. Individuals with PTSD feel numb and detached from their emotions and no longer trust either their physical or their social environments. This phenomenon leads to social isolation and a loss of potentially protective social support. IPT helps patients to re-attune their emotions and to use their feelings to rebuild relationships and regain social support.

This is how I would introduce IPT when I would meet David for our first session. An IPT therapist always aims for transparency in discussing therapy, presenting the approach clearly and intelligibly, so the patient can partner in formulating treatment goals. This would be important for David, who would enter a new therapy experience haunted by past traumas, still enduring a debilitating set of symptoms, and possibly disheartened by his past therapy experience. For many years, David kept his symptoms largely to himself, and avoided seeking the treatment recommended for his condition. When he finally did seek it, the treatment did not alleviate his distress. Unsurprisingly, then, David might be skeptical of engaging in a treatment approach that shifts the focus from his trauma experiences, the presumptive focus of his previous treatment, to his interpersonal world. On the other hand, David might be relieved that his current interpersonal world would be a distinct focal point, rather than his having to concentrate on the feared trauma itself: Avoiding anything related to the trauma is common in PTSD; thus David might feel he could agree to the intervention and still stay out of harm's way.

David's condition has been chronic: the nearly 40 years since the Yom Kippur War account for almost his whole adult life. Therefore, he is likely to view PTSD as an intractable part of himself and may have a bleak outlook regarding any possibility of recovery. Thus, it would be important to explore David's reaction to his previous therapy and therapist: what he found helpful, what he disliked, and how long the therapy lasted, before imposing any new set of aims or goals. Part of the IPT treatment of chronic PTSD, as for chronic depression (Markowitz, 1998), would involve helping him distinguish chronic symptoms from whom he is. Ultimately, I would need to keep in mind David's path leading to our initial session: the experiences along the way that marked progress, along with any obstacles which blocked his growth. Whether David embraces IPT from the onset, or is initially impervious to any prospect of change, he will need a therapist who understands his story and can offer an unthreatening relationship and environment, where planning and pacing is tailored to this unique individual.

Initial Phase of IPT

The therapist uses the first few IPT sessions to form an alliance, assess current symptoms, and obtain history including an Interpersonal Inventory, which gathers information from the patient about interpersonal functioning: his social past, his present relationships, and his hopes for the future (Weissman, Markowitz, & Klerman, 2000; Markowitz & Weissman, 2012). Sessions have flexibility, so that patients have room to reflect on and engage in the emotions and interpersonal elements essential to their own story, and to tailor the therapy individually. In the IPT-PTSD protocol (Bleiberg, K.L., Markowitz, J.C., 2005) obtaining the inventory involves recounting the outlines of the trauma history, but it emphasizes how the traumatic events have affected interpersonal functioning.

In building David's inventory, I would want to hear more about his relationships with his parents (particularly since his father may have had PTSD); the type of attachment he formed with each of them in his earlier years, other important friends, confidants, family members; and the period he described as "the best years of his life":

> Who was in your family? What was it like growing up with them? To whom were you closest?
> Tell me more about your childhood friendships?
> What made your friendship with Ruben special, unique?

How did you support and encourage each other in your friendship?
Describe any conflicts you had and how they were resolved. How do you get angry?
What was dating like? How did you first meet your wife?
What were some favorite ways you and friends passed the time together?
Before the war, how close did you get to other people? How did they see you? What have your relationships been like since?
Do you see any patterns in your relationships with other people?

Such open-ended questions elicit narratives that range from typical everyday memories to extraordinary milestones. These can open windows into David's past and clarify the interpersonal experiences that had been rewarding and supportive for him.

Recounting these past social experiences will trigger in David the intense feelings that accompany them. Remembering lost loved ones can evoke complex feelings: pain, guilt, sadness, and hopelessness. There may be reminiscences of pleasant times spent with these close friends alongside recollection of incidents that provoked anger or disappointment. David would be encouraged to "stay with" these feelings rather than avoid them, with an understanding that tolerance of his full range of emotions is healthy. The intention here is not exposure *per se*, but rather to help the patient understand the connection between his feeling state and life experiences.

Once David has described past relationships, I would gently guide him to the present, asking about the important people in his life today:

What do you like about the relationships in your life now?
How often do you see them?
How do you spend time together?
How does being with them affect your mood?
Are there any ways in which you'd like current relationships to be different?
How would you like them to be in the future?

The IPT therapist focuses on patterns in relationships, and particularly on current relationships that might be the source of interpersonal dispute or of social support.

Having explored David's constellation of friendships, support networks, and patterns of interpersonal behavior, I would then work on a case formulation, aiming to synthesize the details of his life stories and highlight specific problem areas he currently appears to be having with interpersonal functioning. The formulation would link David's clinical diagnoses to these problem areas, rather than present them as any shortcoming of his. This is a standard IPT position: the IPT model links life circumstances to the patient's current symptoms and offers goals for addressing and resolving them. This stance holds particular power when working with the diagnosis of PTSD, as there is such a clear external explanation for the syndrome. I would present the formulation to David towards the end of the initial sessions (usually around session 3), obtain feedback about his understanding of it, and work with him towards crafting it into a concise statement that will help focus and organize the remainder of therapy.

Another aspect of this formulation process would be to provide David with a clear, explicit definition and explanation for his diagnosis. I would explain to him that he is suffering from PTSD and major depression, both treatable illnesses related to his past traumas. Over the course of this therapy, he will learn to recognize and monitor symptoms, but I will urge him not to blame himself either for the symptoms or for their impact on his relationships. This process is referred to in IPT as "assigning the sick role" (Weissman et al., 2007).

IPT-PTSD might focus on a Role Transition, Role Dispute, or Grief as a problem area. Most PTSD cases involve an evident role transition: patients talk about the new roles (e.g., "a victim", "a survivor") they acquired post-trauma and often have complicated feelings about lost pre-traumatic roles. Such role transitions are present in David's case, and he also reported role disputes—i.e., interpersonal conflicts he experienced as anger outbursts, possibly due to "having a short fuse." Still, what appears most prominent in David's presentation is a complicated grief reaction.

Of the three IPT problem areas, complicated grief may at times most resemble exposure-based treatments for PTSD: after all, mourning the loss of another involves evoking a narrative that helps to uncover the sources of the current distress and suffering. Exposure-based techniques would use these data to help the patient actively confront past feared situations. For the IPT therapist, however, the purpose of such an exploration would be to encourage David to reconstruct his relationship with Ruben and explore in more depth how and why this particular loss hurt so much. Who was Ruben, what did David love about him and their relationship, and why does he miss him? What may have been troublesome or frustrating in their relationship?

David displays signs of an interrupted grieving process, a phenomenon that may affect patients who have suffered multiple losses. The interruption to the natural process of grief most likely started in the context in which David's losses occurred—namely, the Yom Kippur War in which he himself was a combatant, and where he experienced multiple traumas. He had to bear the shock of three consecutive near-death experiences; he witnessed horrific images of death and injury on the battlefield. But the worst trauma by far for David was leaving behind his best friend when their tank was under fire and being unable to rescue him. Although logically one could argue that he wasn't responsible for Ruben's death, he nevertheless was left with profound survivor's guilt. The way he lost his best friend must have been so charged with anger, pain, and guilt that David probably could not bear to mourn the event at the time, to feel the intense distress any form of processing the event would endure. The case history describes David as having PTSD and complicated grief. In essence these two findings are one and the same. The greatest traumatic episode of his life was the ultimate loss he suffered, and the impossible task he faced of, as he put it, "enjoying life without him."

Thus, I would suggest that our therapy focus on **grief**. If David agreed, we would enter the middle phase of treatment. Here's an example of an IPT case formulation (Markowitz & Swartz, 2007):

> You've given me some helpful history. Tell me whether I've understood you: You've been through some terrible things: nearly being killed in the war, but perhaps worst of all having your best friend Ruben die and being unable to save him. That kind of awful situation can be overwhelming, and its awful events like these that bring on posttraumatic stress disorder and depression. Neither the PTSD nor the depression is your fault, and even though they've been really debilitating, they're treatable.
>
> PTSD makes the whole world feel unsafe. It's hard to know whom you can trust, hard to risk getting close to anyone. Like many people with PTSD, you've pulled back and withdrawn from people around you. You've kept your feelings to yourself, but they're overwhelming. I suggest that we spend the next 11 weeks talking about your feelings about Ruben's loss,

> helping you to make sense of them in order to deal with your terrible grief. I'm not going to ask you to relive the burning tank, but rather to think about what you loved about Ruben and your relationship with him, what you've lost with his death. If you can process your feelings, you'll come to see that they're painful but powerful, but not dangerous.
>
> We'll also work to rebuild the supportive relationships in your life, because we know that having connections with trustworthy people really helps with PTSD and depression. Unfortunately, you can't bring Ruben back to life, but one way to keep his memory alive is to talk with other people about him—something you missed out on when you were in the hospital. Does that make sense to you?

This case formulation needs to be clear and concise, presented in a language that speaks directly to David's condition and circumstances. He has the opportunity to reexamine his own narrative within the context of IPT and its principles, and consider this "unconventional" approach to treating PTSD.

Middle Phase of IPT

In the middle phase, the IPT therapist shifts gears from assessment to intervention, using the case formulation as a bridge. These sessions help David monitor his symptoms, restore his interpersonal functioning, and mobilize social support. The IPT therapist listens for specific problems with communication, interaction with others, and affects regulation, and helps the patient to explore options for improvements.

> How have things been since we last met?

In the first session of the protocol, the therapist describes IPT, making certain that the patient understands the approach and its application. The therapist invites the patient into each subsequent session with one uncomplicated question: "How have things been since we last met?" This question focuses the therapist and the patient on current feelings and life events related to the problem area, and elicits concrete examples of the patient's interactions with others.

By the middle phase of treatment, the patient expects this question. However, some may struggle with the notion of staying in the "here and now." I would encourage David to think of events to discuss from his week, even if he feels his week is devoid of encounters and that there is little to recount. For even within the slightest interpersonal incident in which David interacts, comes the opportunity to re-attune to emotions from which he has presumably been detached for years. These modest moments from his week are not insignificant; over time, David can build upon them and may even find that he has spontaneously stopped avoiding the people and places he had connected to past traumas.

At the start of treatment, we know little about David's feelings towards the war itself, whether or not he was a willing combatant, whether he had spoken with fellow soldiers about his feelings around the death of his best friend—either when it happened or later, or whether his hospitalization disrupted that opportunity. Did he attend shivas? Annual memorials? Unit reunions? The answers to these questions, along with a better understanding of his general communication of grief and anger over the years, would shed light on whether David would be able to express even small levels of anger and frustration at the start of treatment. If he has not had much opportunity to express intense feelings since the war, he would probably have a difficult time conveying any feelings without a severe emotional reaction.

Assuming this is so, David may have dealt with people as little as possible over several decades, restricting his range of emotional responses. I would blame this on his PTSD and major depression, and spend time normalizing his emotions in daily current encounters. I would take the time to normalize his experience and choices: he's been through a multitude of overwhelming events and has feelings to match. It will understandably be difficult to tolerate the intense ones. To start, he can simply share recent interpersonal events, and become familiar with any feelings that emerge. When negative or intense emotions surface, I will assure David that he can tolerate them. If he can experience these feelings in the therapy room rather than shutting them off, he will see that even the most painful of emotions can pass.

Moreover, the IPT approach is to help him recognize his "negative" emotions as helpful social cues: anger means someone is bothering him; sadness is a response to separation or loss. Detachment from these emotions is part of what makes the world feel unsafe: it's hard to know what's going on when you're not in touch with your emotions. He's experienced events that have made such emotions feel overwhelming, but he may benefit from reconnecting to them and seeing that such feelings, while potent, also pass.

In all likelihood, events in the "here and now" will bring David back to those pockets of time past that he has tried so hard to forget. For example, if there are opportunities for meeting or spontaneous encounters with surviving corp members, friends of those who died in the war, and Ruben's family members, David might easily feel overwhelmed. Up until now, he most likely steered clear of any such encounters, for they would only raise fear, anger, guilt, or terror. Such behavior would be directly linked to avoidance symptoms that are so common in PTSD profile. However, IPT will allow him the opportunity to experience complex feelings, survive their intensity, and recognize feelings as simply feelings that inform these encounters. We could then work on interpersonal options he has for verbalizing and expressing these feelings to others: how can he use how he feels to understand and influence the outcome of social encounters? We would role play options in sessions to help him gain comfort in expressing himself. David would not be expected to practice any exercises at home; IPT does not assign homework.

Traumatized patients may avoid social situations for fear of the intense and negative feelings that may surface. Additionally, patients experiencing complicated grief may be so preoccupied with their lost relationships that the thought of new ones would be simply overwhelming. Yet social support has clinical benefits (Markowitz et al., 2009). Thus, once David has some foundation in identifying and labeling his feelings, I will encourage him to begin approaching interpersonal situations, to resume old friendships, and to engage in new social activities. He will probably experience discomfort: guilt that he is somehow betraying his lost best friend, irritation when communication is more effortful than he may remember, or simply overwhelming sadness as new events remind him of his past. For this reason, when working with complicated grief, IPT aims to help the patient process the lost relationship in conjunction with developing new skills.

One of these skill-based techniques is Communication Analysis, which helps the patient more effectively understand and deal with interpersonal incidents by unpacking the events which precipitated the incident, and reflecting on one's own actions. If, for example, David were to describe one of the anger outbursts mentioned in the case presentation, I would suggest we reconstruct the event, ensuring that we process it together without judgment or criticism of any past behavior. Below is a brief illustration of how the technique could be applied in David's case:

> Let's review this incident again, David. This time, we'll analyze it together, step by step, in order to understand the feelings it brought up for you, and whether you would like to discuss some alternatives to handling the situation. It will be as if we are putting this interpersonal incident under a microscope, so we can notice any and all details that might help us better understand your experience.

To help David increase clarity and directness in his communication, I would ask him to focus on all details, big and small, when reenacting each stage of the incident (*What did you say? What did she/he say? Then what happened?*). As David recalls the event, I would listen for how he felt, for specific statements that convey affect, both at the time of the event and during the present reenactment (*How did you feel? Could you tell her/him how you felt? Was that the message you wanted to convey? How do you feel now while re-telling the story?...*), and for discrepancies between David's emotional reactions and his expression of them. To further appreciate the complex range of emotions that may have accompanied the incident, I would also assess his tone of voice, body language, and gestures he may have exhibited during the exchange. This would help both of us to understand the impact David may have had on the other person, both nonverbal and verbal. Finally, I would find any opportunity to respond empathically, and with explicit acknowledgment of David's feelings (*Of course you felt angry*), normalizing them for him, while also connecting any difficulties in communication back to his current symptom functioning (*Irritability is a symptom of PTSD. It makes sense that you would have a hard time handling your anger in such a stressful situation*). From this point, David might be ready to consider alternative ways to handle the incident, and possibly even rehearse them through role-play, to prevent future anger outbursts.

I would listen to David's communication style and work with him to develop a deeper understanding of his feelings and intents at critical points during interpersonal events. David may be unaware of how his way of speaking or interaction affects others; ambiguous, indirect, or nonverbal communication, for example, could lead to false impressions or misunderstandings. He may also be filtering messages from others inaccurately, as is often the case when someone is depressed. David therefore may need direction and guidance on how to communicate his own needs and feelings more directly and how to interpret social situations more appropriately.

Having encouraged David to embark on such forms of interpersonal communication, the therapist is well aware that this feels like quite a risky journey, full of uncertainty and apprehension. As part of PTSD, David learned to avoid emotional signs and signals, and he is now being asked to respond to those very cues. These techniques will help him accept certain emotional truths: for example, anger arises when someone bothers or frustrates you; memories of loved ones can trigger a range of feelings from sorrow to delight to resentment. Feelings are unavoidable, but can be used as a useful indicator—with comfortable and effective communication now on his side. Alas, what options might David have to express his feelings? Did he attend memorials for fallen soldiers in his past? If so, what was the experience and how might he attend one differently today? This could be a time to approach friends and soldiers, to sort out confused feelings that were covered up for too long. And what of other friends who may have been close before, but were distanced over time? Perhaps, when ready, David could even draw Rubin's family near so as not to remain so alone in missing his best friend. At each step, I would engage David in the process, asking what it might be like to act on some of these "what ifs," to even rehearse through role play what to say, how to sound, and how to ensure the content he meant to share was communicated effectively.

In the remainder of the middle phase, David could practice being more assertive and express emotions without precipitating conflict or confusion. He could rehearse verbal exchanges he anticipates having in new social situations. He may even choose to role-play a conversation with the lost loved ones, to bring thoughts and feelings that were halted to a close. In each case, David would be encouraged to develop a stronger awareness of how he is communicating his own needs and feelings with others.

As the middle session comes to a close, I would convey to David a key distinction. The important people whom he has lost can never be replaced, that would prove impossible, but the complicated grief which ensued can be resolved. He now has the confidence, strength, and tools to embrace present day meaningful social interactions, and the potential for new relationships, new sources of pleasure and fulfillment. This will not "replace" Ruben, but it is possible to have new meaningful relationships and a new direction in life. What would that direction be? For David, sadness, anger, and distress about the losses will likely continue to surface: grief continues, but it changes over time.

Thus, the focus of intervention in IPT focuses on David's outside world. In fact, this interpersonal focus on the patient's existence *beyond* the therapist's office is one facet that distinguishes IPT from psychodynamic therapies (Markowitz, Svartberg, & Swartz, 1998). Rather than turning to introspection, or transference in order to develop insight, as psychodynamic therapy might, I would actively support David's efforts towards connections with those people who make up his own history, and are present throughout his day. His interpersonal behaviors in-session are certainly informative, and the connection, rapport, and trust between us are crucial, but even more important is David's development of kinship and unity amongst his actual contemporaries. He might, for example, want to do something to memorialize his lost friend and tank mates, or seek support from other veterans who know firsthand the torment and affliction he has had to undergo. For in IPT, the notion is that it is not sufficient to stop and remember. David must learn to stop remember, and look forward.

The Final Phase of IPT: Termination

The final sessions focus on termination, an important interpersonal event in its own right, and one anticipated from the start of the 14-week, 50-min session time-limited therapy. Here I would review the course of treatment, reinforce David's progress, and address his feelings about ending the therapy. Why is he better? The IPT therapist emphasizes gains in understanding and expressing emotions: David's bravery in tolerating his grief, and gains he may have made in establishing new relationships. Although the focus of IPT treatment lies primarily with David's relationships outside of the therapeutic relationship, I would be curious about the patient's views, positive and negative, of the therapeutic relationship itself, and believe that feelings that surface in the treatment are important to understand.

It is difficult to predict the outcome of the termination phase without an actual sample of treatment sessions, but it is important to attend to the patient's experiences vis-à-vis the therapist as a reflection of real-life relationship patterns. David's feelings about loss and abandonment will likely raise strong emotional responses to the ending of the therapeutic relationship. I would suggest to David that our ending will allow him the opportunity to have meaningful and supportive closure, to recognize the difference between sadness (an interpersonal signal of separation) and depression, and remind him that he now has developed useful skills for communicating his feelings. This ending may even offer a gratifying sense of completion, a finishing point that marks growth and recovery. Grief continues well beyond the 14 weeks of acute IPT, but it will hopefully have been transformed into more tolerable and bearable grief that can proceed "normally."

Conclusion

In IPT, PTSD is considered a medical condition, with symptoms that can subside if and when the patient's affect tolerance and interpersonal functioning are stronger. Typically, individuals suffering from such symptom clusters tend to distance themselves from distressing feelings; detachment and numbness offer safety from the painful memories of past traumas. Thus, embracing the goal of reconnecting with such feelings, to ultimately see them as useful rather than "bad" or dangerous, involves courage and effort. The IPT therapist must provide reassurance, facilitate affect development, and offer helpful and relevant strategies that will enable stronger interpersonal ties. The reintegration of feelings seems to help patients with PTSD feel under better internal control, a necessary first step to clinical improvement. Indeed, a difference between IPT for depression and IPT for PTSD is that the latter often requires the therapist spend a good portion of the early sessions on reestablishing affective awareness and tolerance before proceeding with the more usual IPT maneuvers. (Markowitz & Milrod, 2011).

David's presentation of complicated grief makes him a good candidate for IPT, as there is strong evidence to support the treatment of this as a problem area (Law, 2012; Weissman et al., 2000). Recent studies point to the necessity of specific and targeted interventions that work directly on the cluster of symptoms that make up complicated grief, namely an extreme focus on the loss and reminders of the loved one, intense longing for the deceased, problems accepting the death, preoccupation with sorrow, and bitterness about the loss (Shear, Frank, Houck, & Reynolds, 2005a, 2005b). David presents with a complex profile of comorbid symptoms: Depression with complicated bereavement and PTSD. In contrast to other evidence-based therapies for PTSD, IPT has been well tested for the treatment of depression with complicated bereavement (Weissman et al., 2007; Law, 2012).

In contrast, applying IPT to the treatment of PTSD has only recently been a focus of clinical trials (NIMH-funded randomized controlled trial, grant MH079078 from the National Institute of Mental Health, J. Markowitz, Principal Investigator). There have been some promising preliminary findings (Krupnick et al., 2008; Bleiberg and Markowitz, 2005), yet no clear evidence enables us to compare IPT to extant efficacious cognitive behavioral treatments for PTSD.

Thus, we must acknowledge potential benefits with caution, and consider liabilities to applying IPT to the case of David. IPT differs from other available treatments for PTSD by not focusing on exposure to trauma reminders, not assigning homework. It may be friendlier and gentler for patients who do not want to relive traumas. However, David might possibly respond better to an exposure-based protocol that argues for his confronting his trauma head on—if he can tolerate such treatment. Perhaps David would be willing to reenter the burning tank and heal by confronting those horrific images directly. There is certainly evidence to show that exposure-based treatment is effective.

We have noted that IPT for complicated grief is more similar to exposure-based treatments than work on a role transition or role dispute. Yet it still differs considerably. Although mourning the loss of Ruben and exploring why it hurts so much involves confronting his past losses, in IPT, David would not be asked to repeatedly relive the events within the burning tank, but rather to reconstruct his relationship to Ruben and what was lost. This might also involve discussing frustrations David had with Ruben which he now feels too guilty to address post mortem. There would be no systematic retelling of the narrative in order to induce habituation and extinction.

For many years, David's symptoms have denied him the chance to rebuild a life filled with new and meaningful interpersonal connections. His symptoms keep him detached from intense feelings, which he believes would only cause him more distress and anguish. IPT would offer him the strategies to address interpersonal problems areas that may otherwise seem hopeless. This approach can give David a chance to change his life situations, and to mourn past traumas without the torture and anguish that made the process unbearable. This could in turn allow him the chance to foster and nourish new and meaningful life connections, relationships that can lead to healthier and happier living.

Therapy for a Chronic Combat PTSD Veteran

Case Discussion: Utilizing Virtual Reality and DCS

The patient presented in Nacasch, Rachamim, and Foa (this volume) would appear to be a perfect candidate for prolonged imaginal therapy (PE). He clearly avoided talking about the events during the Yom Kippur War, especially when the tank was attacked and his comrades, including his boyhood friend Ruben, were killed and he was severely burned. He engages in active avoidance of malls, crowded places, barbecues (because of the smell of the smoke and the sight of the burning meat), and closed places such as elevators, airplanes, and any room with the door closed. His complicated bereavement would also be expected to be aided by exposure to the war memories as well as memorabilia of Ruben and their time together.

In PE, we usually begin with the most traumatic memory. It would seem that would be the tank attack when his fellow soldiers and Ruben were killed. This will naturally be expected to trigger a powerful grief response, which would be very painful for the patient and possibly the therapist. In such cases, the pain in the room is almost palpable. If he has been avoiding reminders of Ruben, they would be introduced either in session or for homework. This might include photos, videos, or other memorabilia. Other in vivo exposures would include his currently avoided situations, such as malls, crowded places, barbecues, and closed places such as elevators, airplanes, and any room with the door closed. He would be instructed to remain in the situation long enough for his anxiety to decrease and to not allow himself to feel relief upon leaving the situation so he can teach his brain and his body that these situations pose no increased threat. Behavioral activation items that would enhance his quality of life such as engaging in social activities could also be placed on this list. Clinically, many exposure therapists prefer sessions twice weekly to move patients up the hierarchy quickly and not allow as much of their usual avoidance in between sessions.

He would not be a candidate for virtual reality (VR) exposure therapy for the simple reason that, as far as this author is aware, there is no VR simulation that matches an Israeli tank from the Yom Kippur War. If there were a VR scenario that would match closely enough, it might be useful for him in that he is so very avoidant. Although the randomized controlled trials comparing VR to PE for PTSD are currently under way, so we have no empirical data on which treatment to recommend for which patient, our clinical experience suggests that as VR presents a very potent stimulus, it is difficult to engage in active avoidance while in VR. It is also a very different stimulus for most patients, so the novelty might have some value in engaging them in the traumatic memory. The VR would need to be modified to at least match his traumatic incident enough that it helped engage him. It is not mandatory that it match 100 %, but at least that it places him back in the 1973 Yom Kippur War setting. He does not need to be able to enter a tank, but it would be useful to have a tank represented. The fire in the tank does not need to be represented, but the patient should be instructed to engage in imaginal exposure to that memory while immersed in the Yom Kippur War scenario. Just like in PE, this exposure should be repeated over and over, in as much detail as possible, and tape-recording it for exposure homework. The therapist should match in the VR what the patient is recounting. Hot spots should be identified and recounted repeatedly until distress is decreased. As in PE, this would be likely to engender a strong grief reaction, and this should be encouraged, as painful as it is likely to be. Also as in PE, twice weekly sessions would be preferable.

Currently, the adjunctive use of D-Cycloserine (DCS) with exposure therapy is considered experimental, so we are cautious about recommending its use clinically. With DCS, less is more, so if it is used, sessions should be conducted once weekly so that the DCS is not dosed too frequently. The patient should be asked to come to the clinic 30 min prior to his appointment to take the medication. One strategy could involve just treating with exposure therapy (PE or VRE) monotherapy first and if the patient does not seem to be responding, add DCS. Another strategy is to add DCS for the first few exposure therapy sessions and observe the patient's response.

In all of the exposure therapy, the processing following the exposure will be important to help him with his grief and the guilt. This processing first focuses on his response to the exposure, for example, if his distress was decreased with repeated recountings, if he remembered more details, etc. Later sessions will sound similar to CPT in identifying unhelpful thoughts and assisting him through Socratic questioning in modifying them.

References

Bleiberg K. L., Markowitz J.C. (2005). Interpersonal psychotherapy for posttraumatic stress disorder. *American Journal of Psychiatry, 162*, 181–183.

Brewin, C. R., Andrews, B., & Valentine, J. D. (2000). Meta-analysis of risk factors for posttraumatic stress disorder in trauma-exposed adults. *Journal of Consulting and Clinical Psychology, 68*, 748–766.

Chard, K. M. (2005). An evaluation of cognitive processing therapy for the treatment of posttraumatic stress disorder related to childhood sexual abuse. *Journal of Consulting and Clinical Psychology, 73*, 965–971.

Chard, K. M., Schumm, J. A., Owens, G. O., & Cottingham, S. P. (2010). A comparison of OEF and OIF veterans and Vietnam veterans receiving cognitive processing therapy. *Journal of Traumatic Stress, 23*, 25–32.

Krupnick, J. L., Green, B. L., Stockton, P., Miranda, J., Krause, E., & Mete, M. (2008). Group interpersonal psychotherapy for low-income women with posttraumatic stress disorder. *Psychotherapy Research, 18*(5), 497–507.

Law, R. (2012). Complicated grief. In J. C. Markowitz & M. M. Weissman (Eds.), *Casebook of interpersonal psychotherapy*. New York: Oxford University Press.

Markowitz, J. C. (1998). *Interpersonal psychotherapy for dysthymic disorder*. Washington, DC: American Psychiatric Press.

Markowitz, J. C., & Milrod, B. (2011). The importance of responding to negative affect in psychotherapies. *American Journal of Psychiatry, 168*, 124–128.

Markowitz, J. C., Milrod, B., Bleiberg, K. L., & Marshall, R. D. (2009). Interpersonal factors in understanding and treating posttraumatic stress disorder. *Journal of Psychiatric Practice, 15*, 133–140.

Markowitz, J. C., Svartberg, M., & Swartz, H. A. (1998). Is IPT time-limited psychodynamic psychotherapy? *Journal of Psychotherapy Practice and Research, 7*, 185–195.

Markowitz, J. C., & Swartz, H. A. (2007). Case formulation in interpersonal psychotherapy of depression. In T. D. Eells (Ed.), *Handbook of psychotherapy case formulation* (2nd ed., pp. 221–250). New York: Guilford Press.

Markowitz, J. C., & Weissman, M. M. (Eds.). (2012). *Casebook of interpersonal psychotherapy*. New York: Oxford University Press.

Monson, C. M., Schnurr, P. P., Resick, P. A., Friedman, M. J., Young-Xu, Y., & Stevens, S. (2006). Cognitive processing therapy for veterans with military-related posttraumatic stress disorder. *Journal of Consulting and Clinical Psychology, 74*, 898–907.

Nacasch, N., Foa, E. B., Fostick, L., Polliack, M., Dinstein, Y., Tzur, D., et al. (2007). Prolonged exposure therapy for chronic combat-related PTSD: A case report of five veterans. *CNS Spectrums, 12*, 690–695.

Nacash, N., Foa, E. B., Huppert, J. D., Tzur, D., Fostick, L., Dinstein, Y., et al. (2010). Prolonged exposure therapy for combat and terror- related posttraumatic stress disorder: A randomized control comparison with treatment as usual. *Journal of Clinical Psychiatry, 72*, 1174–1180.

Ozer, E. J., Best, S. R., Lipsey, T. L., & Weiss, D. S. (2003). Predictors of posttraumatic stress disorder and symptoms in adults: A meta-analysis. *Psychological Bulletin, 129*, 52–73.

Rauch, S. A. M., Defever, E., Favorite, T., Duroe, A., Garrity, C., Martis, B., et al. (2006). Prolonged exposure for PTSD in a veterans health administration PTSD clinic. *Journal of Traumatic Stress, 22*, 60–64.

Resick, P. A., Galovski, T. E., Uhlmansiek, M., Scher, C. D., Clum, G. A., & Young-Xu, Y. (2008). A randomized clinical trial to dismantle components of cognitive processing therapy for posttraumatic stress disorder in female victims of interpersonal violence. *Journal of Consulting and Clinical Psychology, 76*, 243–258.

Resick, P. A., Monson, C. M., & Chard, K. M. (2010). *Cognitive processing therapy: Veteran/military manual*. Veterans Administration.

Schnurr, P. P., Friedman, M. J., Engel, C. C., Foa, E. B., Shea, M. T., Chow, B. K., et al. (2007). Cognitive behavioral therapy for posttraumatic stress disorder in women: A randomized controlled trial. *The Journal of the American Medical Association, 297*, 820–830.

Shear, K., Frank, E., Houck, P. R., & Reynolds, C. F., 3rd. (2005a). Treatment of complicated grief: A randomized controlled trial. *Journal of the American Medical Association, 293*(21), 2601–2608.

Shear, K., Frank, E., Houck, P. R., & Reynolds, C. F. (2005b). Treatment of complicated grief: A randomized controlled trial. *The Journal of the American Association, 293*(21), 2601–2608.

Tuerk, P. W., Yoder, M., Grubaugh, A., Myrick, H., Hamner, M., & Acierno, R. (2011). Prolonged exposure therapy for combat-related posttraumatic stress disorder: An examination of treatment effectiveness for veterans of the wars in Afghanistan and Iraq. *Journal of Anxiety Disorders, 25*, 397–403.

Weissman, M. M., Markowitz, J. C., & Klerman, G. L. (2000). *Comprehensive guide to interpersonal psychotherapy*. New York: Basic Books.

Weissman, M. M., Markowitz, J. C., & Klerman, G. L. (2007). *Clinician's quick guide to interpersonal psychotherapy*. New York: Oxford University Press.

Chapter 21
Matching Treatment to Patients Suffering from PTSD: What We Know and Especially What We Don't Know

Helene S. Wallach

The major goals of this volume were to answer the dilemmas regarding prevention, diagnosis, and treatment of PTSD. In this chapter, I will attempt to "pull" together the wealth of treatment information detailed in this book, and help untangle the age old dilemma of choosing the best treatment for our clients.

Matching Treatment to Client

In 1969 Paul asked "What treatment, by whom, is most effective for this individual, with that specific problem, under which set of circumstances, and how does it come about?" (Paul, 1969, p. 62). Although we have advanced significantly since Paul posed this question, we are still far from answering this question. In the beginning, research and practice attempted to tailor treatment to diagnostic classification. These studies found "modest differences between treatment methods that are largely independent of other factors influencing outcome" (Shapiro & Shapiro, 1982, p. 598). We now know that comparisons between treatment approaches yield only minor differences. For example, Cuijpers et al. (2008) conducted seven meta-analyses in which seven major types of psychological treatment for depression were examined and conclude that "There was no indication that 1 of the treatments was more or less efficacious…. This study suggests that there are no large differences in efficacy between the major psychotherapies for mild to moderate depression" (p. 909).

Tailoring treatment appropriate to diagnosis requires accuracy in our diagnostic systems. However, both major diagnostic systems (DSM and ICD) ignore etiology, intrapsychic conflicts, family and social networks, and ego strengths. This neglect

H.S. Wallach, Ph.D. (✉)
Department of Psychology, University of Haifa, Aba Khoushy 199, Mount Carmel, Haifa 3498838, Israel
e-mail: helenwa@yahoo.com

M.P. Safir et al. (eds.), *Future Directions in Post-Traumatic Stress Disorder*,
DOI 10.1007/978-1-4899-7522-5_21

may affect treatment selection. In addition, since the diagnosis is determined on the basis of the appearance of a set of symptoms from a larger possible number, heterogeneity among patients in each diagnostic category is huge. In order to diagnose PTSD employing the DSM, a patient must display one of five symptoms from criteria B, three of seven from criteria C, and two of five from criteria D—yielding 49 different manifestations of the disorder. It is not possible to tailor a treatment that will be equally effective with all 49 manifestations of the disorder. A partial solution might lie in subdividing the diagnostic category in order to make it more homogeneous, for example, into three subcategories: behavioral, cognitive, and physiological PTSD, i.e., PTSD with primarily cognitive manifestations of guilt, anger, hopelessness, etc., PTSD with primarily avoidant behavior, and PTSD with increased arousal, etc. This may aid in choosing the most appropriate therapy. For lack of a better system, this approach will be discussed later on in this chapter. However, this division may not be sufficient. It is important to examine patient characteristics which do not appear in the diagnosis, but may also influence treatment choice.

In order to choose patient characteristics, an accepted model which would guide the researcher/clinician to choose relevant patient variables is required. To date, no such accepted model exists, rendering this task unattainable. Single variable models which match treatment to patient abound, for example, on the basis of attributions, self-control, hemisphere dominance, etc. These models are somewhat helpful, but far from satisfying. Several multivariate models have been proposed as well; for example, the model developed by Beutler and Clarkin (1990) which takes into account patient, therapist, and therapy variables, as well as the evolving nature of the therapeutic process. I attempted to employ their model in a paper published in 2000 (Wallach, 2000). It was a very interesting exercise, which taught me humility. I found that the more I thought I knew and understood about the therapeutic process, the more I discovered that I still needed to learn. The model turned out to be very illuminating as a post (therapy)-mortem, but irrelevant as a guide to choosing therapeutic interventions.

Patient Treatment Matching in PTSD

PTSD is a complex disorder. It affects all aspects of the individual's life—social, familial, marital, work, sleep, physical, affective, and more. As detailed elsewhere in this book (Echterling, Stewart, & Field, 2013), diagnosis has evolved through the years, and we are now able to make a precise diagnosis as who suffers from PTSD, and who does not, as well as length and depth of the disorder. We also are able to trace and map the neurological underpinnings, as described in other chapters of this book (Gilboa, 2013; Richter-Levin, 2013). Two main effective therapies have been developed to treat PTSD—Prolonged Exposure, developed in the mid 1980s by Edna Foa and colleagues, and described in this book (Foa, Nacasch, & Rachamim, 2013), and Cognitive Processing Therapy developed by Patricia Resick and colleagues in the 1990s and described in this book (Chard & Walter, 2013).

Recently, Interpersonal Therapy has been successfully applied to PTSD as well and is described in this book (Klein Rafaeli & Markowitz, 2013). In addition, in recent years, modifications to these various therapies have been successfully employed: adding D-Cycloserine (Burton, Youngner, McCarthy, Rothbaum, & OlasovRothbaum, 2013) and using Virtual Reality (Garcia Palacios, Botella, Banos, Guillen, & Vicenta Navarro, 2013; Rizzo, 2013). Karen Seal and her group (Seal, 2013) have also attempted to locate the treatment in a general healthcare facility to reduce stigma and other barriers to therapy.

Thus we can see that there have been a number of therapeutic approaches that are currently employed to treat PTSD. All appear to be equally effective. However, all report large dropout rates and only modest success rates. Thus, the main question remains unanswered: which approach to use for the client we are attempting to treat. I will try to sketch several decisive factors to employ to match treatment to our PTSD client.

Appropriate or inappropriate patient choice may influence motivation and dropout rate, as reported by Zoellner, Feeny, and Bittinger (2009). Zoellner et al. developed path models of treatment preference for psychotherapy or pharmacotherapy, following which they conducted confirmatory analyses of these models. They found that treatment-related beliefs (credibility and personal reactions) were the strongest predictors of treatment preference. In addition, severity of depression reduced likelihood of choosing psychotherapy, and severity of PTSD increased likelihood of choosing pharmacotherapy. However, appropriate treatment rationale can influence patient choice (Wallach, 1988). I compared somatic and cognitive treatment for dysmenorrhea, giving participants a detailed treatment rationale prior to therapy. The rationale differed between the groups, and it was evident that following the rationale, women changed their treatment expectations.

An additional treatment dilemma is that of secondary gains. We must consider that patients who overcome PTSD may lose compensation and other secondary gains that accrue from the disorder. Thus some patients may have low or mixed motivations regarding treatment. One possible solution is to give patients the choice to wait for treatment following the compensation board's evaluations, or to begin treatment with the possibility of receiving reduced compensation.

In addition problems of comorbidity should also be addressed. For example, clinical depression may complicate therapy. Therefore, we must conduct an appropriate and focused case formulation and then address comorbidity prior to treatment of PTSD. In cases of comorbidity, additional treatment sessions may be necessary to achieve sufficient improvement than were provided in the original treatment protocol.

And finally, some patients over-engage. Various solutions can be provided for over-engagement—introducing medication to reduce symptoms and over-engagement, or using graduated VRPE in these cases.

In another section of this book (Case Discussion), a case was presented by Nacasch, Rachamim, and Foa. We asked several of the authors to determine whether their main therapeutic approach was appropriate or not to this client. We also asked them to focus on the patient or case characteristics which helped them to come to their conclusions.

PE was presented by Nacasch, CPT by Chard, VR and DCS by Rothbaum, and IPT by Klein-Rafaeli. We hoped that this would enable us to identify the patient characteristics that therapists from different orientations focus on to determine which therapy approach is best suited to the client. We are not sure that we have managed to reach that goal. It appears that the same client may be successfully (or unsuccessfully) treated with all these different approaches. So, we have reached an impasse. However, the following suggestions may help.

CPT may be most appropriate with patients who are sophisticated, intelligent, and verbal, but have cognitive distortions. Patients suffering from increased anger and or guilt seem to be specifically suited for CPT. CPT is less successful with patients with low education, individuals who are homeless, minorities, and immigrants as they may have difficulty articulating, and may be uncomfortable with writing assignments.

PE may be more appropriate with patients whose primary problem is that of avoidance, those whose executive functions such as concentration are impaired, and those with cognitive distortions, but who experience difficulties in articulation. In addition, homework assignments in PE are more demanding than the other therapies; therefore it may be less suited to those who experience difficulty in homework assignments. In these cases, in vivo exercises in PE can be conducted with a co-therapist. However, for some avoiders in-vivo exercises will not help as they don't do home work and/or skip sessions and/or don't engage in therapy; thus, they may not benefit from PE.

VRPE like PE is also well suited for those who are high on avoidance. Unlike PE it is also well suited for those who over- or under-engage in therapy. In addition, dropout rates are reduced and there are increases in treatment response in comparison with conventional PE. VRPE also builds resilience for future traumas. VRPE facilitates treatment more than PE as memories are triggered without efforts to recall. It is also useful for those that do not engage in conventional PE.

DCS—adding DCS can increase treatment benefits and is especially suited for over and under engagers.

IPT appears to be the treatment of choice when there are multiple interpersonal problems, as patients are unable to focus on PE or CPT.

When do we want to combine more than one approach? If we have a client with severe PTSD as well as existential issues, we may want to combine PE and CPT. Kathy Shear (2012) developed a protocol to treat complicated grief using the combination of PE and CPT and IPT. Perhaps this may be applied to chronic PTSD as well. Borderline Personality Disordered patients do not fare well in "conventional" treatments. Therefore, perhaps with these patients, a DBT like therapy should be employed. Lisa Najavits (2012) developed a DBT protocol for PTSD which includes emotional regulation. Azucena Garcia Palacios and her team are collaborating with Edna Foa to develop a protocol for BPD patients using DBT first and then "conventional" PE PTSD treatment.

References

Beutler, L. E., & Clarkin, J. F. (1990). *Systematic treatment selection: Toward targeted therapeutic interventions*. New York: Brunner-Mazel.

Burton, M. S., Youngner, C. G., McCarthy, A. J., Rothbaum, A. O., & OlasovRothbaum, B. (2013). Enhancing exposure therapy using D-Cycloserine (DCS). In M. P. Safir, H. S. Wallach, & A. Rizzo (Eds.), *Future directions in post traumatic stress disorder: Prevention, diagnosis and treatment*. New York: Springer.

Chard, K., & Walter, K. H. (2013). Cognitive processing therapy: Beyond the basics. In M. P. Safir, H. S. Wallach, & A. Rizzo (Eds.), *Future directions in post traumatic stress disorder: Prevention, diagnosis and treatment*. New York: Springer.

Cuijpers, P., van Straten, A., Andersson, G., & van Oppen, P. (2008). Psychotherapy for depression in adults: A meta-analysis of comparative outcome studies. *Journal of Consulting and Clinical Psychology, 76*, 909–922.

Echterling, L., Stewart, A. L., & Field, T. (2013). Evolution of DSM diagnosis for PTSD. In M. P. Safir, H. S. Wallach, & A. Rizzo (Eds.), *Future directions in post traumatic stress disorder: Prevention, diagnosis and treatment*. New York: Springer.

Foa, E., Nacasch, N., & Rachamim, L. (2013). The psychopathology and evidence-based treatment for post-traumatic stress disorder: PE. In M. P. Safir, H. S. Wallach, & A. Rizzo (Eds.), *Future directions in post traumatic stress disorder: Prevention, diagnosis and treatment*. New York: Springer.

Garcia Palacios, A., Botella, C., Banos, R., Guillen, V., & Vicenta Navarro, A. (2013). A rationale for the use of VR in the treatment of PTSD. In M. P. Safir, H. S. Wallach, & A. Rizzo (Eds.), *Future directions in post traumatic stress disorder: Prevention, diagnosis and treatment*. New York: Springer.

Gilboa, A. (2013). Functional neuroanatomy of PTSD: Developmental cytoarchitectonic trends, memory systems and control processes. In M. P. Safir, H. S. Wallach, & A. Rizzo (Eds.), *Future directions in post traumatic stress disorder: Prevention, diagnosis and treatment*. New York: Springer.

Klein Rafaeli, A., & Markowitz, J. C. (2013). Interpersonal therapy for PTSD. In M. P. Safir, H. S. Wallach, & A. Rizzo (Eds.), *Future directions in post traumatic stress disorder: Prevention, diagnosis and treatment*. New York: Springer.

Najavits, L. M. (2012). Extracted August 21, 2012. http://www.seekingsafety.org/

Paul, G. (1969). Behavior modification research: Design and tactics. In C. M. Franks (Ed.), *Behavior therapy: Appraisal and status* (pp. 29–62). New York: McGraw-Hill.

Richter-Levin, G. (2013). Post-traumatic stress or post-traumatic depression? In M. P. Safir, H. S. Wallach, & A. Rizzo (Eds.), *Future directions in post traumatic stress disorder: Prevention, diagnosis and treatment*. New York: Springer.

Rizzo, A. (2013). Virtual reality applications for anxiety disorders and PTSD: The first ten years and the next! In M. P. Safir, H. S. Wallach, & A. Rizzo (Eds.), *Future directions in post traumatic stress disorder: Prevention, diagnosis and treatment*. New York: Springer.

Seal, K. (2013). Mental health problems and treatment utilization of Iraq and Afghanistan Veterans enrolled in department of Veterans affairs healthcare. In M. P. Safir, H. S. Wallach, & A. Rizzo (Eds.), *Future directions in post traumatic stress disorder: Prevention, diagnosis and treatment*. New York: Springer.

Shapiro, D. A., & Shapiro, D. (1982). Meta-analysis of comparative therapy outcome studies: A replication and refinement. *Psychological Bulletin, 92*, 581–604.

Shear, K. (2012). Extracted August 21, 2012. http://www.complicatedgrief.org/about/profile/katherine-shear-m.d/

Wallach, H.S. (1988). *Dysmenorrhea – Clients' expectations and psychological therapy*. Doctoral Dissertation, University of Western Ontario, London, ON, Canada

Wallach, H. S. (2000). Patient treatment interaction: Where are we and how do we proceed. *The Israel Journal of Psychiatry and Related Sciences, 37*, 51–63.

Zoellner, L. A., Feeny, N., & Bittinger, J. N. (2009). What you believe is what you want: Modeling PTSD-related treatment preferences for sertraline or prolonged exposure. *Journal of Behavior Therapy and Experimental Psychiatry, 40*, 455–467.

ERRATUM TO

Chapter 20
Case Presentation of a Chronic Combat PTSD Veteran

Nitsa Nacasch, Lilach Rachamim, and Edna B. Foa

M.P. Safir et al. (eds.), *Future Directions in Post-Traumatic Stress Disorder*,
DOI 10.1007/978-1-4899-7522-5_20

DOI 10.1007/978-1-4899-7522-5_22

Each case discussion mentioned in the chapter "Case Presentation of a Chronic Combat PTSD Veteran" was written by different authors. Only the first discussion on Prolonged Exposure (PE) was written by Nitsa Nacasch, Lilach Rachamim, and Edna B. Foa.

The authors of the three additional sections were inadvertently omitted from their analyses in the published chapter and also in the book table of contents. Herein the title of each section appears with the discussion section title followed by the authors' names.

This Erratum serves to provide the authors credit on the table of content, and the section titles within chapter 20 should reflect as follows:

The online version of the original chapter can be found at
http://dx.doi.org/10.1007/978-1-4899-7522-5_20

M.P. Safir et al. (eds.), *Future Directions in Post-Traumatic Stress Disorder*,
DOI 10.1007/978-1-4899-7522-5_22

Index

M.P. Safir et al. (eds.), *Future Directions in Post-Traumatic Stress Disorder*,
DOI 10.1007/978-1-4899-7522-5

E

F

G

FSC
www.fsc.org
MIX
Papier | Fördert
gute Waldnutzung
FSC® C083411

Kolibri 360 GmbH
Ferdinand-Jühlke-Straße 7
99095 Erfurt, Deutschland
produktsicherheit@kolibri360.de